NURSING in TODAY'S WORLD

Trends, Issues, and Management

Janice Rider Ellis, RN, PhD, ANEF
Nursing Education Consultant
Shoreline, Washington
Professor Emeritus
Shoreline Community College
Seattle, Washington

Celia Love Hartley, RN, MN, ANEF
Nursing Education Consultant
Camano Island, Washington
Professor Emeritus
College of the Desert
Palm Desert, California

Illustrations by Tomm Scalera

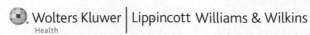
. Wolters Kluwer | Lippincott Williams & Wilkins
Health
Philadelphia · Baltimore · New York · London
Buenos Aires · Hong Kong · Sydney · Tokyo

Acquisitions Editor: Hilarie Surrena
Product Manager: Helen Kogut
Editorial Assistant: Zachary Shapiro
Design Coordinator: Joan Wendt
Illustration Coordinator: Brett MacNaughton
Manufacturing Coordinator: Karin Duffield
Prepress Vendor: SPi Global

10th edition

Library of Congress Cataloging-in-Publication Data
Ellis, Janice Rider.
    Nursing in todays world : trends, issues & management / Janice Rider Ellis, Celia Love Hartley;
Illustrations by Tomm Scalera.—10th ed.
        p. ; cm.
    Includes bibliographical references and index.
    ISBN 978-1-60547-707-7
  1. Nursing. 2. Nursing—Practice. 3. Nursing—United States. I. Hartley, Celia Love. II. Title.
    [DNLM: 1. Nursing—trends. 2. Legislation, Nursing. 3. Nursing Care—organization & administration.
4. Nursing Care—trends.   WY 16.1]
    RT82.E45 2012
    610.73—dc23

                                                                                        2011013528

LWW.com

CCS0913

This book is dedicated to all those students who have used the previous editions and are now practicing nurses. We value their contribution to nursing and to the health of our communities.

Janice Rider Ellis
Celia Love Hartley

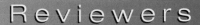

Virginia L. Byer, RN, MSN, CS
Assistant Professor
Community College of Baltimore County
Catonsville, Maryland

Eileen R. Chasens, RN, DSN
Assistant Professor
University of Pittsburgh
Pittsburgh, Pennsylvania

Darlene Clark, RN, MS
Senior Lecturer in Nursing
The Pennsylvania State University
University Park, Pennsylvania

Laura A. Conklin, RN, MSN, MSA
Nursing Faculty
Wayne County Community College District
Detroit, Michigan

Kim D. Cooper, RN, MSN
Dean, School of Nursing
Ivy Tech Community College
Terre Haute, Indiana

Karen Cummins, PhD, CRNP, FNP-BC, CNE
Professor of Nursing
Carlow University
Pittsburgh, Pennsylvania

Janis Guilbeau, RN, MSN, FNP-BC
Instructor of Nursing
University of Louisiana at Lafayette
Lafayette, Louisiana

Karen Jagiello, RNC, MSN
Instructor
James Madison University
Harrisonburg, Virginia

Beverly Kawa, RN, MS
Instructor of Nursing
Morton College
Cicero, Illinois

Ronnalee Netteburg, BSN, MS
Assistant Professor
Columbia Union College
Takoma Park, Maryland

Valerie O'Dell, RN, MSN
Assistant Professor
Youngstown State University
Youngstown, Ohio

Laurie J. Palmer, RN, MS, AOCN
Associate Professor of Nursing
Monroe Community College
Rochester, New York

Theresa L. Piekut, RNC, MSN, CCE
Professor of Nursing
Community College of Allegheny County
West Mifflin, Pennsylvania

Cynthia Rubenstein, RN, PhD, CPNP-PC
Assistant Professor
James Madison University
Harrisonburg, Virginia

Reviewers

Luise Speakman, RN, PhD
Chair, Health Sciences Department
Coordinator, Nursing Program
Cape Cod Community College
West Barnstable, Massachusetts

Kathy S. Taydus, RN, MSN, BSN
Assistant Professor of Nursing
Jamestown Community College
Jamestown, New York

Mildred Yarborough, RN, MSN
Assistant Professor of Nursing
Coppin State University
Baltimore, Maryland

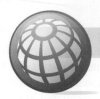

*N*ursing in Today's World: Trends, Issues, and Management, 10th edition focuses on the nonclinical aspects of the professional nursing role. Much of this content is just as critical to practicing safely as is competence in the performance of clinical skills. As nursing steps up to play a major role in the changes brought about by healthcare reform, knowledge of the profession and its place in the healthcare environment has never been more important. We have endeavored to keep the content of this textbook current by revising and updating each chapter with the latest information on the delivery of care, the structure of the healthcare milieu, roles performed by the variously prepared caregivers, the impact of technology, and the changing financial picture. Additionally, we have made every effort to be responsive to suggestions provided by our readers and reviewers. Thus, the 10th edition provides background information to help the reader understand the changes that are occurring and suggestions for moving from the role of the student into that of a contributing professional in today's healthcare setting. And we have retained in a concise and readable format, the content that is basic to a textbook that has the nursing profession as its focus. Here is what you will find.

TEXT ORGANIZATION

We consistently have attempted to design a textbook that provides a flexible approach to instruction with the intention that each chapter be able to stand alone, with references occurring throughout that will lead the reader to related content appearing in other areas of the book. This goal has been maintained so that content can be reordered if so desired. For example, instructors who prefer to skip the historical development of nursing as a profession and move directly to leadership and management are encouraged to adapt their use of the various chapters to match this preference. Thus, you might order your syllabus to first present the content found in Unit III (Accepting Greater Responsibility for Nursing Practice), which focuses on the nurses' role in working with others in the management of care. Another approach would be to begin with Unit II (Understanding Healthcare in Today's Society) and present information about the healthcare environment, its financing, and its legal and ethical aspects. Similarly, some content areas might be combined or perhaps eliminated if they appear elsewhere in the curriculum of your program.

This textbook is organized into three major units of study.

- Unit I: Moving Into the Profession of Nursing

  Chapters 1 through 5 focus on nursing itself. Students will learn about the development of the profession and the challenges to its professional standing in Chapter 1. By understanding these origins and challenges and by exploring the various educational avenues providing entry into the profession of nursing, students will be better prepared to participate in the nonclinical activities and discussions that are part of nursing. The diverse educational paths that prepare graduates for registered nurse licensure are presented in Chapter 2. Issues discussed include the controversy that exists regarding the form of educational preparation deemed most appropriate for entry-into-practice, the implementation of differentiated practice, and whether continuing education should be mandatory or voluntary. Chapter 3 delves into the credentialing of nurses with a discussion of the history of licensing in the United States, explains the process of obtaining and retaining a license, and speculates on the future of licensure in the United States. Chapter 4 provides a discussion of employment opportunities today, employer expectations of new graduates, and steps to be taken to realize career goals. The Unit concludes with Chapter 5 presenting information related to understanding organizational structures, especially those that provide healthcare. This chapter also discusses patterns of care delivery and collective bargaining.

- Unit II: Understanding Healthcare in Today's Society

Chapter 6 begins this unit with a discussion and description of the various healthcare facilities that provide care to individuals and their families and the evaluation and accreditation of those facilities. It explores the various methods and sources of funding for that care and how power is distributed within the system. Chapter 7 deals with the legal responsibilities for practice and includes legal issues common in nursing, malpractice, and the role of the nurse as a witness. Chapter 8, devoted to ethics, provides a foundation for ethical decision making, including a broad discussion of ethical issues that impact nursing and nursing practice. Chapter 9, focused on bioethics, challenges students to consider the many controversial facets of stem cell research, gene therapy, and the human genome project, as well as other topical issues. Reports released by the Institute of Medicine on errors that have resulted in death or increased hospitalization and cost to patients have highlighted the need for greater safety in the delivery of care. In answer to this need, a new chapter, *Safety Concerns in Healthcare,* has been added to this edition. Chapter 10 presents common errors and the necessary steps to reduce their occurrence. Unit II concludes with a discussion of community-based nursing and the nurse's role in that environment in Chapter 11. Health promotion and disease prevention are included in the content with a discussion of Healthy People 2020 and alternative and complementary approaches to healthcare.

- Unit III: Accepting Greater Responsibility for Nursing Practice

The book concludes with five chapters devoted to the nurses' professional role in the various aspects of healthcare. Chapter 12 provides a basis for understanding leadership and management and the importance of communication in the process of directing the activities of others. Concepts of power, time management, and performance evaluation are also included. Chapter 13 is devoted to management skills: team building, coaching, motivating others, delegating, leading change, and managing conflict. It is followed by Chapter 14 with a discussion of the challenges found in today's workplace: reality shock, burnout, and workplace safety for nurses. Chapter 15 addresses the nurse and the political process and discusses the relevance of the political process to nurses. It concludes with a description of the various nursing organizations. The final chapter, Chapter 16, looks to the future and is devoted to an overview of nursing research and the importance of evidence-based practice. Also included is a discussion of the use of information technology in healthcare.

PEDAGOGICAL FEATURES

- **Learning Outcomes** introduce each chapter and guide learning efforts.
- **Key Terms** used in the chapter discussion are listed to help focus the reader.
- **Critical Thinking Activities** interspersed throughout each chapter help students critically process possible applications of the content.
- **Communication in Action** emphasizes the role of effective communication in every aspect of the nursing role.
- **Examples** provide a vignette of real-life experiences to assist students in understanding difficult concepts presented in the chapter.
- **Key Concepts** summarize each chapter and aid retention of the content.

SPECIAL FEATURE

The engaging cartoons in the 10th edition of *Nursing in Today's World* provide an eye-catching and provocative interpretation of concepts presented in each chapter. The cartoon feature, always a hallmark of this text, complements the easy reading style and logical approach of this textbook. Over the years, nurses have grown in their ability to find humor in many aspects of the profession. We believe that a little humor keeps us healthier and we hope that you, too, will appreciate this aspect of the text.

STUDENT AND INSTRUCTOR RESOURCES

A variety of teaching and learning resources are available for students and instructors. Visit thePoint at *http://thePoint.lww.com/Ellis10e* to access journal articles related to each chapter, relevant Web sites with direct links, and more!

YOUR INPUT IS WELCOMED

We continue to appreciate the comments and suggestions of colleagues, friends, and students. We encourage you to review this text critically and to advise us of ways in which we can make it better meet classroom needs. We thank the many educators who continue to select *Nursing in Today's World* as the textbook for their class. In this competitive market, we know there are many texts from which to choose. We appreciate your support and strive to bring to you the book that will continue to best meet your needs.

Janice Rider Ellis
Celia Love Hartley

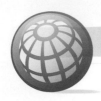

Acknowledgments

We are always appreciative of the help and support that we enjoy from the fine staff at Lippincott Williams & Wilkins, particularly that of product manager Helen Kogut, and the editorial assistants, who saw us through a series of changes. We have enjoyed working with Tomm Scalera, who is responsible for capturing our concepts in the colorful illustrations, and Arin Ceglia and Fred Burns of O'Donnell & Associates, who worked with us as the project managers. Janice continues to value the support of her husband Ivan. His encouragement and good humor about all the crises, both small and large, that occur with any project provide solid grounding. Celia celebrates the contributions of her late husband, Gordon. His loss is deeply felt and his contribution sorely missed.

Janice Rider Ellis
Celia Love Hartley

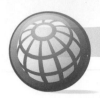

Contents

4   Making Professional Goals a Reality   121

5   The World of Healthcare Employment   155

UNIT II   Understanding Healthcare in Today's Society   193

6   Understanding the Healthcare Environment and Its Financing   194

7   Legal Responsibilities for Practice   244

8 Ethical Concerns in Nursing Practice 287

9 Bioethical Issues in Healthcare 331

10 Safety Concerns in Healthcare 372

11 The Nursing Profession and the Community 397

UNIT III Accepting Greater Responsibility for Nursing Practice 425

12 Initiating the Leadership and Management Role 426

13 Working With Others in a Leadership Role 460

14 Facing the Challenges of Today's Workplace 504

15 Valuing the Political Process 529

16 Applying Research and Technology to Nursing Practice 563

Index 593

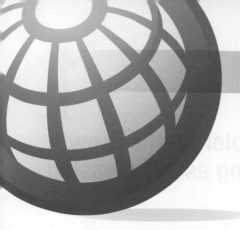

Moving Into the Profession of Nursing

You are entering the nursing profession at a time when it is being affected by a number of sociological issues. As we see in the country at large, there is a graying of the profession with the number of nurses over age 45 increasing. The recession affected retirements and job opportunities. The healthcare environment is rapidly changing, and the forces of healthcare reform may create even more change. The purpose of Unit I is to help you understand nursing as it is today by increasing your perception of the events affecting its development.

Learning about the history and development of the profession can help you to appreciate the heritage of the discipline, understand the events that resulted in nursing offering the opportunities and challenges that it provides today, and interpret the changes occurring now. Chapter 1 begins with a history of nursing that describes its growth from early times to an era when preparation for nursing existed as apprentice-type training to a profession that now encompasses doctoral and postdoctoral education. Many believe that nursing is a young profession. Others note that nursing has always existed in some form, while some question whether nursing should be considered a profession at all. This unit considers those debates and addresses the results of the studies that were conducted about nursing and their impact on the development of the profession.

The educational processes by which we prepare nurses continue to experience revision, modification, refinement, and innovation in response to changes that occur in the broader educational environment as well as in the healthcare delivery system. Chapter 2 discusses these as well as the various routes to educational preparation for a nursing career, including a history of the different avenues. You will learn about some of the individuals who made significant contributions to the profession.

Throughout the healthcare system, accreditation of institutions and the licensure and certification of individual professionals serve to safeguard the public. Understanding the various mechanisms by which approval is given helps you to develop your personal career goals and select the organizations where you wish to be employed. As you move into your career as a professional nurse, you will first need to pass examinations that qualify you for a nursing license and may then seek further credentials attesting to your expertise. The various approaches to credentialing are presented in Chapter 3 of this unit.

Once licensed, you will be concerned with finding employment. Chapter 4 focuses on your beginning job search. Information is provided about the competencies needed for the wide variety of opportunities available to nurses today. The various career opportunities in nursing are outlined as well as the expectations of employees. Helpful strategies for seeking that special first job are provided, including writing resumes and composing letters of application and letters following up on interviews.

The final chapter in this unit provides information on the basic structure underlying the healthcare environment, including the mission and/or vision statement, organizational charts, chains of command, and approaches to governance. Also discussed are the forms of nursing care delivery and some major areas of nursing practice in which negotiation occurs, including collective bargaining. Thus, you are moved through the history of the profession into your first role as a practicing professional.

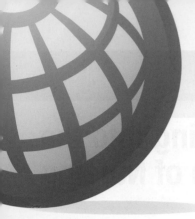

1

Exploring the Growth of Nursing as a Profession

LEARNING OUTCOMES

After completing this chapter, you should be able to:

1. Discuss the early origins of nursing and factors influencing nursing's development as a profession.
2. Describe Florence Nightingale's contribution to nursing and to the growth and improvement of nursing education.
3. Discuss the development and characteristics of the early nursing schools.
4. Analyze the impact wars and conflicts have had on nursing and nursing education.
5. Analyze the challenges of defining nursing and formulate your personal definition of nursing.
6. Identify the major differences between nursing and medicine.
7. Describe the seven characteristics against which social scientists have evaluated professions, and analyze how these can be applied to nursing.
8. Compare and contrast the terms "profession" and "professional" and explain why the issue is of significance to nursing.
9. Describe some of the traditions in nursing and explain why the nursing profession has embraced them.
10. Discuss the history of the image of nursing in the United States and why it is important for nursing to have a positive image within society.
11. Analyze areas of nursing about which studies have been conducted and explain why each is important.
12. Explain how a universal language for nursing that includes the North American Nursing Diagnosis Association International (NANDA-I), Nursing Outcomes Classification (NOC), and Nursing Interventions Classification (NIC) systems of nursing classification supports the growth of nursing as a profession globally.
13. Discuss the ultimate goal of specific documentation systems for nursing and describe how the use of these systems might affect nursing practice.

KEY TERMS

Characteristics of a profession
Classification systems
Committee for Nursing Practice Information Infrastructure (CNPII)
Florence Nightingale
Folk image
International Classification for Nursing Practice Project (ICNPP)
Military influence
Minimum Data Set for Nursing Home Resident Assessment and Care Screening (MDS)
National Information and Data Set Evaluation Center (NIDSEC)

North American Nursing Diagnosis Association-International (NANDA-I)
Nursing Interventions Classification (NIC)
Nursing nomenclatures
Nursing Outcomes Classification (NOC)
Omaha System
Profession
Professional
Religious image
Servant image
Taxonomy

Nursing as a profession is, and will continue to be, responsive to and influenced by the society it serves. Thus, the major activities occurring within the nursing field are also a reflection of what is happening in the society as a whole. Understanding this interrelationship and the progression of nursing as it has developed will help you to evaluate issues arising while you are in practice. Placing the concepts found within this chapter into the broader framework of society may serve to help make the background of nursing more relevant, easier to understand, and more memorable. Throughout the chapter, we mention some of the eras of nursing.

There is no particular date or time period when nursing came into being. While nursing as we know it today may go back less than 150 years, the early origins of nursing, like those of medicine, are intertwined with the ancient civilizations and cultures of the world. With little recorded history, our best speculations regarding the origins of nursing are tied to our knowledge of the varied cultures that existed in the past and to the contributions that these cultures left for future generations. They reflected the events and developments that characterized each period in history.

HEALTHCARE IN ANCIENT CULTURES

Primitive societies and ancient cultures were nomadic out of necessity. Well-defined groups, built around the nucleus of family relationships, wandered in search of food, warmth, and an environment that supported life. Solidarity among these scattered groups, organized for the convenient management of human affairs, existed for purposes of mutual protection. Anthropologists believe that primitive groups originated in Africa and migrated across the world. Ice ages in the northern latitudes may have driven these groups back to the warmer climates found around the Mediterranean Sea, in India, and in China, where civilizations developed.

In early human history, the regions around the Mediterranean Sea were thought to occupy the center of the earth, with all areas to the east known as "eastern" and all those to the west known as "western" (Donahue, 2010). The sophistication of healthcare practices varied considerably from one culture to another and was based largely on the ingenuity of the group. Consistent among most of the groups were strong beliefs in the power of gods, with sickness and suffering attributed to the presence of evil spirits. These evil spirits were dealt with in various ways: performing incantations and dances, making offerings and sacrifices, and working with medicine men who performed magic to drive away the demons. Health rules were often part of the religious codes which gave them authority. A sound theory of disease was absent from most early cultures. The healthcare practices of some of the early cultures are summarized in Table 1.1.

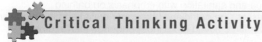

Critical Thinking Activity

Study Table 1.1. Because of the lack of organized nursing and healthcare in the early societies, how do you believe the people of the early cultures were cared for and by whom? How did they know what to do? How was this knowledge shared and from whom did they learn the skills they used? What was the quality of that care?

Table 1.1 **Summary of Healthcare Practices of Selected Early Civilizations***

SOCIETY & APPROXIMATE TIME PERIOD	CHARACTERISTICS AND CONTRIBUTIONS
Egypt 3000 BC	Provided the earliest medical records, dating back as far as 3000 BC, which included more than 700 classified drugs
	Developed a system of community planning that helped avoid public health problems
	Established strict rules regarding cleanliness, food, drink, exercise, and sexual relations
	Was credited with being one of the healthiest of the ancient civilizations
Ancient Israel 1900 BC	Developed the Mosaic Code under the leadership of Moses, which included an organized method of disease prevention
	Isolated people with communicable diseases, differentiated clean from unclean, and established dietary rules such as not eating meat past the 3rd day after slaughter, monitored by priest–physicians who functioned as health inspectors
	Shared knowledge with other cultures
Babylonia 2100 BC	Credited with being skilled mathematicians and astrologers: Many beliefs were based on study of nature, beliefs in the potency of numbers, and observations of the movement of stars and planets
	Believed illness was a punishment for sin and used incantations and herbs for purification; surgery was more advanced than internal medicine
	Developed Code of Hammurabi, which perhaps represents the first sliding scale for payment based on class
Assyria 745–635 BC	A group with strong instruments of war, had severe laws, and made frequent use of mutilation and death as punishments
	Believed in good and evil spirits, magic, and superstition, and in many gods; ill health was viewed as a punishment for sin
Persia 600–300 BC	An extensive empire whose people followed the preaching of Zoroaster, who introduced the concept of two creators: one good, one evil
	Adopted many of the medical practices of the lands they conquered
	Established early schools for priest-physicians, from which evolved three types of physicians: those who healed by the knife, those who healed with herbs, and those who healed through exorcism
Greece 800–300 BC	Society with beliefs in the power of a wide array of gods who had human characteristics
	Divination of the future and animal sacrifice to seek healing were common
	Placed much emphasis on healthy bodies; founded the Olympic games
	Built exquisite temples where learning and healing occurred
	Built institutions to care for sick and injured called *xendochium; iatrion* were built to offer ambulatory care
	The home of Hippocrates, born about 400 BC, who became known as the Father of Modern Medicine
	Hippocrates stressed natural causes for disease, a patient-centered approach, and the necessity of accurate observations and record keeping
Rome 800 BC to 476 AD	Borrowed medical practices from the countries they conquered; physicians were often slaves
	Had a pantheon of gods similar to the Greeks with different names
	Used both sacrifice and herbs when faced with illness
	Practiced advanced hygiene and sanitation with emphasis on bathing
	Society divided into two classes: the patricians (the upper class) and the plebeians (the common people); women enjoyed more independence than in other comparable societies

SOCIETY & APPROXIMATE TIME PERIOD	CHARACTERISTICS AND CONTRIBUTIONS
India (3000–1500 BC)	Early civilizations highly developed, with systems of sanitation, bathrooms, public baths, and other amenities Vedic age (1500 BC) characterized by worship of Brahma (Brahmanism or Hinduism), which resulted in segregation of society into four castes and sacrifice to satisfy gods Sacred book, the Vedas, a source of information about health practices and considered some of the oldest known written material Emphasized hygiene and prevention of sickness and described major and minor surgery, children's diseases, and diseases of the nervous and urinary systems
500 BC	Buddhism emerged about 500 BC; and during this period, an advanced understanding of disease prevention, hygiene and sanitation, medicine, and surgery was developed Prenatal care was emphasized for mothers, and public hospitals were constructed which were staffed with nurses (mostly men)
China 3000–249 BC	Followed the teachings of Confucius emphasizing the value of knowledge Patriarchal rule dominated with emphasis on the whole family; women considered vastly inferior to men Developed concept of yin and yang and had elaborate materia medica, identifying many drugs still used today Developed acupuncture skills still in practice today, studied circulation, and developed approach to examination: look, listen, ask, feel Baths used for reduction of fever, bloodletting to release evil spirits from the body
Arabia 570 AD	Populated by nomadic people who lived a difficult life in the hot, dry desert Muhammad, born about 570 A.D., developed the religion of Islam. Muhammad's teachings established strict rules of living, dictating habits of cleanliness, eating, and human interaction
The Americas	Civilization may have begun 10,000 to 20,000 years ago, with nomadic early inhabitants coming from Central Asia
Mayan and Aztec civilizations 2000–1000 BC	The great civilizations that created cities and far-flung empires were in Central and South America Sun god of particular significance; health viewed as a balance between man, nature, and the supernatural Rites, ceremonies, herbal treatments, charms, and perhaps human sacrifice contributed to healing practices Medicine men (known first as shamans and later as priests) were responsible for curing ills of body and mind

*Compiled from Donahue (2010).

HISTORIC PERSPECTIVES AND EARLY IMAGES OF NURSING

Although ancient cultures developed medicine as a science and a profession, writings about early healthcare make little or no mention of nursing or nurses. One might assume that a family member, particularly the wife or mother, provided the needed care. The possible exceptions to this were the male attendants in early Buddhist hospitals in India and midwives who had an established role in several cultures. It was not until the early Christian period that nursing as we think of it today began to develop.

Nursing has carried forward three heritages from the past that some believe impeded the development of nursing as a profession. They are the **folk image** of the nurse brought forward from primitive times, the **religious image** of the nurse inherited from the medieval period, and the **servant image** of the nurse created by the Protestant-capitalist ethic from the 16th to 19th century (see Fig. 1.1). Whether they hampered progress, these concepts of the nurse have certainly had an impact. A summary of these images is provided in Table 1.2.

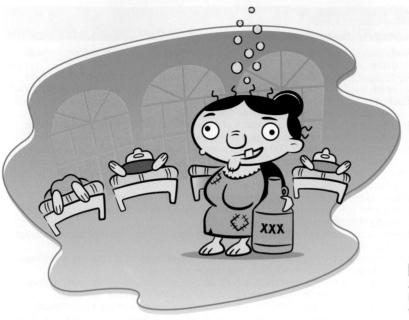

FIGURE 1.1 From the Middle Ages to the 19th century, nursing was often left to "uncommon women."

Table 1.2   **Nursing Heritages From the Past**

The folk image of the nurse	Primary responsibilities focused on nourishing and nurturing children, caring for the elderly, and caring for aging family members. Skills were learned through trial and error and passed from one generation to another. This image presents the nurse as a "caring" person who uses common sense to help the sick individual.
The religious image of the nurse	Groups were organized in conjunction with the establishment of churches in the Christian era with their primary concern focused on care for the sick, the poor, orphans, widows, the aged, slaves, and prisoners. These groups included the deaconesses of the Eastern Christian Church, the Order of Widows and the Order of Virgins, and monastic orders including the Benedictines, which still exist. The first hospitals were also developed at this time, being located close to monasteries. The Crusades (1096–1291) witnessed the founding of military nursing orders, such as the Knights Hospitallers of St. John, the Knights Templars, and the Knights of the Teutonic Order. Nurses in this setting were expected to devote their lives to caring and to exhibit selfless commitment based upon their religious faith.
The servant image of the nurse	The Reformation, which began in Germany in 1517, brought with it a change in the role of women, limiting it to the confines of the home. Duties were those of bearing children and caring for the home. Hospital care was relegated to uncommon women, a group consisting of prisoners, prostitutes, and drunks (Fig. 1.1) who had no status in society and were treated as servants who did distasteful tasks. This began what may be called the "Dark Ages" of nursing reflected in Charles Dickens's (1936) description of Sairey Gamp and Betsy Prig in his book *Martin Chuzzlewit*. This image may have greatly influenced the development of nursing as a profession as many capable and desirable persons were unwilling to enter nursing while it had this image.

THE BEGINNING OF CHANGE

During the 17th century, social reform began in Europe. Several nursing groups were organized. These groups gave money, time, and service to the sick and the poor, visiting them in their homes and ministering to their needs. Their activities established many of the early images that were carried forth in nursing, particularly the religious image. Some of these groups and their work are presented in Table 1.3.

Critical Thinking Activity

Knowing what you do about the history and early image of nursing, how will you, as a nurse of the future, advance the image of nursing? What characteristics do you believe are most critical? Who are the people who most need to be influenced? How do you think young people can best be encouraged to select nursing as a career?

Table 1.3   Early Providers of Nursing Care

Sisters of Charity in France and the United States	Founded in Paris in 1633 and receiving help from St. Vincent de Paul, the Sisters of Charity recruited and educated intelligent young women to care for abandoned children as well as provide hospital care. In 1809, the Sisters of Charity established a nursing order in the United States under the direction of Elizabeth Bayley Seton.
Sisters of the Holy Cross in France and the United States	Founded in 1839 in Le Mans, France and in the United States in Bertrand, Michigan in 1844, the Sisters of the Holy Cross provided care to the sick in hospitals and orphanages.
Catholic Religious Orders in Mexico and South America	Following the Reformation, several Roman Catholic religious groups traveled to the Americas. In 1524, the first hospital on the American continent, the Hospital of Immaculate Conception (Hospital de Nuestra Senora O Limpia Concepcion) was built in Mexico City, and mission colleges were founded. The first medical school in America was founded in 1578 at University of Mexico and the second at the University of Lima before 1600.
Ursuline Sisters in Canada	Accompanied Augustinian nuns from France to Quebec, Canada in 1639 to staff the Hotel-Dieu-de-Quebec (a hospital which opened that year), and organized the first training of nurses on the North American continent, teaching the native women to care for their families during a smallpox epidemic.
Deaconesses at Kaiserwerth, Germany and Pittsburgh, Pennsylvania	Led by Theodore Fliedner (1800–1864) with the assistance of his first wife, the Christian deaconess movement was revived in Germany in 1836 and a training institute was reestablished. Deaconesses cared for the sick, made visitations, worked in the parish, and taught. In 1849 Pastor Fliedner traveled to the United States to help establish the first Motherhouse of Kaiserwerth in Pittsburgh, Pennsylvania. The Deaconesses managed Pittsburgh Infirmary, which later became Passavant Hospital, the first Protestant hospital in the United States.
Nursing Sisters in England and Ireland	Institute of Nursing Sisters, a secular group, was organized in England by Elizabeth Fry (1780–1845). Sisters of Mercy: A Roman Catholic group formed in 1827 by Catherine McAuley (1787–1841). Irish Sisters of Charity: A Roman Catholic group formed in 1815 by Mary Aikenhead (1787–1857).

THE NIGHTINGALE INFLUENCE

As we look back to the middle of the 19th century, we encounter a world in the throes of an industrial revolution. Factories were built, schools were established, and travel and communication took giant leaps. The telegraph had revolutionized communication, making the happenings on a far-flung battlefield immediately available to the newspaper-reading public. The first rumblings regarding women and their right to vote occurred in England. This is the period in which nursing as a profession was born.

During this time, one woman dramatically changed the form and direction of nursing and succeeded in establishing it as a respected field of endeavor. This outstanding woman was **Florence Nightingale**.

Born May 12, 1820, the second daughter of a wealthy family, she was named after the city in which she was born—Florence, Italy. Because of her family's high social and economic standing, she was cultured, well traveled, and educated. By the age of 17, as the result of tutoring from her father, she had mastered seven languages and mathematics and was extremely well read. This was very unusual for a woman of her time, as she was expected to select a desirable husband from the influential people she met, marry, and assume her place in society, and therefore, further education was deemed unnecessary for her role in life.

Florence Nightingale had other ideas, however. She wanted to become a nurse, but this aspiration was unthinkable to her family because of the terrible conditions of the hospitals at that time and what we now refer to as the "servant image" of nursing. She continued to travel with her family and their friends and, in the course of these travels, met Sidney Herbert and his wife, who were interested in hospital reform. At the time, the public health movement and concerns about hospital reform were growing across England. Inspired, she began collecting information on public health and hospitals and soon became recognized as an important authority on the subject.

Through friends, she learned about Pastor Fliedner's institute at Kaiserwerth where care was provided and nurses were trained. She visited Kaiserwerth briefly in 1850. Because it was a religious institution under the auspices of a Protestant church, her parents would permit her to go there, although she could not go to English hospitals. In 1851, at age 31, she spent 3 months studying at Kaiserwerth.

In 1853, she began working with a committee that supervised an "Establishment for Gentlewomen During Illness." She eventually was appointed superintendent of the establishment, a position she held from August 1853 to October 1854. As her knowledge of hospitals and nursing reform grew, she was consulted by reformers and physicians who were beginning to see the need for trained nurses.

After the Crimean War began in March 1854, war correspondents communicating through the newly developed telegraph wrote about the abominable conditions in which the British Army cared for sick and wounded soldiers. Florence Nightingale, by then a recognized authority on hospital care, wrote to her friend Sir Sidney Herbert, who was then Secretary of War, and offered to take a group of 38 nurses to the Crimea. (At the same time, he had written a letter proposing that she assume direction of all nursing operations at the war front. Their letters crossed in the mail.) Her tireless efforts in the Crimea resulted in greatly reduced mortality rates among the sick and wounded. There is a museum in her honor in the barracks where she worked in what is now part of Istanbul, Turkey.

When the war ended in 1856, Florence Nightingale returned to England as a national heroine. Her next major project involved working to change the entire approach to health for the British soldier. These activities included constructing hospitals and improving basic hygiene and public health measures for the army. Her focus was on providing cleanliness, wholesome food, fresh air, and separation of people from garbage and sewage both for living environments and for hospital construction. These simple public health measures were revolutionary in the late 1800s.

After her return from the Crimea, she experienced ongoing health problems. Much has been written of her illness. Some authorities indicate that her symptoms were consistent with chronic brucellosis, a not uncommon disease of the time; others have expressed the view that it was, to a large degree, a neurosis; and more recently, some declare that it was posttraumatic stress disorder.

Early writers suggested that she retreated to her bedroom and, for the next 43 years, conducted her extensive involvement in healthcare from her secluded apartment. However, more recent research indicates Florence Nightingale had a greater personal involvement in nursing in her later years including providing care to the villagers at Lea Hurst (a family summer home). In addition to her ongoing public health work, she cared for her mother, sister, and extended family members; provided nursing to Holloway villagers; and reformed nursing at Buxton Hospital where her patients were admitted (MacQueen, 2007).

Throughout her lifetime, Florence Nightingale wrote extensively about hospitals, sanitation, health, and health statistics (creating the first pie chart), and especially about nursing and nursing education. Among her most popular books is *Notes on Nursing*, published in 1859. She crusaded for and brought about great reform in nursing education. Her reform of the nursing system and nursing education eventually spread to many nations.

In 1860, she devoted her efforts to the creation of a school of nursing at St. Thomas' Hospital in London, financed by the Nightingale Fund, established to honor her work in the Crimea. The basic principles on which Miss Nightingale established her school included the following:

- Nurses would be trained in teaching hospitals associated with medical schools and organized for that purpose.
- Nurses would be selected carefully and would reside in nurses' houses designed to encourage discipline and form character.
- The school matron would have final authority over the curriculum, living arrangements, and all other aspects of the school.
- The curriculum would include both theoretic material and practical experience.
- Teachers would be paid for their instruction.
- Records would be kept on the students, who would be required to attend lectures, take quizzes, write papers, and keep diaries.

In many other ways, Florence Nightingale advanced nursing as a profession. She believed that nurses should spend their time caring for patients, not cleaning; that nurses must continue learning throughout their lifetime and not become "stagnant;" that nurses should be intelligent and use that intelligence to improve conditions for the patient; and that nursing leaders should have social standing. She had a vision of what nursing could and should be. Further discussion of Florence Nightingale's definition of nursing occurs later in this chapter.

Florence Nightingale received many honors from foreign governments, and in 1907, she was recognized by the Queen of England, who awarded her the British Order of Merit. It was the first time it was given to a woman.

Florence Nightingale died in her sleep at the age of 90 on August 13, 1910. The week during which she was born is now honored as International Nurses Week. The enthusiastic student is encouraged to learn more about this fascinating woman in Mark Bostridge's biography *Florence Nightingale: The Making of an Icon (2008)* or by pursuing the topic of Florence Nightingale through the Internet.

THE BEGINNING OF NURSING EDUCATION IN THE UNITED STATES

After the establishment of the Nightingale School in England, nursing programs flourished, and the Nightingale system spread to other countries. In the United States, much of the push for nursing education occurred shortly after the Civil War, during which the lack of trained nurses presented a serious concern.

The Establishment of Early Schools

As with many other significant events that have evolved from a variety of influences, it is difficult to pinpoint the first nursing program in the United States. As early as 1798, a pioneer physician, Dr. Valentine Seaman, is said to have initiated the first system of instruction for nurses at New York Hospital. A society was formed in 1839 under Quaker influence, called the Nurse Society of Philadelphia, and a combined Home and School were opened. Historical records show that before 1850, some intermittent preparation was provided to individuals who cared for the sick. A plan of instruction also had been developed for women who would supply maternity service in the home, under the guidance of Dr. Joseph Warrington, who was the obstetric physician for the Philadelphia Dispensary for the Medical Relief of the Poor (Donahue, 2010).

In 1850, a commission of the Massachusetts legislature recommended that institutions be formed to educate nurses. A plan for educating nurses was included in the formation of the *New England Female Medical College*, and a few nurses were educated through this institution. Other hospitals operated training programs, although the course of studies lasted only 6 months. The *Woman's Hospital of Philadelphia*, which operated under the direction of two female physicians, opened a training school in 1861, but it made little progress until it was endowed in 1872. Despite these efforts, the nursing services provided by most hospitals during the 1860s were disorganized and inadequate. In many cases, nursing care was provided by women who had been recruited from among the poor who were sheltered in almshouses or from those who had been arrested for drunkenness or disorderly conduct and who were serving out 10-day sentences. The better hospitals benefited from the work of Catholic sisters or Protestant deaconesses, although most of them also were untrained (Kalisch & Kalisch, 2004, p. 60–61).

In 1869, responding to the impetus given to nursing during the Civil War, the American Medical Association established a committee to study the issue of training for nurses. The committee, chaired by Dr. Samuel D. Gross (1805–1884), was charged with identifying the best possible method to organize and manage institutions for training nurses. Its report concluded that every large hospital should have a nursing school, emphasized that the union between religious exercises and nursing would be conducive to the welfare of the sick, and recommended that schools be placed under the guardianship of county medical societies (Donahue, 2010).

The *New England Hospital for Women and Children* is often credited with being the first hospital to establish a formal 1-year program to train nurses in 1872. It operated under the guidance of a female physician, Susan Dimock, who had received her medical education in Europe and had some knowledge of the work of Florence Nightingale. Five probationers started the program on September 1. It was from this school that Melinda Ann (Linda) Richards graduated in 1873, to become America's first trained nurse. This school was also the alma mater for the first black nurse graduate, Mary Eliza Mahoney, in 1879.

By 1873, three additional schools had opened: the *Bellevue Training School* in New York City, the *Connecticut Training School* in New Haven, and the *Boston Training School*. Typically, these schools did not admit men. In 1888, the *Mills School of Nursing* at Bellevue Hospital opened to train male nurses for patient care. Separate schools to educate black nurses also opened; among them were *Spelman Seminary* in Atlanta in 1886, *Hampton Institute* in Virginia and *Providence Hospital* in Chicago in 1891, and *Tuskegee Institute* in Alabama in1892 (Kalisch & Kalisch, 2004). Table 1.4 identifies some of the early schools.

Similar movements to establish nursing schools occurred in other countries. In 1868, a school was organized in Sydney Hospital, Australia. In Edinburgh, Scotland, a program was started at the Royal Infirmary. The *Mack Training School* in St. Catharines, Toronto, Canada, was started in 1884 (Kalisch & Kalisch, 2004).

Table 1.4   Early North American Training Schools for Nurses*

DATE	NAME AND PLACE	COMMENTS
1798	New York Hospital—New York	Dr. Valentine Seaman initiated a system of instruction for nurses. His lectures covered the topics of anatomy, physiology, maternal nursing, and care of children.
1839	Philadelphia Dispensary—Philadelphia	Dr. Joseph Warrington provided obstetric training to a group of women who would work with families who would otherwise not receive care. The Nurse Society of Philadelphia grew out of this training.
1861	Bellevue Hospital—New York	Dr. Elizabeth Blackwell converted Bellevue Hospital into a training center for nurses. About 100 women were trained to provide care during the Civil War in an intensive 4-week course.
1861–1862	Woman's Hospital of Philadelphia—Philadelphia	Opened a training school, but it progressed slowly until 1872, when it became endowed—the first endowed school of nursing in America. Organized and conducted by two female physicians.
1862	New England Hospital for Women and Children—Boston	Dr. Marie Zakrzewska, a colleague of Dr. Blackwell's, offered a 6-month program to nurses.
1872	New England Training School—Boston	An expansion of the New England Hospital Program was identified as the first formal school for nurses, directed by Dr. Susan Dimock. The first graduate was Linda Ann Richards. Mary Mahoney, the first black nurse to graduate from a nursing school, also attended this school.
1873–May	Bellevue Training School—New York	First of a trio of schools modeled after the Nightingale model—Lavinia Dock was one of the early graduates.
1873–October	Connecticut Training School—New Haven	Second of the trio of schools started in 1873—introduced first textbook, *New Haven Manual of Nursing*, written by a committee of nurses and physicians.

(table continues on page 12)

Table 1.4   **Early North American Training Schools for Nurses*** (continued)

DATE	NAME AND PLACE	COMMENTS
1873–November	Boston Training School—Boston (attached to Massachusetts General)	Third of the trio—Linda Richards became superintendent of nurses in November 1894. Idea for school initiated by the Woman's Educational Association. Medical staff did not support initiation of the school.
1874	St. Catharine's General and Marine Hospital—Ontario, Canada—later called the Mack Training School	Patterned after the Nightingale schools, this program included instruction in the art of nursing, chemistry, sanitary science, physiology, and anatomy.
1877	Training School of the New York Hospital—New York	Offered an 18-month course to prepare graduates for nursing.
1878	Boston City Hospital Training School—Boston	Required graduates to complete a 2-year program of study.
1884	Toronto General Hospital—Toronto, Canada	Mary Agnes Snively became superintendent of this school, which had early beginnings in 1877.
1884–1885	Farrand Training School for Nurses—Harper Hospital, Detroit	Considered one of the better schools, students had two annual series of lectures, approximately 20 hours totally.
1886	Spelman Seminary—Atlanta	The first separate school to educate black nurses, who were often denied admission to other schools.
1888	Mills School of Nursing at Bellevue Hospital—New York	First school established for male nurses. Prepared them to give general patient care.
1889	Johns Hopkins School of Nursing—Baltimore	Program opened under direction of Isabel Hampton Robb. Mary Adelaide Nutting graduated in 1891.
1890	Montreal General—Montreal, Canada	Although wanting a nursing program as early as 1835, hospital conditions would not allow. Nora Gertrude Livingstone established the school in 1890.

*Compiled from Donahue (2010), and Kalisch and Kalisch (2004).

Characteristics of the Early Schools

The life of the nursing student at the turn of the century was not an easy one. The strong militaristic and religious influences over nursing were embodied in the expectations held for nursing students. The nurse in training was expected to yield to her superiors and demonstrate the obedience characteristic of a good soldier with actions governed by the dedication to duty derived from religious devotion (Kalisch & Kalisch, 2004).

The typical nursing student was about 21 years of age, single, and female. The first weeks or months of their education were spent as probationers, or "probies," and their duties, although helping with the operation of the hospital, did little to educate them as nurses. For example, they spent much of their time washing, scrubbing, polishing, folding, stacking, and the like. Rules of conduct were rigid and unforgiving; early superintendents saw it as their responsibility to discipline pupils, ensuring that they possessed good morals and were honest, conscientious, obedient, respectful, loyal, passive, and devoted to duty. Nursing students were expected to be unselfish, thinking not of themselves but of the happiness and well-being of others (Fig. 1.2). This is in keeping with the "religious image" of the nurse.

Initially, nursing education was largely an apprenticeship and resulted in students providing much of the workforce of hospitals. The workday was long and arduous, often starting at 5:30 AM and ending with nursing prayers very late at night, and consisted primarily of work

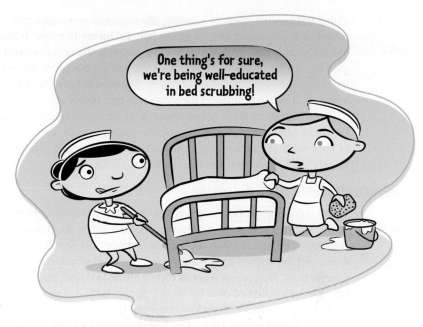

One thing's for sure, we're being well-educated in bed scrubbing!

FIGURE 1.2 The duties assigned to probationers may have helped operate the hospital but did little to educate the nurse.

on the hospital wards. The superintendent or her assistants provided instruction. There was no standardization of curriculum and no accreditation. The few lectures that were part of the program were usually given by physicians and scheduled at 8 or 9 PM after a long day of work. A 7-day workweek was the standard, and the help needed on the hospital units took precedence over the education of the young women. Lectures were canceled if students were needed to care for patients.

As schools developed, facilities to house nursing students became necessary. Although some of the early programs provided sleeping quarters in the hospital, nursing students usually were housed in a building next to the hospital, often referred to as the "nurses' dormitory." A "housemother" often controlled the nurses' residence. In religious affiliations, a deaconess or Sister served the same purpose. Housemothers ensured that codes of behavior were adhered to and that curfews were enforced. Violations usually resulted in expulsion from the program or the loss of a part of the uniform, such as a cap or the bib section of an apron. This signified to all that some infraction had occurred. Young women, who were attracted to nursing because of the imagined glamour of wearing a long, crisp, white apron and ministering to sick (though handsome) young men, often became discouraged with the severe duties and routine. The attrition rate was high in the early schools.

From about 1900 to 1920, nursing in Western Europe, Canada, and the United States was beginning to establish itself with the growth of schools, the publication of journals and textbooks, and the formulation of organizations for nursing (see Chapter 15). For both society and nursing, it was an era of great growth. Schools proliferated, as even small hospitals established nursing programs, recognizing the valuable commodity available in students who provided the majority of care given. As early as 1905, early pioneers and advocates for nursing, concerned about the proliferation of schools, championed programs that offered a sound educational foundation and reasonable working hours. During the time Isabel Hampton was principal of the Johns Hopkins Training School (a position she accepted in 1889 and continued until her marriage to Dr. Robb in 1894), she arranged for a regular period of 2 hours of free time during a day that was limited to 12 hours. She would have liked to limit the workday to 8 hours, however. Time was allowed for recreation and for meals.

Although there were some changes in the curriculum—work hours were decreased, the length of study was increased, and the theory component was organized into specific areas of care such as medical, surgical, and obstetric nursing—hospital-based programs remained largely unchanged through the 1940s and 1950s.

Early Textbooks and Journals

There were few textbooks before 1900, a factor that complicated the learning process. Many of the lectures presented by physicians were given from notes they had taken while medical students. The first nursing textbook was reportedly the *Hand-book of Nursing for Family and General Use*, written by a committee composed of physicians and nurses associated with the *Connecticut Training School* at New Haven Hospital and published by Lippincott in 1878. Other books followed over the next 2 years. Table 1.5 describes some of the early textbooks.

Nursing journals also appeared toward the end of the 19th century. Five journals for nurses were published before 1901. The first appeared in 1886 and was entitled *The Nightingale*. In 1889, under the direction of Mary E. P. Davis, a company was formed with 550 cash subscriptions, and a new journal called the *American Journal of Nursing* made its debut in October 1900 (Kalisch & Kalisch, 2004, p. 106). The journal continues to be published today.

Critical Thinking Activity

Imagine that you are an instructor in an early nursing program. There are no textbooks. There are no nursing journals from which you can assign reading. Computers and the Internet were unheard of. How would you go about teaching the students for whom you are responsible? What would you see as the major concerns? How would the classes differ from those you attend today?

Table 1.5   Early Nursing Textbooks*

YEAR	AUTHOR	TITLE
1878	A committee of physicians and nurses	*Hand-book for Family and General Use*
1885	Clara Weeks Shaw	*A Textbook of Nursing for the Use of Training Schools, Families and Private Students*
1890	Lavinia Dock	*The Textbook on Materia Medica for Nurses*
1893	Diana Kimber	*The first anatomy book for nurses, Anatomy and Physiology*
1889 (about)	Isabel Hampton	*Nursing: Its Principles and Practices for Hospital and Private Use*
1894 (about)	Isabel Hampton Robb	*Nursing Ethics*

*Compiled from Donahue (2010), and Kalisch and Kalisch (2004).

THE MILITARY INFLUENCE

Through her experience in the Crimean War, Florence Nightingale first brought attention to nursing as a career and profession and to needed changes in the healthcare delivery. Similarly, other wars have brought advances in how care is provided. In war and after war, nurses have provided care, expanded the role of nursing, and created new nursing techniques. In the following section, we highlight some of those areas of **military influence**; however, it is impossible, in the context of this book, to provide more than just an overview.

The American Revolution

All of the English colonies scattered along the Atlantic Coast of the United States were involved in the American Revolution. The hastily organized army existed without the benefit of a medical corps or trained nurses. The nuns of the Catholic Church, who also cared for those who were ill with epidemic diseases, such as scarlet fever, dysentery, and smallpox, nursed wounded soldiers. Women who had followed their husbands to the battlefield often cared for soldiers. Homes and barns near the battles were turned into hospitals. Other women contributed to the cause by making clothing and bandages or by helping to feed the soldiers from their own pantries.

When the war ended, the usual type of poverty existed, and invalids and the disabled needed care. However, the colonies were not sufficiently developed to have such services available. In response, a new type of institution evolved, which is perhaps the forerunner of today's clinic or hospital outpatient department. In 1786, the Philadelphia Dispensary was established, and volunteer physicians treated those needing care at no charge. These dispensaries later became a major site for controlling disease. Vaccination against smallpox was one of the earliest preventive treatments offered there.

The Civil War

The Civil War broke out in the United States in 1861. Although social reform was on the rise, the nursing profession was still in an embryonic, unorganized stage. There was neither an army nurse corps nor an organized medical corps. There were no ambulance services or hospital units. Responding to the nursing needs created by the war, in which it is estimated that 618,000 men died (Donahue, 2010), many men and women volunteered to help. After a brief training course, they performed nursing duties on behalf of the Union. The poet Walt Whitman is one of the better known individuals who became nurses during this time. Many religious orders also volunteered and provided service. A steamer, captured from the Confederates, was converted into a floating hospital and anchored near Vicksburg, Mississippi. Considered the first Navy hospital ship, the *Red Rover* was staffed through the volunteer efforts of the Catholic Sisters of Mercy, who became the first "Navy" nurses. An account of some of the contributions of nurses during the Civil War and afterward is found in Table 1.6 The serious need for trained nurses created by the Civil War was undoubtedly a significant factor in the development of nursing in the United States.

The Spanish–American War and the Boer War

These two wars occurred at about the same time in history. The United States entered the Spanish–American War in 1898, and the British battled the second Boer War in South Africa in late 1899. By this time, the Red Cross, founded by Clara Barton, a New England

Table 1.6   **Nurses of the Civil War and Their Contributions***

NURSE	CONTRIBUTION
Sojourner Truth (1797–1883)	Born into slavery and named Isabella, this African American was sold three times by the time she was 13, the last time for $300. She married an older slave and bore him five children, some of whom were also sold into slavery. In 1843 she changed her name to Sojourner Truth. She nursed Union soldiers, worked for improvement in sanitary facilities, and sought contributions of food and clothing for black volunteer regiments. She supported her travel from sales of her *Narrative* of *Sojourner Truth: A Northern Slave* (1850), dictated to Olive Gilbert because she was illiterate. She continued her work as a nurse/counselor for the Freedmen's Relief Association after the war (Whitman, 1985, pp. 814–816).
Dorothea Lynde Dix (1802–1881)	A Boston schoolteacher already known for her humanitarian efforts on behalf of the mentally ill, she was commissioned as Superintendent of Women Nurses for All Military Hospitals during the Civil War when she was over 60 years of age. Her authority was often challenged by the physicians.
Mary Ann Ball Bickerdyke (1817–1901)	Called "Mother" Bickerdyke by the troops, this Illinois woman challenged the work of lazy, corrupt medical officers. She served under fire in 19 battles. Her efforts were recognized by the government in the launching of the hospital ship, the *SS Mary A. Bickerdyke* in 1943.
Walt Whitman (1819–1892)	A well-respected poet, who worked as a volunteer in hospital wards after searching for a brother who had been wounded. Dressed wounds, wrote letters, read to soldiers, brought gifts and food. Later wrote about the war and suffering of soldiers.
Harriet Ross Tubman (1820–1913)	An abolitionist sometimes called "Conductor of the Underground Railroad," this black nurse was commended for caring for the sick and wounded without regard for color.
Mary Livermore (1820–1905)	Another untrained nurse of the Civil War, she later became a suffragist and advocated education for all women. Addressing the 6th annual convention of the Nurses' Associated Alumnae, she described the activities of the Civil War nurses.
Clara Barton (1821–1912)	Served as a Volunteer with the Sixth Massachusetts Regiment. Independently operated a large-scale relief operation. Was instrumental in founding the American Red Cross in 1882. Called "little lone lady in black silk" (Donahue, 2010).
Kate Cummings (1828–1909)	A volunteer in the Southern army, her diaries chronicled the work of the "matrons" who served in the Confederate hospitals.
Louisa May Alcott (1832–1888)	Served as a volunteer nurse during the Civil War. From these experiences she wrote a small book entitled *Hospital Sketches,* which described the work of the volunteer nurses of the Civil War. The nurse character of the book was Miss Tribulation Periwinkle.
Jane Stuart Woolsey (1830–1891)	One of three sisters from a cultivated and elite northeastern family with colonial ancestry, Jane served the Union Army as supervisor of the nursing and cooking department. She provided much narrative to describe the conditions of the day, authoring a book entitled *Hospital Days.* Later, she served as the directress of the Presbyterian Hospital in New York.
Abby Howland Woolsey (1828–1893)	A sister of Jane, she too served as a volunteer nurse for the Union Army and fought diligently for the abolition of slavery. Helped found the Bellevue Hospital Training School for Nurses and wrote one of the first books on the organization of nursing schools— *A Century of Nursing with Hints Toward the Organization of a Training School* (1876) (Whitman, 1985, pp. 904–906).
Georgeanna Muirson Woolsey (1833–1906)	Another Woolsey sister involved in war efforts, she benefited from a month-long nursing training experience in New York when selected by the Woman's Central Association of Relief as one of a group of 100 for leadership potential. She wrote of her war experiences in a book entitled *Three Weeks at Gettysburg.* She later helped found the Connecticut Training School for Nursing in New Haven, enjoying the support of her husband, Dr. Francis Bacon (Whitman, 1985, pp. 903–906).
Susie King Taylor (1848–1901)	Born into slavery, as a young girl she secretly learned to read and write. While serving as a volunteer nurse for the Union Army, she also worked as a teacher.

*Compiled from Kalisch and Kalisch (2004), except as otherwise noted.

schoolteacher, had been organized. The United States, Canada, and Great Britain all had nursing schools to prepare young women for nursing roles.

In the early days of the Spanish–American War, little attention was given to the selection of nurses to care for the wounded. Volunteers, both men and women, included nurses with training, those partly trained, and the untrained. The entire system lacked organization; needed supplies were seriously deficient. These conditions attracted the attention of both the government and the people. Among groups addressing the concern was the Nurses' Associated Alumnae of the United States and Canada, who offered to develop a process through which better skilled nurses might be secured. The management of the chosen nurses was given over to the Red Cross, which retained this role throughout the war.

Nursing occurred in the military camps, where problems such as inadequate water facilities, lack of laundry and laundry services, and inadequate medical supplies were encountered. Many nurses became ill with typhoid fever. A memorial in Arlington National Cemetery honors the memory of the women who gave their lives as Army nurses in the Spanish–American War. It was erected by the Society of Spanish–American War Nurses.

When the war ended, nurse leaders exerted pressure to secure legislation to ensure an efficient army nursing service. A bill establishing the Army Nurse Corps was passed in 1901, and in 1908, the Navy Nurse Corps was established. At about this time, the Red Cross began a complete reorganization. William Howard Taft, who also became president of the United States during this time, served as its president for 8 years.

In South Africa, the situation was much the same as in the United States—the need for more efficient and educationally prepared nurses was apparent. The British Army Nursing Service, organized in 1881 as a result of the Crimean experience, recruited nurse volunteers who functioned in tented field hospitals but not at army lines. Britain soon learned that it needed a group of nurses who could be called upon in an emergency, and, in March 1902, the Queen Alexandra's Imperial Military Nursing Service (QAIMNS) replaced its predecessor the British Army Nursing Service. It is recognized today as Queen Alexandra's Royal Army Nursing Corps (QARANC, 2006).

World War I

Following a number of diplomatic clashes, in 1914, war broke out in Europe. On April 6, 1917, the United States joined forces with Britain, Russia, and the French Empires against Germany, Austria–Hungary, and Italy. In 1914, Austria–Hungary declared war on Serbia; Germany invaded Belgium and France; and England became involved in the conflict. The United States joined them in what was also called The Great War on April 6, 1917. Through QAIMNS, England was prepared to meet the emergency needs for care. Navy and Air Force branches were added to that of the Army, and an organized Voluntary Aid Detachment composed of laypersons was organized. In the United States, the Army and Navy Nurse Corps had been created in 1901 and 1908; thus, when the United States joined the conflict, nurses from these groups were ready to provide care to the wounded; other experienced nurses were recruited and enlisted. It is estimated that 30,000 nurses served in World War I. The impact of this figure is made more impressive when one remembers that women did not have the right to vote until 1919. In fact, President Woodrow Wilson is said to have been won over to the suffragist's position by the contribution of nurses during the war.

Despite continuous efforts to provide an adequate supply of nurses in both civilian and army hospitals, the lack of qualified nurses became more marked as time went on. The influenza epidemic of 1918 was of major proportions; pneumonia and typhus also claimed many lives, including those of doctors and nurses. In this time of great national need, the Army Nursing Corps finally agreed to admit black nurses, although the war had ended before they began their service. Recognizing the demand for a long-term supply of military nurses, the Army School of Nursing was organized in 1918. In 1938, a statue sculpted by Francis Rich from Tennessee marble, titled "Spirit of Nursing," was erected at Arlington National Cemetery among the graves of nurses who had served their country. The only one of its kind to honor nurses in all the services, it was rededicated in 1971 (The Nurse's Memorial, 2007). Students who wish to learn more about nurses' contributions during the war are encouraged to visit the Web site *http://www.spartacus.schoolnet.co.uk/FWWwomen.htm*.

The experiences of the war also pointed to the serious need for uniformity in methods of nursing education. In response, England founded the Royal College of Nursing in 1916. Inspection and accreditation of schools became one of this group's major concerns.

World War II

In response to Germany's invasion of Austria and Poland, England declared war against Germany and Italy in September 1939. The United States entered the war after Japan attacked Pearl Harbor on December 7, 1941. Thus began a conflict that was to be known as a "total war" because it affected every nation in the world. In the United States, the National Nursing Council for War Service was organized in July 1940 to help meet the increasing need for individuals at all levels of preparation who could care for the sick and wounded. The U.S. Cadet Nurse Corps was established under the Bolton Act, which was authorized in June 1943 and lasted until 1948. Under this program, more than 124,000 women graduated from the Cadet Nurse Corps with over 1,100 of the nation's nursing schools participating (O'Neil, 2008). It provided funds for tuition, a monthly allowance, uniforms, and other expenses for women who would enter nursing and, upon completion of their education, serve in the military service (Fig. 1.3). Unfortunately, no state or federal benefits have been established for nurses who served in the military service via the Cadet Nurse Corps route. Volunteer nurse aides were given short, intensive training so that they might assist nurses in hospitals.

In World War II, nurses were given commissions as officers and had military rank, something that had not been true previously. This gave them a level of status and authority that supported their work. Nurses who were assigned to war zones, as opposed to working in military hospitals, often found themselves facing a serious dilemma. The Army had done nothing to prepare them for battlefield medicine or for life in the field. Wounded men were treated in field hospitals close to battle lines with supplies and equipment that might be inadequate, while bombs dropped around them. Although they were in the Army, the nurses considered themselves healers, not soldiers. Elizabeth Norman (1999) poignantly describes the situation in her book *We Band of Angels*:

Then the shooting started, and they found themselves confronting as much danger and deprivation as any dogface in the field. The men who worked with them—doctors, medics, orderlies and attendants—were no longer "colleagues" and "staff," they were comrades in arms now, and "the girls," as so many referred to them, were no longer anomalies in the ranks, they were a military unit in the middle of battle. They were women at war. (p. 39) (Note: "dogface" was a slang term for the ordinary soldier.)

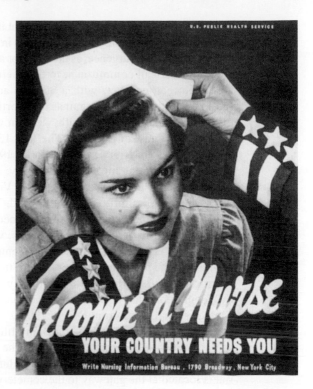

U.S. PUBLIC HEALTH SERVICE

become a Nurse

YOUR COUNTRY NEEDS YOU

Write Nursing Information Bureau , 1790 Broadway , New York City

FIGURE 1.3 Nurses were widely recruited for service in the military.

During this time, flight nursing came into existence, as nurses were taught to assist with the air evacuation of sick and wounded soldiers and at ground medical installations. Nurses in these roles worked under extremely dangerous circumstances because the planes used to transport patients also were used to transport cargo. Because of this dual activity, the planes were not marked with the Geneva Red Cross or other insignia, and they remained fair targets for enemy fighters.

Meanwhile, the United States experienced an industrial boom as defense plants mushroomed in response to military needs. Public health nurses moved into industry to carry out preventive health education and programs. Industrial nursing evolved on a national scale, with nurses employed in all types of manufacturing plants.

All of these activities left the country desperate for nurses. Serious shortages were felt in civilian hospitals and military situations. Nursing students began to carry much of the workload in hospitals that had nursing education programs.

After the war, the nurses who returned to civilian life had the benefit of the GI bill for education. As former officers in the military, they were accustomed to taking responsibility and leading. They entered bachelor's and master's degree programs and began to enlarge the cadre of college-educated nurses.

The Korean and Vietnam Conflicts

On June 25, 1950, the Korean Conflict broke out. Once again, nurses were called into military service. Learning from the experiences of World War II, treatment centers located close to the front lines were established—the Mobile Army Surgical Hospital (MASH). Triage care evolved, made more effective by advances in antibiotics and medical technology. Flight nursing saw a significant resurgence, as the need for air evacuation of the wounded reached new heights.

The American commitment to the Vietnamese government began about the same time as the Korean conflict, with a 35-man advisory team sent by President Truman to aid the French in their fight against the North Vietnamese. By 1963, approximately 15,000 military advisers were in South Vietnam working with Vietnamese troops in their battles against the Viet Cong troops. The first 13 nurses were placed on the staff at the Eighth Field Hospital in Nha Trang in March 1962 (Kalisch & Kalisch, 2004). Recruitment of nurses was once again a major activity; extraordinary incentives were offered because of widespread lack of support for the Vietnam conflict. Due to the guerrilla tactics of the Viet Cong, no military front existed. The country was partitioned into separate field zones, and semipermanent, air-conditioned hospitals were constructed. Fixed installations were assigned to area-support missions, with ground evacuation of the wounded almost impossible. Terrain and climate were tremendous obstacles. Advances in medical technology, however, permitted far better care than during any other combat situation. The contribution of nurses during this conflict was recognized publicly in a sculpture, designed by Glenna Goodacre, of three nurses and a wounded soldier erected near the Vietnam Memorial in Washington, DC, in 1993.

On October 18, 1997, the Women in Military Service for America memorial was dedicated at the Arlington National Cemetery as the only major national memorial honoring women who have served in our national defense during all eras. This marble, stone, and glass memorial is located at the gateway to the cemetery.

The Gulf War

The Iraqi Republican Guard invaded Kuwait on August 2, 1990, and seized control of that country. In an effort to protect Kuwait and deter any invasion of Saudi Arabia, Kuwait's oil-rich neighbor, the United States mounted Operation Desert Shield, the code name of the military action to eject the Iraqi army from Kuwait. When no withdrawal occurred, as mandated in a United Nations ultimatum, a US-led coalition launched air and ground attacks against Iraqi targets, thus initiating the first Gulf War.

Again, nurses were deployed to the area of battle, setting up MASH units in conditions quite different from anything they previously had experienced. Often equipped with protective gas masks to combat any chemical warfare that might have been present, these nurses endured rocket attacks, cold rains, hot winds, and dust and sandstorms of the Arabian desert. Operating from tents, they mobilized triage areas, assisted with surgery, treated shrapnel wounds, and cared for the innocent Iraqi and Kuwaiti victims of war, many of whom were women and children, as well as wounded soldiers. As in other war situations, a major challenge was found in improvising equipment and techniques to handle emergency situations. If you are interested in learning more about nurses and the Gulf War, an extensive bibliography of articles related to the topic is available at *www.gulflink.osd.mil/gwv_bib/nursing.html*.

The Middle East Conflict

When the conflict began in Iraq in 2003, nurses were again playing critical roles in helping to care for soldiers and civilians. In field hospitals housed in tents and placed close to the front, rapid trauma care was required along with better bandages and ways to stem uncontrolled bleeding. The need to speedily airlift seriously injured soldiers from aeromedical staging facilities in Iraq and Afghanistan to military field hospitals in Germany and then to other countries became critical. Nurses played important roles in air force hospitals preparing patients for aeromedical evacuation from Iraq, assessing conditions before and during transport in what were sometimes referred to as flying intensive care units. Working in expanded roles as nurse practitioners and anesthetists, nurses provided care to American and coalition armed services, merchant marines, Iraqi nationals (including women and children), and Iraqi enemy prisoners of war on the navy hospital ship *USNS Comfort* as a part of Operation Iraqi Freedom and Operation Enduring Freedom missions.

TERRORIST ATTACKS AND NATURAL DISASTERS

Some of the most devastating events calling for skilled nursing actions and leadership behavior occur at times other than wartime. Examples include events such as the terrorist attacks on the World Trade Center or the destruction, damage, and illness that occur as the result of hurricanes, floods, earthquakes, and fires. Being able to respond quickly and decisively in times of national crisis requires preparedness, collaboration, and formalized deployment roles. Human, financial, and technical resources must be maximized.

Critical Thinking Activity

In which of the wartime conflicts described do you believe nurses' roles were most critical? Provide the rationale for your choice, focusing on the factors that resulted in your choosing this conflict.

DEVELOPING A DEFINITION FOR NURSING

When you entered the nursing program in which you are now enrolled, what was your perception of nursing as a profession? Has that perception of nursing been changed by the experiences you have had as a nursing student? Some might ask, "Why spend so much time and effort trying to define nursing?"

Over the years, the profession has worked at establishing a definition of nursing; however, nurses themselves cannot agree on a single definition. A major factor that has made it difficult to define nursing is that it is taught as encompassing both theoretic and practical aspects, but it is pursued (and continues to be defined) primarily through practice, until recently a little-studied area. This failure to chart and study our practices and clinical observations has deprived nursing theory of the uniqueness and richness of the knowledge embedded in expert clinical practice. When attempting to define nursing, we often stumble over theoretical concepts and the practical, hands-on application of nursing and how to combine the distinct and unique aspects of both. Despite the challenges, serious efforts were put into defining nursing in the late 1970s and early 1980s.

Early Definitions of Nursing

A nurse is a person who nourishes, fosters, and protects—a person who is prepared to care for the sick, injured, and aged. In this sense, "nurse" is used as a noun and is derived from the Latin *nutrix,* which means "nursing mother." The word "nurse" also has referred to a woman who suckled a child (usually not her own)—a wet nurse. Dictionary definitions of nurse include such descriptions as "suckles or nourishes," "to take care of a child or children," and "to bring up; rear." In this way, "nurse" is used as a verb, deriving from the Latin *nutrire*, which means "to suckle and nourish." References to "the nurse" can be found in both the Talmud and in the Old Testament, and appear more similar to the wet nurse than to someone who cared for the sick.

Over the centuries, the word "nurse" has evolved to refer to a person who tends to the needs of the sick. Florence Nightingale, in her *Notes on Nursing: What It Is and What It Is Not*, described the nurse's role as one that would "put the patient in the best condition for nature to act upon him" (Nightingale, 1954, p. 133), a definition that often is quoted today.

In the past, nurses undoubtedly were more concerned about carrying out their responsibilities than about defining the role of the nurse. Through the years, we have seen the concept of the nurse grow and evolve from the nurse as mother, nourishing and nurturing children, to the nurse without specific reference to gender, with responsibilities encompassing expanded roles and involved in providing vital services to people needing healthcare.

Not surprising, the development of nursing as a profession, the defining of its role and language for society, and the placing of it among other attractive careers have been inextricably tied to the role of women in society at various times in history and to the forces that have had an impact on society. If we are frustrated at what appears to be the slow development of nursing as a profession, we need to remember that it was 1916 when Margaret Sanger opened the first birth control clinic in the United States. And not until 1919, after 40 years of campaigning, were women in the United States granted the right to vote, through the 19th Amendment to the Constitution.

Distinguishing Nursing From Medicine

The formulation of clear and concise definitions of nursing also has been hindered by the lack of an obvious distinction between nursing and medicine. For example, it is not unusual to hear a prospective nursing student say, "I've always been interested in the medical field, so I decided to go into nursing." Something of an interdependence exists between medicine and nursing, and they have somewhat paralleled one another in historic development. However, anyone who has been involved in the profession of nursing for any period of time will be quick to assure you that distinct differences exist, and more and more the reference is to healthcare rather than to medicine when speaking of the entire field.

The primary differences between nursing and medicine are the purpose and goal of each profession and the education needed to fulfill each role. Further, historically, medicine was perceived as a profession for men and nursing as a profession for women although that situation is much changed today. We can dismiss these stereotypes today, but they had an influence on the development of both professions.

Finally, the subservient role of the nurse in relationship to the physician in the past—often referred to as the handmaiden of the physician—has been significant in shaping the definition of nursing.

In general, medicine is concerned with the diagnosis and treatment (and cure, when possible) of disease. Nursing is concerned with caring for the person from a holistic perspective in a variety of health-related situations. The caring aspects of nursing are well documented in nursing literature (Benner & Wrubel, 1989; Bevis & Watson, 1989; Carper, 1979;

Watson, 1979). We think of medicine as being involved with the cure of a patient and nursing with the care of that patient. The role of the nurse in patient care (client care) also involves teaching about health and the prevention of illness, as well as caring for the ill individual. It also may encompass case management and is increasingly being practiced outside the walls of hospitals. Nursing takes place in the community and the home, hospice centers, ambulatory care environments, schools and day care centers, and rehabilitation facilities. In all environments, nurses play a key role in promoting higher standards of health.

With advancing technology in the healthcare fields, the diverse areas of specialization within those fields, the different routes to educational preparation for nurses, and the distinct practice settings and roles occupied by the nurse, it is critical that nurses provide clear information for themselves and for the public. To state that you are a registered nurse (RN) says little about what you do. It conveys nothing about where you are employed or your educational background. For example, as an RN, you might be employed in a community hospital or in a long-term care facility, have a role in a critical care unit, have earned additional credentials, be working in advanced practice, or be a nurse educator.

Thus, you can see that the words "nurse" and "nursing" have been applied to a wide variety of healthcare activities, in many different settings, performed by people with a variety of educational backgrounds. The old adage "A nurse is a nurse is a nurse" is out of place in a highly technical healthcare delivery system that struggles to keep "high touch" and "high tech" compatible.

Influences on the Definition of Nursing

A number of factors have influenced the definition of nursing. One might first think of technologic advances that have significantly affected the definition of nursing and the role of the nurse. The acute care hospital provides care to patients who are much more acutely ill with conditions from which they would not have survived 25 years ago. Today, recovery is anticipated after careful evaluation and treatment that can require diagnostic imaging, sophisticated laboratory tests, delicate medical procedures, and specialized critical care utilizing a host of variously prepared healthcare providers. Critical thinking skills are essential to the successful performance of the diverse tasks expected of a nurse. Nurses in many positions have been required to assume ever-greater levels of responsibility. Only recently are nurses beginning to receive the official authority, autonomy, and recognition that should accompany those responsibilities.

Another factor influencing the definition of nursing is the work of nursing theorists. As nursing has grown into a profession, many nursing theorists developed definitions of nursing consistent with their conceptual frameworks. Table 1.7 presents the definitions of some of the theorists.

In 1958, Virginia Henderson, a nurse educator, author, and researcher, was asked by the nursing service committee of the International Council of Nurses (ICN) to describe her concept of basic nursing. Hers is still one of the most widely accepted definitions of nursing:

> The unique function of the nurse is to assist the individual, sick or well, in the performance of those activities contributing to health or its recovery (or to peaceful death) that he would perform unaided if he had the necessary strength, will or knowledge. And to do this in such a way as to help him gain independence as rapidly as possible. (Henderson, 1966, p. 15)

Table 1.7   **Definitions of Nursing by Major Theorists**

THEORIST	MAJOR THEME	DEFINITION
Florence Nightingale (1954[1860])	Environment/Sanitation	The goal of nursing is to put the patient in the best condition for nature to act upon him, primarily by altering the environment.
Hildegard Peplau (1952)	Interpersonal process	Nursing is viewed as an interpersonal process involving interaction between two or more individuals, which has as its common goal assisting the individual who is sick or in need of healthcare.
Faye Abdellah (1960)	Nursing problems	Nursing is a service to individuals, families, and society based on an art and science that molds the attitudes, intellectual competencies, and technical skills of the individual nurse into the desire and ability to help people cope with their healthcare needs, and is focused around 21 nursing problems.
Ernestine Wiedenbach (1964)	Nursing problems model	Nursing is a helping, nurturing, and caring service rendered with compassion, skill, and understanding, in which sensitivity is key to assisting the nurse in identifying problems.
Virginia Henderson (1966)	Development/Needs	Nursing's role is to assist the individual (sick or well) to carry out those activities … he would perform unaided if he had the necessary strength, will, or knowledge.
Myra Levine (1969)	Conservation and adaptation	Nursing means the nurse interposes her/his skill and knowledge into the course of events that affect the patient. When influencing adaptation favorably, the nurse is acting in a therapeutic sense. When the nursing intervention cannot alter the course of adaptation, the nurse is acting in a supportive sense.
Ida Orlando Pelletier (1972)	Interpersonal process	Nursing's unique and independent role concerns itself with an individual's need for help in an immediate situation for the purpose of avoiding, relieving, diminishing, or curing that individual's sense of helplessness.
Jean Watson (1979–1988)	Caring	The essence and central unifying focus for nursing practice is caring, a transpersonal value. Nurse behaviors are defined as 10 curative factors. Focuses on the spiritual subjective aspects of both the nurse and the patient and the "caring moment" relating to the time when the nurse and patient first come together (LeMaire, 2002).
Dorothy Orem (1980)	Self-care	Nursing is concerned with the individual's need for self-care action, which is the practice of activities that individuals initiate and perform on their own behalf in maintaining health and well-being.
Dorothy E. Johnson (1980)	Systems approach	Nursing is an external regulatory force that acts to preserve the organization and integration of the patient's behavior at an optimal level, under those conditions in which the behavior constitutes a threat to physical or social health, or in which illness is found.
Imogene M. King (1981)	Open systems approach	The focus of nursing is the care of human beings resulting in the health of individuals and healthcare for groups, who are viewed as open systems in constant interaction with their environments.
Rosemarie Rizzo Parse (1981)	Man-Living-Health	Nursing is rooted in the human sciences and focuses on man as a living unity and as qualitatively participating in health experiences. Health is viewed as a process.
Betty Neuman (1982)	Systems approach	Nursing responds to individuals, groups, and communities, who are in constant interaction with environmental stressors that create disequilibrium. A critical element is the client's ability to react to stress and factors that assist with reconstitution or adaptation.
Sister Callista Roy (1984)	Adaptation	The goal of nursing is the promotion of adaptive responses (those things that positively influence health) that are affected by the person's ability to respond to stimuli. Nursing involves manipulating stimuli to promote adaptive responses.

THEORIST	MAJOR THEME	DEFINITION
Martha E. Rogers (1984)	Science of unitary man	Nursing is an art and science that is humanistic and humanitarian, directed toward the unitary human, and concerned with the nature and direction of human development.
Katharine Y. Kolcaba (1992)	Holistic theory of comfort	The immediate desirable outcome of nursing care is enhanced comfort. This comfort positively correlates with desirable health-seeking behaviors.
Sharon Van Sell and Ioannis Kalofissudis (2002)	A Complexity Integration of Nursing Theory	Nursing is an art and a science that can be depicted in mathematical format that shows the relationship among philosophy, science, culture, and the human being in which the socialization of the nurse into nursing is important (Van Sell & Kalofissudis, 2002).

The American Nurses Association (ANA) first defined nursing in its *Social Policy Statement* published in 1980. The definition was significantly expanded in later editions. The third edition of *Nursing's Social Policy Statement: The Essence of the Profession* states,

> Nursing is the protection, promotion, and optimization of health and abilities, prevention of illness and injury, alleviation of suffering through the diagnosis and treatment of human response, and advocacy in the care of individuals, families, communities, and populations (ANA, 2010).

The National Council of State Boards of Nursing has as one of its major responsibilities, the management of licensure of nurses throughout the United States. Through the Model Nurse Practice Act, the NCSBN states,

> The Practice of Nursing means assisting clients to attain or maintain optimal health, implementing a strategy of care to accomplish defined goals within the context of a client-centered health care plan, and evaluating responses to nursing care and treatment (NCSBN, Article II, Section 1, 2006).

Perhaps nothing so affects the definition of nursing as its legal definition found in each state's nursing practice act (see Chapter 3). This legal definition is critical because it provides the foundation and guidelines for education, licensure, scope of practice, and, when necessary, the corrective actions against people who violate the practice act.

No state adopts the exact wording of any recommended definition, but most states include references to performing services for compensation, the necessity for a specialized knowledge base, the use of the nursing process (although steps may carry different names), and components of nursing practice. Several states include some reference to treating human responses to actual or potential health problems. Most states refer to the execution of the medical regimen, and many include a general statement about additional acts that recognize that nursing practice is evolving and that the nurse's area of responsibility can be expected to broaden.

Defining Nursing for the Future

As the profession grows and responsibilities change, undoubtedly we will continue to refine the definition of nursing. By being responsive to changes, nursing has become more closely aligned with professions such as law, theology, and education, in which changing practices have required greater precision and refinement of definitions of the profession.

Critical Thinking Activity

Analyze the definitions of the major nursing theorists. What is similar among them? What is different? What concepts found in those definitions are most closely aligned with your perception of nursing? Develop your own definition of nursing and compare it to those of the theorists and to those of your classmates.

CHARACTERISTICS OF A PROFESSION

The meanings of profession and professionalism as applied to nursing have been a subject of debate for many years. From approximately the 1950s through the 1970s or mid-1980s, nursing periodically was reviewed against the **characteristics of a profession** that had been established in the sociologic literature. Some critics believe that nursing falls short of meeting these criteria. Amid these challenges, nurses have worked to advance the standing of nursing through the development of a code of ethics, standards of practice, and peer review. Table 1.8 outlines the seven major criteria for a profession and briefly discusses how nursing is meeting them or falls short of doing so. This set of characteristics corresponds to those being used by the American Association of Colleges of Nursing (AACN) when they refer to "professional" nursing as requiring a baccalaureate degree in nursing or higher.

Critical Thinking Activity

Select one of the characteristics of a profession that you believe nursing has difficulty meeting. Describe the actions that you believe should occur in the profession that would result in the profession fully meeting that criterion. How would you go about implementing those actions?

Differentiating Between the Terms "Profession" and "Professional"

Nursing involves activities that may be performed by many different caregivers. These people include nursing assistants, practical (vocational) nurses, and RNs prepared for entry into nursing through any of several educational avenues (see Chapter 2). Each of these caregivers contributes to nursing as a profession. To meet the nursing needs of the public, it is essential that caregivers function at various levels of practice. This has led to confusion about the use of the terms **profession** and **professional**. Is there a difference between looking at the practice of nursing in its totality and the "professional" practice of nursing?

Table 1.8 **How Nursing Meets the Traditional Criteria for a Profession***

CRITERION	HOW NURSING MEETS THE CRITERION
• Possession of a Body of Specialized Knowledge	Critics state that nursing borrows from biologic sciences, social sciences, and medical science, and then combines the various skills and concepts. This amalgamation and synthesis may be one of nursing's distinctive qualities. Nursing researchers work to develop an organized body of knowledge unique to nursing along with a specialized language of nursing (discussed later in this chapter). As this body of knowledge expands, this criterion is more nearly met.
• Use of Scientific Method to Enlarge the Body of Knowledge	Much work has been done toward systematically gathering and analyzing data, correctly identifying problems, selecting alternates, and evaluating patient care. Evidence-based practice and evidence-based education are at the forefront of nursing today (see Chapter 16).
• Education Within Institutions of Higher Education	Over time, the settings in which nurses are educated have changed, with most programs under the auspices of colleges or universities. Controversy over the length of nursing programs (associate degree versus baccalaureate degree) and the technical aspects of patient care continues. A few programs continue to be offered by hospitals.
• Control of Professional Policy, Professional Activity, and Autonomy	Today, nurses are responsible for planning, implementing, and evaluating the care patients receive and are accountable for that care. Nursing policies and protocols, standards of practice, and evaluative measures and criteria have been developed by nurses (see Chapter 6). In some settings, nurses are eligible for third-party payment. More collaborative relationships are occurring with other healthcare team members, including physicians.
• A Code of Ethics	The general standard for the professional behavior of nurses in the United States is the ANA *Code for Nurses,* which is periodically revised. The International Council of Nurses also has developed a code for nurses that sets the standards of ethical practice by nurses throughout the world (see Chapter 9).
• Nursing as Lifetime Commitment	Most nurses view themselves as committed to their profession and continue to identify themselves as nurses long after they retire. However, some do leave the profession due to "burnout" and stress. Better educational and clinical pathways encourage continued growth and retention in the profession.
• Service to the Public	Although discussion occurs with regard to altruism, remuneration for services, and collective bargaining (see Chapter 5), there is no question that nursing provides a service to the public.

*The criteria identified in this table are developed from criteria set forth by Bixler and Bixler (1945).

A Profession as Defined by Legislation

In at least one instance, federal legislation has helped to establish a list of the characteristics of a professional. Public Law 93-360 (Labor Management Relations Act, 1947 [amended, 1959, 1974]), which governs collective bargaining activities, defines the professional employee as follows:

(a) Any employee engaged in work (i) predominantly intellectual and varied in character as opposed to routine mental, manual, mechanical, or physical work; (ii) involving the consistent exercise of discretion and judgment in its performance; (iii) of such a character that the output produced or the result accomplished cannot be standardized in relation to a given period of time; (iv) requiring knowledge of an advanced type in a field of science or learning customarily acquired by a prolonged course of specialized intellectual instruction and study in an institution of higher learning or a hospital, as distinguished

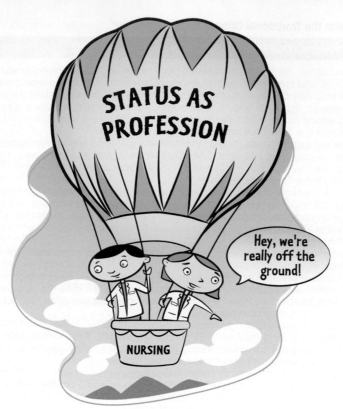

FIGURE 1.4 Some continue to question whether nursing truly can support the title of "profession."

from a general academic education or from an apprenticeship or from training in the performance of routine mental, manual, or physical processes; or

(b) Any employee, who (i) has completed the courses of specialized intellectual instruction and study described in clause (iv) of paragraph (a), and (ii) is performing related work under the supervision of a professional person to qualify himself to become a professional employee as defined in paragraph (a).

Based on this definition, all RNs are considered professionals (Fig. 1.4).

Popular View of a Professional

A popular view of a professional involves the approach a person has to the role that is required. Most professionals approach their activities earnestly, strive for excellence in performance, and demonstrate a sense of ethics and responsibility in relationship to their careers. Such people consider their work a lifelong endeavor rather than a stepping stone to another field of employment. They place a positive value on being termed professional and perceive being termed nonprofessional or technical as an adverse reflection on their status, position, and motivation. Using this definition, we again find that it would apply to all RNs.

Certain people suggest that professionalism has a great deal to do with attitude, dress, conduct, and deportment. The attributes that are considered professional vary according to the personal values and stereotypes of the person doing the evaluation.

TRADITIONS IN NURSING

Because of its history, nursing has developed many traditions. Some of them are being questioned or eliminated, primarily because they are not practical in today's workplace (eg, the wearing of a nursing cap). It is worthwhile, however, to reflect just a little on the development of these traditions and to discuss their relationship to nursing. Many believe that enduring traditions are important; they keep the reality of today connected to the history of the past.

The Nursing Pin

The nursing pin may date back to the time of the Crusades, when Crusaders marched to Jerusalem to recover the Holy Land. Among the Crusaders were the Knights Hospitallers of St. John of Jerusalem. Their uniform, introduced by a man named Gerard, included a black robe with a white Maltese cross. The Maltese cross became a familiar sight on the battlefields of the Holy Land. Following the capture of Jerusalem in 1099, some of the Crusaders noted the excellent nursing care provided by the Hospital of St. John and decided to join the nursing group. The Maltese cross is an eight-pointed cross formed by four arrowheads joining at their points. The eight points of the cross signified the eight beatitudes that knights were expected to exemplify in their works of charity. When the Knights Templars and the Knights of the Teutonic Order were formed, in 1118 and 1190, respectively, this symbol was carried forward, and later, the Maltese cross became a symbol of many groups who cared for the sick, including the United States Cadet Nurse Corps.

The actual symbolism of the pin relates to customs established in the 16th century, when the privilege of wearing a coat of arms was limited to noblemen who served their kings with distinction. In time, the privilege was extended to schools and to craft guilds, and the symbols of wisdom, strength, courage, and faith appeared on buttons, badges, and shields. Perhaps it was this spirit that Florence Nightingale attempted to capture when she chose the Maltese cross as a symbol for the badge worn by the graduates of her first nursing school.

As nursing developed as a profession, each school chose a unique pin, awarded on completion of the program, as a public symbol of work well done. Many of the early schools, particularly those associated with hospitals supported by religious groups, incorporated the cross into their pin. The first Nightingale School of Nursing in the United States was at Bellevue Hospital and is credited with developing the first school badge or pin, which was presented to the class of 1880 (Kalisch & Kalisch, 2004, p. 76). The nursing journal *RN* has collected nursing pins from across the United States and has occasionally created a cover display of pins from that collection.

The Nursing Cap

The history of the nursing cap is less certain. Several explanations of the origin of the cap have been suggested. It probably evolved during the period of time when nursing was greatly influenced by religion. It may have originated in the habit worn by the Sisters of Charity of St. Vincent de Paul, who established the first modern school of nursing in Paris in 1864. Another opinion suggests that the cap was influenced by the Institute of Protestant Deaconesses, founded by Pastor Theodor Fliedner at Kaiserwerth in Germany and the institution where Florence Nightingale studied. The white cap of the deaconesses of the early Christian era and the nun's veil of the Middle Ages have been said to be the forerunners of the nursing cap as we know it today (Mangum, 1994). The veil was modified to become a cap and was associated with service to others. We need to remember, also, that in Florence Nightingale's day, every lady wore a cap indoors. If you look at pictures of Queen Victoria, you notice the cap of plain white stiffened muslin framing her face. It was considered proper for women to keep their heads covered; thus, the cap would be viewed as the proper dress for a young woman of the day. The cap worn by students at Kaiserwerth when Florence Nightingale was a student was hood shaped, had a ruffle around the face, and was tied under the chin. A final conjecture is that the cap originally was designed to cover and help to control the long hair that was fashionable in the late 19th century, when short haircuts were not acceptable for women (Kalisch & Kalisch, 2004).

In the United States and Canada, the head covering became smaller and lost its scarf or veil as women's hairstyles changed and hair was worn shorter. (The hair-covering aspect remained a part of the cap in many areas of Europe.) As nursing education programs developed in hospitals, they each created their own cap, as with their nursing pin, to symbolize that particular hospital and nursing school. Some of these caps were rather frilly and were fashioned after the cloth cone through which ether was dropped. Again, as hairstyles changed, the size of the cap also changed, until it became one of individual taste or preference. A capping ceremony was part of the ritual of the nursing student and is discussed later.

As the role of nurses changed and as high technology became a significant part of the hospital work environment, nurses found that caps were bothersome as they tried to carry out their duties. They were knocked askew by curtains, equipment, and tubing. By the 1980s, many hospitals no longer required the cap as a part of the uniform. Nursing programs responded by dropping the cap as a required article of dress. If students wished to have a cap, it was purchased from a local uniform store and had no particular identification with the program.

The Nursing Uniform

Like the nursing cap, which is actually a part of the early nursing uniform, the requirement for special dress came from the religious and military history of nursing and has always been significant in nursing. This is due to the fact that dress provides a strong nonverbal message about one's image. The nurse attired in a white uniform, at least in the 1950s and 1960s, communicated an impression of confidence, competence, professionalism, authority, role identity, and accountability. As nurses have adopted more casual dress, some of this identity has been lost, and hospital committees, nursing programs, and nurses have spent considerable time discussing appropriate attire.

Early uniforms were long, usually stiffly starched, and had detachable collars and cuffs. A full uniform often included a long cape that would cover the uniform. Kalisch and Kalisch (2004, pp. 75–78) credit the New York Training School for Nurses at Bellevue Hospital with being the first school to adopt a standard uniform for student nurses in 1876. The uniform consisted of a gingham apron worn in the morning and a white apron worn in the afternoon over a dark woolen dress. A well-bred young woman, Euphemia Van Rensselaer, is credited with updating the basic uniform, which students were opposed to wearing. Given 2 days' leave of absence to have a uniform made for herself, she created a tailored uniform consisting of a long gray dress for winter and a calico version for summer, both worn with a white apron and cap. The attractiveness of her appearance resulted in other students accepting the uniform as standard dress. Later, a more easily laundered dress that could be worn throughout the year replaced both dresses.

A regulation uniform became a distinguishing mark of each nursing school by the end of the 19th century. Typically, the uniform consisted of a bodice and skirt of white material, adjustable white cuffs, a stiff white collar, and a white cap. To maintain the feminine hourglass image popular at the time, a tightly laced corset was worn beneath the uniform and ankles were hidden from view. Some suggest that the adoption of a distinctive and attractive uniform played a significant role in developing a professional image for nursing, giving it status, respect, and authority.

By the 1900s, the uniform became more functional, and the hemline was raised. By the mid-1960s, pantsuits became accepted, and nurses in certain settings, particularly psychiatric and pediatric units, challenged the appropriateness of uniforms, especially white uniforms. By 1970, significant changes occurred in uniforms, with the acceptance of styles that were designed to "make the nurse more approachable." In psychiatric settings, "no uniform" became the standard of the day. Today, athletic shoes are acceptable footwear, and scrubs have become the uniform of choice in many institutions. As dress styles have become increasingly casual, many hospitals have been forced to institute dress codes that restrict dangling jewelry, message T-shirts, body piercing, and fake fingernails. With all these changes, often, the nurse is no longer identifiable by dress; only a hospital badge provides information regarding a caregiver's preparation for the role.

Controversy over the appropriate attire for nurses continues. Some hospitals are instituting dress codes that require a return to white attire in an effort to restore professionalism to the job (Glanton, 2005), while others argue that what nurses wear matters less than what they know and that there are ways to differentiate hospital workers other than returning to a white uniform.

Ceremonies Associated With Nursing Programs

Long-standing traditions embraced by nursing include the ceremonies that mark various points along the educational paths of nursing students. Primary among these are the capping and the pinning ceremonies.

Few schools have capping ceremonies today because most nurses and nursing students no longer wear caps. Traditionally, the cap was awarded to students after they completed a certain part of the program. In hospital schools, it may have been awarded on completion of the probationary period, but more often, it was given after the completion of the first year. Often held in a nearby church, a special ceremony was planned, to which students invited family and others who were interested in their progress. The director of the school, assisted by other school dignitaries and faculty, solemnly placed the cap on the head of each student. Students proudly wore the cap throughout the remainder of the program. Often, a stripe was added to one corner of the cap to signify completion of the second year of study, and a black band was added at the time of graduation. At least one baccalaureate program, believing in the value of tradition, has replaced capping with the awarding of a stethoscope to students beginning their nursing studies, the ceremony conducted in an environment similar to that in which capping occurred (Transforming Traditions in Nursing, 2009).

DISPLAY 1.1 The Nightingale Pledge

I solemnly pledge myself before God and in the presence of this assembly:

To pass my life in purity and to practice my profession faithfully;

I will abstain from whatever is deleterious and mischievous and will not take or knowingly administer any harmful drug; I will do all in my power to maintain and elevate the standard of the profession, and will hold in confidence all personal matters committed to my keeping and all family affairs coming to my knowledge in the practice of my calling;

With loyalty I will endeavor to aid the physician in his work, and devote myself to the welfare of those committed to my care.

Agnes, G. Deans & Anne L Austin, *The history of the Farrand Training School for nurses* (Detroit, MI: Alumnae Associate of the Farrand Training School for Nurses, 1936) p. 58, as cited in Kalisch and Kalisch (2004).

The second traditional ceremony in nursing, the pinning, was of even greater significance and is continued by many schools today. The pinning heralded the completion of the program. Amid much pomp and circumstance, family and friends gathered to watch as the nursing director ceremoniously pinned the school pin on each new graduate. Graduates often recited, in unison, the Nightingale Pledge (Display 1.1) written in 1893 by Lystra E. Gretter, superintendent of Farrand Training School for Nurses at Harper Hospital School in Detroit and a small committee of nurses (Kalisch & Kalisch, 2004). This tradition is often repeated in nursing schools today, although a modified version of the original pledge is often used. Some schools include additional tradition through the "passing of the lamp." A representative of the graduating class hands a lamp (symbolizing the lamp carried by Florence Nightingale) to a representative of the next graduating class, thus reinforcing the concept of the continual caring represented in nursing.

As nursing education moved into institutions of higher education, some of the traditional ceremonies were discontinued. Some argue that the ceremony recognizing program completion in the collegiate environment is the college commencement, and that special celebrations for students of particular areas of study are not appropriate. However, in many large universities, the various disciplines now have separate ceremonies or an additional ceremony for their members. In other cases, the tradition is continued, although there is some tendency for graduates not to purchase a pin.

Critical Thinking Activity

Review the traditions established in nursing. Which is the most meaningful to you, and why? Which is the least meaningful to you, and why? Do you believe traditions should be continued in nursing? Provide a rationale for your answer.

THE IMAGE OF NURSING TODAY

During the late 1970s and early 1980s, much time and energy were invested in studying the image of nursing, with much of this work done by Beatrice and Philip Kalisch, who have written prolifically about the topic. Their writing focuses on segments of an overall study of the image of the nurse in various forms of mass media, including radio, movies, television, newspapers, magazines, and novels. They believe that popular attitudes and assumptions about nurses and what nurses contribute to a patient's welfare can greatly influence the future of nursing. It is their contention that since the 1970s, the popular image of the nurse not only has failed to reflect changing professional conditions but also has been based on derogatory stereotypes that have undermined public confidence in and respect for the professional nurse. Nurses should be concerned about negative or incorrect images because such images can influence the attitudes of patients, policy makers, and politicians. Equally important, negative attitudes about nursing may discourage many capable prospective nurses, who will choose another career that offers greater appeal in stature, status, and salary. This issue is of great concern today as we deal with a shortage of nurses.

Although some might argue that nurses have better things to do than to worry about how the nurse is portrayed in the media, a consistently misrepresented image can negatively affect how the public views nurses. Therefore, nurses have responded to television advertisements or programs that portray nurses and nursing in a negative light with letters and telephone calls. Boycotts on the purchase of products that present nurses poorly in advertisements as well as organized written protests have proved to be an effective way to bring about change.

NURSING'S IMAGE AND THE NURSING SHORTAGE

Although the economic climate has temporarily eased the nursing shortage of the past few years, authorities believe this is a short-term change and that the shortage will become more serious within 10 years (Buerhaus, Auerbach, & Staiger, 2009). Even now, the shortage still affects some areas of nursing such as critical care and the supply of nursing faculty.

A number of factors are suggested as contributing to the long-term shortfall of RNs. First of all, nurses are getting older. In the United States, the average age of a nurse is 47 years, with many anticipating retirement within the next decade. Forty-five percent of nurses were over the age of 50 when this (the latest) survey was conducted (HRSA Health Professions, 2010). Another concern centers on the fact that members of the baby boom generation are beginning to enter their senior years, thus increasing the need for nurses in the healthcare system. New nurses often enter nursing as a career change in midlife. They will have fewer years in the profession than those who entered as young adults.

However, a factor that demands serious consideration relates to the fact that nursing has always been a female-dominated profession. Women today have more educational and occupational alternatives. Many other careers may seem more attractive than nursing in terms of salary, the working conditions, and the prestige given to the role.

The past and future shortage is of such importance that various groups that command respect for their work have decided to study the issue or take action to try to encourage more individuals to choose nursing as a career. The Robert Wood Johnson Foundation and Johnson and Johnson have both funded endeavors to increase the attractiveness of nursing as a career. Across the United States, the National Forum of State Nursing Workforce Centers has been established with 29 states participating. Within each state, the nursing shortage is addressed with efforts made to assure an adequate supply of qualified nurses to meet healthcare needs. This is accomplished by supporting and advancing workforce initiatives, collecting and analyzing data, publishing reports and information, and making recommendations for changes needed to resolve the nurse shortage (NCSBN, 2009).

Another factor affecting the nursing supply is the limited number of spaces in nursing programs. Because nursing education is costly, many educational institutions have not been able to increase the size of their programs in the past decade. As applications increase, further efforts will be needed to increase the number of individuals who can be admitted. Some states have instituted major efforts to increase the available spaces for nursing students. The National Council of State Boards of Nursing is maintaining a Web site with information on efforts across the country to increase the nursing supply (*www. ncsbn.org/176.htm*).

To provide advice and recommendations to the Secretary of Health and Human Services and Congress on policy matters relating to the nursing work force, the National Advisory Council on Nurse Education and Practice (NACNEP) was established. In 2001, this group focused on the shortage of nurses in practice; and throughout its existence has addressed the shortage of nursing faculty.

Serious concern has been voiced by educational institutions and organizations supporting educational efforts, such as the National League for Nursing, regarding the supply of educationally prepared nursing faculty. Again, in conjunction with Johnson & Johnson, scholarships have been made available in some geographic areas to nurses who would like to prepare for faculty positions.

Another aspect of any nursing shortage is the retention of current nurses. Some states have identified that there are a large number of RNs not currently working in the profession. Many experts have pointed to working conditions such as mandatory overtime, heavy workloads, and lack of respect in the workplace as reasons for people leaving. The ANA is focusing on actions that will improve the work environment and thus increase retention as means of addressing the nursing shortage.

 ## Critical Thinking Activity

Interview five of your friends who are not nurses. What is their image of nursing? What do they understand of the role of the nurse? Do they view nursing positively? What recurrent information is mentioned?

COMMUNICATION IN ACTION

Affecting Your Image as a Nurse

Susan Williams and her friend Johanna Ireland were about to graduate and were shopping for uniforms to wear to their first jobs. Susan commented, "I really like these scrubs with the pink bunnies. They are really cute and lighthearted." Johanna replied, "I want something that doesn't make me look like a young girl. I'm going to feel a bit unsure of myself as a new graduate and I want to at least look mature and responsible. I am thinking of something plain with a white lab coat that would make me look more like an RN—the real nurse, you know!" "Wow, I never thought of that—Maybe I should look for something more professional too." replied Susan.

STUDIES FOR AND ABOUT NURSING

Early in the 20th century, the quality of many nursing schools and their graduates was poor; many of Florence Nightingale's admonitions regarding nursing education had been forgotten or ignored. Nurses, doctors, friends, and critics of nursing became concerned that the preparation being offered was inadequate. Before the problem could be corrected, it was necessary to learn more about the programs and how nurses were being used in the employment market. To accomplish this, studies about nursing and nurses were initiated.

As you read about the studies that have been conducted, you will recognize recurring themes with which we continue to grapple today. Our discussion is limited to those studies that looked at the profession as a whole and does not include any of the myriad studies conducted each year, primarily clinical in focus, that form the basis for evidence-based practice and for the expansion of the body of nursing knowledge.

Although the first nursing studies were not begun until the early 1900s, the number of studies since the 1950s has been voluminous. It is impossible to look at any professional nursing publication and not find mention of some new study in progress. Efforts were made to classify and catalog references to these studies and to report them. One of the first was completed by Virginia Henderson, who prepared *A Nursing Studies Index*. In 1952, a group of nurses, under the sponsorship of the Association of Collegiate Schools of Nursing, launched a new journal called *Nursing Research*, which was designed to disseminate information about nursing research.

A single individual often conducted many of the early studies, typically with a particular purpose in mind. Through the years, studies frequently took the form of a report by a special group of individuals, often appointed by a governmental or professional agency. Although by no means inclusive of all studies and reports, Table 1.9 highlights some of the major significant studies of nursing that have provided benchmarks to the profession, identifies the primary investigator/sponsor, and briefly discusses the focus and recommendation(s) associated with each study.

Critical Thinking Activity

Identify at least three areas in nursing that you believe need further study, and describe how you would begin to conduct those studies. Whom would you involve and why? How and to whom would you like to see the results and recommendations disseminated?

DEFINING A LANGUAGE FOR NURSING

For many, the development of a special language for nursing is an exciting new development. Structured nursing vocabularies allow nurses to use the acquired information to guide evidence-based clinical decisions, manage information in an electronic format, retrieve information for research, and compare clinical outcomes across settings. It also provides a common means of communication (Display 1.2).

Table 1.9 **Major Studies About Nursing**

DATE	NAME OF STUDY	PRIMARY INVESTIGATOR/SPONSOR	FOCUS AND RECOMMENDATION
1912	The Educational Status of Nursing	M. Adelaide Nutting/U.S. Bureau of Education	What and how students were being taught and conditions under which they were living. Began to establish nursing as a profession.
1923	Winslow-Goldmark Report on Nursing and Nursing Education in the United States	Josephine Goldmark/Rockefeller Foundation	The educational preparation of students including public health nurses, teachers, and supervisors. It pointed out fundamental faults in hospital training schools and resulted in the establishment of the Yale University School of Nursing.
1923	Committee on the Grading of Nursing Schools—a 3-part study	Francis Payne Bolton and contributions of thousands of nurses	
1923	(1) Nurses, Patients, and Pocketbooks	May Ayres Burgess/statistician	An inquiry into the supply and demand for nurses. Demonstrated that there was an oversupply of nurses.
1934	(2) An Activity Analysis of Nursing	Ethel Johns and Blance Pfefferkorn	Looked at the activities that constitute nursing as a basis for improving curricula.
1934	(3) Nursing Schools Today & Tomorrow	Ethel Johns	Described the nursing schools of the period and made recommendations about professional schools.
1937	A Curriculum Guide for Schools of Nursing—not truly a study of nursing, but often referred to as one because of its far-reaching effects	National League for Nursing Education	A revision of a 1917 publication, it outlined the curricula for a 3-year course, emphasizing sound educational teaching procedures. Followed by many schools of the time.
1948	Nursing for the Future	Esther Lucille Brown/Carnegie Foundation, the Russell Sage Foundation, and the National Nursing Council	Done to determine society's need for nursing. Described inadequacies in nursing schools. Resulted in recommendations that nursing education be placed in universities and colleges and encouraged recruitment of large numbers of men and members of minority groups into nursing schools.
1948	The Ginzberg Report or A Program for the Nursing Profession—a report of the discussions of the Committee on the Functions of Nursing	Eli Ginzberg/Columbia University	Reviewed problems centering around the shortage of nurses. Recommended that nursing teams consisting of variously educated nurses be developed.
1950	Nursing Schools at the Mid-Century	Margaret Bridgman/National Committee for the Improvement of Nursing Services—Russell Sage Foundation	Studied the practices of more than 1000 nursing schools (including organization, costs, curriculum, clinical resources, and student health) and stimulated improvement in baccalaureate schools.
1955	Patterns of Patient Care	Francis George and Ruth Perkins Kuehn/University of Pittsburgh	Assessed the amount of nursing service needed by a group of medical/surgical patients and determined how much of that care could be delegated to nursing aides and other nonprofessional people.
1958	Twenty Thousand Nurses Tell Their Story	Everett C. Hughes/ANA and American Nurses Foundation	Looked at nurses, what they were doing, their attitudes toward their jobs, and job satisfaction. Formed basis for development of nursing functions, standards, and qualifications.

Year	Title	Author/Source	Description
1959	*Community College Education for Nursing*	Mildred Montag/Institute of Research and Service in Nursing Education—Teachers College, Columbia University	Reported the findings of a 5-year study of eight 2-year nursing programs. Led to the establishment of more associate degree programs.
1963	*Toward Quality in Nursing: Needs and Goals*	W. Allen Wallis—Consultant Group or Nursing—a panel of nurses in the health field/U.S. Public Health Service	A report requested by the U.S. Surgeon General to determine funding priorities. Advised on the need for nurses, recruitment concerns, need for nursing research, and improvement of nursing education.
1970	*An Abstract for Action* (a report of the National Commission on Nursing and Nursing Education)	Jerome Lysaught/ANA, ANF, NLN, Mellon and Kellogg Foundations	Looked at current practices and patterns of nursing. Suggested joint practice committees, master planning for nursing education, and funding for nursing education and research
1979	*The Study of Credentialing in Nursing*	Inez Hinsvark/ANA	A review of credentialing—especially of nursing. Resulted in the appointment of a Task Force. Supported a freestanding credentialing center for nursing.
1983	*National Institute of Medicine Study*	Katherine Bauer/DHHS	Required by the Nursing Training Act of 1979, determined the need for continued outlay of federal money for nursing education. Resulted in 21 specific recommendations. Found that the shortage of nurses of the 1960s and 1970s no longer existed, that federal support of nursing education should focus on graduate study, and that the federal government should discontinue efforts to increase "generalist nurses."
1988	*Secretary's Commission on Nursing*	Lillian Gibbons/DHHS	Responded to serious nursing shortage. Validated the shortage. Recommended increased financial support of education and improved status and working conditions for nurses
1990	*Secretary's Commission on the National Nursing Shortage*	Caroline Burnett/DHHS	Appointed for 1 year to advise on implementation of 1988 report. Had three main foci: recruitment and retention, restructuring of nursing service, and use of nursing personnel and information systems.
1991	*Report of the National Commission of Nursing Implementation Project (NCNIP)*	Vivian De Back/ANA, NLN, AACN, AONE, Kellogg Foundation	Looked at nursing education, practice, management, and research, and developed recommendations for the future of nursing.
1993	*Health Professions Education for the Future*	E.H. O'Neill/Pew Health Professions Commission—Pew Charitable Trusts	Reinforced the belief that the education of health professions was not adequate to meet the health needs of America. Identified competencies for 2005 and emphasized the need for nurse-midwives, nurse practitioners, and the role of nurses in health promotion.
1995	*Reforming Health Care Workforce Regulation*	Pew Health Professions Commission	Had as its mission assisting schools preparing health professionals to understand the changing nature of healthcare, the needs for the future, and how to design and implement the programs preparing these workers. Recommended reform of the licensing process, specifically elimination of exclusive scopes of practice.

DISPLAY 1.2 Rationale for the Development of a Classification for Nursing

- Permits recognition and communication with others by giving a name to the things nurses do
- Provides a uniform legal record of care
- Supports clinical decision making
- Lays the groundwork for nursing research
- Captures the cost of nursing services for billing and accounting purposes
- Generates a structured retrieval database for quality assurance

The development of nursing languages began as an effort to build a set of terms that would describe the clinical judgments made by nurses that are not in medical language systems. As early as 1909, nurses with a perceptive view of the future recognized that nursing would one day need a language of its own. Ninety years ago, Isabel Hampton Robb wrote the following after attending a meeting of the newly formed ICN:

> While attending a special meeting of the ICN in Paris, I was naturally at once struck by the fact that the methods and the ways of regarding nursing problems were … as foreign to the various delegations as were the actual languages, and the thought occurred to me that … sooner or later we must put ourselves upon a common basis and work out what may be termed a "nursing Esperanto" which would in the course of time give us a universal nursing language. (Hampton-Robb, 1909) (Note: Esperanto was a language developed in 1887 with the goal of being a universal language that could be taught as the second language throughout the world, thus enabling improved communication among peoples.)

Defining a language for nursing primarily involves the development and refinement of **nursing nomenclatures** and **classification systems** that communicate information and guide data collection about nursing activities. The term "nursing nomenclature" refers to the words by which we name or describe phenomena in nursing. A "classification" is the systematic arrangement or a structural framework of these phenomena. As we move toward an international network of healthcare, the development of a language unique to nursing is viewed as critical to communication and decision making. Proponents of a specialized language for nursing emphasize the need for objective, science-based information to use in decision making. These data also provide the basis for accountability and the documentation-supporting processes and outcomes of care. The data can be used further to answer research questions about nursing and nursing actions. In the age of information technology, uniform, accurate, and automated patient care data are required to conduct analyses that will result in improving the quality of care and costing out that care. At present, the language of nursing primarily addresses nursing diagnoses, implementation activities, and nursing outcomes. Some would suggest that the existing systems are not adequate to reflect the entire scope of nursing practice and urge further development; for example, at the present time, none reflects the intensity of nursing practice.

The Approval Process Established for Nursing Languages

The **Committee for Nursing Practice Information Infrastructure (CNPII)** is a committee established by ANA to review material submitted for consideration to determine that it meets established criteria. To date, the committee has accepted 13, one of which has since been retired. Submission of language for recognition is a voluntary process. Criteria used to determine eligibility are periodically updated (Rutherford, 2008).

Another committee, the **National Information and Data Set Evaluation Center (NIDSEC)** evaluates the implementation of the terminology by a vendor. The recognition is valid for 3 years. Some groups have copyrighted their work; others have not.

Here we discuss the four systems that are currently most popular; these and others that are approved by the ANA are listed in Display 1.3.

 DISPLAY 1.3   **Major Nursing Classifications Approved by the American Nurses Association**

Title & Web Site	What It Is
NANDA International (formerly North American Nursing Diagnosis *www.nanda.org*	Provides taxonomy of nursing diagnoses. Defines a nursing diagnosis as a clinical judgment about an individual, family, or community responses to actual or potential health conditions/life processes. A nursing diagnosis provides the basis for selection of nursing interventions to achieve outcomes for which the nurse is accountable (NANDA-I, 2009).
Nursing Intervention Classification *www.nursing.uiowa.edu/cnc*	Provides a comprehensive standardized language, describing treatments that nurses perform in all settings and in all specialties (Dochterman & Bulechek, 2004).
Clinical Care Classification (CCC) Version 2.0 (previously Home Healthcare Classification Diagnoses and Interventions) *www.sabacare.com*	Adapted, revised, and expanded NANDA to include additional home healthcare nursing diagnostic conditions. Now used to assess, document, and classify patient/client care across all settings and is being used in Electronic Health Records (Saba, 2004–2008).
The Omaha System *www.omahasystem.org/overview.html*	A system of client problems, interventions, and client outcomes referred to as the Problem Classification Scheme, the Intervention Scheme, and the Problem Rating Scale for Outcomes (The Omaha System, 2010).
Nursing Outcomes Classification *www.nursing.uiowa.edu/cnc*	Defines a nursing outcome as a variable concept that represents a patient or family caregiver state, behavior, or perception that is measurable along a continuum and responsive to nursing interventions (Moorhead, Johnson & Mass, 2004).
Nursing Management Minimum Data Set(NMMDS) *www.nursing.umn.edu/ICNP/ USANMMDS/home.html*	Provides resources nurse executives need to make informed decisions and manage nursing services delivery and care coordination.
Patient Care Data Set (PCDS) *www.ncvhs.hhs.gov/990518t3.pdf*	Codifies patient problems and actions delivered by all caregivers during a hospital stay (Ozbolt, 1998).

(display continues on page 40)

DISPLAY 1.3 **Major Nursing Classifications Approved by the American Nurses Association** (continued)

Title & Web Site	What It Is
Perioperative Nursing Data Set (PNDS) *www.aorn.org/A*	Standardized language for documenting and evaluating perioperative nursing care (Association of Perioperative Registered Nurses, 2010).
Systematized Nomenclature of Medicine (SNOMED) *http://www.ihtsdo.org/snomed-ct/*	Comprehensive system for indexing the entire medical record, including signs and symptoms, diagnoses, and procedures (SNOMED, 2005).
Nursing Minimum Data Set (NMMMDS) *www.cms.hhs.gov/ NursingHomeQualityInits/*	Identified the four elements of nursing diagnosis, nursing interventions, nursing outcomes, and nursing intensity (Terminology, 2006).
International Classification of Nursing Practice *www.icn.ch/icnp.htm*	Collaborative project under the auspices of the International Council of Nursing for classifying nursing phenomena (diagnoses, interventions, and outcomes). Includes definitions and provides unifying framework to enable comparison of data internationally (Coenen, 2003).
Alternative Billing Codes Developed by ABC Coding Solutions *www.ABCcodes.com*	Identifies alternative medicine, nursing, and other integrative healthcare services and related products that facilitate measuring, validating, managing, and reimbursing for care (ABC Coding Solution, 2009).

NANDA-International

The group originally called the National Group for the Classification of Nursing Diagnosis and then North American Nursing Diagnosis Association (NANDA) and now **NANDA International (NANDA-I)** became a formal organization after its fifth conference in 1982. The Association has two main purposes: to develop a diagnostic classification system (also known as **taxonomy**) and to identify and approve nursing diagnoses. The list of nursing diagnoses (concepts that are given word labels) continues to grow as nurses encounter diagnoses in clinical practice that have not been included and submit these to NANDA-I for consideration. As a student, you have some familiarity with nursing diagnoses from the nursing care plans you develop for patient care and in the case studies you discuss in your classes. The following is the definition of a nursing diagnosis accepted by NANDA-I:

> Nursing diagnosis is a clinical judgment about individual, family, or community response to actual or potential health problems/life processes. Nursing diagnoses provide the basis for selection of nursing interventions to achieve outcomes for which the nurse is accountable. Approved at the 9th conference, 1990, (NANDA-I, 2009)

Nursing Interventions Classifications

Started in 1996 at the University of Iowa, the **Nursing Interventions Classification (NIC)** is a comprehensive, standardized language that describes actions nurses perform in all settings and in all specialties, and includes both physiologic and psychosocial interventions. The interventions are numbered to facilitate computerization and are organized into classes, and the classes are assigned to domains. The domains are functional health, physiologic health, psychosocial health, health knowledge and behavior, perceived health, family health, and community health. Each intervention has been linked with NANDA-I nursing diagnoses and with the **Nursing Outcomes Classification (NOC)** below and with Omaha system problems. Many institutions have adopted NIC as a standardized terminology for use in computerized documentation systems. An overview of NIC is available online (*http://www.nursing.uiowa. edu/excellence/nursing_knowledge/clinical_effectiveness/index*), and a detailed presentation of the entire system is available in print (Dochterman & Bulechek, 2004).

Nursing Outcomes Classification

Also developed at the University of Iowa, the NOC was first published in 1997. An outcome is defined as a variable concept representing a patient or family caregiver state, behavior, or perception that is measurable along a continuum and responsive to nursing interventions. Project developers believed that stating the outcomes as variable concepts rather than goals would allow the identification of positive or negative changes (or no changes at all) in the patient's status. Each outcome has a definition, a list of indicators that assist in evaluation of patient status, a rating scale for evaluation, and a suggested target rating. Listed in alphabetical order, the outcomes are grouped into classes and use the same domains as NIC. Both NIC and NOC are continuing in development. An overview of the NOC is available online (*http://www.nursing. uiowa.edu/excellence/nursing_knowledge/clinical_effectiveness/index*), and the detailed system is available in print (Moorhead, Johnson, & Maas, 2004). A presentation of the linkages among NANDA, NIC, and NOC (Johnson, Bulechek, Butcher, et al., 2006) is a useful tool for those seeking a better understanding of how the three systems can be coordinated.

The Omaha System

The **Omaha System**, another example of classification efforts, is a research-based taxonomy designed to document client care from admission to discharge. It was designed as a three-part, comprehensive yet brief approach to documentation and information management for multidisciplinary healthcare professionals who practice in community settings. It offers terms and codes to classify the client's health-related concerns or problems, the interventions that nurses and other healthcare professionals use, and the client's outcomes (The Omaha System, 2010). Client problems can be identified for individuals, families, and groups. The interventions describe both plans and interventions for specific client concerns. The outcome scales evaluate a client's health-related changes through the use of problem-specific knowledge, behavior, and status ratings. The Omaha System has been recognized by the ANA since 1992 and has been translated into numerous languages. Automation and technology advances and healthcare delivery changes have markedly expanded its use nationally and internationally. Users represent a broad continuum of care with location, size, organization, types of service, and employees becoming increasingly diverse. An overview of the Omaha System is available online (*http://omahasystem.org/index.htm*).

Other Classification Systems

Currently, 12 Data Element Sets and Terminologies are recognized by the ANA (ANA, 2009). All of these are presented in Display 1.3 with a brief description of each and a Web site where more information is provided.

The Minimum Data Set for Nursing Home Resident Assessment and Care Screening

Although not referred to in terms of nursing language, the **Minimum Data Set for Nursing Home Resident Assessment and Care Screening (MDS)** bears some mention here. When the Omnibus Budget Reconciliation Act was passed in 1991, it required assessment of long-term care facility residents. This assessment, done on admission and every 3 months thereafter, must be standardized, comprehensive, accurate, and reproducible. It must be transmitted electronically to data centers in each state. Whenever problems are identified during the assessment, Resident Assessment Protocols (RAPs) must be instituted. The RAPs lists factors that might be associated with the problem, clarifying information to be considered in making a diagnosis and describing the environment that will help reduce the symptoms. Complete documentation of the situation, including nature of the problem, complications, risk factors, referrals, and rationale for action, is required of nurses. The MDS is used as the basis for determining payment to long-term care facilities. The implementation of the MDS nationwide has resulted in a significant collection of data that can be used as a basis for improving the care of the elderly. The MDS 3.0 has been developed for implementation in October, 2010, and an overview is available on the Centers for Medicare & Medicaid Services (CMS) Web site (CMS, 2009).

The International Classification for Nursing Practice Project

The **International Classification for Nursing Practice Project (ICNPP)** is an effort of the ICN to establish a unified nursing language system. It is a compositional terminology for nursing practice that facilitates the development of and the cross-mapping among local terms and existing terminologies (ICN, 2009a) In addition, ICNPP is a classification of nursing phenomena, nursing actions, and nursing outcomes.

Although the United States has been involved in the development of classification and information systems for some time, the need for a unified language is now recognized internationally. Because cultural and language differences exist, many of the classification systems currently employed in the United States are not useful in other countries. For example, the concept of self-care reflects the cultural values and norms of American society but may be perceived quite differently in other cultures. In 1989, the ICN was asked to encourage member National Nurses Associations to become involved in developing information and classification systems and nursing data sets that could be used by nurses in all countries to identify and describe nursing. The project began a year later. In 1996, an alpha version of the Classification of Nursing Phenomenon and Nursing Interventions was field tested, and a beta version was launched in June 1999 at ICN's Centennial Conference. The ICNPP Programme has established a formal evaluation and review process to advance the project. ICNP Version 2 is now available on the ICN Web site (ICN, 2009b.)

 Critical Thinking Activity

Analyze the history of the development of a classification and nomenclature specific to nursing. Describe possible future developments, and provide a rationale for your answer. What do you see as major impediments and why? What do you believe will be the long-term benefits and why?

KEY CONCEPTS

- In its development as a profession, nursing has struggled with its definition, its image, and its role in the healthcare delivery system, due in part to its history and the fact that it has both theoretical and practical aspects. The role of the nurse in the healthcare delivery system has probably never been more important than it is today.

- Florence Nightingale dramatically changed the form and direction of nursing. She set down standards for nursing education and made significant recommendations for changes in how hospitals operated and how nursing was practiced. Many of her recommendations are valid today.

- Early schools of nursing were established shortly after the Civil War with curricula fashioned much like the Nightingale School in England. Early programs were primarily apprenticeships, with long hours during which students provided much of the workforce of the hospital with little time left for study.

- The wars in which the United States have been involved have had a significant impact on nursing. Nurses have always played an important role in the care of the wounded and dying and, over the years, have taken increasingly important roles.

- Nursing is distinct from medicine. Medicine deals with diagnosis and treatment of disease, and nursing is concerned with caring for the person.

- The position nursing occupies as a profession is often judged against sociologically developed characteristics or standards of a profession. Not everyone agrees that nursing meets those standards.

- The standards of a profession typically include seven requirements: (1) possess a well-defined and well-organized body of knowledge, (2) enlarge a systematic body of knowledge and improve education, (3) educate its practitioners in institutions of higher learning, (4) function autonomously in the formulation of policy, (5) develop a code of ethics, (6) attract professionals who will be committed to the profession for a lifetime, and (7) compensate practitioners by providing autonomy, continuous professional development, and economic security.

- Nursing also has struggled with the terms "profession" and "professional." At times, the characteristics of the professional become confused with the formal concept of a profession.

- Nursing as a profession has many traditions, some of which are challenged today, while others are much honored and valued. Among the traditions are the pin, the cap, the uniform, and nursing ceremonies.

- Nursing has struggled with its image. Various groups have waged campaigns to improve the image of nursing and thus make it a more attractive profession. The image of nursing today is viewed as a critical issue because of the nurse shortage. A positive image is needed to attract qualified individuals into the profession.

- Since the beginning of the 20th century, nursing has been a much-studied profession. Early studies dealt with nursing education; later studies dealt with the image of nursing, nurses themselves, and with nursing's role in healthcare delivery.

- As nursing has developed as a profession, more attention has been directed to establishing a unique classification and nomenclature for nursing. Efforts are being made to do this on an international basis.

RELEVANT WEB SITES

Web sites relevant to this chapter can be found at thePoint accessed through *http://the Point. lww.com/Ellis10e* and by entering the code found on the inside cover of your text.

REFERENCES

ABC Coding Solutions. (2009). *About us.* Retrieved September 7, 2009, from www.abccodes.com/ali/about_us

Abdellah, F. G. (1960). *Patient-centered approaches to nursing.* New York: Macmillan.

American Nurses Association. (2010). *Nursing's social policy statement: The essence of the profession* (3rd ed.). Silver Spring, MD: Author.

Association of Perioperative Registered Nurses. (2010). *Perioperative nursing data set (PNDS) and syntegrity standardized perioperative framework (SPF).* Retrieved June 27, 2010, from http://www.aorn.org/PracticeResources/PNDSAndStandardizedPerioperativeRecord

Benner, P., & Wrubel, J. (1989). *The primacy of caring.* Menlo Park, CA: Addison-Wesley.

Bevis, E. O., & Watson, J. (1989). *Toward a caring curriculum: A new pedagogy for nursing.* New York: National League for Nursing.

Bixler, G. K., & Bixler, R. W. (1945). The professional status of nursing. *American Journal of Nursing, 45*(9), 730.

Bostwick, M. (2008). *Florence Nightingale: The making of an icon.* New York: Farrar, Straus and Giroux.

Buerhaus, P. I., Auerbach, D.I., & Staiger, D.O., (2009). The recent surge in nurse employment: Causes and implications, *Health Affairs, 28*(4), w657–w668. Retrieved September 10, 2009, from http://content.healthaffairs.org/cgi/content/abstract/hlthaff.28.4.w657

Carper, B. A. (1979). The ethics of caring. *Advances in Nursing Science, 3,* 11–19.

Centers for Medicare & Medicaid Services. (2009). *MDS 3.0 for Nursing Homes.* Retrieved September 10, 2009, from *http://www.cms.hhs.gov/NursingHomeQualityInits/25_NHQIMDS30.asp.*

Coenen, A. (2003). The international classification for nursing practice (ICNP) programme: Advancing a unifying framework for nursing. *Online Journal of Issues in Nursing* Retrieved September 10, 2009, from www.nursingworld.org/MainMenuCategories/ANAMarketplace/ANAPeriodicals/OJIN/TableofContents/Volume82003/No2May2003/ArticlesPreviousTopics/TheInternationalClassificationforNursingPractice.aspx

Dochterman, J., & Bulechek G. (Eds.). (2004). *Nursing interventions classification* (4th ed.). St. Louis, MO: Mosby.

Donahue, M. P. (2010). *Nursing: The finest art* (3rd.). St. Louis, MO: CV Mosby.

Glanton, D. (2005). White garb returning to hospitals. *Nursing opportunities: Northwest edition, 4,* 1, 6.

Hampton-Robb, I. (1909). *Report of the third regular meeting of the International Council of Nurses.* Geneva: ICN.

Henderson, V. (1966). *The nature of a science of nursing.* New York: Macmillan.

HRSA Health Professions. (2010). *National sample survey of registered nurses.* Retrieved October 15, 2010, from http://bhpr.hrsa.gov/healthworkforce/rnsurvey/

International Council of Nurses. (2009a). International classification for nursing practice.—About—Definition. Retrieved August 30, 2009, from www.icn.ch/icnp_def.htm

International Council of Nurses. (2009b). International classification for nursing practice. Version 2. Retrieved September 10, 2009, from http://www.icn.ch/icnp.htm

Johnson, D. (1980). The behavioral system model for nursing. In J. P. Riehl & C. Roy (Eds.), *Conceptual models for nursing practice* (2nd ed., pp. 207–216). East Norwalk, CT: Appleton-Century-Crofts.

Johnson, M., Bulechek, G., Butcher, H., Dochterman, J. M., Maas, M., & Moorhead, S., et al. (2006). *NANDA, NOC, and NIC Linkages: Nursing Diagnoses, Outcomes, & Interventions.* St. Louis, MO: Mosby.

Kalisch, P. A., & Kalisch, B. J. (2004). *The advance of American nursing* (4th ed.) Philadelphia: Lippincott Williams & Wilkins.

King, I. M. (1981). *A theory for nursing: Systems, concepts, process.* New York: John Wiley & Sons.

Kolcaba, K. Y. (1992). Holistic comfort: Operationalizing the construct as a nurse-sensitive outcome. *Advances in Nursing Science, 1,* 1–10.

Labor Management Relations Act (1947) as amended by Public Laws 86–257 (1959) and 93–360 (1974), Section 2 [On-line]. www.nlrb.gov/publications/nlrb4.pdf. Accessed September 28, 2005.

LeMaire, B. (2002). Jean Watson, on her theory of caring. *Nurse Week (Mountain West Edition), 3*(40),7.

Levine, M. E. (1969). *Introduction to clinical nursing.* Philadelphia: F. A. Davis.

MacQueen, J. S. (2007). Florence Nightingale's nursing practice. In P. D'Antonio (Ed.), *Nursing history review – Volume 15* (pp. 29–49). New York: Springer Publishing Company.

Mangum, S. (1994). Uniforms and caps: Do we need them? In O.L. Strickland & D.J. Fishman, *Nursing issues in the 1990s* (pp. 46–66). Albany, NY: Delmar Publishers.

Moorhead, S., Johnson, M., & Maas M. (Eds.). (2004). *Nursing outcomes classification* (3rd ed.). St. Louis, MO: Mosby.

NANDA-I. (2009). *Glossary of terms.* Retrieved September 18, 2009, from http://www.nanda.org/DiagnosisDevelopment/DiagnosisSubmission/PreparingYourSubmission/GlossaryofTerms.aspx

National Council of State Boards of Nursing, Inc. (2006). *Model nursing act and rules.* Retrieved September 7, 2009 from www.ncsbn.org/regulation/nursingpractice_nursing_practice_model_act_and_rules.asp

National Council of State Boards of Nursing, Inc. (2009). *Workforce data*. Retrieved September 7, 2009, from www.ncsbn.org/176.htm

Neuman, B. (1982). *The Neuman System model: Application to nursing education and practice*. East Norwalk, CT: Appleton-Century-Crofts.

Nightingale, F. (1954). *Notes on nursing: What it is, and what it is not*. [An unabridged republication of the first American edition, as published by D. Appleton and Company in 1860]. New York: Dover Publications.

Norman, E. M. (1999). *We band of angels*. New York: Random House.

O'Neil R. F. (2008). *U.S. Cadet Nurse Corps*. Retrieved September 1, 2009, from http://www.cga.ct.gov/2008/rpt2008-R-0014.htm

Orem, D. (1980). *Nursing: Concepts of practice* (2nd ed.). New York: McGraw-Hill.

Orlando, I. J. (1972). *The discipline and teaching of nursing process*. New York: G. P. Putnam's Sons.

Ozbolt, J. G. (1998). *Patient Care Data Set*. Nashville, TN: Vanderbilt University Medical Center. Retrieved September 10, 2009, from www.ncvhs.hhs.gov/990518t3.pdf

Parse, R. R. (1981). *Man-living-health: A theory of nursing*. New York: Wiley.

Peplau, H. E. (1952). *Interpersonal relations in nursing*. New York: G. P. Putnam's Sons.

QARANC. (2006). History of the QARANC. Retrieved August 31, 2009, from *www.qaranc.co.uk/history.php*.

Rogers, M. E. (May 1984). *Science of unitary human beings: A paradigm for nursing*. Paper presented before the International Nurse Theorist Conference, Edmonton, Alberta.

Roy, C. (1984). *Introduction to nursing: An adaptation model* (2nd ed.). Englewood Cliffs, NJ: Prentice-Hall.

Rutherford, M.A. (2008) Standardized nursing language: what does it mean for nursing practice. *The Online Journal of Issues in Nursing*. Retrieved September 7, 2009, from http://nursingworld.org/MainMenuCategories/ANAMarketplace/ANAPeriodicals/OJIN/TableofContents/vol132008/No1/Jan08/ArticlePreviousTopic/StandardizedNursingLanguage.aspxl

Saba, V. (2004–2008). *Clinical care classification system*. Retrieved August 31, 2009, from www.sabacare.com

SNOMED. (2005). SNOMED International [On-line]. www.snomed.org/index.html. Accessed September 28, 2005.

Terminology: Nursing Minimum Data Set. (2006). Retrieved September 7, from http://www.nursingworld.org/npii/nmds.htm

The Forum of State Workforce Centers. (2009). *Who we are*. Retrieved September 7, 2009, from http://www.nursingworkforcecenters.org/AboutUs.aspx

The Nurse's Memorial. (2007). Retrieved August 31, 2009, from www.arlingtoncemetery.net/nurse-memorial.htm

The Omaha System. (2010) Retrieved June 27, 2010 from www.omahasystem.org.overview.html

Transforming Traditions in Nursing. (2009). Retrieved September 6, 2009, from www.musc.edu/nursing/old/traditions.htm

Van Sell, S. & Kalofissudis, I. (2002), *The evolving essence of the science of nursing: A complexity integration of nursing theory*. Retrieved September 7, 2009, from http:www.nursing.gr/Complexitytheory.pdf

Watson, J. (1979). *Nursing the philosophy and science of caring*. Boston: Little, Brown.

Whitman, A. (1985). *American reformers*. New York: H.W. Wilson Co.

Wiedenbach, E. (1964). *Clinical nursing: A helping art*. New York: Springer Publishing Co.

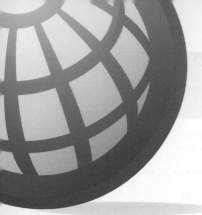

2

Educational Preparation for Nursing

Unlike most professions that provide a single route for the educational preparation of its practitioners, nursing offers three major types of educational programs as well as less common ones that prepare graduates to write the National Council Licensure Examination (NCLEX) for registered nursing. These circumstances have resulted in options and opportunities for prospective students, and the multiple-entry points are viewed by some as one of nursing's strengths.

Despite this acknowledged strength, the existence of multiple-entry points has resulted in confusion for both healthcare consumers and employers. Those consumers often find it difficult to understand the various nursing credentials—and probably have little interest in credentials as long as they receive satisfactory care. Employers may have difficulty differentiating among the three major types of RN graduates who, at least initially, enter the work environment performing similar activities. This confusion led to a recommendation from the Pew Commission that nursing distinguishes between the practice responsibilities of the graduates educated in each of the different educational environments (Pew Health Professions Commission, 1995). This task has proven difficult at best.

Some nurse educators, charged with the responsibility of graduating a "safe" practitioner, are not entirely clear about how the various educational routes to professional preparation should differ in purpose, structure, and outcome. Certainly, there are basic skills and understandings that all beginning nurses must master to ensure safe patient care. Nursing leaders frequently debate aspects of the educational preparation of nurses, such as where it should take place, what content should be included in which programs and to what depth, which tests should measure the various competencies, and which credentials should be awarded.

The three traditional educational avenues that prepare men and women for registered nursing are hospital-based diploma programs, associate degree programs (primarily found at junior and community colleges), and baccalaureate programs (offered at 4-year colleges and universities). It is also possible for students to begin their nursing education in programs that culminate in a master's degree, and several programs now exist in which a student can earn a doctorate before being eligible to write the state licensing examination for registered nursing.

At least two other groups of caregivers are identified with nursing: the nursing assistant, who may be certified, and the practical (vocational) nurse, who is licensed through a separate and different examination from that taken by the RN. We begin with a discussion of those roles.

THE NURSING ASSISTANT

For years, individuals called nursing aides or assistants have provided care to patients in hospitals and long-term care facilities. In the past, these caregivers were hired without formal preparation for their responsibilities and were provided on-the-job training. The use of the nursing aides likely started during World War I and certainly was reinforced during World War II, when approximately 150,000 trained volunteer nursing aides served in wartime hospitals. Nursing aides or assistants have always provided the majority of care in nursing homes. Nursing assistants are within a group that is often referred to as **unlicensed assistive personnel (UAP)**.

In 1987, Congress passed the Omnibus Budget Reconciliation Act, which regulates agencies receiving federal funds and includes an amendment regulating the education and certification of **nursing assistants** who work in nursing homes. The amendment stipulated that by October 1, 1990, all people working as nursing assistants in nursing homes (hospitals and assisted living units were not included) would be required to complete a minimum of 75 hours of theory and practice and pass both a theory and practice examination to be certified. Certification falls under state jurisdiction but is guided by federal regulations. In many states, the hours of preparation required exceed the 75 hours established by federal law. Following the federal legislation, the National Council of State Boards of Nursing Inc. [NCSBN] developed the National Nurse Aide Assessment Program, which identifies the minimum skills a nursing assistant must attain and can be used to guide programs registering or certifying nursing assistants. Currently, 24 jurisdictions use the examination to certify nursing assistants. The examination has two components, written or oral and a skills demonstration portion. It is administered in both English and Spanish. Both components must be successfully passed in order to be listed as a certified nursing assistant (CNA) (NCSBN, 2009). The state agency responsible for certifying and maintaining the list of nursing assistants varies from state to state; most commonly, it is the board of nursing or the state department of health services.

The CNA—referred to as the nursing assistant or patient care assistant in some states—functions under the direction of the RN or the LPN. Each state determines the skills that may be performed by the nursing assistant. Typically, these include basic nursing skills, such as changing bed linens; measuring temperature, pulse, respirations, and blood pressure; bathing patients and helping with personal care; helping patients with eating, walking, and exercise programs; and supporting patients when they are allowed to get out of bed. The preparation of the CNA emphasizes the importance of a safe environment and includes instruction in patients' rights and the use of side rails and restraints. A number of states also require a designated number of hours per year of continuing education.

There are no national regulations governing the educational preparation and scope of practice of nursing assistants in areas other than long-term care, although some states have legislation to regulate the practice of those in other settings. Typically, training in hospitals or other agencies occurs under the sponsorship of the employing facility and without formal certification; student backgrounds may vary from less than a high school diploma to advanced degrees. For example, some physicians licensed in foreign countries but who cannot secure licensure in the United States may work as UAPs in healthcare settings.

A number of states have a category of UAP, known as unlicensed medication administration personnel. Many of these workers are employed within the primary school system and routinely dispense medications to students; in other instances, these individuals are employed in assisted living and similar facilities. In a few states, CNAs may receive additional instruction and become certified medication aides and are allowed to give medications in a nursing home. The criteria for hospital accreditation established by The Joint Commission (formerly the Joint Commission on Accreditation of Healthcare Organizations) now require that hospitals ensure the competence of all employees, including nursing assistants. This has led many hospitals to the practice of hiring only those who were certified as nursing assistants in long-term care facilities and to the development of courses to prepare individuals as nursing assistants for acute care settings. States vary in their requirements for hospital nursing assistants. Many states expect the hospitals to determine what their requirements will be and to then provide their own training.

The **home health aide** is prepared to assist individuals with basic care in their home; thus, a program of instruction includes content related to shopping for groceries, cooking, and doing laundry. Some long-term care nursing assistant programs offer an additional period of training and education for roles as home health aides to those who have completed their nursing assistant program. Other states have a shorter program without a certification examination for home health aides. In some states, there is no standardized certification requirement for those who work in homes.

Training for the various types of nursing assistant occurs in many settings, including high schools, long-term care facilities, hospitals, community colleges, regional occupational programs, and privately operated programs. Some consider this preparation the first rung on the ladder of nursing education, and, in some states, the nursing assistant may be exempt from certain classes required in LPN programs. Some registered nursing programs establish certification as a nursing assistant as an admission requirement.

The employment of UAPs has been of concern to nursing. Some state boards have issued a list of tasks that may be performed by UAPs, and both the ANA and the NCSBN have issued definitions and guidelines for the use of UAPs. More discussion of UAPs in healthcare occurs in Chapter 13.

PRACTICAL NURSE EDUCATION

The **practical nurse** (titled **vocational nurse** in Texas and California) is no newcomer to the healthcare delivery system. In the past, the practical nurse was the family friend or community citizen who was called to the home in emergencies. This person, usually self-taught, learned by experience which procedures were effective and which were not. The practical nurse would perform basic care procedures, such as bathing, and also would cook and perform light housekeeping duties for the family, much like the home health aide does today. Although controls on the licensing of practical nurses and the accreditation of their curricula were slower to evolve than those regulating professional nursing, states gradually enacted licensure laws governing practical nursing. By 1945, 19 states and one territory had licensure laws, but licensure of the practical nurse was mandatory in only one state (Kalisch & Kalisch, 2004). Most, if not all, of these people are now retired from nursing practice. By 1955, all states had licensure laws for practical nurses.

It is not clear when formal preparation for practical nursing began. The most widely accepted view is that the first programs were initiated through the YWCA in Brooklyn, New

DISPLAY 2.1   History of the Development of Practical Nursing

1892	YWCA in Brooklyn, New York, establishes a program in practical nursing named after Lucinda Ballard, who provided the funding for it.
1907	Thompson School is founded in Brattleboro, Vermont.
1908	The American Red Cross founds a practical nursing program.
1918	The Household Nursing Association School of Attendant Nursing begins in Boston.
1938	New York becomes the first state to require licensure for the practical nurse.
1941	The Association of Practical Nurse Schools (APNS) is founded.
1942	Membership in the APNS is opened to practical nurses and the name changed to the National Association of Practical Nurse Education and Service (NAPNES). The first planned curriculum for practical nursing is developed.
1945	NAPNES establishes and accredits service for schools of practical nursing; this program was discontinued in 1984.
1949	The National Federation of Licensed Practical Nurses (NFLPN) is organized.
1957	Working with the American Nurses Association, NFLPN seeks to clarify the role and function of the practical nurse. The National League for Nursing (NLN) establishes the Council on Practical Nursing.
1966	The Chicago Public School Program becomes the first practical nurse program to be accredited by the NLN.
1979	The NLN publishes a list of competencies of graduates of practical/vocational nursing programs.
1996	The National Council of State Boards of Nursing (NCSBN), working with NAPNES, offers a certification examination for licensed practical nurses in long-term care.

York, around 1892. The school established through the YWCA was known as the Ballard School, after Lucinda Ballard, who provided the funding to operate it. The course of study lasted approximately 3 months, and the students, called "attendants," were trained to care for invalids, the elderly, and children in a home setting.

A YWCA may seem a strange place for a practical nursing program. But YWCAs were an important source of inexpensive housing for many young women who, in the late 1890s and early 1900s, traveled from their homes to large cities in search of new careers and better lives. Because most of these women were untrained and had no marketable skills, the YWCA was a natural site for a school. Display 2.1 outlines some of the significant history in the development of practical nursing.

The general curriculum for practical nurses, which typically takes 1 year to complete, varies considerably from state to state and even from school to school. In some states, the education is measured in clock hours instead of credit hours. Most of today's practical nursing education programs stress clinical experience, primarily in structured care settings such as hospitals and long-term care facilities. Basic therapeutic knowledge and introductory content from biologic and behavioral sciences correlate with clinical practice; usually one third of the time is spent in the classroom and two thirds in clinical practice.

The educational preparation of the practical nurse takes place in a variety of settings. High schools, trade or technical schools, hospitals, junior or community colleges, universities, or independent agencies may offer programs. If the rules and regulations of the state board(s) of nursing allow it, practical nursing and associate nursing degree programs can be incorporated in the community college as part of a **career ladder** approach to nursing education. These programs sometimes are referred to as one-on-one programs: 1 year of preparation for practical nursing, followed by one more year qualifying the graduate to take the licensure examination for registered nursing. All nursing students in these colleges are grouped together for core courses, including basic nursing content, during the first academic year. At the end of this time, a student has the option of stopping the educational program to seek licensure as a practical nurse or continuing for an additional year to be eligible to write the NCLEX-RN. Many students opt to do both. Graduates of these core programs in practical nursing usually have a broader and more in-depth understanding of the biologic sciences and sometimes the social sciences (also a part of the core curriculum), especially if these are college-level courses that are transferable to a 4-year institution. Because issues related to educational mobility and articulation between programs have received much attention (discussed later in this chapter), these combined programs have become popular.

Graduates of practical nursing programs take the NCLEX-PN; if they pass the exam, they use the title "licensed practical nurse" (LPN) or, in California and Texas, the title "licensed vocational nurse" (LVN). Their scope of practice focuses on meeting the healthcare needs of clients in hospitals, long-term care facilities, clinics, and the home. Typically, LPNs or LVNs working in acute and long-term care facilities care for clients whose conditions are considered stable, giving direct patient care; observing, recording, and reporting; administering treatments and medications; and assisting in rehabilitation procedures. They also work in clinics and urgent care centers. They receive direction from an RN or a licensed physician.

As with the associate degree and hospital-based diploma programs for RNs, the educational preparation for practical nurses and the future of practical nursing are topics of much discussion. Some advocate two levels of nurses: the practical nurse prepared with an associate degree and the RN prepared with a baccalaureate degree. Others would eliminate practical nursing altogether. In 1987, North Dakota passed legislation that required all candidates taking the licensure examination for practical nursing to have completed an associate degree in practical nursing. In 2003, this requirement was rescinded, and the state moved back to requiring a minimum of 1 year of study for practical nurse licensure and a minimum of 2 years of study for RN licensure.

The nursing shortage has had a major impact on the practice of practical nurses. In many nursing homes, positions that would have been filled with RNs are being filled with LPNs. The effects of this are not clear, with the concern that in some instances LPNs may be asked to practice beyond the scope for which they were originally prepared. With the "graying" of the United States, and the growing need for nurses in home healthcare and in long-term care facilities, practical nurses will continue to play a significant role in healthcare delivery.

PROGRAMS THAT PREPARE GRADUATES FOR RN LICENSURE

A number of different avenues of education now prepare individuals for licensure as RNs. The most traditional of these are diploma programs, associate degree programs, and baccalaureate programs. Innovative programs that offer generic masters and doctoral educational routes in nursing are also available (to be discussed later in this chapter).

Diploma Education

The earliest type of nursing education in the United States took place in **diploma programs** administered by hospitals, also referred to as **hospital-based programs**. The early development of these schools is synonymous with development of nursing as a whole.

Development of Hospital-Based Diploma Nursing Programs

The first hospital with a nurse training school was the New England Hospital for Women, which accepted five probationers on September 1, 1872 (Kalisch & Kalisch, 2004). The characteristics of these early schools were discussed in detail in Chapter 1.

By the late 1940s and early 1950s, many hospital-based nursing schools had affiliated with nearby colleges and universities; these schools adopted general education requirements, such as anatomy, physiology, sociology, and psychology, as part of the curriculum. During this time, the National League of Nursing Education—later to become two organizations, the National League for Nursing (NLN) and the National League for Nursing Accrediting Commission (NLNAC)—assumed an active role in curriculum guidance and accreditation. Nursing programs gained a stronger educational foundation because they were required to align themselves more closely with other types of postsecondary education, that is, education occurring after the completion of high school.

Hospital-Based Programs Today

Thus, diploma schools in operation today have educational programs that meet the criteria necessary for accreditation. They employ qualified faculty who have developed clinical learning experiences that meet the student's learning needs rather than the hospital's service needs (which often took priority in the past). These programs vary in length from 27 to 36 months. Many diploma schools are affiliated with a college or university so that college credit can be awarded formally. Graduates are provided with a foundation in the biologic and social sciences and may have taken some courses in the humanities. There is a strong emphasis in diploma programs on client experiences. The course of study includes experience in nursing management (eg, being in charge of a nursing unit). Graduates work in acute, long-term, and ambulatory healthcare facilities, fulfilling the responsibilities established by the scope of practice for RNs as defined by the state in which they are licensed.

Before the 1970s, diploma schools were a popular avenue to nursing education with over 800 schools in operation: fewer than 100 are in operation today (Get Your Nursing Diploma or Associate's Degree, 2002–2009). Diploma programs comprise less than 10% of all basic RN education programs (American Association of Colleges of Nursing [AACN], 2010a). As more nursing education programs were moved to institutions of higher education, many hospital-based schools elected to discontinue their programs. Some merged with a local community college or university that assumed administrative responsibility for managing the nursing program and awarded an associate or baccalaureate degree when graduation requirements were satisfied.

The elimination of hospital-based programs has occurred because hospitals could not sustain the costs of supporting the programs and because students became more attracted to programs located in colleges and universities. Long-standing programs in some areas of the United States (predominately the east) have continued due to financial support from strong endowments and private funding and community traditions that encourage student enrollment.

Associate Degree Nursing Education

The movement toward **associate degree education** began in 1952. Today, associate degree nursing programs prepare more graduates for licensure as RNs than do any of the other programs and comprise over one half of all students enrolled in prelicensure RN programs (NLN, 2009). Associate degree programs have helped to solve the nursing shortages of the 1960s, 1980s, and today.

Development of Associate Degree Education

Four events undoubtedly influenced the beginning of associate degree nursing education. First, these programs followed in the wake of the organization and growth of 2-year community colleges in the United States, which are located in the community, offer the first 2 years of a traditional 4-year college program as well as technical and vocational programs and make some form of college education accessible to everyone. Second, the cadet nurse program, which was created during World War II (see Chapter 1), demonstrated that qualified students could be educated adequately in less than the traditional 3 years of the diploma program. Third, the development of associate degree education was influenced by the studies conducted on nursing education in the United States, as discussed in Chapter 1. The final factor influencing the development of associate degree education was the critical national nursing shortage of the 1950s, which occurred because nurses employed during World War II returned home to raise families. It was anticipated that the 2-year program would put graduates into the work market more quickly, thus helping to reduce the shortage of nurses while, at the same time, helping to move nursing education into the overall system of higher education in the United States.

Associate degree in nursing (ADN) programs have the distinction of being the first (and, to date, the only) type of nursing education established on the basis of planned research and experimentation. They were initiated through the Cooperative Research Project in Junior and Community College Education for Nursing at Teachers College, Columbia University. The original 5-year research project, which was directed by Mildred Montag, included seven junior and community colleges and one hospital school, located in six regions of the United States. Students graduating from these programs received an associate degree and were eligible to take the RN licensing examination. ADN programs have expanded from these seven programs in 1952 to more than 980 in 2009 (Associate Degree in Nursing Schools and Programs, 2008–2009).

Characteristics of Associate Degree Education

Accrediting groups ensure that ADN programs are an integral part of the college in which they are housed, that faculty and students have the same rights and privileges as their counterparts in other fields of study, and that the curriculum is sound.

In a typical program, approximately 40% of the credits needed for the associate degree must be fulfilled by general education courses such as English, anatomy, physiology, speech, psychology, and sociology; the rest are to be fulfilled by nursing courses. Clinical learning experiences are carefully selected to correspond with the content delivered in classroom lectures; the preconferences and postconferences help to reinforce the relationship between the two. Some modifications in this structure are occurring, as associate degree educators strive to meet the expectations of employers and the community while remaining true to the concept of associate degree education.

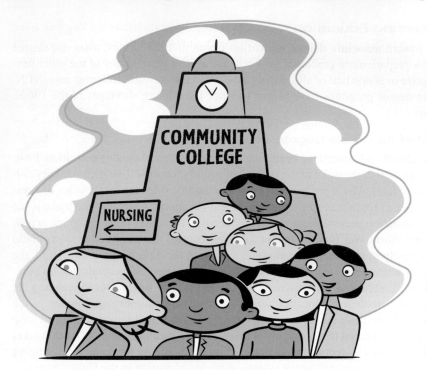

FIGURE 2.1 Associate degree programs attract older people, married women, minorities, men, and students with a wider range of educational experiences and intellectual capabilities.

Traditionally, nursing students were a homogeneous group—typically single white women, ranging in age from 18 to 35, who graduated in the upper third of their high school classes. The advent of associate degree education in nursing increased diversity in the students who enroll in nursing programs attracting older students, married women, minorities, men, and students with a wider range of educational experiences and intellectual abilities (Fig. 2.1). People who already possess baccalaureate or higher degrees in other fields sometimes seek admission to an associate degree program, often because it can be completed in a shorter period of time than would be needed to earn another baccalaureate degree. Additionally, community college programs tend to be more geographically accessible than baccalaureate programs in 4-year colleges and universities, which are characteristically located in major urban areas.

Challenges to Associate Degree Education

Associate degree education, like other educational programs, has experienced change. With these changes have come some challenges.

Pressure to Increase Credits. As programs have developed, there has been a growing tendency to increase the number of nursing credits. Faculty members, who may be struggling to define essential content, often try to comply with requests from advisory committees for graduates who will need shorter orientation programs and possess greater knowledge in certain specialty areas (eg, coronary care). The push to recognize all nurses as managers has led to the addition of management content in most programs. Changes that some colleges have made in the basic requirements for all associate degrees have increased the number of nonnursing credits nursing students must complete; the concept of "core courses" that are taken by all students who graduate from a college has become popular.

The recent shift to community-based practice also offers a challenge to associate degree educators who struggle with decisions regarding allocation and balance of time devoted to content and supervision of community experiences for students. Faculty members who have spent the greater part of their clinical nursing careers in acute care settings are often reluctant to divert even an hour from the time students spend on acute care hospital units. In general, most schools try to adhere to the standard of 108 quarter hours or 72 semester hours for the associate degree.

The Selective Admission Process. Another concern with which educators struggle is the processes used in selecting students for a nursing program. This challenge becomes greater when the number of students seeking admission either increases dramatically or drops significantly, a phenomenon many programs have experienced during the past 15 to 20 years. In response to this problem and in an effort to select students who can realize success in their endeavors, many programs have developed selective admission processes. Although this is common in 4-year schools and colleges, it is a departure from the open-door policy of most community colleges. Some nursing programs use a waiting list, which honors the concept of first come, first served. Other schools use systems similar to a lottery. Also popular are point systems that award numeric scores for courses completed, past work experience, cumulative grade point average, or a combination of all of these, with the students acquiring the greatest number of points being selected for the next class. These factoring systems often require that a student spends at least a year in college to secure a position in the beginning nursing class, resulting in what began as a 2-year program extending to at least 3 years.

Misunderstandings About Associate Degree Education

For many years, associate degree education was poorly understood by employers, the public, and, to some extent, nursing educators in baccalaureate and higher degree programs. Although this route to nursing education is now firmly established as credible preparation for a nursing career, it continues to receive some opposition. The controversy regarding "entry into practice" and the preparation needed for "professional" nursing (which is discussed later in this chapter) is renewed from time to time. Thus, faculty, graduates, and advocates for associate degree education continue to find themselves clarifying facts such as the actual number of nursing credits and the focus on critical thinking and decision making, as well as technical skills, and emphasizing the contributions made by graduates of the programs.

Baccalaureate Education

Baccalaureate degree nursing education occurs in a 4-year college or university and is championed by many to provide the minimum educational preparation for professional practice.

Development of Baccalaureate Education in Nursing

The first school of nursing to be established in a university setting was started at the University of Minnesota in 1909 as a quasi-autonomous branch of the university's school of medicine. The program was not very different from the 3-year hospital-based program operating at that time; nothing was required in the way of higher general education, and graduates were prepared for the RN certificate only. Education took place predominantly through apprenticeship, and students provided service to hospitals in exchange for education. However, nursing education did become a part of an academic organization, with 16 colleges and universities developing programs by 1916.

Many of the early programs offering a baccalaureate degree in nursing extended over a 5-year period. This allowed for 3 years of nursing school curriculum similar to that of the hospital-based programs and for an additional 2 years of liberal arts. While the increase in the number of schools was not rapid, in 1924, the Yale School of Nursing became the first to be established as a separate department within a university; Annie W. Goodrich was its dean.

Although the development of baccalaureate education for nurses may not seem like a major step to young people today, remember that it was not until 1920 that the 19th Amendment to the Constitution of the United States granted women the right to vote. Many people considered nursing to be a less than desirable occupation: vocational in its orientation; overshadowed by militaristic, religious, and technical characteristics; and confined to women. Liberal education, scholarship, and knowledge were thought to be incompatible with the female personality and capable of interfering with marriage—for many years, nursing students generally were not allowed to marry (Kalisch & Kalisch, 2004). The nursing curriculum, with its emphasis on the performance of skills rather than on the philosophic and theoretic approaches used in the humanities, was not well accepted by universities. Opposition to collegiate education for nurses also came from physicians, who argued that nurses would be overtrained. Physicians were not certain that a sound knowledge base was as important as the technical skills and manual dexterity that could be acquired with brief training at the bedside and argued that a baccalaureate education would make nursing services too expensive.

Many nursing leaders advocated for baccalaureate education as the minimum educational preparation for supervisory and administrative nursing roles. Baccalaureate education also provides the background needed for addressing the community as a client and incorporating research into practice, and the educational base for entry into graduate education in nursing. In 1965, the ANA recommended baccalaureate preparation in nursing as the minimum educational preparation for entry into professional nursing practice, an issue discussed later in this chapter.

Characteristics of Baccalaureate Education

A baccalaureate nursing program is termed a basic or **generic program** when it is a prelicensure program leading to eligibility to take the NCLEX-RN. It includes an upper division (junior and senior years) nursing major that is built upon 2 years of liberal arts and science courses taken during the freshman and sophomore years.

Nine essential components have been identified by the AACN as critical to professional nursing education. They include a liberal education; organizational and systems leadership; scholarship for evidence-based practice; information management and application; healthcare policy, finance, and regulatory environments; interprofessional communication and collaboration; clinical prevention and population health; profession and professional values; and baccalaureate generalist nursing practice (AACN, 2008).

Applicants to such programs must meet the entrance and graduation requirements established by the university and those of the nursing school. The admission requirements usually specify academic preparation at the high school (or preadmission) level, including courses in foreign language and higher level mathematics and science, and a high cumulative grade point average. Relatively high scores on college admission tests also may be required.

During the freshman and sophomore years, students who pursue a nursing education take humanities, social, life, and physical science courses with college students who are preparing for other majors. The number of required liberal arts and science courses may vary from program to program but usually constitutes about one half the total number of credits specified for graduation—typically 120 semester credits or 180 quarter credits. Students usually begin their study of nursing content during their junior year, thus the term "upper-division major" in nursing. Nursing theory can be taught so that it builds on an understanding of the physical and biologic sciences and liberal arts studied the previous 2 years.

Students in baccalaureate nursing programs learn basic nursing skills. They also learn concepts of health promotion and disease prevention at an individual and population level. Supervisory and leadership theory and skills are taught, along with an introduction to research. Clinical course work includes experience in community health settings, and leadership responsibility. Emphasis is placed on developing skills in critical decision making, exercising independent nursing judgments that call for broad background knowledge, and working in complex nursing situations in which the outcomes often are not predictable. These call for the application of current evidence into one's practice. Acting as a client advocate, the graduate with a baccalaureate degree in nursing collaborates with other members of the healthcare team in structured and unstructured settings and supervises those with lesser preparation. Baccalaureate graduates often work with groups as well as with individuals. Knowledge and skills in managing information and patient care technology are also essential components of baccalaureate education. The roles of the baccalaureate graduate are defined as provider of care, designer/manager/coordinator of care, and member of the profession (AACN, 2008).

Changes in Baccalaureate Education

In recent years, the nature of baccalaureate education has changed. Many baccalaureate nursing programs have taken steps to respond to the need for more RNs prepared for licensure at the baccalaureate level. Innovative methods include the development of accelerated programs and external degree programs. These are discussed in detail later in this chapter.

Table 2.1 provides a comparison of these traditional major avenues to RN licensure.

Master's and Doctoral Prelicensure Programs

Our discussion of the various educational programs for registered nursing would be incomplete without mention of the generic master's program. The first generic master's degree in nursing was opened at Yale University in 1974, and other schools soon followed. Students are admitted with a baccalaureate degree in another discipline and are granted a master's degree in nursing after completing an established 2-year program of study that prepares them for RN licensure. Case Western Reserve University initiated the first program in which a student may earn a doctorate in nursing (ND) before being eligible to take the licensing examination. Most of the graduates of these programs are engaged in teaching and research.

Such programs reflect the thinking of some nursing leaders that the minimum preparation for professional nursing should be the master's degree. The programs also provide a higher degree to those people who possess basic baccalaureate preparation in another area of study

Table 2.1   **Basic Educational Opportunities for Registered Nursing: A Comparison**

	DIPLOMA	ASSOCIATE DEGREE	BACCALAUREATE
Location	Is usually conducted by and based in a hospital	Most often conducted in junior or community colleges, occasionally in senior colleges and universities	Located in senior colleges and universities
Length of study	Requires generally 24–30 months but may require 3 academic years	Requires usually 2 academic or sometimes 2 calendar years—with prerequisites completed before nursing courses, up to 3 years	Requires 4 academic years
Requirements for admission	Requires graduation from high school or its equivalent, satisfactory general academic achievement, and successful completion of certain prerequisite courses	Requires that applicants meet entrance requirements of college as well as those of program	Requires that applicants meet entrance requirements of the college or university as well as those of program
Program of learning	Includes courses in theory and practice of nursing and in biologic, physical, and behavioral sciences that may be taken at a local college or university	Combines a balance of nursing courses and college courses in the basic natural and social sciences with courses in general education and the humanities.	Combines courses in the liberal arts as well as the behavioral and physical sciences taken in the first 2 years with concentration of courses in the theory and practice of nursing in the junior and senior years
Clinical component	Clinical component completed in large part in the hospital offering the program.	Requires as a significant part of the program supervised clinical instruction in hospitals and other community health agencies	Includes courses in community health, leadership, and research as part of the nursing curriculum as well as clinical instruction in a variety of settings
Opportunity for educational advancement	Little or no transferability of courses unless affiliated with a community college or university	Is structured so that some credits may be applied to baccalaureate degree	Provides the basic academic preparation for advancement to higher positions in nursing and to master's degree
Competency on graduation	Graduate is prepared to plan for the care of patients with other members of the healthcare team, to develop and carry out plans for the care of individuals or groups of patients, and to direct selected members of the nursing team. Has an understanding of the hospital climate and the community health resources necessary for the extended care of patients.	Graduate is prepared to plan and give direct patient care in hospitals, nursing homes, or similar healthcare agencies and to participate with other members of the healthcare team, such as LPNs, nurses aides, physicians, and other registered nurses, in rendering care to patients	Graduate is prepared to plan and give direct care to individuals and families, whether sick or well, to assume responsibility for directing other members of the healthcare team, and to take on beginning leadership positions. Practices in a variety of settings and emphasizes comprehensive healthcare, including preventive and rehabilitative services, health counseling and education, and care in acute and long-term illnesses. Has necessary education for graduate study toward a master's degree and may move rapidly to specialized leadership positions in nursing as teacher, administrator, clinical specialist, nurse practitioner, and nurse researcher.
Licensure	Must successfully complete licensing examination	Must successfully complete licensing examination	Must successfully complete licensing examination

and are making a career change. With increasing emphasis on the need for a baccalaureate degree for professional practice, this type of program provides a credible opportunity to those with baccalaureate degrees in another area of study. When programs of this type are not available, many students with degrees in other disciplines choose to pursue a 2-year ADN.

Nontraditional Prelicensure Programs

Throughout the years, various adaptations have been made in the traditional ways of educating nurses. These innovative approaches have occurred primarily because of the need to educate more individuals to become nurses, the need to prepare nurses with higher degrees in nursing, shifts in the economy, and the desire among young people to find work that will make a difference while at the same time making a living.

Accelerated Programs

Accelerated programs prepare students at both the baccalaurcate and the master's level. Building on previous learning experiences, they are designed to transition adults with baccalaureate and graduate degrees in other fields into nursing. Baccalaureate programs may be completed in 11 to 18 months including prerequisites, and master's degree programs generally take about 3 years to complete. Accelerated baccalaureate programs make this the fastest route to licensure as an RN (AACN, 2010b). Instruction is intense with all courses offered full-time with no breaks between sessions. These fast-track programs have proliferated over the past 15 years with programs available in 43 states plus the District of Columbia and Puerto Rico—more are in the planning stages.

Typical students, referred to as **second-degree students**, are motivated, older, competitive, and have high academic expectations. Admission standards are high, typically requiring a minimum of a 3.0 GPA. Programs are geared to students who have already demonstrated an ability of succeed at a senior college or university. Students receive the same number of clinical hours as the counterparts in the traditional programs (AACN, 2010b). More detailed information on accelerated programs can be obtained at *www.aacn.nche.edu/Publications/issues/Aug02.htm*.

External Degree Programs

The concept of an **external degree** is not new to education in general. Universities in Australia, the Soviet Union, and England have long recognized independent study validated by examination. The University of London has awarded college degrees earned in this fashion since 1836. The major difference between the external degree and the traditional educational experience is that students awarded an external degree are not required to attend classes or follow any prescribed methods of learning (however, they may choose to take some classes).

Learning is assessed through highly standardized and validated examinations. This approach to education was not developed in the United States until about the mid-1950s and then only in selected areas. New York's Empire State College and the University Without Walls consortium were the first schools in the United States to recognize the value of self-directed learning. Now known as Excelsior University, the New York Regents External Degree Program of the University of the State of New York has become part of this movement.

The nursing program, like other external degree programs in arts, science, and business, uses an assessment approach and is primarily—although not exclusively—designed for those with some experience in nursing. It is philosophically based on principles of adult learning, which advocate flexible and learner-oriented education. Specifically, the responsibility for demonstrating that learning has occurred is placed on the student, and the responsibility for identifying the content to be learned and objectively assessing that this has occurred rests with the faculty. The nursing major is divided into cognitive and performance components. Cognitive learning is documented through nationally standardized and psychometrically valid written examinations. Clinical skills are evaluated through criteria-referenced performance examinations at regional performance assessment centers throughout the country.

There are some limitations on the use of external degree programs. Some states do not accept Excelsior degrees for initial licensure because their laws mandate that the educational process include supervised clinical practice. Some states will admit to the licensure examination for RNs only those external associate degree graduates who were LPNs and therefore have had supervised clinical practice in addition to clinical examinations. Despite objections, alternative and nontraditional avenues to nursing education appeal to the learner, and these programs continue to evolve. Nursing education, like nursing care, should be tailored to fit the consumer's needs.

COMMUNICATION IN ACTION

Dealing With Educational Challenges

Alice Mason, a recent graduate from an associate degree nursing program was working on a unit with a new baccalaureate graduate. On several occasions, the baccalaureate graduate made comments such as, "I just don't know how you could learn all you need to know in just two years." Alice invited her colleague to join her for coffee. She initiated the conversation by saying, "From some of your remarks, I don't believe you understand the scope of associate degree nursing education, and I'd like to explain a bit about it." Calmly, she further explained, "In an associate degree program, we have the same science requirements as in a baccalaureate program in this state. We do take fewer credits in general education, but we are required to take two full years of nursing courses, often using the same texts used by programs such as yours. Although sometimes we earn fewer credits in some of those classes. My understanding is that you have spent time studying the community as a client, which I did not, and that you have more time devoted to statistics, nursing research, and leadership. Although I took a nursing management course, I believe it, too, was fewer credits. In order to complete my bachelor's degree, I will need to take the general education courses I do not have, plus 20 semester credits of nursing." She then said, "Tell me more about your program." Her colleague began to share details of her program, and they both felt they more clearly understood one another's education.

SIMILARITIES AMONG TRADITIONAL ENTRY-LEVEL PRELICENSURE PROGRAMS

Currently, there are as many similarities in the various avenues to nursing education as there are differences. These similarities may be grouped into several broad classifications, including academic standards, administrative concerns, and areas relating to students.

Academic Similarities

The most obvious similarity is that all programs must academically prepare graduates to pass the NCLEX for registered nursing in their state at the same minimum standardized score used across the nation. All schools must meet criteria established for state board approval in their respective state.

Administrative Similarities

Adequate financial support is a major concern for many programs because they are relatively expensive to operate. Lower student-to-teacher ratios, expensive laboratories, and limited federal and state funding for nursing education affect the economics of the programs. Another administrative concern focuses on securing appropriate learning experiences. Schools often compete with one another for clinical spaces in hospitals and healthcare facilities. Certain experiences, such as maternal, child, and psychiatric nursing, may be especially difficult to secure. Developing and maintaining curricula that prepare graduates for current practice often present a challenge. Demographic changes, with people living longer, technological advances—especially in the area of informatics—changes in venues of care, bioethical concerns, and myriad other changes leave faculty struggling to construct and teach state-of-the-art curricula. Not the least of the administrative similarities is the recruitment and retention of qualified faculty, which has become intensified in recent years. More lucrative salaries in other positions and the aging and retirement of the present faculty both affect this concern.

Similarities Relating to Students

Similarities also exist among students. First of all, recruitment and selection is a major task. Although some schools must turn students away (often because they are unable to find faculty to teach them), at the same time, schools must be responsive to an increasingly diverse population that may enter school unprepared for college-level studies. This has resulted in the development of selective admission policies that must be scrutinized carefully by school officials and, in some areas, reviewed by the school's attorney for correct legal form and legal ramifications before being accepted by the school's policy-making group.

Programs are caught up in more legal concerns than in the past because applicants and students are seeking their rights as individuals and challenging admission, progression, and dismissal policies. Another legal concern relates to malpractice coverage for students. Some collegiate programs, now removed from the umbrella coverage of the hospital, ask that students purchase malpractice insurance as protection against any lawsuits that might arise as the result of errors committed in the learning process.

There is greater diversity in the student body. Programs are receiving more applications from men, minorities, older adults, and persons who possess degrees in other fields of study. Students with English as a second language present new challenges to nursing faculty in all types of programs. Special courses and other forms of assistance are being developed to enable students with academic challenges to succeed in nursing.

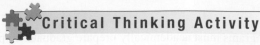

Critical Thinking Activity

Imagine that you could restructure nursing education for an ideal world. Where would you begin? How many levels of nursing education would you incorporate into your model? Would each level be terminal or articulated with others? Where would general education fit into your model? How would you see the graduate of each program functioning on the healthcare team? How would you see each level reimbursed for services?

NURSING EDUCATION AT THE GRADUATE LEVEL

The critical need for nurses with additional preparation to work in educational settings, in supervisory roles, as clinical specialists and to fulfill the expanded role of the nurse has resulted in more programs at the graduate level.

Master's Preparation

As indicated in our earlier discussion of master's education in nursing, there are a variety of models. Some less-traditional approaches include outreach programs, summers-only programs, RN-to-MSN tracks (that provide a direct route to the master's degree for RNs who have graduated from diploma or associate degree programs), programs taught primarily on-line, and programs for students with different educational backgrounds (such as RNs with nonnursing baccalaureate degrees or foreign graduates). Some schools offer off-campus classes, at times rotating sites, and some deliver core content by way of television or through other distance learning technology.

Most programs require at least a full year for completion, and many have been expanded to 2 years. Master's programs in nursing are found in senior colleges and universities that have baccalaureate programs in nursing. They have the option of seeking voluntary accreditation from the NLNAC or from the Commission on Collegiate Nursing Education (CCNE).

Master's preparation is recommended for leadership positions in nursing, for clinical specialization, and is generally the minimum preparation required to teach nursing. The AACN has outlined roles for graduates at the various educational levels. Their vision is for a generalist at the baccalaureate level and an advanced generalist at the master's level that includes the clinical nurse leader (CNL) (see Chapter 14). The CNL oversees the care coordination of a distinct group of patients and actively provides direct patient care in complex situations (AACN, 2007).

Further identified is advanced specialty nursing education with a Doctor of Nursing Practice (DNP) or a research-focused program (PhD, DNS, or DNSc).

Doctoral Studies

The number of requests for admission to doctoral study in nursing has increased greatly since the early 1980s. The impetus for this movement stems from the need for advanced study for academic advancement or tenure in the educational setting and reflects the need in nursing research for the advancement of the profession as a whole.

Before doctorates in nursing were offered, doctoral study in other fields allowed nurses to benefit from post-master's preparation. A doctorate outside the area of nursing was often the only doctorate available to persons seeking further education; doctorates in nursing are relatively new to the educational milieu, as opposed to such degrees in psychology, sociology, anthropology, or physiology. Certainly, nursing can benefit and has benefited from other disciplines.

Doctoral programs in nursing offer various degrees, such as the doctor of nursing science DNS), the doctor of science in nursing (DSN), the doctor of nursing education (DEd), and the more traditional doctor of philosophy in nursing (PhD). Nonnursing doctorates are available to nurses, such as the doctor of education (EdD) and the doctor of public health (DPH).

In 2004, the AACN proposed a doctor of nursing practice degree (DNP). The DNP is designed for nurses seeking a terminal degree in advanced nursing practice, as opposed to working in research (AACN, 2006a). The DNP was developed with the premise that the challenges of today's healthcare demanded a higher level of preparation for advanced practice nurses (APNs) who could design and assess care and provide leadership. Some universities are changing their nurse practitioner programs from master's degree programs to this type of clinical practice doctorates. The difference in the preparation and function of graduates possessing the various degrees is confusing. Typically, the nurse with a doctorate assumes a leadership role in education, often serving as a faculty member or the dean or director of a nursing program. These nurses also may choose to be involved in the research and development of a body of nursing knowledge.

Critical Thinking Activity

If nurse practitioners are to work collaboratively with physicians, and as primary care providers, what type and level of education do you believe they should complete? How would you ensure that this would occur? What standards regarding continuing education should be mandated for those involved in advance practice? Should it be more stringent than that required at the RN level? Defend your position.

OTHER FORMS OF NURSING EDUCATION

A number of factors have fostered the development of other forms of education for nurses. Most of these are seen in the changing role of the nurse in healthcare delivery and the need this creates for more adequate education to meet the requirements of that role. Another contributing aspect is the continuing push to make nursing truly professional and prepare nurses to complete research. A third significant reason for advancing nursing education relates to the need for leadership in nursing administration and education. Thus, RNs seek baccalaureate, master's, and doctoral degrees to support the complex roles into which they move.

Registered Nurse Baccalaureate Programs

Enrollments continue to increase in **registered nurse baccalaureate (RNB) programs** (AACN, 2010a). These programs are designed for RNs with either a diploma or an associate degree who wish to return to school to complete a baccalaureate degree in nursing.

Some schools also have added programs designed to admit the LPN, who will emerge with a baccalaureate degree in nursing and be eligible for RN licensure. These programs carry different names in different parts of the country, including baccalaureate registered nurse programs, two-on-two programs, and, in the Midwest, capstone programs.

There are many reasons for the increase in this form of nursing education, several of which have been discussed. In addition, many highly qualified young men and women enter associate degree programs because of cost and time factors and plan for more education several years after completing the original program. The nursing profession is endeavoring to increase the number of nurses prepared with baccalaureate and higher degrees.

The RNB programs vary greatly throughout the United States. In some instances, they exist in universities that already offer the generic baccalaureate program. The students may be completely integrated with generic baccalaureate students, partially separated from them, or in a totally separate program. Some are distance education programs discussed below.

Another form of RNB preparation is the two-on-two approach, in which RN students transfer into the college or university with junior standing and complete an additional 2 years of upper-division nursing classes. In some instances, this is the only nursing program offered by a college or university; that is, the college may not offer a basic program that prepares a graduate for licensure. Credits in the natural and biologic sciences, and in basic courses such as psychology and sociology, earned at junior and community colleges or other 4-year colleges are transferred in. Often, transfer of credit is allowed for nursing courses (eg, 45 quarter credits or 30 semester credits), or the courses may be challenged by examination. Distribution requirements as well as any minimum residency credits of the particular college or university must be satisfied, and upper-division nursing courses must be completed in such areas as physiologic nursing, community health, understanding nursing research, and supervision. A minimum of 2 years usually is required for completion of the program, although the time may be shorter or longer, depending on the number of requirements satisfied at the time of entry.

Today, RNB education and two-on-two educational programs flourish. Schools with both generic and RNB programs may report more graduates from the RNB program. At least four factors are responsible for the change in attitude toward RNB education. First, the ANA Commission on Nursing Education has provided a push to increase the availability of baccalaureate programs for RNs. Nursing educators are challenged to create and accept more innovative educational strategies.

The second factor comes from pressure within each state. Several states have enacted legislation, sometimes in response to the nursing shortage, which requires the development of a statewide plan for articulation between various types of nursing education programs. In most instances, the legislation establishes a date by which the plan will be implemented.

The third factor influencing the development of RNB programs has been a call for increased educational mobility from organizations in the healthcare arena. The American Medical Association House of Delegates has suggested career mobility as one way to alleviate the nurse shortage. The Pew Commission recommended strengthening existing career ladder programs to make movement through these levels of nursing as easy as possible (de Tornyay, 1996). Some of the RNB programs currently in operation provide for part-time study or for studies completed through evening courses. The desirability of such approaches for nurses who must work to support their education is obvious. Other innovative RNB programs provide baccalaureate education to people living in areas geographically remote from colleges or universities. These programs use new technologies for distance learning, including the electronic transmission of information.

A final factor influencing the development of RNB programs relates to the allocation of federal dollars to assist students who seek to advance their preparation in nursing. Major nursing groups such as the ANA and NLN are lobbying Congress for additional funds directed toward nursing education including the creation of grants to provide scholarships to assist disadvantaged students and individuals entering or seeking advanced education in nursing.

Articulated Programs

Another approach to nursing education is found in programs that are articulated. **Articulation** indicates that the two programs at different levels have well-defined links enabling the student to move from one educational level to the next. This can be seen at various levels of nursing education. The major difference between these programs and the ones mentioned earlier is that the curricula are designed so that maximum credit is awarded for work completed earlier.

Today, as increasing numbers of graduates seek education beyond the associate degree or diploma, the career ladder concept in nursing education, mentioned earlier, is growing in popularity. Programs have been developed that provide direct articulation between lower level and higher level programs. As mentioned earlier, in some states, legislation has been passed strongly encouraging, and in some instances mandating, articulation plans.

The purpose of an articulated program is to facilitate opportunities for students to start nursing education, stop when some goal is reached or degree awarded, or keep moving up the educational ladder. Statewide articulation plans exist in most states. Many of the plans allow most of the work completed at the lower level to meet the requirements of the next degree. Some have been mandated as part of legislation, some are statewide agreements, and others are school-to-school articulation agreements (AACN, 2006b). Similar plans exist for articulation between practical (vocational) nurse programs and associate degree programs, and some associate degree programs allow credit for nurse assistant preparation or require it for admission. Again, the articulated program allows students to move up the career ladder from practical nurse to associate degree nurse to the nurse with a baccalaureate degree. Students in an articulated LPN/associate degree program spend a year preparing to be an LPN, and another year completing the associate degree. If they want to continue after this 2-year period, they can earn a baccalaureate degree at another institution after 2 more years of study. Some schools have established LPN-to-baccalaureate degree programs. From that point, a student may continue to work toward a master's degree (Fig. 2.2).

The multiple-entry, multiple-exit programs are not without problems. Initially, they are difficult to develop because of the tremendous amount of joint planning required. Questions develop regarding granting upper degree credit (course work with 300 and 400 numbers) for studies completed with 100 and 200 numbers in the community college. Understanding what has been taught and determining how to evaluate current knowledge are important. This is particularly relevant to articulation between practical nurse programs and RN programs, where graduates of the practical program may know how to perform many of the nursing skills but may lack the theory base of RNs. Educators need to speak the same language and develop mutual respect.

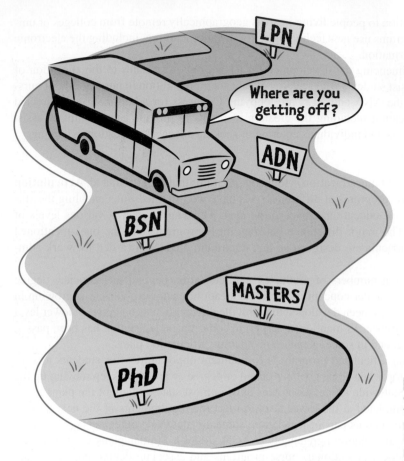

FIGURE 2.2 Among innovations occurring in nursing education over the past decade are programs that provide direct articulation between lower-level and higher-level programs.

▶ *EXAMPLE*

An Articulated Approach to Nursing Education

Hannah Bledsoe began her nursing education in a practical nursing program. Located in a community college, this program was articulated with an associate degree program. Because of financial concerns, Hannah worked as an LPN for 2 years following completion of the practical nurse program. Eager for more knowledge and the career opportunities it provided, Hannah sought admission to the associate degree program, was admitted, and completed the program. The program she chose had a written articulation agreement with a local 4-year university. On graduation from the associate degree program and successful completion of the RN licensing examination, Hannah was hired at the University Hospital. This employment allowed her to continue to take six credits of study per quarter toward a baccalaureate degree in nursing tuition-free. Working and studying worked well for Hannah, and within a few years, she had earned a baccalaureate degree in nursing. She is now considering enrolling in a master's degree program.

Distance Education

Distance education is being used by a variety of universities and other educational entities to make attaining a baccalaureate or master's degree more accessible. This approach focuses on making education available through a variety of distance technologies including online strategies, video broadcasting to distant sites, and courses taught in areas distant from the campus. A wide variety of approaches and methods are used, including courses that are Internet-enabled, Web-based, computer-mediated, on-line, synchronous, and asynchronous.

Students may participate in clinical learning through a relationship with a mentor or preceptor in a local clinical setting. These clinical experiences follow prescribed procedures leading to specified outcomes and receive academic credit. Part-time study is welcomed. Some programs have brief, intensive times when all students in a cohort gather at the institution for 1 to 2 weeks in order to foster interaction between students and faculty and enhance the educational experience. Students benefit because they can continue to work while attending school and experience reduced travel costs. The RN who wishes to obtain a baccalaureate or higher degree from such an institution may take some courses, such as general education requirements, at a local college, attain credit by examination for some nursing courses, and enroll in still other courses on-line, with all accepted as credit by the university granting the degree.

For on-line courses, sometimes referred to as a **virtual university**, students register for a class and are given passwords and access to the system. They work with an instructor and other class members, discussing issues, sharing ideas, and testing theories without the need to gather physically, although that also may occur in some programs.. Often individuals in the group share a mailbox, which serves as an electronic classroom, facilitating a group forum among students. Research material is available through an electronic library. Students usually concentrate on one subject at a time, with courses being sequenced but offered outside the constraints of established times. Students may sign on at any hour, day or night. The instructor may have posted a short lecture and provided discussion questions. Students complete reading and written assignments as in traditional learning situations, except that the written assignments are sent to the instructor, graded, and returned on-line. Computer conferencing allows the students to participate in class discussion, ask questions, and receive feedback. After completing one course, the students move to the next until degree requirements are met.

Although these programs offer much flexibility to students, they also demand a great deal of discipline on their part. A single course may require as much as 15 to 20 hours of study time per week. A student attempting such a program needs to be an independent learner. Sufficient faculty time also must be provided for students to receive effective feedback regarding their efforts. Library resources are always a concern for distant learners, and colleges need to provide access to appropriate learning resources for distance learners. Mechanisms for evaluating the learning must be developed thoughtfully to ensure the integrity of resulting credentials.

OTHER POSTLICENSURE EDUCATIONAL OPPORTUNITIES

Several opportunities for continued growth and career advancement are available to registered nurses. Some assist the graduate to move into a professional role, some support continued competence, and others are geared to a particular role development but may not culminate in an advanced degree.

Residencies and Structured Orientation for the New Graduate

When nursing education moved from hospital-based diploma programs into higher education, a new problem arose. Employers of the new graduates expected these graduates to function as experienced and qualified professionals on the day after graduation and complained that the graduates were not prepared to assume staff nurse positions within their institutions.

As nursing education moved into institutions of higher education, all clinical time was recognized in credit hours. If students worked on hospital units on weekends, they did so as hospital employees, not as a requirement of their education. As a result, students spend less time in the clinical area. Many graduates of diploma schools in the 1950s would have had as much as 4,000 clock hours of clinical experience, albeit more as apprenticeship and service to the hospital than as a planned learning experience. Graduates of associate and baccalaureate degree programs, with integrated curricula and outcome-based learning experiences, join the work world with clinical learning time of 800 or fewer clock hours. Hospital-based programs also decreased their clinical hours as curricula were reorganized. Students in all programs receive their clinical experience in a variety of settings as opposed to one primary healthcare facility where they become very familiar with policies, procedures, and the physical plant.

All of this results in new graduates needing orientation to the work facility and their new role, and time to become proficient in using their newly learned skills. Although few would question the need for internships and residencies for new physicians, the need for similar experiences for new nursing graduates has not been readily accepted. New graduates, when unable to live up to expectations placed on them, often become frustrated and discouraged; some opt for less stressful situations, sometimes even outside nursing. Nursing educators, in defending the education provided, cite other professions, such as law and engineering, in which graduates need time to adapt to the world of work.

As a result of efforts to address this concern, orientation programs, **internships**, and **residencies** for new graduates have been instituted by hospitals. The programs are intended to ease the transition from the role of student to that of staff by providing the opportunity to increase clinical skills and knowledge as well as self-confidence. These programs can last from several weeks to a year and are designed for graduates of all nursing programs—associate degree, diploma, and baccalaureate. They often include rotations to various units in the hospital, including specialty areas, and they accommodate different shifts. Usually, some formal class work is associated with the experience, but the majority of the time is spent in direct patient care, often under the supervision of a preceptor.

Institutions receive some direct benefits from such programs in addition to securing a better-prepared employee who remains employed. Inadequacies in policies and procedures have been uncovered and, as a result, rewritten. Performance evaluation tools that are more objective in format have emerged. Nursing practice throughout some agencies has become more standardized. Job satisfaction has increased. It is no longer unusual for hospitals to advertise planned orientation and internships as benefits offered to the new graduate seeking employment, a strong recruitment tool in times of nurse shortages.

The major disadvantage voiced by hospitals is the cost of operating such programs. When cost containment is crucial, hospitals may not be eager to deal with these additional costs. Another problem is that some employees who benefit from such programs may resign from their positions soon after completing an internship. This has resulted in hospitals stipulating a period of required employment following the orientation or internship.

Continuing Education

Continuing education in nursing is defined as

> planned learning experiences beyond a basic nursing educational program. The learning experiences are designed to promote the development of knowledge, skills, and attitudes for the enhancement of nursing practice, thus improving healthcare to the public. (ANA, 1974)

Continuing education programs are widely publicized in today's nursing literature. They often are presented just before and during major nursing conventions. Some professional meetings carry continuing education credit. Other continuing education programs exist as extensions of nursing programs at colleges and universities.

Like so many other areas of nursing, continuing education is not new. In an article entitled "Nursing the Sick," written around 1882, Florence Nightingale wrote:

> Nursing is, above all, a progressive calling. Year by year nurses have to learn new and improved methods, as medicine and surgery and hygiene improve. Year by year nurses are called upon to do more and better than they have done. It is felt to be impossible to have a public register of nurses that is not a delusion. (Nightingale, as cited in Seymer, 1954, p. 349)

The first continuing education courses for nurses probably would be considered postgraduate instruction today. In 1899, Teachers College at Columbia University instituted a course for qualified graduate nurses in hospital economics. Nursing institutes and conferences were first offered to nurses in the 1920s; often these were given to make up for deficiencies in basic nursing curricula. The first hospital inservice classes or staff development programs were discussed in nursing literature around this time. Today most hospitals employ someone who is responsible for the staff education program. By 1959, federal funds became available for short-term courses, giving much thrust to continuing education. In 1967, the ANA published Avenues for Continued Learning, its first definitive statement on continuing education; and in 1973, the ANA Council on Continuing Education was established. The Council, which is responsible to the ANA Commission on Education, is concerned about standards of continuing education, accreditation of the programs, transferability of credit from state to state, and development of guidelines for recognition systems within states. In 1974, the first edition of *Standards for Continuing Education in Nursing* was published by the ANA, and the federal government altered the Nurse Traineeship Act of 1972 to include an option that would provide continuing education as an alternative to placing more students into programs receiving federal capitation dollars.

By the 1970s, most nursing publications had something to say about continuing education for nurses. Practically, all states were organizing or planning to organize some method by which the nurse could receive recognition for continued education. These systems were called continuing education approval and recognition programs, or continuing education recognition programs, and most state systems followed the guidelines and criteria prepared by the ANA.

The **continuing education unit** (CEU) became a rather uniform system of measuring, recording, reporting, accumulating, transferring, and recognizing participation in nonacademic credit offerings. The National Task Force on the Continuing Education Unit, which

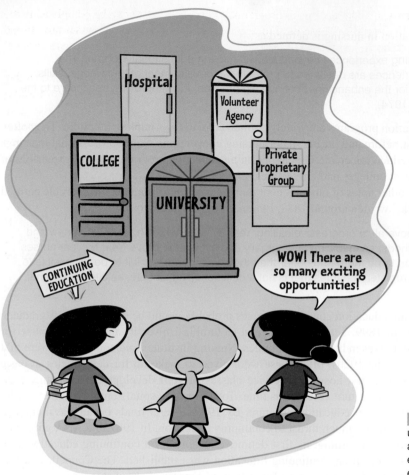

FIGURE 2.3 Today, colleges, universities, hospitals, voluntary agencies, and private proprietary groups all offer continuing education courses to nurses.

represented 34 educational groups, developed the definition of a CEU. Although nursing was not one of the groups, the profession has accepted the definition. Ten hours of participation in an organized continuing education experience under responsible sponsorship, with capable direction and qualified instruction, is equal to one CEU. Many states and organizations, however, simply report clock hours of instruction. Following a system for accreditation and approval of continuing education in nursing that was developed and implemented by the ANA in 1975, programs or individuals offering courses for continuing education now receive authority to do so from a recognized body, thereby ensuring quality programs and standardization in their approach.

Today, colleges, universities, hospitals, voluntary agencies, and private proprietary groups all offer continuing education courses to RNs (Fig. 2.3). The cost of this education varies tremendously. Nurses can earn continuing education credits for merely attending meetings and conferences. Attempts to assess whether learning has occurred vary tremendously.

Professional journals include sections of programmed instruction that can be completed in the comfort of one's living room. These have an evaluation mechanism. Telecourses are offered by television. Workshops, institutes, conferences, short courses, and evening courses abound. Additionally, courses are available on the Internet.

However, some nurses do not feel the need to keep up with these offerings. An issue today is whether continuing education should be mandatory or voluntary. **Mandatory continuing education** affects licensure, meaning that any nurse renewing a license in a state requiring (mandating) continuing education will have to satisfy that requirement. **Voluntary continuing education** is not related to relicensure. Government agencies and state legislatures are exerting pressure on nurses, as they have on physicians, attorneys, dietitians, dentists, pharmacists, and other professionals, to provide evidence of updated knowledge before license renewal.

A position supporting mandatory continuing education raises some questions. How should the learning be measured? Who should accredit the programs? How can quality be ensured? By whom and where should records be retained? Who should bear the cost? What should be the time frame for continuing education? How many hours, courses, and credits should be required?

You can contact any state board of nursing for information on specific requirements for that state.

Advanced Practice Preparation

Specialized programs have been developed to help individuals prepare for roles of increased breadth and scope. Programs may be incorporated into the preparation leading to a particular degree, exist as part of a school's continuing education program, or result in certification after examination.

Recent healthcare reform has resulted in an increased emphasis on the role of **advanced nursing practice** in healthcare delivery and more demand for educational programs to prepare these practitioners. An APN is an umbrella term that includes nurse practitioners, clinical nurse specialists, certified nurse–midwives (CNM), and certified registered nurse anesthetists.

The RN anesthesia and midwifery programs both award a certificate after completion of a standardized and rigorous course of study lasting from 18 months to 2 years. At one time, admission requirements stipulated RN licensure only; however, a baccalaureate degree in nursing is now required for admission to schools of anesthesia, with a master's degree awarded on completion. The American College of Nurse Midwives has taken a position establishing a master's degree as required for completion of a CNM program by 2010. Some states require a master's degree for the nurse anesthetist or nurse–midwife.

Other programs offer nurse practitioner and nursing specialist preparation in areas of nursing practice such as pediatrics, gerontology, family health, genetics, and women's healthcare. In the 1990s, the Pew Commission encouraged growth in the number of master's level nurse practitioner training programs, and many more were developed (de Tornyay, 1996). Programs that prepare nurse practitioners concentrate study in specific areas during a period lasting from several months to a year or more. Requirements for admission vary tremendously. Most programs require a bachelor's degree in some field and a current RN license to enter and award the master's degree on completion. Still others require that the education occur at the post-master's degree level or be part of the new ND. The ANCC requires the master's degree for all those seeking initial nurse practitioner certification, and some states now require the master's degree for those seeking initial licensure as a nurse practitioner.

The development of new APN programs has been so great that a complete listing is impossible. A student interested in pursuing such preparation is encouraged to write to the college or university of choice for information about available programs.

 Critical Thinking Activity

Do you believe continuing education should be a mandatory requirement for the renewal of one's license? Why or why not? If your answer is no, how would you ensure competence? If you believe it should be mandatory, what kind of record keeping would you require? Who do you believe should keep the records?

FACTORS BRINGING ABOUT CHANGES IN NURSING EDUCATION

During the 20th century, society experienced tremendous change. Nursing, as a part of that society, has also experienced enormous change. A number of factors influenced nursing education.

The Brown Report

In 1948, Esther Lucille Brown, who was not a nurse, conducted one of the important early studies of nursing. She was concerned that young women were not choosing nursing as a profession and believed, as a result of her study, that the majority of nursing schools failed to provide a professional education. In *Nursing for the Future*, Brown (1948) recommended that nursing education move away from the system of apprenticeship that predominated at the time (see earlier discussion of hospital-based programs in Chapter 1) and move toward a planned program of education similar to that offered by other professions. She recommended that the schools be operated by universities or colleges, hospitals affiliated with institutions of higher learning, medical colleges, or independently. She also recommended that programs periodically be examined or reviewed and that a list of accredited schools be published and distributed.

The Brown report attracted the attention of many nursing leaders, who shared her concerns about recruiting qualified women into nursing. The study took place shortly after World War II, and nurses who had been involved in the military had a new sense of autonomy and independence that they were not willing to leave behind. Committees were formed to respond to the suggestions put forth in the Brown study, particularly those related to the accreditation of programs. At the same time, the National League for Nursing Education (NLNE), later to become the NLN, recommended that hospital schools of nursing consider transferring control and administration of their programs to educational institutions. The NLNE also urged that federal grants be provided to nursing schools to allow for their improvement.

Development of a National Examination Standard

Along with the push for the improvement of nursing education, licensing authorities were pressured to establish a uniform licensing examination. The development of the State Board Test Pool Examination, which gradually expanded until all states required that same examination, helped all schools to focus on common goals and laid the foundation for interstate endorsement of licenses. The test required to obtain licensure is now known as the NCLEX for Registered Nursing (or Practical Nursing for practical nursing program graduates) (see Chapter 3).

National Accreditation of Nursing Programs

By 1952, the NLN had a temporary accreditation program in place and was helping schools to find ways to improve their programs of instruction. Accreditation of all kinds requires that the institution studies its own practices in relationship to standards. Peers, prepared as accreditation visitors, then examine the institution and a determination is made as to whether the school meets the standards. The **accreditation** of programs had a noticeable effect on standards of nursing education. As a result of accreditation activities, schools were forced to look at the educational preparation of faculty, the workload of faculty and students, the structure of clinical teaching, withdrawal rates, the self-evaluation of the program, and the state board examination scores. This system of program assessment enhanced the quality of education; graduation from a nationally accredited school meant added opportunities for advanced education or certain types of employment. Today accreditation of nursing programs is carried out by the NLNAC for practical, associate degree, baccalaureate, and master's programs in nursing. For baccalaureate and master's programs, accreditation is also available through the CCNE (see Chapter 3).

Changes in Nursing Service

While changes were occurring in the education of nurses, nurses in the workplace also experienced significant changes. With the advent of antibiotics, major advances in medical protocols and medical technology that allowed treatment of very serious conditions but resulted in patients who were in more critical condition, the public received care in hospitals rather than treatment in the home. Births that previously took place at home now occurred in hospitals. Federal funds were allocated for the construction of hospitals. Increased hospitalization drove the need for qualified nurses to a new high. Hospitals were desperate to find nurses to fill needed positions, and nurses represented half of all hospital personnel. Today RNs constitute the largest healthcare occupation, with a reported 3.1 million nurses (Health Resources and Services Administration, 2010).

The role of the nurse changed in response to changes in the workplace. Nursing staff began assuming responsibilities formerly associated with physicians. Unfortunately, they also assumed responsibilities that could have been assumed by housekeeping, dietary, laboratory, and pharmacy departments. Nurses began spending more time managing personnel, delegating responsibilities, and carrying out other administrative duties. Nurses at higher levels in the organization needed higher levels of education (ie, baccalaureate and master's degrees).

The Report of the Surgeon General's Consultant Group

In 1961, the Surgeon General of the U.S. Public Health Service appointed a group to advise him of the federal government's role in providing adequate nursing services to the country. This group was known as the Surgeon General's Consultant Group on Nursing, and they published their report in 1963.

The report emphasized the need for more nurses and identified the lack of adequate financial resources for nursing education as a major problem. Several other major concerns also were reported. Of critical importance were the reports that too few schools were providing adequate nursing education, that too few college-bound young people were being recruited into the profession, and that more nursing schools were needed in colleges and universities. (By now, you are recognizing this as a recurrent theme regarding nursing.) Educational preparation at the baccalaureate degree level was recommended as the minimum preparation for nurses assuming leadership roles (U.S. Public Health Service, 1963).

The Surgeon General's Consultant Group on Nursing also recommended that federally funded low-cost loans and scholarships be made available to students in both professional and practical nursing programs. It advocated the use of federal funds to construct additional nursing school facilities and to expand educational programs. The Nurse Training Act of 1964 was an outgrowth of these recommendations.

The American Nurses Association Position Paper

In the early 1960s, the educational preparation of nurses became a major concern of the ANA. The ANA believed that the improvement of nursing practice and the profession as a whole depended on the advancement of nursing education. After studying the issue for 3 years, *A Position Paper on Educational Preparation for Nurse Practitioners and Assistants to Nurses* was published in December 1965. In 2000, the ANA reaffirmed this position (ANA, 2000). The positions of the paper are listed in Display 2.2. It resulted in the **entry into practice** controversy.

No other single action or position has affected nursing more or has there been any issue that has been more divisive or contentious than the ANA position paper. For 45 years, the profession has been plagued with the issues it brought forth. A basic concern related to the fact that the roles, functions, and responsibilities (competencies) of programs offering three different routes to preparation for registered nursing were not clearly differentiated for graduates. All graduates took the same examination and performed similar activities when hired as new graduates in acute care facilities.

Associate degree nursing programs in community colleges and hospital-based diploma programs took serious exception to the paper. To this group, not being considered professional was unacceptable, and they were unwilling to compromise title or licensure. Because of the dissension the position paper created among nursing groups, little immediate action followed although four states—Oregon, Montana, Maine, and North Dakota—were chosen as focus

DISPLAY 2.2 **Four Major Positions of the ANA Position Paper on Educational Preparation**

1. The education of all those who are licensed to practice nursing should take place in institutions of higher education.
2. Minimum preparation for beginning professional nursing practice at the present time should be baccalaureate degree education in nursing.
3. Minimum preparation for beginning technical nursing practice at the present time should be associate degree education in nursing.
4. Education for assistants in the health service occupations should be short, intensive preservice programs in vocational education institutions, rather than on-the-job training programs.

American Nurses Association. (1965) American Nurses Association's first position on education for nursing. *American Journal of Nursing*, 65(12), 106–107.

states for early adoption. However, groups slowly began to take action regarding the paper, with many nursing organizations supporting the position, and others adamantly opposed to it. The controversy continues today, which would support the belief that the historical lack of internal cohesion within the nursing community has been a major impediment to progress (Smith, 2009).

Problems Associated with Changing Educational Requirements for Licensure

Several problems are associated with making any changes in educational requirements for licensure. Four major problems are related to titling, scope of practice, grandfathering, and interstate endorsement.

Titling. One of the most controversial problems associated with changing requirements for licensure involves **titling**, or the use of titles. The RN title has a long history and is clearly recognizable to the public and to the healthcare community. Currently, graduates of all nursing programs preparing graduates for registered nursing use this title if they pass the NCLEX-RN. If a differentiation were to be made among those with a baccalaureate degree, those with associate degrees, and those prepared in hospital-based programs, which graduates would use the title Registered Nurse? What alternate titles would be available for graduates from the other programs currently preparing individuals for licensure?

Scope of Practice. Of equal concern is the description and delineation of the **scope of practice** for the two levels of caregivers. The scope of practice (discussed in Chapter 3) is that section of the Nurse Practice Act that outlines the activities a person with a particular license may legally perform. This would mean the separate testing of each level as it currently exists between the RN and the practical nurse licensure examination. This problem might be of less concern if the nursing profession could agree on an approach to differentiated practice. In some suggestions for two levels of practice, the process of making nursing diagnoses and developing nursing care plans was at times included in the scope of practice of the baccalaureate-prepared nurse only, a position totally unacceptable to associate degree advocates. Again, the diploma graduate was left out of the discussion.

The Grandfather Clause. The application of a grandfather clause presents another challenge to nurses. Traditionally, when a state licensure law is enacted, or if a current law is repealed and a new law enacted, a grandfather clause has been a standard feature that allows persons to continue to practice their profession or occupation after new qualifications have been enacted into law. The legal basis for the process is found in the 14th Amendment to the U.S. Constitution, which declares that no state may deprive any person of life, liberty, or property without due process of law. The Supreme Court has ruled that the license to practice is a property right. A grandfather clause is not new to nursing; for example, it was applied when psychiatric nursing became a requirement of all programs. Nurses who were licensed without psychiatric nursing experiences were grandfathered into the new role. In other words, they continued to practice as RNs without taking a formal course in psychiatric nursing and without being required to write a psychiatric examination to maintain their licenses. If nursing began to require a baccalaureate degree for individuals using the RN title, under the provisions of a grandfather clause, all associate graduates licensed before the implementation date for the change would continue to use the title "registered nurse." Those licensed after the change would use whatever new title was established. Although this serves to protect the title of currently licensed nurses, it does not prevent employers from writing job descriptions stipulating a baccalaureate degree as the minimum educational preparation acceptable for a particular position.

Complicating this matter is the fact that some nurses believe a grandfather clause should be conditional. If it were conditional, nurses licensed before the changes in the licensure law would continue to use their current title for a stipulated period of time—for example, 10 years. At the end of that period, if they had not completed the education mandated in the changes (or any other conditions that might have been added), they would have to use the title stipulated in the new law for nurses with their educational preparation. Because of the complexity and the difficulties associated with implementation, it is unlikely that conditional grandfathering will ever become a reality.

Interstate Endorsement. A fourth concern is that of **interstate endorsement**. Nursing is one of the few professions to have developed a process whereby national examinations with standardized scores are administered in each state or jurisdiction, thus allowing a nurse who has passed the licensing examination in one state to move to another state and seek licensure without the need to retake and pass another examination. (However, with the exception of those states participating in the licensure compact [see Chapter 3], they do need to secure licensure in each state in which they practice.) Because nurses can be highly mobile, this has been a great advantage. As the profession examines multistate licensure, this issue takes on new dimensions.

The Position Paper and Nursing Today

Because the initial thinking and work on the **position paper** occurred 45 years ago, nursing leaders are raising questions about its relevancy today. The education of nurses has changed greatly with less than 10% of the new graduates coming from diploma programs and greater than 60% completing associate degree programs, many of which have articulation agreements with baccalaureate schools. If one views the position paper as a move to close hospital-based programs and place all nursing in colleges and universities, certainly that goal has been realized. However, two thirds of the graduates still possess less than a baccalaureate education, resulting in the majority of registered nurses being the least educated of all health professionals.

The AACN (an organization of baccalaureate and higher degree nursing programs) has taken a position on licensing of associate degree graduates. Its Web site (*www.aacn.nche.edu*) clearly states that it does not advocate changing licensure for associate degree nurses (ACCN, 2002). It recognizes the valuable role of associate degree nurses in healthcare and encourages articulation and continued education. It does support the baccalaureate degree as entry into "what the organization holds to be professional-level nursing practice." At the spring 2000 meeting, the ANA board of directors reaffirmed the long-standing position that baccalaureate education should be the standard for entry into professional nursing practice (ANA, 2000).

Some nursing groups target a specific year for requiring the baccalaureate in nursing as the educational preparation for entry into practice as an RN (both New York and New Jersey have legislation pending regarding entry into practice). It becomes clear that this contentious issue is not one of the past but, rather, is one with which the nurses of tomorrow will continue to grapple.

More recently AACN has focused attention on two different propositions that will transform graduate education: CNL and the DNP. This serves to shift attention to advanced practice and raise the education bar (Donley & Flaherty, 2008).

Critical Thinking Activity

Take a stand on the ANA position on nursing education. Provide a rationale for the position you have taken. What do you see as outcomes of the position paper? How would your position be implemented in the future? What implications might it have for nursing practice? Do you believe the salaries of nurses educated at different levels and practicing at differentiated levels should differ? Why or why not? If so, how?

DIFFERENTIATED PRACTICE

In the 1990s, some nursing leaders began to reassess the entry-into-practice issue. Although the nursing shortage of the late 1980s and the push toward cost cutting in the 1990s may have encouraged its reevaluation, the review also may reflect a new thinking regarding the role of nurses and nursing and the role of all education in the United States. Many nursing leaders encouraged recognition of the need for different types of practitioners, prepared with different types of education, or differentiated practice. **Differentiated nursing practice** can be defined as "the practice of structuring nursing roles on the basis of education, experience, and competence" (Boston, 1990, p. 2).

Many groups support the concept of differentiated practice. The report of the Pew Health Professions Commission (1995) advised that nursing distinguish between the different levels of nursing. The Commission recommended associate degree preparation for the entry-level hospital setting and nursing home practice, baccalaureate degree preparation for hospital based care management and community-based practice, and master's degree preparation for specialty practice in the hospital and independent practice as a primary provider. The National Commission Nursing Implementation Project also strongly supported differentiated practice.

The AACN and the American Organization of Nurse Executives established a Task Force on Differentiated Competencies for Nursing Practice; the group was later expanded to include representatives from The National Organization for Associate Degree Nursing. A joint publication of these three organizations, titled *A Model for Differentiated Nursing Practice*, is available at *www.aacn.nche.edu* (click on "Publications"). It recognizes that nurses with differing educational preparation bring different capabilities to the patient care system. With all this said, most of the serious work toward differentiated practice occurred from about the mid-1990 until about 2005.

Competency Expectations and Differentiated Practice

The task of describing and differentiating the **competencies** and the scope of practice of nurses graduating from various types of programs is one of the major challenges facing nursing today. The NCLEX RN taken by graduates of all programs preparing for registered nurse licensure is designed to ensure minimum safe practice, thus failing to recognize the broad range of functions in nursing, and the potential for improving the quality of care given, if different roles and responsibilities were identified. In the work environment of acute and long-term care facilities, little differentiation exists in beginning staff nurse positions.

If developed and implemented, realistic statements about competencies of each level or category of nursing education will facilitate the effective and efficient use of each category of graduate within the healthcare delivery system. Validated competencies also will provide a basis for the development of curriculum patterns to ensure adequate preparation of each category of caregiver, without running the risk of overeducating or undereducating at any one level. The competencies also can serve as a foundation for educational mobility patterns in the profession, job descriptions in the healthcare system, and responsive reimbursement packages.

The Work of Organizations in Defining Competencies

Some work has been done toward describing the competencies of graduates of different programs in nursing. The Council of Associate Degree Programs (CADP) of the NLN developed a document, *Educational Outcomes of Associate Degree Nursing Programs: Roles and Competencies in 1978*. In 1990, the CADP revised this document and identified three roles that are still in use by many associate degree nursing programs: provider of care, manager of care, and member within the discipline of nursing (NLN, 1990).

The *Characteristics of Baccalaureate Education in Nursing*, revised by the Council of Baccalaureate and Higher Degrees of NLN in 1994, was an initial approach to describing a standard for baccalaureate education. In 2008, the AACN revised earlier publications and published *Essentials of Baccalaureate Education for Professional Nursing Practice*. This document includes the role of the baccalaureate-prepared nurse, professional values for baccalaureate nursing education, an outline of essential curriculum content, baccalaureate core competencies and knowledge, as well as suggested teaching strategies (AACN, 2008).

Similarly, the Council of Diploma Programs and the Council of Practical Programs of NLN developed competencies for graduates. Since 1999, all the educational councils of NLN have been merged into one group, and there has been no further activity in the area of role definition.

In 1986, and every 3 years following that, the NCSBN has conducted several studies aimed at role delineation and job analysis of entry-level RNs for the purpose of validating the NCLEX-RN (this process is discussed in Chapter 3). In 1999, it published the *Role Delineation Study*, which describes the similarities and differences in the roles of nurse aides, LPNs, RNs, and APNs.

Some of the most recent work related to defining competencies has come from the Pew Health Professions Commission's final report. The fourth report, which continued the theme of reforming health professions, addressed skills needed to function in healthcare in the 21st century. Twenty-one competencies were identified as critical to practice (Display 2.3)

Special Projects to Differentiate Practice

Several projects have been conducted throughout the United States in an effort to achieve a regional consensus among nursing service persons and educators on differentiated statements of scope of practice for each level of graduate. Some of these include the Midwest Alliance in Nursing Projects, the first project funded by the W. K. Kellogg Foundation and the second project by a grant from the Division of Nursing of the Department of Health and

DISPLAY 2.3 Competencies Defined by the Pew Health Professions Commission

1. Embrace a personal ethic of social responsibility and service.
2. Exhibit ethical behavior in all professional activities.
3. Provide evidence-based clinically competent care.
4. Incorporate the multiple determinants of health in clinical care.
5. Apply knowledge of the new sciences.
6. Demonstrate critical thinking, reflection, and problem-solving skills.
7. Understand the role of primary care.
8. Rigorously practice preventive healthcare.
9. Integrate population-based care and services into practice.
10. Improve access to healthcare for those with unmet health needs.
11. Contribute to continuous improvement of the healthcare system.
12. Advocate for public policy that promotes and protects the health of the public.
13. Continue to learn and help others learn.
14. Practice relationship-centered care with individuals and families.
15. Provide culturally sensitive care to a diverse society.
16. Partner with communities in healthcare decisions.
17. Use communication and information technology effectively and appropriately.
18. Work in interdisciplinary teams.
19. Ensure care that balances individual, professional, system, and societal needs.
20. Practice leadership.
21. Take responsibility for quality of care and health outcomes at all levels.

Bellack & O'Neil (2000). Recreating nursing practice for a new century. *Nursing and Health Care Perspectives, 21(1)*, 14–21.

Human Services (Primm, 1987); the Healing Web Project, composed of representatives of nursing education and practice from six Midwestern and western states; and the Sioux Falls Experience, a detailed project implemented to differentiate educational design.

Other states have developed sets of recommendations to enable differentiated practice. For example, in 1988, the Colorado Experiment recommended a statewide plan to facilitate articulation of nursing education programs and called for a differentiated model of nursing practice that would facilitate appropriate use of nurses with varying educational credentials and degrees of experience. This would be accompanied by a differentiated pay scale, to allow appropriate compensation of nursing personnel as career advancement or growth occurred. Movement from one role to another required completion of the appropriate additional degrees, although growth within each role was possible without acquiring formal education. Wide-scale implementation of this model has not yet occurred.

In 1995, the AACN, working with the AONE and the National Organization for Associate Degree Nursing, published *A Model for Differentiated Nursing Practice*. This document outlined a model for differentiated learning and practice, identifying separate and distinct roles that could be delineated for associate degree nursing, BSN, and master's of science in nursing levels, with each needed and valued for comprehensive healthcare delivery (AACN, 1995). Another approach focused on the development of competency models. These models were frequently the outgrowth of the work of one of the 20 colleagues in caring projects throughout the United States that were funded by the Robert Wood Johnson Foundation. Frequently incorporated into the models were ANA's standards of care or the levels of practice identified by Benner (1984) of novice, advanced beginner, competent, proficient, and expert. One such model, originating in New Jersey, was developed for two levels of practice and licensure. Other states, including California, Mississippi, New Mexico, Alaska, South Dakota, Arizona, and South Carolina, initiated pilot projects for differentiated practice (Ellis & Hartley, 2009). The Oregon Consortium for Nursing Education has created a curriculum for both the associate degree and the baccalaureate degree that is based on a differentiated practice model.

All the above points to the fact that, despite interest and desire, the implementation of differentiated practice is slow in coming. If it is to be realized, it will continue to take high levels of commitment and perseverance.

Critical Thinking Activity

Given the situation we have today, with three routes to preparation for registered nursing, how would you suggest that the skills of the graduate of each program be differentiated? How should that influence nursing practice? How would you implement differentiated practice on a unit on which you were working? Do you believe that there should be a difference in salary? What is the rationale for your answer?

FORCES FOR CHANGE IN NURSING EDUCATION

As the nursing profession advances and education remains responsive to the changes that occur, it is imperative that nursing education undergoes modifications. A discussion of some of the most significant challenges follows.

Incorporating Computer Technology in Nursing Education

It is safe to say that in the past 10 years nursing education has experienced no transformation more dramatic than the incorporation of computer technology into all aspects of teaching, learning, and healthcare. These changes encompass activities covering everything from entire degrees that can be earned via on-line courses to separate courses that are taught on-line to the incorporation of computer technology in the classroom and learning laboratory. In the healthcare setting, computers are used for patient records, business functions, and increasingly as a support to effective decision making.

Computer Technology in the Classroom

The computer plays a major role in nursing education and is as essential to the operation of colleges and universities as it is to the operation of hospitals. Additionally, it is an important instructional tool. The computer offers a variety of approaches to instruction that are appealing and helpful to a diverse student population. Classroom teaching is augmented by computer-assisted instruction in the form of interactive and linear video programs, patient simulations, drill and practice routines, problem-solving programs, and tutorials, to name a few examples. Faculty also use computers for word processing, literature review, and the development and scoring of tests. Some faculty use computers in the classroom to enhance their lectures and discussions through PowerPoint presentations, response "clickers," and other computer technology. E-mail and the Internet are also a part of most teaching environments. Some instructional programs are delivered to sites far from the main campus through distance learning modalities using computer technology. At the end of their program of study, all students demonstrate their ability to practice safely on computerized licensing examinations in the form of computerized adaptive testing. In the nursing skills laboratory, mannequins that can blink their eyes, have dilating pupils, breathe, and have a heartbeat and a pulse assist students in the process of learning about heart attacks, diabetic shock, and other emergencies.

Computer literacy among students and faculty is no longer an issue—they possess computer skills. Nursing educators express concern about the initial cost of the equipment and programs needed for this instruction, as well as the increasing cost of keeping both equipment and programs current. For example, the mannequin mentioned above carries a price tag of $215,000. At a time when the budgets of educational institutions are experiencing severe cuts, people responsible for purchasing supplies and equipment increasingly must find creative ways to acquire needed items. Another challenge to faculty is finding time to evaluate the existing software and integrate it into the approved curriculum.

Computers in the Hospital Environment

Today's healthcare settings could not operate without computers and computerized equipment. Computers are used for business operations, medical records, and collection of clinical data, such as vital signs and hemodynamic values. Computers may be voice activated for charting at the bedside, for use with nursing care plans, for communication from the physicians' office to nursing stations, for regulating the administration of medications, and for many other facets of operation and patient care. Most of the equipment used in today's modern hospital is computerized. New graduates move into a highly technical world when they seek their first nursing positions. The education they receive to prepare them for these positions also must include the skills necessary to work in this highly computerized environment.

Distance Learning Options

Many students who are geographically bound and unable to relocate to a community offering a baccalaureate or master's education in nursing have found distance learning convenient and flexible. It also appeals to the nurse who cannot quit work to attend school. Essentially, distance learning refers to a teaching/learning situation in which the student and the teacher are not present in a classroom together and was discussed earlier in this chapter.

Establishing Programs That Provide for Educational Mobility

The concept of **educational mobility** in nursing has been discussed earlier in this chapter in the section dealing with articulation. In current times, it certainly must be included as one of the forces for change in nursing education. The National Advisory Council on Nurse Education and Practice urged that at least two thirds of the nurse workforce hold baccalaureate or higher degrees in nursing by 2010. Only 50% of nurses are prepared with this education today (AACN, 2010c).

Increasing Community-Based Practice Experiences

Another significant change in nursing practice is the trend toward community-based practice. Most nursing programs, especially hospital-based and associate degree programs, have a history of being strongly oriented toward the hospital as the primary clinical teaching environment. "Community," as the term was used in nursing education, was associated with public health nursing and was to be found in baccalaureate education only.

Earlier hospital discharge to the home and an increasing emphasis on prevention have created new demands on nursing. Nurses are expected to provide care in clients' homes, the workplace, schools, nursing homes, community health agencies, clinics, shelters, and community gathering places. As the arena in which nursing is practiced begins to shift, nursing educators are challenged to define what part of the nursing curriculum should be taught in a community setting. Often this requires different clinical teaching strategies and approaches. Some faculty, reticent to shorten any time in acute care facilities, are uncertain how a community experience should be provided and evaluated and about the legal ramifications associated with having students in many different environments and in less-controlled situations. Tremendous strides have been taken in developing innovative approaches to community-based nursing; more will follow.

Increasing Emphasis on Research

As the nursing profession continues to grow, one of the areas receiving more emphasis is nursing research. It is difficult to open any nursing journal today without learning more about evidence-based practice and nursing decisions (see below).

Other research, that of nursing theorists, received much attention in the 1980s until the beginning of the 21st century when attention was diverted to evidence-based practice. Many curricular patterns responded to the work of nursing theorists. Most approval bodies, state and national, stipulate that a nursing program must have a coherent organizing or conceptual framework around which the program of learning is developed. Some programs have chosen to select the approach of a particular nursing **theorist** and structure the program of learning around that theorist's work. The program in which you are enrolled may reflect this trend. Perhaps one of the hospitals to which you are assigned for clinical experience also uses the principles of a nursing theory to structure the delivery of care, although this is less common than using a theory in curriculum development.

A **theory** is a "scientifically acceptable general principle which governs practice or is proposed to explain observed facts" (Riehl & Roy, 1974, p. 3). Because nursing as a developing profession is seriously involved in research, theories are valuable to use in building a sound body of nursing knowledge. They provide the bases for hypotheses about nursing practice. They make it possible for us to derive a sound rationale for the actions we take. If the theories are testable, they allow us to build our knowledge base and to guide and improve nursing practice.

Today, there are many published nursing theories. In an attempt to structure and organize those theories, various authors have categorized or classified them. Not all are classified similarly. Included are general classifications such as the art and science of humanistic nursing, interpersonal relationships, systems, and energy fields. Other categories include growth and development theories, systems theories, stress adaptation theories, and rhythm theories.

Examples of growth and development theories with which you are probably familiar are those of Maslow, Erikson, Kohlberg, Piaget, and Freud discussed in most basic nursing texts. The theories are so named because they focus on the developing person and arrange this development in stages through which a person must pass to reach a particular level of development. They allow nurses to monitor progress through the stages and evaluate the appropriateness of that progress. These theories are not truly theories of nursing, however, because they were not developed for the purpose of explaining, testing, and changing the practice of nursing. They represent some of the borrowed knowledge around which we build our profession.

Most nursing theories are developed around a combination of concepts. Among these concepts, four approaches usually include those directed to the human person, health and illness, the environment (or society), and nursing.

Nursing theories usually are classified according to the structure or approach around which they are developed. Theories that speak to the art and science of humanistic nursing were among the earliest pure nursing theories developed. Some authors have looked back at the contributions of Florence Nightingale and have included her work in that grouping. Among others are Virginia Henderson and her *Definition of Nursing*, Faye Abdellah and the *Twenty-one Nursing Problems* (which is often cited as one of the early attempts at classification of nursing behaviors), Lydia Hall and her *Core, Care, and Cure* model, and Madeleine Leininger's *Transcultural Care Theory*.

Interpersonal process theories deal with interactions between and among people. Many of these theories were developed during the 1960s. Included in this grouping could be Hildegard Peplau's *Psychodynamic Nursing*, Joyce Travelbee's *Human to Human Relationship*, Ernestine Wiedenbach's *The Helping Art of Clinical Nursing*, and Imogene King's *Dynamic Interacting Systems* model, although the last also could be classified as a systems theory.

Systems theories are so named because they are concerned with the interactions between and among all the factors in a situation. A system usually is viewed as complex and in a state of constant change. It is defined as a whole with interrelated parts and may be a subsystem of a larger system as well as a suprasystem. For example, a person may be viewed as a system composed of cells, tissue, and organs. The person is a subsystem of a family, which in turn is a subsystem of a community. In a systems approach, the person usually is considered as a "total" being, or from a "whole" being viewpoint. Systems theories also provide for input into the system and feedback within the system. The systems approach became popular during the 1970s. Included in this group of theorists are Dorothy Johnson, Sister Calista Roy, and Betty Neuman.

Stress adaptation models are based on concepts that view the person as adjusting or changing (adapting) to avoid situations (stressors) that would result in the disturbance of balance or equilibrium. The adaptation theory helps to explain how balance is maintained and therefore directs nursing actions. One often finds Sister Calista Roy's adaptation model and Betty Neuman's work included in this group, but both also may be considered systems models, as mentioned above.

One of the most recent classifications of theories is by energy fields. These theories, although developed earlier, received growing recognition during the 1980s. Included in this group are the works of Myra Levine, Joyce Fitzpatrick, Margaret Newman, and Martha Rogers.

Humanistic models are also fairly recent. These focus on man's humanness and needs for love, caring, personal meaning, and living in concert with the environment. Theorists noted

Table 2.2   **Nursing Theories and Theorists**

THEORIST	THEORY OR MODEL
Lydia Hall	Viewed illness and rehabilitation as learning experiences in which the nurse's role was to guide and teach the patient through personal caregiving. Role involves therapeutic use of self (core), the treatment regimen of the healthcare team (cure), and nurturing and intimate bodily care (care).
Dorothy Johnson	A behavioral systems approach that focuses on health viewed as a state of equilibrium that the nurse assists in maintaining or balancing.
Imogene King	A model in which three open systems interact with the environment: personal, individual, and social. Nurse's role is to assist individual to perform daily activities and includes health promotion and maintenance. Involves goal attainment.
Madeleine Leininger	Focused on a caring model that must be practiced interpersonally. Emphasized a transcultural approach.
Myra Levine	Developed around the four concepts of conservation of energy, structural integrity, personal integrity, and social integrity. Supports a holistic approach to nursing based on recognition of the total response of the person to the interaction between the internal and the external environment.
Betty Neuman	A systems model influenced by Gestalt theory, stress, and level of prevention. Employs lines of resistance and lines of defense in creating a healthy being. Nurses are to identify the stressors and assist the individual to respond. Involves primary, secondary, and tertiary prevention.
Dorothea Orem	Recognized as a self-care theory of nursing, supports the concept that each person has a need for the provision and management of self-care actions to achieve "constancy." When the individual is unable to provide these, a self-care deficit exists. The role of the nursing system is to help eliminate the self-care deficit through wholly compensatory, partially compensatory, or supportive–educative actions.
Martha Rogers	Includes complicated approaches to health that involve helicy, resonancy, and complementarity. The holistic individual moves through time and space as part of an expanding universe with potential states of maximum well-being. Nurses act to promote symphonic interaction between man and environment by repatterning the human and environmental fields.
Sister Calista Roy	Identified as an adaptation model that conceives of the individual as being in constant interaction with a changing environment, thus requiring adaptation. Four adaptive modes, or ways in which a person adapts, are identified through (1) physiologic needs, (2) self-concept, (3) role function, and (4) interdependence relations. The nurse's role is to assess a patient's adaptive behaviors and the stimuli that may be affecting the person to manipulate the stimuli in such a way as to allow the patient to cope or adapt.

for developing these theories include Jean Watson, Rosemarie Rizzo Parse, and Margaret Newman.

It is not our purpose to discuss and critique the many approaches to nursing theory. The student who wants to pursue nursing theorists further is encouraged to consult the section on further reading at the end of the chapter or visit enursescribe.com and click on research and theory. Table 2.2 outlines the approaches of several recognized nursing theorists.

Critical Thinking Activity

Select one nursing theorist. Describe what you find interesting and attractive about that person's nursing theory. Give a rationale for your decision, and describe how using that theory might affect your practice of nursing.

Education Supporting Evidence-Based Practice

The term **evidence-based practice** has a variety of definitions and interpretations. Evolving from evidence-based medicine, it generally refers to the integration of the best evidence available into expert nursing care. It requires that nurses and other healthcare providers have access to the latest research, expert opinion, and understandings of cultural and personal values as a basis for planning and delivering nursing care. Evidence-based practice is discussed in detail in Chapter 16.

KEY CONCEPTS

- Educational programs prepare nursing assistants and LPNs for roles in the healthcare delivery system. As these programs have grown, greater oversight of the programs by approval bodies has occurred. The education of UAP can vary tremendously.

- Three major avenues to preparation for licensure as a registered nurse exist in the United States: the hospital-based diploma, the college-based baccalaureate degree, and the associate degree (usually offered in community colleges). Many similarities exist among these programs. In addition, various nontraditional approaches to nursing education have evolved.

- The nursing shortage of the late 1980s and 1990s, coupled with recommendations or mandates from important groups, has resulted in greater creativity and collaboration in educational approaches. Articulated programs exist in most states created through the pressure of legislation or agreement between schools.

- Master's and doctoral programs that prepare nurses for leadership positions in the profession continue to grow, with more emphasis on the master's degree for advanced practice. The actual degree awarded at the end of doctoral studies varies. A variety of new educational approaches to higher degrees in nursing have evolved.

- One of the most rapidly growing areas is that of advanced practice; this growth was accelerated by healthcare reform. Recommendations from major commissions have urged continued expansion of advanced practice programs and the educational qualifications for such positions.

- Continuing education, whether further education that results in a higher degree or rather in the form of classes, seminars, or workshops that update and increase expertise, is being encouraged by more and more organizations. Staying current in practice is critical to safe client care.

- Nursing education has been influenced by the ANA position on nursing education that advocated the baccalaureate degree as the minimum educational preparation for professional practice. Many nursing educators, particularly those in diploma and associate degree programs, disagreed with this position. This issue may take on new life in the 21st century.

- Models for differentiated practice that recognize and use graduates according to the competencies inherent in the program from which they graduated have been encouraged.

- Many changes are occurring in nursing education. These include more emphasis on articulation and career ladder programs and a shift in educational settings from acute care facilities to community-based experiences.

- No change has affected nursing education as greatly as has the computer age. Entire programs can be completed on-line. Computer technology has changed the structure of the typical nursing classroom, and instructors prepare graduates who will be able to function in a healthcare environment that makes heavy use of computerized services.

- Nursing theories continue to influence nursing and nursing education. Nursing theories assist us in building a body of nursing knowledge and describing and defining nursing practice.

- The advent of evidence-based practice is impacting the curricula of nursing education programs.

RELEVANT WEB SITES

Web sites relevant to this chapter can be found at thePoint✳ accessed through *http://the Point. lww.com/Ellis10e* and by entering the code found on the inside cover of your text.

REFERENCES

American Association of Colleges of Nursing. (1995). *A model for differentiated nursing practice.* Washington, DC: Author.

American Association of Colleges of Nursing. (2002). *Associate degree in nursing programs and AACN's support for articulation.* Retrieved June 27, 2010, from www.aacn.nche.edu/Media/Fact SheetsADNFacts.htm

American Association of Colleges of Nursing. (2006a). *DNP Roadmap Task Force Report.* Retrieved October 5, 2009, from www.aacn.nche.edu/DNP/pdf/DNProadmapreport.pdf

American Association of Colleges of Nursing. (2006b). *Articulation agreements among nursing education programs.* Retrieved June 27, 2010, from www.aacn.nche.edu/Media/FactSheets/AA.htm

American Association of Colleges of Nursing (2007). *White Paper on the Role of the Clinical Nurse Leader.* Retrieved March 31, 2011, from www.aacn.nche.edu/Publications/WhitePapers/ClinicalNurseLeaer.htm

American Association of Colleges of Nursing. (2008). *The essentials of baccalaureate nursing education for professional nursing practice.* Washington, DC: Author.

American Association of Colleges of Nursing. (2010a) *Fact Sheet: Nursing Fact Sheet.* Retrieved June 27, 2010, from http://www.aacn.edu/Media/FactSheets/nursfact.htm

American Association of Colleges of Nursing. (2010b). *Fact sheet: Accelerated baccalaureate and master's degrees in nursing.* Retrieved June 27, 2010, from www.aacn.nche.edu/Media/FactSheets/AcceleratedProg.htm

American Association of Colleges of Nursing. (2010c). *Fact sheet: The impact of education on nursing practice.* Retrieved June 27, 2010, from http://www.aacn.nche.edu/Media/FactSheets/ImpactEdNP.htm

American Nurses Association. (1965). American Nurses Association's first position on education for nursing. *American Journal of Nursing, 65(12),* 106–107.

American Nurses Association. (1974). *Standards for continuing education for nursing.* Kansas City, MO: American Nurses Association.

American Nurses Association. (2000). *ANA reaffirms commitment to BSN for entry into practice-supports new certification program to be offered by ANCC.* Retrieved December 7, 2010, from http://www.nursingworld.org/FunctionalMenuCategories/MediaResources/PressReleases/2000/CommitmenttoBSN.aspx

Associate Degree in Nursing Schools and Programs—Your Path to Becoming a Nurse (2008–2009). Retrieved October 3, 2009, from http://www.associatedegreenursing.com

Bellack, J. P., & O'Neil, E. H. (2000). Recreating nursing practice for a new century. *Nursing and Health Care Perspectives, 21(1),* 14–21.

Benner, P. (1984). *From novice to expert.* Menlo Park, CA: Addison-Wesley.

Boston, C. (1990). Differentiated practice: An introduction. In C. Boston, *Current issues and perspectives on differentiated practice* (pp. 1–3). Chicago, IL: American Organization of Nurse Executives.

Brown, E. L. (1948). *Nursing for the future.* New York, NY: Russell Sage Foundation.

de Tornyay, R. (1996). Critical challenges for nurse educators. *Journal of Nursing Education, 35(4),* 146–147.

Donley, R., & Flaherty, M. J. (2008, April 30). Revisiting the American Nurses Association's first position on education for nurses: A comparative analysis of the first and second position statements on the education of nurses. *OJIN: The Online Journal of Issues in Nursing, 13(2).* Retrieved June 28, 2010, from http://www.nursingworld.org/search.aspx?SearchMode=1&SearchPhrase=Entry into Practice&SearchWithin=2&PageIndex=1 - select from list of articles http://www.nursingworld.org/MainMenuCategories/ANAMarketplace?ANAPeriodicals/OJIN/TableofContents/vol132008/No2May08/ArticlePreviousTopic/EntryIntoPracticeUpdate.aspx

Ellis, J. R., & Hartley, C. L. (2009). *Managing and coordinating nursing care* (5th ed.). Philadelphia, PA: Lippincott Williams & Wilkins.

Get Your Nursing Diploma or Associate's Degree (2002–2009). Retrieved October 3, 2009 from http://www.allnursingschools.com/faqs/nursing-diploma-associates.php

Health Resources and Services Administration (2010, March 17). *HRSA study finds nursing workforce is growing and more diverse.* Retrieved December 7, 2010 from http://www.hrsa.gov/about/news/pressreleases/100317_hrsa_study_100317_finds_nursing_workforce_is_growing_and_more_diverse.html

Kalisch, P. A., & Kalisch, B. J. (2004). *American nursing: A history* (4th ed.). Philadelphia: Lippincott Williams & Wilkins.

National Council of State Boards of Nursing. (2009). *National Nurse Aide Assessment Program.* Retrieved September 30, 2009 from http://www.ncsbn.org. Click on NNAAP 7 MACE Examinations.

National League for Nursing (Council of Associate Degree Programs). (1990). Educational outcomes of associate degree nursing programs: Roles and competencies (Publication No. 23-2348). New York, NY: Author.

National League for Nursing. (2009, Spring). *NLN Annual Nursing Data Review Documents Application, Admission, Enrollment, and Graduation Rates for All Types of Prelicensure Nursing Programs. The NLN Report.* New York, NY: Author

Pew Health Professions Commission. (1995). *Critical challenges: Revitalizing the health professions for the twenty-first century.* San Francisco, CA: UCSF Center for the Health Professions.

Primm, P. L. (1987). Differentiated practice for ADN- and BSN-prepared nurses. *Journal of Professional Nursing, 3*(4), 218–225.

Riehl, J. P., & Roy S. C. (1974). *Conceptual models for nursing practice.* New York, NY: Appleton-Century-Crofts.

Seymer, L. R. (1954). *Selected writings of Florence Nightingale.* New York, NY: Macmillan.

Smith, T. G. (2009, October 5). A policy perspective on the entry into practice issue. *OJIN: The Online Journal of Issues in Nursing,* 15(1). Retrieved October 7, 2009 from http://www.nursingworld.org/MainMcnuCategories/ANAMarketplace/ANAPeriodicals/OJIN/TableofContents/Vol152010/No1Jan2010/Articles-Previous-Topic/Policy-an-Entry-iinto-Practice.aspx, http://www.nursingworld.org/search.aspx?SearchMode=1&SearchPhrase=Entry into Practice&SearchWithin=2&PageIndex=1. Select from list of articles.

U.S. Public Health Service. (1963). *Toward quality in nursing: Needs and goals. Report of the Surgeon Generals' Consultant Group on Nursing.* Washington, DC: U.S. Government Printing Office.

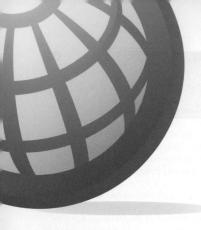

3

Credentials for Healthcare Providers

LEARNING OUTCOMES

After completing this chapter, you should be able to:

1. Define and discuss the concept of credentialing for health professionals.
2. Describe how each of the following types of credentials differs: diploma, certificate, certification, and license.
3. Outline the purposes of accreditation and the general process for seeking accreditation.
4. Identify and analyze the major elements addressed by nursing practice acts.
5. Outline the role of the state boards of nursing or other state regulatory authority.
6. Differentiate between licensure by examination, licensure by endorsement, and mutual recognition of licensure.
7. Discuss personal strategies to avoid violating the provisions of the nursing practice acts and encountering the disciplinary process.
8. Discuss issues in licensure, including ensuring continued competence, multistate licensure, and licensure for graduates of foreign nursing schools.
9. Explain the various uses of certification in nursing.
10. Discuss current trends in credentialing within the healthcare workforce.

KEY TERMS

Accreditation
Administrative law
Advanced practice registered nurse (APRN)
Certification
Computerized adaptive testing (CAT)
Credentials
Disciplinary action
Enacted (statutory) law
Grandfathering
Home state
Injunctive relief
Licensure by endorsement

Licensure by examination
Mandatory licensure
Mutual recognition of licensure
NCLEX-PN
NCLEX-RN
Nurse Practice Act
Party state
Remote state
Revocation
Rules and regulations
State board of nursing
Telenursing

Credentials provide information regarding qualifications and whether standards have been met. Credentials for organizations or institutions are awarded by bodies (either professional or governmental) that set standards for specific type of organizations (such as hospital or nursing homes). Approval or accreditation from one of these bodies demonstrates to the public that the healthcare organization adheres to accepted standards. Credentials for individuals communicate to others the nature of the person's competence and provide evidence of preparation to perform in a specific capacity. Credentials for individuals include certificates, degrees, and diplomas awarded by educational institutions; legal licenses awarded by a government body; and recognition by a professional organization usually termed certification. Members of health professions have supported the need for credentials of all kinds to protect the public; those who are engaged in careers in health occupations want to be assured that the standards of practice in their discipline and in healthcare organizations remain high. All these types of credentials are discussed below.

APPROVAL AND ACCREDITATION OF INSTITUTIONS AND PROGRAMS

Institutions are approved by government bodies to operate within their state borders. States have varying standards and processes for approval of educational institutions such as technical institutes, colleges, and universities. The approval of most educational institutions is carried out by a state board of education or similar educational authority. States also have approval processes for programs that provide education for licensed health professions. These are most commonly carried out by professional boards.

Accreditation of Educational Institutions

"**Accreditation** is a process of external quality review created and used by higher education to scrutinize colleges, universities, and programs for quality assurance and quality improvement" (Eaton, 2009). Educational institutions and programs may voluntarily seek this type of accreditation for both their general education and specialized programs.

Organizations that have the authority to offer this type of national or regional accreditation of educational institutions must be approved by the Council on Higher Education Accreditation of the US Department of Education. Some accreditations recognize the entire educational institution, such as the accreditation offered by regional bodies for colleges and universities. If an institution's programs meet standards developed and published by that regional body, it is awarded accreditation. In many instances, educational credentials such as degrees and certificates are accepted by the public, employers, or other educational institutions only if offered by an accredited educational institution. Although a nonaccredited institution might award a degree, there is no guarantee that the school meets educational standards; therefore, the degree might not be accepted as an adequate evidence of qualifications. Similarly, only course work completed at an accredited institution may be accepted for transfer to another accredited institution. You may have experienced the need for this type of accreditation if you transferred academic credits from one college to another. Accreditation is also necessary for the institution and its students to have access to federal funds (Eaton, 2009). Some academic accreditation is specialized, applying only to a particular program in an institution. Specialized accreditation is voluntary and requires that the specific program meets professional standards for excellence established by a specialized accrediting agency. Specialized accreditation for nursing is discussed below. An educational institution might have general accreditation for its degrees but still not have specialized accreditation. Certain educational organizations are not degree-granting institutions and therefore are not eligible for general accreditation, but they are still eligible for specialized accreditation. This is true of hospital-based diploma schools of nursing.

Government Approval of Nursing Programs

For its graduates to be eligible to take the National Council Licensure Examination (NCLEX) in any state, a nursing program should be approved by a state board of nursing or another designated state government department. In most states, this is called approval, but in a few states, it is called accreditation (a term most commonly associated with a voluntary process described above).

In most states, the approval/accrediting activities for nursing programs are carried out through the state board of nursing. After registration laws were passed, state boards of nursing began to emerge for the purpose of licensing nurses and protecting the public. Inspectors from the boards began making program visits for approval. Through the American Nurses Association (ANA), the Council of State Boards of Nursing was created to have a common forum for state boards of nursing. In 1978, the National Council of State Boards of Nursing, Inc., (NCSBN) was formed to replace the ANA Council. NCSBN provides the mechanism for state boards of nursing to collaborate in terms of licensing examinations and other issues of importance to the regulation of nursing practice.

When a new nursing program is to be initiated, it must provide preliminary information to the appropriate state government department while in the planning phase. The nursing program must be approved prior to admitting students to assure prospective students that they will be eligible to become licensed upon graduation. Each state also has a designated time frame to renew its approval of existing nursing programs. This often involves a comprehensive evaluation study, done by the program/school and submitted to the state. Representatives of the state approval authority then visit the program. In some jurisdictions, a school that has received specialized accreditation is exempted from a separate governmental review (see below).

Accreditation of Nursing Education Programs

The specialized accreditation of nursing education programs arose from concerns about the quality of nursing education among nurses. Accreditation helps to strengthen uniform national standards for nursing education. Some employers and educational institutions offering additional education require graduation from a nursing program that has specialized accreditation. In 1893, the American Society of Superintendents of Training Schools for Nurses was established to develop and maintain a universal standard for nursing education. It was renamed the National League for Nursing Education in 1912, and in 1917, it released the first Standard Curriculum for Schools of Nursing. Throughout the first half of the 20th century, the National League for Nursing Education continued to provide guidance for quality in nursing education. In 1952, seven organizations combined into one and became the National League for Nursing (NLN), which assumed responsibility for accrediting nursing education programs. In 1997, in response to the Department of Education's expectations for greater separation of the membership organization (NLN) and the accrediting process, the NLN formed the NLNAC as an independent subsidiary to provide accreditation of nursing programs. The NLNAC accredits nursing programs at all levels: practical nursing, hospital diploma nursing education, associate degree nursing education, and baccalaureate and higher-degree education programs.

In 1999, the Council on Collegiate Nursing Education, a subsidiary of the American Association of Colleges of Nursing, began offering accreditation for baccalaureate and higher-degree nursing programs only. Advanced practice nursing organizations such as the American Association of Nurse Anesthetists provide specialized accreditation for institutions offering advanced practice/nurse practitioner programs.

Voluntary accreditation has a process similar to that of mandatory approval. Accreditation is based on a systematic self-study and evaluation by the nursing program itself that focuses on the standards and criteria for accreditation. Peer evaluators from the accrediting organization visit the nursing program, review the self-study, and provide an independent evaluation. Their visit includes meetings with officials throughout the institution, faculty, and students, as well as a review of records and documents. The report and recommendations of the visiting evaluators, along with the self-study document, are submitted to a panel in the organization composed of peer educators. A nursing program may be granted accreditation, granted accreditation with conditions that must be remedied, placed on a warning status for being deficient, or denied accreditation. A program that is accredited has met the national standards of the organization for quality in nursing education. Accreditation exists for limited period of time and must then be renewed.

COMMUNICATION IN ACTION

Jerry Wilson was a student in an associate degree nursing program. His program was being evaluated for reaccreditation, and an evaluator visited his clinical site. As part of the process, the evaluator interviewed Jerry. The evaluator said, "Please tell me about your objectives for today's clinical experience." Jerry was nervous but pleased to be able to be prepared to respond. "I am working on my neurological assessment skills today," he said. "Although I have performed them in the lab, this is my first opportunity to use those skills with a patient and to interpret their meaning in a real-life situation. This assignment is also giving me an opportunity to increase my abilities to relate to the family as well as the patient, because a family member is always with the patient." The evaluator then asked, "Would you give me some feedback on the adequacy of this clinical site in providing opportunities for the learning that you need?" Jerry responded, "This unit has provided an exceptionally good learning environment. The nurses are very helpful and supportive. They go out of their way to help us find good learning experiences. I am always able to find patients that will help me meet the course objectives." Jerry's communication was clear, direct, and provided important information to the evaluators.

Accreditation of Continuing Education Programs

The American Nurses Credentialing Center, which is best known for providing certification for individual nursing specialties (discussed later in this chapter), also provides an accreditation mechanism for institutions or organizations that want to be approvers or providers of nursing continuing education programs. State nurses associations and specialty organizations often seek accreditation as *approvers of programs*. These organizations then approve specific continuing education offerings as meeting appropriate standards for content and process. Accreditation as a *provider of a program* assures the nurse consumer that the specific continuing education offering meets appropriate standards.

Many of the states that require continuing education for renewing a nursing license require that the offering be approved or accredited by some official group. This ensures that the continuing education is of high quality and will be meaningful for a nurse. Some states operate their own approval systems. When evaluating continuing nursing education offerings, it is important to know whether that class, workshop, or course has been approved and by whom.

CREDENTIALS FOR INDIVIDUALS

Individuals may hold multiple types of credentials. As people progress in their careers, they are likely to attain additional credentials.

Diplomas, Degrees, and Certificates of Completion

A school or business offering instruction awards a diploma or certificate to those who complete a designated program of study. A business that provides instruction in using computer programs might present certificates to those who complete the course. Licensed practical nursing (LPN) programs offer a certificate of completion. Hospital-based programs preparing registered nurses (RNs) offer a diploma. College-based nursing programs offer academic degrees, such as the associate, baccalaureate, or master's degree, which require the fulfillment of certain general education courses and course work specific to a particular career, such as nursing. The value of a diploma or educational certificate or degree is related to the quality of the educational institution or program, as well as to the actual title of the certificate or degree. So, when deciding which institution to attend, check on both the approval of the institution and the specific accreditation of the program.

Licensure

A license is a legal credential awarded by an individual state that grants permission to an individual to practice a given profession. Most states require licensing only of those who have more direct contact with clients. Physicians, dentists, pharmacists, and nurses are licensed in all states. The licensing of other healthcare workers varies. An individual state or province determines eligibility for licensure and the type of testing required for that profession within that state. Each state develops and enforces its own practice act, which includes the scope of practice for the profession the license represents. We will discuss the nursing practice act later in this chapter.

Certification

For some groups, a standard credential is available in the form of **certification** provided by a nongovernmental authority, usually a professional organization. Workers with this credential are referred to as "certified" or "registered." This type of credential should not be confused with a legal license or a simple certificate of completion (nursing is an anomaly in that the term "registered nurse" was adopted early in this century and refers to legal licensure). Certification usually is granted on completion of an education program and the passing of a standardized examination. The program usually has been approved by the professional organization and the organization that administers the examination. Certification does not include a legal scope of practice. Scope of practice will be discussed later in this chapter.

While some professional organizations conduct their own certification, in most instances they have established an independent national affiliated organization whose sole purpose is credentialing. By having an independent organization that focuses all of its efforts on certification, they better ensure objectivity and enhance the confidence of others in the process.

Some organizations provide certification for several related occupational groups. One such organization is the National Accrediting Association for Clinical Laboratory Sciences. Members of the various professional groups involved in laboratory science cooperated in setting up this association. This organization awards a credential to those who have met the educational standards and passed the certification examination for each of seven laboratory science occupations. All groups in the field of laboratory science recognize these as professional credentials. Some states have made certification by this body the required criterion for practice in clinical laboratory sciences.

One of the concerns regarding certification is the potential for confusion that exists because regulatory agencies (such as state boards of nursing) and professional associations may use the term "certification" differently and in different contexts. In nursing, certification is used for identifying licensed RNs who have specialized or advanced competence in a specific area of nursing. Certification in nursing will be discussed after the information on basic licensure.

Critical Thinking Activity

Choose an allied health occupation found in a healthcare facility in which you have clinical practice. Investigate the credentials needed for that occupation and how they would be obtained in your state. Analyze a way in which you could work collaboratively with an individual in this health occupation.

NURSING LICENSURE IN THE UNITED STATES

Nursing leaders historically have maintained an ethical position that accountability to the public for quality nursing care is essential. The public, however, often has no method for evaluating the competence of an individual nurse. Therefore, the nursing profession has tried to ensure that nurses have credentials that can be recognized by everyone. Legal licensure provides a standard mechanism for judging competence and therefore protects the safety of the public (Fig. 3.1). Through the efforts of nurses working collectively, a licensure process was developed and state agencies were established to regulate the practice of nursing.

The History of Licensure in Nursing

Recognizable credentials were not always available for nurses. Before the Nightingale schools became prevalent in England and nursing schools were established in the United States, little training was available to those who wanted to provide nursing care. Nurses with some training and those without typically worked side by side. After schools of nursing became common, a rudimentary means of identifying the qualifications of a caregiver was the certificate of completion issued by the nursing school. This was the first true nursing credential. However, because the quality of education offered in the nursing schools varied greatly—programs varied in length from 6 weeks to 3 years— it became apparent that a completion certificate was not an adequate guarantee of competence.

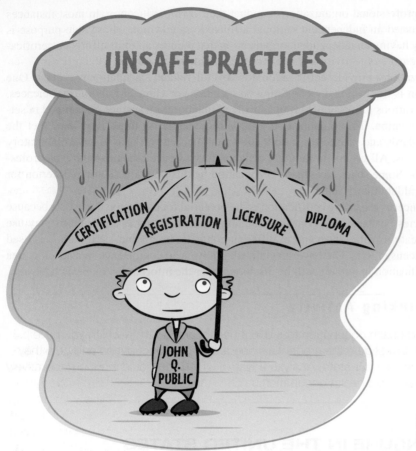

FIGURE 3.1 Various forms of credentialing ensure the public of qualified caregivers.

England first debated the issue of self-regulation versus legal regulation. Florence Nightingale did not support individual licensure for nurses because she believed the focus should be on the societal/moral standards of the professional nurse. She believed that only continuing education and practice could ensure competence and that a license approved at one time could not. While England debated whether to initiate some form of registration, it was instituted in South Africa in 1892, followed by Natal (1899) and New Zealand (1901). Great Britain initiated registration in 1902 (Kalisch & Kalisch, 2004, p 178). Similarly, Canada began to regulate nurses in the early 1900s.

Meanwhile in the United States, the Nurses' Associated Alumnae of the United States and Canada was created in 1896. This organization later evolved into the ANA. One of the major concerns of the association was the establishment of legal licensure for nurses. The ANA campaigned vigorously for the adoption of state licensing laws. Nurses, legislators, and the public had to be educated about the value of licensure for the profession and encouraged to support it. The set of laws regulating the practice of nursing is termed the **Nurse Practice Act**.

The early laws provided for permissive licensure. **Permissive licensure** is a voluntary system whereby an individual could choose to become licensed to provide evidence of competence, but a license was not required to practice. The requirements for permissive licensure included graduating from a school that satisfied certain standards established in the practice act for that state and passing a comprehensive examination. Only those who had met these standards could use the title RN; others used the title "nurse." Under this system, no one was required to have a license to practice nursing, and variability in standards from one state to another continued.

North Carolina passed the first permissive licensure law in 1903, followed by New York, New Jersey, and Virginia. However, the early laws did not define the scope of practice; New York first did this in 1938 (NCSBN, 2004). By 1923, all the existing 48 states had permissive licensure laws. Alaska and Hawaii passed licensure laws while they were still territories, and continued to recognize these laws when they became states.

After permissive licensure laws came into being, nurses' activity regarding licensure became less intense because most individuals graduating from nursing schools sought and received licenses to practice. However, there was still concern that some individuals were practicing nursing without having demonstrated skill and knowledge. The majority of those functioning without licenses were nursing school graduates who had failed the licensing examinations; they were referred to as "graduate nurses," rather than RNs. Other nurses who practiced without licenses included individuals who had been educated as nurses in other countries.

To end this situation and provide greater protection to the public, many nurses began to call for **mandatory licensure**. Mandatory nursing licensure requires that all persons who wish to practice nursing meet the established standards for education, pass standardized examinations, and secure a license to practice in the state, province, or territory in which they wish to work.

The first mandatory licensure law took effect in New York in 1947. Today, mandatory licensure is the standard in the United States, Canada, and most other countries. Therefore, if you wish to work as a nurse in any state, territory, province, or other country, you must obtain a license that is valid in that jurisdiction before you begin working (see Display 3.1 for the chronology of nursing licensure).

Although the terms "RN" and "LPN" (or licensed vocational nurse [LVN], as used in Texas and California) were protected in law, the more general term "nurse" has not been protected traditionally. Many individuals describe themselves as nurses, when their roles in healthcare are assistive. Their employers also may refer to them as nurses to support those individuals' status. Some states (eg, Washington) have made "nurse" a protected term. In these states, only RNs or LPNs may use the title nurse. Others, such as certified nurses' aides/assistants and medical assistants, may use only their specific title.

Current Nursing Licensure Laws

The authority for establishing a licensure law lies with the legislature of each jurisdiction. A proposed change in the law enters the legislative process through an elected member of the legislature who has been persuaded that the change is in the best interest of the public. That individual introduces a bill (see Chapter 7 for an overview of how a bill becomes a law). A group, such as the nurses association, wishing to instigate this action may spend months preparing and planning the content for a bill and gaining the support of legislators who might introduce the legislation.

DISPLAY 3.1   The History of Nursing Licensure

1867	Dr. Henry Wentworth Acland first suggested licensure for nurses in England.
1892	American Society of Superintendents of Training Schools for Nurses organized and supported licensure in the United States.
1901	First nursing licensure in the world: New Zealand
1903	First nursing licensure in the United States: North Carolina, New Jersey, New York, and Virginia (in that order)
1915	ANA drafted its first model nurse practice act.
1919	First nursing licensure in England
1923	All 48 states had enacted nursing licensure laws.
1935	First mandatory licensure act in the United States: New York (effective 1947)
1946	Ten states had definitions of nursing in the licensing act.
1950	First year the same examination used in all jurisdictions of the United States and its territories: State Board Test Pool Examination
1965	Twenty-one states had definitions of nursing in the licensing act.
1971	First state to recognize expanded practice in the nursing practice act: Idaho
1976	First mandatory continuing education for relicensure: California
1982	Change to nursing process format examination: National Council Licensure Examination for Registered Nurses (NCLEX-RN)
1986	Only state to require baccalaureate degree for initial RN licensure and associate degree for licensed practical nurse licensure: North Dakota (effective 1987 and rescinded in 2003)
1994	Computer-adapted testing initiated nationwide
1998	Mutual Recognition Nurse Licensure Compact finalized. Utah is the first state to become part of the Compact.
2008	Consensus reached on a model for Advanced Practice RN education and practice

During the legislative process, individuals and organizations may affect the content of the proposed legislation by influencing the legislators to amend the bill. Amendments to a bill may change the content dramatically and cause the original supporters of the bill to reconsider their support. Once the appropriate legislative body passes a bill, it becomes the **enacted** or **statutory law**. This law cannot be changed without another vote of the legislative body.

The government agency that has the legal authority to regulate nursing is usually named the board of nursing (although some states use different titles). This body establishes the administrative rules and regulations regarding practice and enforces the provisions of the statute as well as the rules and regulations.

Rules and Regulations

Each state has its own set of administrative **rules and regulations** to carry out the provisions of laws regulating nursing. These rules are considered **administrative law**. Most states require that public hearings be held regarding proposed rules and regulations, but the board has the authority to make the final decision. The rules and regulations must be within the scope outlined by the legislation that was passed. Those that are accepted by the appropriate board have the force of law unless they are challenged in court and are found not to be in accord with the legislature's intent.

In some states, the Nurse Practice Act is detailed and specifies most of the critical provisions regarding licensure and practice. In other states, the practice act is broad, and the administrative body is given a great deal of power to make decisions through rules and regulations. Both the Nurse Practice Act and state rules and regulations govern nursing in every state.

Nursing Licensure Law Content

In the early 1900s, the ANA, assuming its leadership role in nursing licensure, formulated a model nurse practice act to be used by state associations when planning legislation. The last ANA revision of this model was in 1990 by the ANA Congress for Nursing Practice (ANA, 1990). When the responsibility for overseeing the licensure process shifted to the NCSBN, that group also developed a model nursing practice act. In addition, it wrote the model nursing administrative rules. The NCSBN updated its entire model act and model rules and regulations in 2009 (NCSBN, 2009a). This document includes model law provisions and model regulations in a side-by-side format to facilitate understanding of their reciprocal nature.

Carefully read the Nurse Practice Act for the state in which you will practice. A copy of the Act may be obtained from the state board of nursing (check the NCSBN Web site, *www.ncsbn.org*). Many states make these documents available online. In some states, one act includes both practical nursing and registered nursing; other states have separate, but similar, acts. Historically, the role of the nursing assistant was not outlined in nursing laws. As federal legislation mandating classes and certification for nursing assistants in long-term care took effect, some states modified laws and rules and regulations to address the role of the nursing assistant. In other states, regulations governing nursing assistants rest within a different department of the state government.

The following general topics usually are covered in state licensure laws for nursing.

Purpose

The purpose of regulating the practice of nursing is twofold: Regulations protect the public and make individual practitioners accountable for their actions. Note that the protection of the status of the licensed individual is not the reason for licensure. With this in mind, you can better understand the inclusion of some other topics in the act.

Definitions and Scope of Practice

All of the significant terms in the act are defined for the purpose of carrying out the law. This is where the legal definition of nursing and the scope of practice are spelled out. The NCSBN has given the following definition:

> Nursing is a scientific process founded on a professional body of knowledge; it is a learned profession based on an understanding of the human condition across the lifespan and the relationship of a client with others and within the environment; and it is an art dedicated to caring for others. The practice of nursing means assisting clients to attain or maintain optimal health, implementing a strategy of care to accomplish defined goals within the context of a client-centered health care plan, and evaluating responses to nursing care and treatment. Nursing is a dynamic discipline that is continually evolving to include more sophisticated knowledge, technologies, and client care activities (NCSBN, 2009a).

The document then proceeds to distinguish between RN and LPN practice.

No state adopts the exact wording of any recommended definition, but many states include references to performing services for compensation (which has been deleted from the NCSBN definition), the necessity for a specialized knowledge base, the use of the nursing process or its parts (although steps may be named differently), and components of nursing practice. Several states include some reference to treating human responses to actual or potential health problems; this was first addressed in New York State's license law and was later incorporated in the ANA's first Nursing: A Social Policy Statement (ANA, 1980). Most states refer to the execution of the medical regimen, and many include a general statement about additional acts that recognize that nursing practice is evolving and that the nurse's area of responsibility can be expected to broaden.

Definitions of practical nursing are more restrictive and usually state that the individual must function under the direction of an RN or a physician, in areas demanding less judgment and knowledge than is required of the RN. In the NCSBN model act, this is referred to as "a directed scope of nursing practice" (NCSBN, 2009a). Practical nurse standards usually focus on data collection rather than comprehensive assessment, and they specify that the practical nurse contributes to the plan and evaluation of care rather than being accountable for them.

The scope of practice for any profession includes those activities, processes, and skills that are part of that profession and is directly tied to the legal definition. The education of the professional provides the basis for scope of practice and therefore differs for RNs, advanced practice nurses, and LPNs. The scope of practice also differentiates those activities that are nursing actions from those that are a part of other professions.

Because the definition of nursing in the law is written in broad terms, it is sometimes difficult to determine whether a specific action is permitted as part of the scope of practice. Figure 3.2 provides a decision-making process to help you examine whether any action is within your scope of practice as an RN. In some instances, when the issue is very complex, an advisory opinion regarding whether a specific action is within a nursing scope of practice may be sought from the state board of nursing.

Healthcare facilities employ a variety of nursing assistants, in the way of mental health technicians, nursing assistants, or medication technicians. The preparation and scope of practice for these individuals are a matter of serious concern to the public. Laws regarding educational requirements and legal definitions of scope of practice have been adopted for nursing assistant practice. Through the Omnibus Budget Reconciliation Act of 1987 regulations for long-term care facilities, a nationwide standard was established for the training and certification of nursing assistants employed in these facilities. Each state administers the regulations and is free to raise the standards but may not lower them.

Qualifications for Licensure Applicants

The most common basic requirements for licensure are completion of an application, payment of fees, graduation from an approved educational program, and proficiency in the English language. Some states make the educational requirements more specific—requiring, for example, high school graduation and either an associate or baccalaureate degree, or a diploma in nursing, for the RN applicant. Many include a provision that the applicant report any mental illness, criminal convictions, drug or alcohol dependence, or disciplinary action taken in regard to another professional license that will then be evaluated by the board of

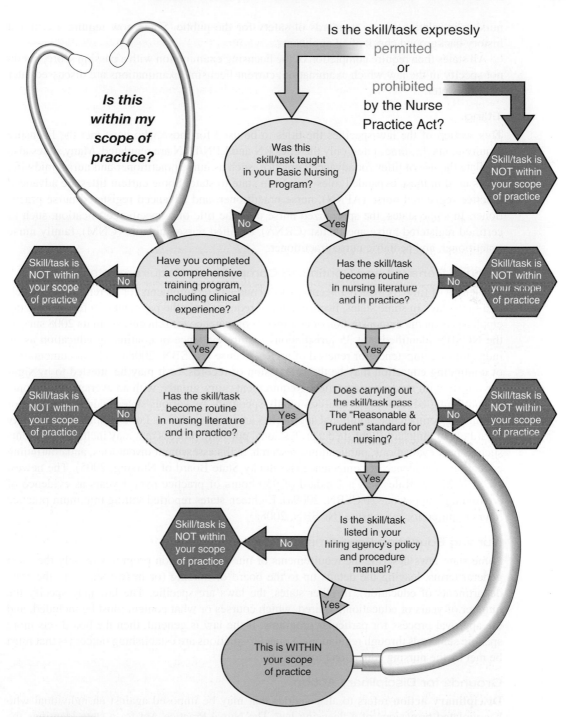

FIGURE 3.2 Nursing scope of practice: a decision-making model (Decisioning Model, 2004, with permission of South Dakota Board of Nursing).

nursing in relationship to standards of safety for the public. Some now require a criminal history background check of all applicants.

All states then require completion of the licensing examination with a passing score, but do not specify in the law which examination; current licensing examinations are discussed later in this chapter.

Titling

This section of the law specifies the titles to be used for those who have met the licensure requirements. In some states, only the titles RN and LPN/LVN are regulated. Many states also regulate the use of titles for advanced practice, such as nurse practitioner and nurse–midwife. Titles used in these expanded roles vary from state to state. Some current titles are advanced practice registered nurse (APRN), nurse practitioner, and advanced registered nurse practitioner. In some states, the specialized nurse uses the title of a specific certification, such as certified registered nurse anesthetist (CRNA), certified nurse–midwife (CNM), family nurse practitioner, and pediatric nurse practitioner.

License Renewal and Continuing Competence Requirements

The length of time for which a license is valid and any requirements for its renewal are specified in the law. In some states, license renewal requires only the payment of a fee. A growing emphasis is on the demonstration of continued competence for relicensure. In its 2008 survey, the NCSBN identified that 35 jurisdictions require evidence of continuing education as an indicator of competence for renewal of an RN license (NCSBN, 2008a). The documentation of continuing education may be the submission of records, or it may be attested to by signing a form with random verification. Requirements vary greatly, with an average of 15 hours of continuing education per year commonly specified. As various states address the issue of continuing competence, additional approaches are being included. For example, the Kentucky Board of Nursing has established a professional portfolio process that may include documents such as peer evaluations, publications, research, skills assessment inventories, and continuing education as evidence of competence (Kentucky State Board of Nursing, 2005). The newest NCSBN Model Rules sets a standard of 960 hours of practice over 3 years as evidence of continuing competence (NCSBN, 2009a). Eighteen states reported setting minimum practice hours required for relicensure (NCSBN, 2008a).

Nursing Education Programs

Some state laws describe the requirements of nursing education programs in only the most general terms, leaving the details up to the board of nursing (or in two states, to the state departments of education); in other states, the laws are specific. The law may specify the number of years of education required, which courses or what content must be included, and the approval process for particular programs. If the law is general, then the board sets more specific standards through regulations. Some jurisdictions are establishing outcomes that must be met by the nursing education program.

Grounds for Disciplinary Action

Disciplinary action refers to all penalties that may be imposed against an individual who has violated provisions of a licensing law. The Nurse Practice Act for a state identifies the basis for disciplinary action, and the board is empowered to prosecute those who violate the law. Disciplinary actions may include fines, reprimands, restrictions on practice (such as working only under supervision), suspension of a license for a specified period, or **revocation** (removal) of a license. The board may be authorized to ask a court to halt a specific practice that it believes is contrary to the law until a full hearing can be held. This is called **injunctive relief**. This term refers to the court order called an injunction that requires an individual or organization to stop a particular activity. The board also may immediately suspend a license, pending investigation, if the situation holds a serious threat to the public.

Disciplinary action can only be taken based on criteria stated in the law (Fig. 3.3). Most courts have supported revocation of a license only when the offense was related in some way to practice issues that affected public safety. Thus, most modern nurse practice or disciplinary acts contain specific concerns such as the following:

- Fraud or deceit in obtaining a license
- Criminal conviction
- Unethical conduct
- Drug diversion
- Unsafe or unprofessional practice (including practicing while chemically impaired)
- Practicing outside the scope of practice

Some states also have clauses that call for license revocation for individuals who default on government-sponsored education loans or on agreements regarding service in return for scholarship aid.

Exceptions

Certain provisions may allow those who are not licensed to act as nurses in specific situations. The primary exception is usually for those performing as a student enrolled in a nursing

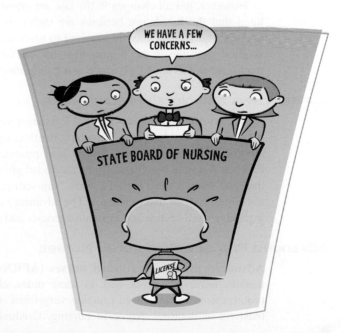

FIGURE 3.3 A nursing license may be revoked by the State Board of Nursing.

program. Those who care for family members or friends without pay are also exempted from license regulations. Those who practice nursing in a federal agency, such as a military hospital, are exempted from seeking a license in the state where they are stationed as long as they maintain a current license in another state. Some states are adopting exceptions for self-directed care by the disabled. In these situations, a paid care provider may perform certain care that is usually considered nursing when directed to do so by the mentally competent, physically disabled client. This includes administering medications in the home and carrying out specific care procedures, such as catheterization.

Administrative Provisions

Each law requires administrative specifications detailing when the law will become effective and when a previous act will no longer be in force. Although the Nurse Practice Act itself usually does not specify the fees to be charged for obtaining or renewing a license, general authority for setting fees is provided.

All states charge a fee for processing an application for licensure, for taking the licensing examination (which is paid to the company that prepares and scores an examination), and for license renewal. For specific information about current fees, contact your state board of nursing or visit its Web site.

Grandfathering

When a new law is written, it usually contains a statement specifying that anyone currently holding a license may continue to hold that license if and when requirements for the license change. This is termed **grandfathering**. Without this provision, the enactment of a new law would require individuals who are currently licensed to reapply and to show that they meet the new standards.

However, not all changes in the law are grandfathered. When new requirements are instituted that the legislature believes are important for the safety of the public, all currently licensed individuals may be required to meet the new standards within a given time period. A good example is the requirement for continuing education for relicensure. When this requirement was added, all applicants had to meet the requirement by a specific date.

Sunset Laws and Nurse Practice Acts

Most laws remain in effect until the legislature votes to rescind or replace them. Because this has resulted in archaic laws remaining in effect for many years, some states have passed what are known as "sunset laws." Sunset laws provide that any regulatory act, such as the Nurse Practice Act, will automatically be rescinded after a predetermined length of time if not reauthorized. Nurses must identify when "sun-setting" will occur and work in advance to sustain the current law or make changes. The advantage of sunset laws is that they guarantee that the legislature will review and evaluate agencies and programs.

Advanced Practice Registered Nurses

Advanced practice registered nurses (APRNs) include nurse practitioners, nurse anesthetists, nurse–midwives, and, in some states, clinical nurse specialists (CNSs). Licensure requirements for advanced practice vary from state to state. Most, but not all, require the master's or doctoral degree in nursing. Gradually, states are moving toward the master's degree as the minimum standard. None of the states administers a state licensing examination for advanced practice nursing.

Certification for advanced practice forms the basis of legal approval of APRN qualifications. The certification may be from the American Nurse Credentialing Center (ANCC) or a nursing specialty organization (see section on certification later in the chapter). Contact the board of nursing in the state in which you are interested for information about advanced practice.

The NCSBN has adopted the position that the licensing of nurses in advanced practice is an appropriate responsibility of the legal jurisdiction governing nursing practice and that methods to facilitate movement between states would enhance public health by providing healthcare professionals where needed. Based on this, a variety of task forces and committees within the NCSBN have worked to develop models that can be used in the regulation of advanced nursing practice. The document *Consensus Model for APRN Regulation: Licensure, Accreditation, Certification & Education* (NCSBN, 2008b) provides a basis for states to move toward greater symmetry in licensing and scope of practice.

Recommendations of the consensus model include titles. All are termed APRN with one of four roles: CRNA, CNM, certified nurse practitioner, or CNS. Within these roles, the individual will also have a population focus of family/individual across the life span, adult/gerontology, neonatal, pediatrics, women's health/gender related, or psychiatric mental health. Education for all of these roles would be in an accredited master's or doctoral degree program, or in a postgraduate certificate program. These programs would have to meet broad-based expectations that include pathophysiology, pharmacology, and physical assessment as well as significant clinical practice. Certification by an appropriate organization that includes both review of education and a sound examination would be required. Specialization for a specific practice such as oncology would not be part of licensure but would be a postlicensure professional designation. APRNs would be licensed as independent practitioners without requirements for collaboration or supervision (NCSBN, 2008b). A plan for an APRN compact for multistate licensing has been developed but not yet implemented.

Advanced practice nurses have the skills and abilities to help meet the needs of the millions of individuals expected to enter the system through the healthcare reform process. State regulations that do not allow APRNs to practice within the full scope of their abilities create a barrier to their being able to make this contribution. The 2010 Institute of Medicine report *The Future of Nursing: Leading Change, Advancing Health* recognizes the contributions of APRNs and the work that still needs to be done to ensure their full utilization to meet the healthcare needs of the public.

The Role of the State Board of Nursing

The **state board of nursing** (or its equivalent) is the administrative department of the government legally empowered to carry out the provisions of the Nurse Practice Act. Each state board must operate within the framework of its own state law regarding the practice of nursing, but all cooperate through the NCSBN. For example, state boards acting together through the NCSBN contract with the company that prepares the licensing examinations for RNs and practical nurses that are used throughout the United States. They also cooperate with other organizations, such as the ANA, the NLN, and the NLNAC, in some matters, but maintain the separation that is required of a group whose focus is protection of the public through effective licensure of nurses.

The board of nursing typically performs the following functions:

1. Establishes standards for licensure
2. Examines and licenses applicants
3. Provides for interstate endorsement
4. Renews licenses, grants temporary licenses, and provides for inactive status for those already licensed who request it
5. Enforces disciplinary codes
6. Provides rules for revocation of license
7. Regulates specialty practice
8. Establishes standards and curricula for nursing programs
9. Approves nursing education programs

Some or most of these duties may be performed by a centralized state agency acting in that capacity for all licensed occupations. When a centralized agency has the majority of the responsibility, the board of nursing may act in an advisory capacity in regard to issues.

Board membership, the procedures for appointment and removal, and the qualifications of board members are determined by the Nurse Practice Act. The governor of the state usually appoints the members of the board. The law specifies the occupational background of the candidates; nominations may be made by nurses' organizations and other interested parties. North Carolina is the only state in which the RN members of the state board are elected by the RNs in the state.

Most states have a single board for RNs and LPNs. In some states, separate boards exist. Each state board has a paid staff that usually is headed by an RN with advanced education who is employed as the executive director of the state board of nursing. The executive director is responsible for administering the work of the board, for seeing that rules and regulations are followed, and for working with the NCSBN and other state boards.

OBTAINING A NURSING LICENSE

There are two procedures for obtaining a nursing license. The first is used for obtaining an initial license and is termed **licensure by examination**. The second is for obtaining a license when the nurse is already licensed in another jurisdiction and is called **licensure by endorsement**. In both instances, the applicant for licensure must meet all provisions of the law (such as educational preparation, language proficiency, and legal residency status) in the state where he or she seeks licensure. In the initial licensure process, the applicant must take and pass the NCLEX. When seeking licensure by endorsement, the applicant is not required to take another examination—the licensing examination results from the initial state are accepted as proof of minimum safe practice—but other requirements must be met. This process is discussed later in the chapter.

Licensure by Examination

The establishment of a licensing examination was an important part of early efforts to achieve a professional standard for the RN. When each state adopted a licensing law, it also established a mechanism for examining license applicants. A major achievement in the history of nursing licensure was the formation of the Bureau of State Boards of Nurse Examiners, which eventually led to the use of an identical examination in all states in 1950. The original examination, called the State Board Test Pool Examination, was prepared by the testing department of the NLN, under a contract with the state boards. Although each state initially determined its own passing score, eventually all states adopted a common passing score. The current examination, called the **NCLEX-RN** for registered nursing and the **NCLEX-PN** for practical nursing, is used in all states and territories of the United States. Beginning in October 2002, Pearson Professional Testing of Minnesota was granted the contract for preparing and administering all NCLEX.

Content of the Examination

The NCSBN supports a study called the RN Practice Analysis every 3 years. This is used to guide the development of test questions. There is a similar cycle for studying PN practice. These studies identify nursing behaviors critical to maintaining a safe and effective standard of care. In all of these studies, newly licensed, practicing RNs or PNs are studied to determine both the frequency and the importance of various behaviors. These studies are reflected in the 2010 NCLEX-RN Test Plan (NCSBN, 2009b) and the 2011 NCLEX–PN Test Plan (NCSBN, 2010). The test plans are available for downloading without charge from the NCSBN Web site (NCSBN, 2009b, 2010). The NCLEX-RN questions are organized into client needs and the steps of the nursing process. The four client need categories (safe effective care environment, health promotion and maintenance, psychosocial integrity, and physiologic integrity) and their subcategories form the basis of the exam (see Table 3.1). There are four integrated processes: nursing process, communication and documentation, caring, and teaching/learning. The nursing process is divided into five steps: assessment, analysis, planning, implementation, and evaluation. These client need categories and the integrated processes form a matrix in which each question tests both an integrated process and one category or subcategory of client need.

The NCLEX-PN has a similar construction pattern. A "PN Job Analysis" study is conducted, and then the test plan is developed. The most recent PN Job Analysis was completed in 2009; the newest test plan for the PN was approved in 2008 and implemented in April 2011. A practical nurse is expected to assume a more dependent role in assessment; therefore, that step is titled data collection. Analysis is not part of the test plan. Whereas the RN examination includes management of care, the PN examination focuses on coordination of care. Even when topics are the same, the level of judgment expected of the PN differs from that

Table 3.1   2010 Test Plan for NCLEX-RN

CLIENT NEEDS CATEGORIES/SUBCATEGORIES	PERCENTAGE OF ITEMS
Safe Effective Care Environment	
Management of care	16–22
Safety and infection control	8–14
Health Promotion and Maintenance	6–12
Psychosocial Integrity	6–12
Physiological Integrity	
Basic care and comfort	6–12
Pharmacological and parenteral therapies	13–19
Reduction of risk potential	10–16
Physiological adaptation	11–17

expected of the RN. The newest test recognizes that many LPNs are employed in long-term care settings, with clients older than 65 years of age; therefore, it focuses on the older population (NCSBN, 2010).

Preparing and Administering the Examination

Preparing questions for the examination is a complex process. Nursing educators and RNs who work with new graduates are brought together to write exam questions based on the test plan. Content experts who are also nurses currently working with new graduates review all questions. Another panel of individuals reviews the questions for bias. Each question then is verified for accuracy by using current nursing references; test-construction experts also review the structure of all of the questions. The final versions of all questions are tested by inclusion in a nongraded part of the license examinations being given to new graduates; the questions are evaluated for their level of difficulty and appropriate use as part of a future scored examination.

In addition to assuming responsibility for test preparation, the testing service administers the computerized tests through contracted testing centers, scores the examinations, and reports scores to the state boards. The testing service is authorized to sell statistical information related to the examinations to the states and to individual schools. The entire testing process is explained in the candidate booklet (NCSBN, 2011), which is also available online at the testing Web site www.vue.com/nclex. An overview is presented below.

Computerized Adaptive Testing

All NCLEX (both RN and PN) are now administered through **computerized adaptive testing (CAT)**. CAT consists of a bank of examination questions administered through a computerized system. It was first field tested in 1990, then across the country in 1993, and finally adopted for all testing beginning in April 1994.

In this computerized test, the multiple-choice questions are delivered on a computer screen. The computer contains a large bank of questions, and different individuals may be presented with different questions. The computer program evaluates each response and then selects an appropriate question to present next, choosing a slightly harder question if the previous question was answered correctly or an easier question if the response was incorrect. The computer program ensures that all essential aspects of the test matrix plan are part of every examination. The development of questions and the design of the computer program ensure that all tests are equivalent, even when they're not identical. On the NCLEX-RN, the minimum number of questions that might be administered is 75 and the maximum is 265. The maximum length of time for the examination is 5 hours, but a candidate performing either especially well or very poorly might complete the exam in just 1 hour. One break is required after 2 hours of testing, and others may be taken at the discretion of the applicant. Testing ends when the scoring analysis clearly indicates a pass or fail, the maximum number of questions has been answered, or the maximum time has been completed.

Each candidate for licensure makes an individual appointment at a testing site. Security at the center is tightly monitored using photo identification, a finger print, and a palm vein scan. The computers are located in a quiet room without distractions. No test study materials are allowed at the testing center and no food or drink is allowed in the test environment. An erasable note board is provided for notes or calculations. An optional on-screen calculator is provided.

The multiple-choice questions in the examination typically are based on situations that require a nursing response. They are designed to test judgment and decision making, not simply knowledge of facts. Setting priorities, delegating, and communicating with the health team are aspects of that judgment. In addition to multiple-choice questions, there are several alternative question types that involve computation, short answer, identifying items on the screen, or multiple answers. These are described in the NLCEX-RN Candidate Bulletin (2011). A tutorial on how to use the computer, including the on-screen calculator, along with some practice questions is provided to ensure that the individual understands the process.

Scoring the Examination

The computer calculates the score as the applicant answers questions. Based on the computation made as the applicant progresses, additional questions are presented to clearly determine whether the applicant meets the standards for safe, effective practice in all areas of the test plan. The score used to determine whether a student passed or failed is not a raw score (ie, the number correct), but is derived from a complex statistical process that takes into consideration both the difficulty of a question and whether the response was correct. As soon as the statistical computation provides a prediction with 95% certainty of pass or fail, the test is terminated. If the computerized score has not provided a 95% certainty of pass or fail by the end of the examination (because either time is up or the maximum number of questions are answered), the system identifies whether the estimate of ability is above the standard even if it does not meet the 95% certainty standard. If it meets or is above that standard, the person passes.

Although the computer immediately determines pass or fail (upon the completion of the examination), the individual is not notified of the result at that time. The scoring information is communicated to the testing service, which then notifies the appropriate board. The board of nursing then notifies the individual whether he or she passed or failed. Every 3 years, the NCSBN considers the appropriateness of the passing standards for both the PN and RN examinations and may modify them.

Preparing for the NCLEX

Individuals must determine how best to prepare for the licensure examination based on their background and preferred study style. A review of the knowledge basic to nursing is important for most individuals. This may be done using course notes and texts. Those who become anxious in testing situations may want to focus on exercises to decrease anxiety during the examination. Those who find the process of test taking difficult can gain greater self-confidence by practicing test-taking techniques. This can be done through printed tests in books or computerized test preparation programs.

For both the NCLEX-RN and the NCLEX-PN, many commercial study aids are available. To prepare applicants to take the examination, the NCLEX Candidate Bulletin (NCSBN, 2011) explains the examination, how it is written, and the scoring system, and provides sample questions to familiarize applicants with the way the test is written. Many companies also prepare NCLEX-RN and NCLEX-PN review books, sample examination questions, audiotapes, and computerized practice examinations that are used to prepare for the licensing examinations. Manuals that outline standard nursing practice relative to many different healthcare problems may be useful for reviewing nursing content. Live and videotaped review courses, produced both by individual schools of nursing and by commercial publishers, are available to those who want assistance with preparation. During your preparation, remember that the goal is to solidify your knowledge and skills and to develop your critical-thinking and problem-solving skills. Memorizing answers to test questions presented in study books will not help you with the problem solving in regard to the unique questions presented in the actual examination.

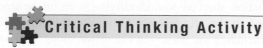

Critical Thinking Activity

A student about to graduate from an RN program in New York plans to live and practice nursing in New Jersey. What options are available to her to become licensed? Investigate the steps she should take to ensure that she may legally practice nursing in New Jersey as soon after graduation as possible.

Licensure by Endorsement

The process of obtaining a nursing license in a new state (while already licensed in another state) is called licensure by endorsement. In licensure by endorsement, each case is considered independently, based on the rules and regulations of the state to which one is applying for licensure. However, due to the uniformity of licensing laws throughout most of the United States and its territories, nurses have enjoyed easy mobility between geographic areas.

Because the same licensure examination and passing standards are used nationwide, no state requires that the examination be retaken. Basic educational and legal requirements of the individual state where a license is sought must be met. Sometimes a nurse moving to a new state must meet the current criteria for new licensure. In other states, a nurse must fulfill only the requirements that were in effect at the time of the original licensure. A state may require a nurse to meet other criteria, such as those for continuing education, before granting licensure by endorsement. In all cases, appropriate paperwork must be completed, necessary fees paid, and a license obtained before a nurse may begin employment.

A temporary license, which allows the applicant for licensure by endorsement to be employed while credentials are being verified and processed, is available in some states. Other states require that a permanent license be obtained before any employment is legal in those jurisdictions.

If a nurse wishes to maintain licensure in more than one state, this may be done by paying the renewal fees and meeting other requirements for continued licensure, such as continuing education, in each state in which a license is maintained. Some nurses hold licenses in several states to be able to work as a traveling nurse or to choose work in different locations. Nurses working close to state lines may need more than one license to be employed by an agency that operates in more than one state. This might also be true of a nursing education program that has clinical sites in two adjacent states or a home care agency with clients in two states.

Critical Thinking Activity

An RN who has been working in San Jose, California, for 10 years decides to relocate to Orlando, Florida. What are the steps that the nurse must take to ensure that she is able to work as an RN in Florida? Where should she seek information about the needed steps?

Mutual Recognition of Licensure

The process of **mutual recognition of licensure** in nursing has been established through the NCSBN based on a multistate agreement called the Nurse Licensure Compact. Mutual recognition of licensure involves an individual receiving an RN license in the state where he or she resides (the home state) and being legally permitted to practice in additional states without obtaining additional licenses for those states. This is sometimes referred to as "multistate licensure." Those states that have entered into the NCSBN Nurse Licensure Compact have all passed legislation adopting the terms of the Compact into their licensure laws (NCSBN, n.d.). At the time of this writing, 23 states have entered the compact agreement, and another state has passed legislation and is planning implementation. For the most current information on states participating, go to the NCSBN Web site and link to Nursing Licensure Compact.

Processes Involved in Mutual Recognition

All of the states that have signed the compact are referred to as **party states**. A person's **home state** is the state in which he or she resides and has a registered nursing license. An individual maintains only one license, the license granted in the home state, but is legally permitted to practice in any party state. When renewing a license, the individual renews in the home state. The individual nurse cannot hold a license in two party states at the same time. When an individual changes residence to a new party state, he or she applies for a new home state license based on residency. Individuals who wish to practice in a nonparty state still need to apply for a license in the nonparty state before practicing nursing.

A **remote state** is a party state other than the nurse's home state where the patient or recipient of nursing practice is located. For purposes of this law, nursing care location is based on where the patient is, not where the nurse is. The individual nurse must comply with the state laws regulating nursing practice in the state in which the client is located. Any party state where nursing care occurs (whether the home state or the remote state) may institute disciplinary action based on appropriate procedures. The home state is notified of the action being taken in the remote state through a coordinated information data bank system called NURSYS. When a remote state institutes disciplinary action, it may revoke a nurse's privilege to practice in that state only. Only the home state may revoke the license itself. If an individual has been assigned to some type of alternative program (such as drug treatment and monitoring) as part of the disciplinary process by any party state, the conditions of the disciplinary process must prohibit the individual from practicing in other states in the compact until the problem is resolved.

NURSYS was completed in 2000. This data bank contains licensure and disciplinary information from approximately 40 states that have chosen to use the system (NCSBN, 2009c). NURSYS provides online access to this computerized data bank for member state boards of nursing. It also provides an effective mechanism for individuals to have their records sent from one state to another when seeking endorsement.

As you can see, the RN who is licensed in a Nurse Licensure Compact state who chooses to work outside the home state must follow the directives contained in the compact and become familiar with the nursing practice act in any state in which clients are located. The state board of any state participating in the compact will provide complete information on the specific requirements to be met.

A separate APRN compact has also been developed. States participating in APRN compact must meet the expectations for education and licensure requirements found in the Consensus Model for APRN Regulation (NCSBN, 2008.)

Reasons Nurses Seek Mutual Recognition of Licenses

Under standard licensing laws, the nurse who practices in more than one state must hold multiple nursing licenses. This is both costly and complex. As the healthcare system grows more diverse, it is not uncommon for a healthcare-providing organization to operate across state boundaries.

Telenursing includes the use of telecommunications technology (eg, telephone, fax, computers, teleconferencing, interactive television, and video phone) to provide nursing services to individuals and groups. A telenurse in one state may care for a client in a distant state, thus raising questions regarding licensure requirements for a nurse who serves clients in more than one state. Does the nurse who provides telephone monitoring and advice for the client in another state need to be licensed in that client's state? Another area of concern is the nurse who works for an agency that serves clients across state borders. This nurse needs to visit clients in more than one state. The nursing case manager may follow clients in several states. All of these situations create a demand for a simpler licensing system for working in multiple states.

Concerns Regarding Mutual Recognition of Licenses

Not all nurses have supported mutual recognition of licenses. The ANA has identified that nurses who have differing requirements for relicensure could be practicing side by side; for example, one home state requires continuing education and another does not. Some state attorneys general have given opinions that it would be unconstitutional in their state to allow another state to control the requirements for practice. Issues of privacy regarding the data stored in the NURSYS system are another area of concern. The mutual recognition of licenses system may save money for the nurse who practices in multiple states because only one license would be purchased. However, if fewer nurses are licensed in the state, but the same number practice in the state, one would expect that disciplinary costs would remain even. The cost of licenses for all nurses, therefore, would have to rise to ensure adequate funds to support disciplinary costs (ANA, 2006).

A major concern is the disciplinary process. Although the board of nursing can investigate nursing practices and enforce its own standards in the state, it cannot change the licensure status of the person whose licensure originates in a different state; this fact is troubling to some boards of nursing. They are concerned that this doesn't allow them to protect the public adequately. A person disciplined in a remote state will still possess what would appear to be a valid home state license, but perhaps would not be able to practice legally in the remote state. For the individual nurse, the differences in licensure regulations could result in the same behavior being the cause of disciplinary action in one state but not in others; however, if the license were removed by the home state, then it would be invalid in all states.

The future not only holds many exciting possibilities for nursing but also poses many potential pitfalls. This is a complex issue, because state licensing agencies are charged with protecting the public and have legitimate concerns regarding such areas as disciplinary action.

REVOCATION OR LIMITATION OF A LICENSE

A license to practice any occupation becomes a property right of the individual once the state has awarded it. As long as the individual renews a license by paying the appropriate fees and meeting any requirements, such as continuing education, the license cannot be revoked without cause. Actions taken to restrict or remove a license are termed **disciplinary action**.

DISPLAY 3.2 Top Ten Reasons for Disciplinary Action Against Nurses

Drug abuse
Drug diversion for self
Other drug related
Failure to maintain minimal standards
Violating a board order
Documentation errors
Other unprofessional practice
Failure to comply with requirements
Medication errors
Felony
(NCSBN, 2009d)

The possible reasons for disciplinary action are spelled out in the law. Display 3.2 lists the top ten reasons for disciplinary action against all licensed nurses (LPN/LVN, RN, and APRN) as identified in a study by the NCSBN (NCSBN, 2009d). The combined violations related to drugs and alcohol constituted 25% of the total violations. Those related to medication administration in some way constituted 7% of the violations. Nine percent of the violations constituted criminal behavior. Unfortunately, the number of total violations has gone up 72% in the 11 years studied.

The procedure for revoking a license includes a fact-finding process and a hearing, which functions in many ways like a court proceeding. The state board or a specially designated hearing board is responsible for conducting the hearing and making a decision. The board may provide a license with conditions, suspend a license until certain conditions are met, or revoke a license completely. For example, a nurse faced with charges of chemical dependency might be directed to enter a treatment program, to refuse employment involving direct responsibility for clients who need controlled substances or access to drugs, and to be monitored for compliance. If these conditions are met, the individual may be allowed to work in a restricted environment and then be reinstated to full rights and privileges of licensure when treatment is completed. The board's decision may be appealed in a court of law in most states. If a board of nursing finds that the individual's actions constitute a felony, the board is obligated to report that to the criminal authorities for prosecution.

The individual being investigated for any violation of the Nurse Practice Act should have an attorney who is knowledgeable about professional disciplinary issues from the time of notification of the complaint. Some nurses fail to take this important action: they may have the mistaken impression that only those guilty of misconduct need an attorney; they may believe that if they made an error they deserve punishment; or they may worry about the cost of an attorney. Just as in a criminal proceeding, the law is complex and a knowledgeable attorney provides direction and support throughout a disciplinary process. Penalties may vary greatly and the naïve nurse may not realize that extenuating circumstances or negotiations may change penalties. Although attorney costs are substantial, a license to practice nursing is extremely valuable to the individual nurse. Some malpractice insurance policies include payment for attorney fees in the case of disciplinary action (see Chapter 7). The state nurses association or the local chapter of the National Association of Nurse Attorneys can often provide referrals of attorneys who are familiar with the disciplinary process.

As a licensed professional, be aware that you are responsible to your clients and to the state in which you practice. You can act to protect your license through maintaining current knowledge and appropriate standards of practice. Also, understand and abide by the scope of practice as described in your individual nursing practice act. If you take a position in a new state, be sure to become informed about that state's Nurse Practice Act.

Critical Thinking Activity

A nurse in your state receives a notification from the board of nursing that a complaint has been lodged with the board regarding his practice. Find out what the process would be in your state for this nurse to respond to the complaint. What resources will this nurse need? What are the possible consequences if the complaint is sustained?

LICENSURE OF GRADUATES OF FOREIGN NURSING SCHOOLS

Many nurses from other countries have immigrated to the United States and sought licensure to be able to work in their new home. Some nurses have come to the United States for additional education and need a license to engage in clinical practice associated with that education. Still others are attracted by the higher salaries and better living conditions for nurses in the United States. During the nursing shortage of the early 1980s, and again in the nursing shortage in the first part of this century, employers in the United States actively recruited foreign nurses, sometimes providing support for travel and relocation expenses.

Several concerns have been expressed regarding the recruitment of foreign-educated nurses to the United States. In many of the countries from which nurses emigrate to the United States, shortages exist. Thus, the United States depletes other countries of an important health resource. Some US nurses believed that overseas recruitment replaces the need to address workplace problems that contribute to the shortage. Nurses educated in other countries may lack understanding of the US healthcare system and the expectations for scope of practice. Further, they may lack English language proficiency.

For the foreign-educated nurse, there are two requirements that must be met in order to work in the United States. The first of these is a visa that permits employment, either a visa granted to a permanent immigrant or one granted to a temporary worker. The employer is required to verify the individual's eligibility for employment in the United States. When the visa is contingent upon employment, the foreign-educated nurse may feel constrained from changing employers if circumstances differ from what was promised during recruitment.

The second requirement is that the foreign-educated nurse must obtain a state license to practice nursing. To obtain a license, all graduates of foreign nursing schools who want to practice nursing in the United States must provide verification to the state licensing authority that their nursing education meets state requirements and they must take the appropriate NCLEX. In the past, institutions would sometimes hire foreign nurses into lower paying positions until they obtained a license. When many did not pass the examination, the nurses felt exploited by the system.

CGFNS International

The U.S. Department of Labor, the Department of Health and Human Services (HHS), the Immigration and Naturalization Service (INS), the ANA, and the NLN are all concerned about the safety of the public and about the well-being of the foreign-educated nurse. To address these problems, these organizations and government agencies collaborated in the development of an independent organization originally called the Commission on Graduates of Foreign Nursing Schools (CGFNS—pronounced "cog-fens") and now titled CGFNS International.

While some nurses who come to the United States possess regular immigrant visas, the majority come on special-preference visas. Special immigration regulations allow a foreign nurse to obtain a special-preference visa from the INS, or a work permit from the U.S. Labor Department because of the need for nurses. To obtain this special-preference visa, an individual nurse must obtain a visa certificate from an HHS-approved agency, such as CGFNS. The Department of Homeland Security ruled in July 2005 that nurses from Mexico and Canada, who were formerly exempted from this requirement under NAFTA, were subject to this same requirement for a certificate.

The CGFNS service *VisaScreen* provides a certificate enabling an individual to apply for a visa. A VisaScreen includes (1) a review of the foreign nurse's education, (2) evaluation of all current and previous licenses to practice, (3) assessment of English language proficiency (Canadian nurses, except those from Quebec province, are exempt from the language assessment), and (4) completion of either the CGFNS Assessment of General Nursing Knowledge Examination or the NCLEX-RN. The CGFNS Assessment is offered around the world for individuals to take before emigrating. Because many foreign-educated nurses still come to the United States without having taken the CGFNS examination, it is also offered in selected cities in the United States. When these requirements have been completed satisfactorily, a certificate is issued that can be presented to the immigration service to obtain a special-preference visa (CGFNS, 2011).

The evaluation of education credentials, which includes course-by-course evaluations, also can be submitted to a licensing board to demonstrate that the individual has an appropriate education for registered nursing practice. Some states require only verification of educational credentials before admitting an individual to the NCLEX-RN. The NCLEX-RN is now administered in select foreign cities. Passing the NCLEX-RN does not provide permission to be employed, but it can be used in place of the CGFNS Assessment. Some states require that a language proficiency examination and CGFNS examinations as well as credential verification be completed prior to admission to the NCLEX. Up to 90.8% of foreign-educated nurses who have obtained CGFNS certification pass the licensing examination on first attempt. Those who failed the CGFNS exam had an NCLEX pass rate of only 40.7% on their first attempt (CGFNS-International, 2007).

International Centre on Nurse Migration

The International Centre on Nurse Migration is a project of the CGFNS and the International Council of Nurses (ICN). The goals of the Centre relate to both effective patient care and the well-being of nurse migrants. To achieve its goals, the Centre works on policies worldwide that affect nurse migration, collects and reports data on nurse migration, and serves as a resource for those working with regulations regarding nurse migration (International Centre on Nurse Migration, 2011). Because there is a worldwide shortage of nurses and a wide disparity of wages and recognition between developing and developed countries, nurse migration will continue to be an important international issue.

NURSING LICENSURE AROUND THE WORLD

Nursing education and nursing licensure differ greatly throughout the world. Additionally, practice patterns and expectations of nursing behaviors may differ between countries. In Australia, nursing education has been moved into university settings, and future applicants for licensure in that country are required to have a university education. In Italy, nursing education is now consolidated under broad, multisite programs administered by university nursing departments. The European Union is moving toward a system that allows freer movement of professionals between its nations. The nations of Eastern Europe have faced many drastic changes in their healthcare systems as they changed internally and formed different relationships with the West. Nursing education was restricted during Soviet domination, and many nurses had limited nursing educational opportunities, with basic nursing education sometimes occurring at the high school level. Nursing in those countries is moving toward contemporary expectations.

Because of educational and practice differences as well as language barriers, nursing credentials are not easily transferred internationally. The ICN has supported the development of effective licensure legislation worldwide. In 1988, it launched a project called "Nursing Regulation: Moving Ahead," which was funded by the W. K. Kellogg Foundation. This ongoing project involved nurses and officials from 77 countries in seminars and studies. To date, nursing licensure laws in the United States have not been affected by this study, but it has supported the development of licensure laws in some parts of the world.

Individuals who are interested in international nursing need to consider both their language proficiency and their educational backgrounds. Organizations actively working in the international health field, such as the World Health Organization and medical relief organizations, usually will provide information on opportunities and licensure requirements in various countries. The ICN in Geneva can provide addresses of appropriate government authorities to contact regarding licensure in other countries. During times of emergency, such as the tsunami in the Indian Ocean, countries may welcome nurses as part of relief groups without requiring licensure in that country. Additionally, there are opportunities for short-term healthcare work in developing countries through charitable agencies and international missions.

CERTIFICATION IN NURSING

As mentioned earlier, certification in nursing is primarily a professional, not legal, credential, and it focuses on knowledge and skills related to a particular area of practice. The definition of certification adopted by the Interdivisional Council on Certification of the ANA (1978) states, "Certification is the documented validation of specific qualifications demonstrated by the individual RN in the provision of professional nursing care in a defined area of practice." Certification is available from many professional nursing and healthcare organizations (Fig. 3.4).

American Nurses Credentialing Center Certification

In 1988, the ANA established the ANCC, which assumed all of the ANA credentialing activities. The ANA invited all other organizations providing credentialing for nurses to join; some joined, but many retained their individual programs.

ANCC certification is a method of recognizing nurses who have special expertise. Applicants must demonstrate current practice and knowledge beyond that required for

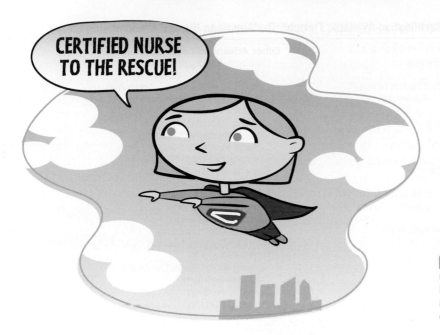

CERTIFIED NURSE
TO THE RESCUE!

FIGURE 3.4 Certified nurses provide an expert level of practice and may serve as a resource to others.

licensure as an RN. After submitting evidence of completing all requirements, a nurse may take the national examination for a specific certification. Certification is granted for a period of 5 years, after which a nurse may renew the certification by submitting new evidence of current practice and ability.

The master's degree currently forms the basis of the requirement for certification as a clinical nurse specialist, a nurse practitioner, or other advanced practice roles but is moving toward the use of the doctor of nursing practice. For specialty certifications, there are requirements for continuing education and hours of practice in the area of specialization. All certifications require passing an examination. See Table 3.2 for a list of ANCC certifications available.

Other Nursing Certifications Available

In 1991, eight national nursing certification programs joined to establish the American Board of Nursing Specialties. These organizations included the ANCC of the ANA, the American Board for Occupational Health Nursing, the American Board of Neuroscience Nursing, the Association of Rehabilitation Nurses, the Council on Certification of Nurse Anesthetists, the National Board of Nutritional Support Certification, the Nephrology Nursing Certification Board, and the Orthopaedic Nurses Certification Board. Since that time, a number of other nursing organizations that provide certification have joined this organization. The goals of this board are to ensure quality in specialty nursing, improve the public's perception of specialty nurses, and provide specialty nurses who bring a consistent standard of education and experience to their practice. This is a major breakthrough in the entire certification process for nursing. This board has established a peer review process for certification organizations that provides evaluation and recognition of the certification granted.

Table 3.2   Nursing Certification Available Through The American Nurses' Credentialing Center

Nurse Practitioners	Other Advanced-Level Specialties
Acute Care Nurse Practitioner	Diabetes Management—Advanced
Adult Nurse Practitioner	Nurse Executive—Advanced
Adult Psychiatric & Mental Health Nurse P	Public Health Nursing—Advanced
Diabetes Management—Advanced	Ambulatory Care Nursing
Family NP	Cardiac Rehabilitation Nursing
Family Psych & Mental Health NP	Cardiac Vascular Nurse
Gerontological NP	Case Management Nursing
Pediatric NP	College Health Nursing
School NP	Community Health Nursing
Clinical Nurse Specialists	General Nursing Practice
Adult Health CNS	Gerontological Nursing
Adult Psychiatric & Mental Health CNS	High-Risk Perinatal Nursing
Child/Adolescent Psych & Mental Health CNS	Home Health Nursing
CNS Core Exam	Informatics Nursing
Diabetes Management—Advanced	Maternal–Child Nursing
Gerontological CNS	Medical–Surgical Nursing
Home Health CNS	Nurse Executive
Pediatric CNS	Nursing Professional Development
Public/Community Health CNS	Pain Management
	Pediatric Nursing
	Perinatal Nursing
	Psychiatric & Mental Health Nursing
	School Nursing

Detailed information on requirements and credentialing process available from ANCC at *www.nursecredentialing.org/*.

There are additional organizations providing certification that are not part of the American Board of Nursing specialties. The American College of Nurse-Midwives certifies for practice as a nurse–midwife. Other nurses seek certification from nonnursing organizations, such as lactation consultants, which are certified by the La Leche League.

 Critical Thinking Activity

An RN with 5 years of general medical–surgical acute care experience is interested in obtaining certification in medical–surgical nursing. Research the requirements for such certification and outline what she will need to do to be eligible to be certified as a medical–surgical nurse.

Certification for Licensed Practical Nurses

Certification for LPNs/LVNs is available for those practicing in long-term care. The National Association of Practical Nurse Education and Service determined that many LPNs have responsible positions in long-term care and that recognition of their abilities through certification would be appropriate. They contracted with the NCSBN to develop and administer a certification examination. Those taking this examination use the title certified in long-term care (CLTC).

THE FUTURE OF CREDENTIALING IN HEALTHCARE

Because credentialing in nursing involves so many aspects of education, licensure, and certification, it has confused the public, nurses, and other healthcare professionals. The ideal credential clearly communicates qualifications and competence; therefore, it is important for nursing to have a credentialing system that can be understood by others. Current changes are moving nursing closer to an effective credentialing system.

Institutional Control of Credentials

Many new healthcare occupations related to new procedures and processes in medical care are being developed as new technology develops. Those who believe the state should take positive action to protect the public continue to exert pressure to license additional healthcare providers. Those who oppose credentialing of additional individual groups of healthcare workers believe that modern-day employers are able to assess workers and to differentiate among them on the basis of competence. Some who oppose credentialing of individual health occupations believe that licensing the institution that hires the employees would be an adequate safeguard for the public.

Another approach to credentialing in healthcare is certifying specific competencies rather than an entire field of practice. Those advocating this approach believe that it would facilitate the development of individuals with a broad range of competencies suited to a particular setting. For example, in a rural area, one individual might be certified as competent to perform certain basic x-ray examinations (such as for simple fractures), basic laboratory studies (such as complete blood count and urinalysis), and some basic client care procedures (such as bathing, toileting, feeding, and positioning). Because more complex procedures are sent to a larger center and there is no need for a full-time person in any of these positions, basic care would be made available in a convenient and low-cost manner. Certification of specific competencies by the employing agency is sometimes referred to as site-based examination and site-based certification. One concern about this method of certifying competencies is its focus on technical skills, without adequately recognizing the knowledge base needed for decision making and judgment. Other concerns are the complexity of keeping track of the many specific competencies and the difficulty with job mobility when competencies are not standardized.

Institute of Medicine Recommendations

In the Institute of Medicine (IOM) report *Health Profession Education: A Bridge to Quality* (2003), the study committee came to some conclusions around the issues confronting health professions education. One concern is the fact that each profession tends to educate, practice, and dialogue within a "silo." These narrowly constructed walls make it difficult for interdisciplinary collaboration to occur. The languages used by the differing groups are a major barrier.

One of the recommendations of the report was that there should be an interdisciplinary focus on building a common language of healthcare with the ultimate aim of creating a set of core competencies for all health professionals. This proposal would seem to run counter to the efforts in nursing to develop *nursing-specific* language to describe the work of nurses.

Another recommendation was that those with responsibility for oversight of the various health professions (approval and accreditation bodies) meet to develop specific core competencies that relate to the following:

- Delivering patient-centered care
- Working as part of interdisciplinary teams
- Practicing evidence-based healthcare
- Focus on quality improvement
- Using information technology

These have been incorporated into accreditation criteria for nursing education and healthcare delivery agencies.

A third recommendation is that accreditation bodies should revise their processes to require outcomes related to these core competencies. Two other recommendations are related to the oversight of continued competence by health professionals. The IOM report recommended that both licensing bodies and specialty certification bodies require health professionals to demonstrate in some way their continued competence in the previously determined core competencies. Again, this has become an accepted practice for most licensing and certification bodies.

The Future of Approval/Accreditation of Nursing Education Programs

As nursing grows and moves forward, the dual expectations of state approval and national accreditation create a substantial workload and cost for the individual nursing program. The NCSBN developed a *White Paper on the State of the Art of Approval/Accreditation Processes in Boards of Nursing* (NCSBN, 2004c). The group preparing this paper investigated the current processes in place for approval and accreditation and identified the models being used. The report noted both benefits and costs of the current system and discussed the value of using interdisciplinary faculty in order to enhance interdisciplinary practice. The report also recommended that future approval processes include the five areas of competence identified by the IOM (IOM, 2003).

KEY CONCEPTS

- Credentials are written proof of qualifications and may include diplomas awarded by educational programs, certification, or registration by professional groups, and legal licenses awarded by governmental agencies.
- Permissive licensure allows for those meeting certain standards voluntarily to be licensed, whereas mandatory licensure requires that all individuals who wish to practice in the field be licensed to practice.

- Nursing leaders began efforts to obtain legal licensure in 1896. The first permissive licensure law was passed in 1903 by North Carolina, and the first mandatory licensure law was passed in New York in 1947.
- Legal rules governing nursing practice are found in the licensure law passed by a legislative body. Further provisions governing nursing are found in the rules and regulations

established by the administrative agency in which the legislation vests authority.

- The state nursing practice acts usually contain a definition of nursing and address qualifications for licensure applicants, use of titles, renewal and continuing competence requirements, grandfathering, financial concerns, nursing education programs, disciplinary action, violations and penalties, administrative provisions, and expanded nursing roles.
- The state boards of nursing (or their equivalent) are the administrative agencies that have the authority to carry out the provisions of the Nurse Practice Act.
- A license to practice nursing must be obtained from the state or province in which you wish to work, except in the case of states that belong to the Multistate Compact. An initial license is termed licensure by examination, and subsequent licenses may be obtained in other jurisdictions through licensure by endorsement.
- Advanced practice nurses are regulated by each state. Most require professional certification in an advanced practice nursing specialty to be licensed in that role.
- Mutual recognition of licensure involves a compact between certain states that allows nurses who are licensed in one of those states to work freely among all the compact states belonging to the Multistate Compact without the need for obtaining additional licenses.
- The NCLEX-RN is administered through a computerized plan that covers the four integrated processes: nursing process, communication and documentation, caring, and teaching/learning, and four areas of client needs, and that identifies competence for entry-level safe nursing care.
- Graduates of foreign nursing schools must have their credentials reviewed and may be required to take the CGFNS examination, which reviews nursing content and a test for English language ability, before being admitted to take the NCLEX.
- A license may be revoked by the state board of nursing, a designated disciplinary board, or a court of law based on specific reasons stated in the Nurse Practice Act.
- Certification provides evidence of specialized clinical knowledge and ability beyond the basic level. Certification as a nurse practitioner may be used as a basis for legal approval for the advanced registered nurse practitioner role.
- Concerns about the future of healthcare worker credentialing include issues of public accountability and continued competence.
- The IOM report on health professions education made a series of recommendations, several of which focus on developing a set of core competencies that could be used for both education and ongoing professional regulation.
- The NCSBN has endorsed the core competencies identified by the IOM and encourages movement toward outcomes assessment as part of approval and accreditation decisions.

RELEVANT WEB SITES

 Web sites relevant to this chapter can be found at **thePoint** accessed through *http://thePoint. lww.com/Ellis10e* and by entering the code found on the inside cover of your text.

REFERENCES

American Nurses Association. (1978). *A study of credentialing in nursing: A new approach, vol. 1, The Report of the Committee*. Kansas City, MO: Author.

American Nurses Association. (1980). *Nursing: A social policy statement*. Kansas City, MO: American Journal of Nursing Co.

American Nurses Association, Congress for Nursing Practice. (1990). *Suggested state legislation: Nursing Practice Act, Disciplinary Diversion Act; Prescriptive Authority Act*. Kansas City, MO: Author.

CGFNS-International. (2007). *The certification program validity study: April 2006–March 2007*. Retrieved September 13, 2009, from http://www.cgfns.org/sections/tools/stats/validity.shtml

CGFNS-International. (2011). *Overview*. Retrieved March 25, 2011, from http://www.cgfns.org/sections/about

Eaton, J. S. (2009), An overview of U.S. accreditation. U.S. Dept. of Education, Council on Higher Education Accreditation (CHEA). Retrieved Sept. 11, 2009 from http://www.chea.org/pdf/2009.06_Overview_of_US_Accreditation.pdf

Institute of Medicine. (2003). *Health professions education: A bridge to quality*. Washington, DC: National Academies Press.

Institute of Medicine. (2010). *The future of nursing: Leading change, advancing health*. Washington, DC: National Academies Press.

International Centre on Nurse Migration. (2011). *Mission, vision, and goals*. New York: Author. Retrieved March 28, 2011, from www.intlnursemigration.org

Kalisch, P. A., & Kalisch, B. J. (2004). *American nursing: A history*. 4th ed. Philadelphia, PA: Lippincott Williams & Wilkins.

Kentucky State Board of Nursing. (2005). Continuing Competency Requirements, 201 KAR 20:215. Retrieved March 26, 2011, from www.kbn.gov/laws

National Council of State Boards of Nursing. (2004). *White paper on the state of the art of approval/accreditation processes in boards of nursing*. Chicago, IL: Author.

National Council of State Boards of Nursing. (2008a), *Member board profiles*. Retrieved September 17, 2009, from https://www.ncsbn.org/983.htm

National Council of State Boards of Nursing. (2008b). *Consensus model for APRN regulation: Licensure, accreditation, certification & education*. Retrieved September 12, 2009, from https://www.ncsbn.org/7_23_08_Consensus_APRN_Final.pdf

National Council of State Boards of Nursing. (2009a). *Model nursing act and rules*. Chicago, IL: Author. Retrieved March 28, 2011, from https://www.ncsbn.org/1455.htm

National Council of State Boards of Nursing. (2009b). *2010 NCLEX-RN test plan*. Chicago: Author. Retrieved September 12, 2009 from https://www.ncsbn.org/1287.htm

National Council of State Boards of Nursing. (2009c). *NCSBN Unveils New Nursys.com Web Site with Enhanced Nurse Licensure Verification Tools*. Chicago, IL: Author. Retrieved September 12, 2009, from https://www.ncsbn.org/1607.htm

National Council of State Boards of Nursing. (2009d). An analysis of NUR*SYS* disciplinary data from 1996–2006. *NCSB Research Brief 39* (June 2009). Chicago: Author. Retrieved September 12, 2009 from https://www.ncsbn.org/09_AnalysisofNursysData_Vol39_WEB.pdf

National Council of State Boards of Nursing. (2010). *2011 NCLEX-PN test plan*. Chicago: Author. Retrieved March 26, 2011, from https://www.ncsbn.org/1287.htm

National Council of State Boards of Nursing. (2011). *2011 NCLEX-RN detailed test plan (candidate version)*. Chicago, IL: Author. Retrieved March 27, 2011, from https://www.ncsbn.org/1287.htm

National Council of State Boards of Nursing (n.d.) *Nurse licensure compact*. Chicago: Author, Retrieved September 12, 2009 from https://www.ncsbn.org/nlc.htm

Making Professional Goals a Reality

4

LEARNING OUTCOMES

After completing this chapter, you should be able to:

1. Describe the various employment opportunities available to nurses today and discuss the educational requirements of each.
2. Describe the competencies needed by the new graduate as outlined by the job analysis study that is the basis for the National Council Licensure Examination (NCLEX).
3. Analyze the eight common expectations employers have of new graduates explaining why each is important and relate them to your own background and education.
4. Develop a list of your personal short- and long-term career goals.
5. Prepare a personal résumé and sample letters of application, follow-up, and resignation.
6. Describe aspects to consider when preparing for an interview.
7. Formulate possible responses to an employment interview.

KEY TERMS

Application letter/cover letter
Competency

Proficiency
Résumé

When you graduate, one of your first goals will be to obtain employment as a registered nurse (RN). You probably look forward to practicing in the nursing role you have spent so long attaining. Although some new graduates have worked as unlicensed assistive staff or practical (vocational) nurses during their education, for others their only contact with healthcare settings may have been as students rather than as employees. You may not have experienced all of the many settings in which RNs are employed. You may have questions regarding employer expectations and your own role as an RN.

Planning a nursing career can be complex and finding that first job may be a challenge. In this chapter, we try to assist you as you survey the RN job market and plan for a successful approach to obtaining that important first position.

EMPLOYMENT OPPORTUNITIES TODAY

The nursing shortage was so great in 2007 that hospitals were recruiting overseas, and nursing programs across the country were being encouraged to increase enrollments. Nursing graduates often had multiple job offers from which to choose and some hospitals were offering incentives for hiring. Then, in 2008, the sudden economic recession affected healthcare institutions as well as every other part of society.

At the time of this writing, positions for new graduate RNs have decreased. This is due in part to the effects of the economic recession—people without insurance put off all care, elective procedures are avoided, hospital census drops, nurses who could retire continue working, and nurses who have been employed part time are accepting full time positions. Orientation programs for new graduates are costly and if experienced nurses can be hired that is the preference.

Although hospital vacancies have decreased in many places, those in long-term care continue to increase. Using 2007 as a baseline, the American Health Care Association (AHCA) predicted that the long-term care environment will need to increase licensed nursing positions by 2% a year as the demand for long-term care services grows (AHCA, 2008). Thus, even if no nurses retired or left their positions (an unlikely scenario), there would still be a rising demand. Unfortunately, long-term care facilities may not offer the same extended orientations to new graduates that are found in acute care settings.

According to the U.S. Bureau of Labor Statistics (2008), the long-term outlook for all nursing positions is excellent with 587,000 new jobs created by 2016. While the decrease in acute care positions is expected to be temporary and the overall nursing shortage is expected to return strongly within 10 years (Buerhaus, Auerbach, & Staiger, 2009), that does not make it easier for the new graduate of today.

In planning a job search in this climate, flexibility will be key. You may find it most productive to consider a range of positions you would like or to examine whether your most desired position would best be obtained by starting in a different position and moving to the desired position after becoming more experienced. You might consider changing your geographical location; some areas have a greater need for RNs than do others.

While just 59% of nursing jobs are located in hospitals (U.S. Bureau of Labor Statistics, 2008), most new graduates choose to begin their careers in structured healthcare settings where planned orientations and mentoring provide support for the novice in making the adjustment to the RN role. This also may result from the fact that many of the noninstitutional positions require expertise and independent functioning. New graduates often seek institutional positions for the orientations and mentoring available. In its trend studies, the National Council of State Boards of Nursing (NCSBN) has identified changes over time in the work environments, employment characteristics, and job activities of newly licensed nurses. The most recent publication includes the data from the 2008 survey (NCSBN, 2009a). Of those responding, over 89% worked in hospital settings. 4.8% worked in long-term care and 4.3% worked in community-based or ambulatory care settings. Only 1.7% indicated that they worked in "other" settings. This study showed that 36.6% of new graduates were employed in critical care and 36.8% were in medical–surgical units.

When reporting the types of clients for whom they care, newly licensed nurses most frequently identified acutely ill clients as the population for whom they cared with 70.7% including this population. 24.2% indicated they cared for clients older than 85 years, 61.3%

indicated caring for those aged 31 to 64, and only 22.8% cared for those aged 18 to 30. Much lower percentages indicated they care for children. Of those working a regular shift, 37.7% reported working day shift and 10.2% evening shift, leaving 37.1% on the night shift. Rotating shifts are less common than a straight shift assignment with 13.3% reporting that they work rotating shifts (NCSBN, 2009a).

The number of positions for RNs in many settings other than those involved in providing direct client care has grown. Healthcare-oriented businesses, such as insurance companies and medical equipment supply companies, have found that it is often easier to teach nurses about business than to teach business people about healthcare. As a result, nurses are being employed in what some individuals see as nonnursing positions. Others argue that these, too, should be considered nursing positions, because the expertise that makes the individual successful is nursing expertise. Although experienced nurses usually hold these positions, moving into such positions may be a part of a career plan of the new graduate.

The number of men in nursing, which remained relatively small for many years, is beginning to grow as society reassesses its attitude toward labeling jobs as women's or men's work. In 2008, the number of men in nursing was estimated at 6.6%—up from 5.4% in 2000 (U.S. Bureau of Health Professions, 2008). Men have been attracted by the career opportunities and improving the economic picture offered by a career in nursing. The number of new graduates who are men is greater than the number of men in the overall nursing population. According to the National League for Nursing (NLN), in the 2008–2009 academic year, 15% of ADN students were men, while 12% of BSN students were men (NLN, 2009). By 2008 6.6% of nurses were men (U.S. Bureau of Health Professions, 2008).

The economic position of the nurse has improved for several reasons. One reason is the extension of laws governing fair labor practices to nonprofit institutions and the advent of collective bargaining (see Chapter 5). Another major reason is the nursing shortage that occurred in the 1980s. The demand for nurses rose faster than the supply; employers began increasing salaries and benefits to attract nurses. This trend was especially notable in urban communities. Nurses comprise one of the largest segments of the US workforce and are among the highest paid with RN salaries averaging $65,130 per year (U.S. Bureau of Labor Statistics, 2010).

All these factors bring you, as a new graduate, into a world of uncertainty, but one also filled with opportunity and promise. We encourage you to look forward to the positive contribution that you can make to patients and to nursing practice.

Critical Thinking Activity

Obtain the Sunday classified advertising section of a local newspaper or examine an online job board for your location. Count the advertisements for RNs. How many employers are represented? Think of all the different healthcare agencies in the community. Do the ads represent most of them, some of them, or only a few of the potential employers of nurses? Of those listed, how many specify background or experience beyond that which a new graduate would have? How many specify the shift or work schedule? If wages are noted, what is the range of wages quoted? Reflect on your own expectations for employment after graduation. How do your expectations compare with what you find in these advertisements?

COMPETENCIES OF THE NEW GRADUATE

Recently, you may have heard the term **competency** used a great deal, especially as it applied to you as a student. Competency, as used here, refers to the ability of the person to effectively and safely perform specified nursing actions, including the application of critical thinking skills. Some have differentiated competency, which is an entry-level expectation, and **proficiency**, which is expected of the experienced nurse (Fig. 4.1).

Competencies Identified by Nursing Organizations

A number of nursing organizations have developed statements regarding the competencies expected of the new graduate. Chief among these organizations is the NCSBN.

National Council of State Boards of Nursing Competencies

The most definitive statements on the competencies needed by the newly licensed practical nurse (PN) and the RN have been developed by the NCSBN based on its job analysis studies, which serve as the basis for the NCLEX-RN and NCLEX-PN.

In these studies, frequency and importance of activities reported by a stratified random sample of newly licensed, entry-level nurses were examined. Both the frequency of the nursing activities and their importance were studied. Importance was scaled from 1 (not important) to 5 (critically important) and was in regard to the maintenance of client safety and/or threat of complications or distress (NCSBN, 2009c). The last published RN study was completed in 2008; the results of that study supported changes to the current test plan for 2010 although the passing score remained unchanged (NCSBN, 2009c). The most recent PN study was

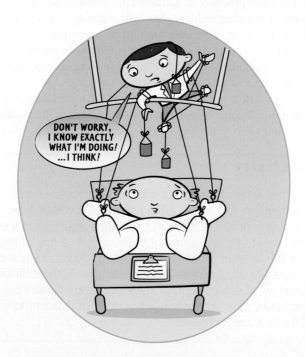

FIGURE 4.1 New graduates are expected to know both their own abilities and when to seek appropriate help.

completed in 2009 (NCSBN, 2009c) with a new test plan initiated in 2011 (NCSBN, 2010). See Chapter 3 for a greater discussion of licensing.

Display 4.1 lists the 10 most frequent activities for new graduates recorded with the most frequent at the top in all groups. The three most frequent activities also were rated in the top 10 most important activities. Activities could be rated important that were seldom performed such as cardiopulmonary resuscitation.

In addition to looking at activities for all new graduates in general, the study also looked at activities in relationship to the care setting. Physiologic and psychosocial integrity were supported by many individual nursing actions. Some, such as assessing vital signs, seemed almost universal. Others, such as monitoring for side effects of radiation therapy, were needed in a minority of settings. Allowing clients to talk about their concerns and assisting them to communicate effectively were almost universal activities.

When recent graduates were surveyed in regard to important postgraduate competencies, they provided a wide array of competencies (NCSBN, 2009b). These were grouped into major categories of

- Juggling complex patients and assignments efficiently
- Intervening for subtle shifts in patients' condition or families' responses
- Possessing interpersonal skills of calm, compassion, generosity, and authority
- Knowing how to work the system
- Demonstrating an attitude of dedicated curiosity and commitment to lifelong learning

National League for Nursing Competencies

In addition to the NCSBN, other organizations have explored the issue of competencies of new nursing graduates. The various educational councils that were previously a part of the NLN structure developed statements regarding competencies of new graduates during the late 1970 through the 1980s.

In 1990, the Council of Associate Degree Programs of the NLN CADP approved a revised set of competencies for the associate degree graduate (NLN, 1990). This clarification of the

DISPLAY 4.1 **Top 10 Nursing Activities Rank Ordered by Average Total Group Frequency**

*Apply principles of infection control (eg, hand hygiene, room assignment, isolation, aseptic/sterile technique, universal/standard precautions)
*Provide care within the legal scope of practice
*Ensure proper identification of client when providing care
Practices in a manner consistent with a code of ethics for registered nurses
Prepare and administer medications, using rights of medication administration
Prioritize workload to manage time effectively
Use approved abbreviations and standard terminology when documenting care
Maintain client confidentiality/privacy
Provide individualized/client-centered care consistent with Standards of Practice
Review pertinent data prior to medication administration (eg, vital signs, lab results, allergies, potential interactions)

*Items also listed in the 10 most important actions (NCSBN, 2009c)

role of the associate degree graduate as provider of care, manager of care, and member of the profession continues to guide the development of many associate degree nursing curricula. All educational councils were eliminated in restructuring of the NLN. In 2010, after a great deal of study and work, the NLN developed a comprehensive statement of the expected outcomes and competencies of each level of nursing education from practical/vocational through the research doctorate in nursing (NLN, 2010.) This document is expected to have wide-reaching influence in nursing education.

Competencies Expressed by Other Groups

In 1998, the American Association of Colleges of Nursing (AACN) developed a document titled, *Essentials of Baccalaureate Education for Professional Nursing Practice,* which was updated in 2008 (AACN, 2008). This document identifies essentials for education that are aimed at developing the competencies needed (see Chapter 2). Additionally, some states have developed statements of competencies for graduates of the nursing programs in those states. This often has been part of a process to improve articulation between programs at different levels.

Similarities and patterns have emerged from all of these statements. The outline of theoretic knowledge and functioning regarding the nursing process seems to be the most consistent. The most divergent opinions seem to be in the area of specific skill or task competency.

Employers' Expectations Regarding Competencies

Employers often ask for further clarification of competence. Does competence mean that the new graduate can function independently, or will some supervision still be needed? Further complicating the picture is the confusion surrounding competencies of the graduates of the three types of nursing education programs that prepare individuals for RN licensure (see Chapter 2). Although statements by several organizations have distinguished among levels of functioning, many employers do not differentiate expectations. Some employers state that new graduates from different types of programs have not clearly demonstrated differences in competencies.

What is expected of the new graduate varies across healthcare agencies and geographic areas. The acuity of the client care load and the types of services offered by an agency also may affect expectations. The Joint Commission has a criterion requiring that accredited institutions monitor and ensure the competence of their staff. This requires that an institution identify expected competencies for staff and then design an assessment method. As institutions move to comply with this standard, most direct their initial efforts toward technical skills because these are more easily identified and assessed. Other competencies are more difficult to assess.

Some general patterns of expectations can be seen:

1. **Possess the necessary theoretic background for safe client care and for decision making.** For example, the new graduate should understand the signs and symptoms of an insulin reaction, recognize the reaction when it occurs, and know what nursing actions to take. The new graduate must know when an emergency or complication occurs and secure medical help for the client. Many employers believe that new graduates today are very competent in their theoretic foundations for practice.

2. **Use the nursing process in a systematic way.** This includes assessment, analysis, planning, intervention, and evaluation. As noted previously, a large percentage of the new graduates' time is spent in activities they would describe as using the steps of the nursing process. New graduates should be able to develop plans of care and follow plans, such as care pathways, that have been developed by the agency.

3. **Recognize own abilities and limitations.** To provide safe care, the nurse must identify when a situation requires greater expertise or knowledge and when assistance is needed. Employers may be able to assist if nurses ask for help and direction but cannot accept the risk to clients created by nurses who do not know or accept their own limitations.

4. **Use communication skills effectively with clients and coworkers.** In every setting, there are clients and families who are anxious, depressed, suffering loss, angry, or experiencing other emotional distress. The nurse is expected to respond appropriately to these individuals and to facilitate their coping and adaptation. Effective communication skills are essential to the functioning of the entire interdisciplinary healthcare team. Often, the nurse is expected to help coordinate the work of others, and this cannot be done without effective communication skills.

5. **Work effectively with assistive personnel, delegating and supervising nursing care tasks in an appropriate manner.** In most settings, assistive personnel are a part of the nursing team. The RN, and in some instances the PN, is expected to identify which nursing activities can be delegated and do so in a way that contributes to appropriate patient care outcomes.

6. **Provide accurate and complete documentation.** Employers generally recognize that the new graduate must be given time to learn the documentation system used in the facility. However, the new graduate is expected to recognize the need for recording data. It is anticipated that the nurse will keep accurate, grammatically correct, and legible written records and complete electronic records that provide the necessary legal documentation of care.

7. **Possess proficiency in the basic technical nursing skills.** This is an area in which a wide variety of expectations may be present. In most settings, proficiency in the basic skills required to support activities of daily living is expected. In some settings, nurses will carry out these tasks, whereas in others they will direct or teach others, such as nursing assistants or family members, to do them. The technical skills or tasks that are reserved for the RN represent the area of widest diversity in the identification of essential skills. The settings in which nurses practice are wide-ranging, and the technical skills needed in one setting may not be required in another. Often, employers are flexible in their expectations, so that it may be acceptable if an individual seems to have competency in a reasonable percentage of the skills required by that agency. Also, there may be a difference between what the employer would wish and what the employer will accept.

8. **Possess basic skills in information technology.** Nurses of today must be able to learn and navigate the computer system in use in a particular facility, manage email communication, seek information resources to support evidence-based care, and use electronic medical records.

In addition to these professional responsibilities performed as a nurse, employers also speak of their concern for worker-related competencies they want to see in all healthcare workers. These include the following:

1. **Demonstrate a commitment to a work ethic.** This means that the employee will take the responsibility of the job seriously and will be on time, take only the allowed coffee and lunch breaks, and will not take sick days unless truly ill. It also means that the new graduate recognizes that nurses may be needed 24 hours a day, 365 days a year, and that this may require sacrifices of personal convenience, including working evening shifts or on holidays.

2. **Function with acceptable speed.** This is another area in which expectations differ greatly. Generally, an orientation period is planned—although, with the pressures on healthcare agencies, this often has been shortened considerably. An acceptable speed of function is reflected by the ability to carry out a typical RN assignment within a shift.

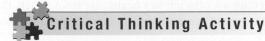

Critical Thinking Activity

Compare your nursing program outcomes with the new graduate expectations. How are they similar, how different? What is the difference in the language used to describe competencies? Translate or interpret the language of your school outcomes to the language found in the NCSBN information.

PERSONAL CAREER GOALS

In caring for clients, you are involved in the process of goal setting. Many nurses recognize the value of this in client care but never transfer the concept to their personal lives. Nursing as a profession offers many career options. Without carefully setting goals, your professional growth may be impeded. As well as the information here, you may want to explore the Web sites listed on The Point that relate to personal goal setting.

Focusing Your Goals

You may want to focus on a broad area of clinical competency, such as pediatric nursing, or on a more restricted area, such as neonatal care. Clinical areas available for concentrated effort become more varied as healthcare becomes more complex. Most of these areas offer certification to individuals who possess the expertise and pass the examinations. Many individuals focus their careers on particular client populations without ever seeking formal certification in that field. However, there may be advantages in terms of salary and recognition to holding specialty certification.

Opportunities for additional education and certification in most clinical specialties are available for any experienced RN, although some require that the individual have a bachelor's or master's degree in nursing. Some specialty positions are in advanced practice, such as the woman's healthcare specialist, the family nurse practitioner, and the pediatric nurse practitioner. These advanced practice specialties require a master's degree for certification. Although some educational programs preparing advanced practice nurses require the bachelor's degree in nursing for entry, many will accept an individual with an ADN combined with a bachelor's degree in another field.

Another approach may be to focus your goals on the setting in which care is delivered, such as acute, long-term, or community care. As healthcare needs expand, these separate realms of care delivery all demand more specialized knowledge. Even within the individual area of focus, differences are present. For example, within the community are ambulatory care settings, public health nursing agencies, occupational health nursing departments, and day care facilities.

Another way of focusing your goals is according to functional categories. Although nurses are initially thought of as direct care providers, they also are needed in many other positions. For example, there is need for those who would move into supervisory and administrative capacities, those who teach, and those who conduct nursing research. Additional education supports the ability to advance into these fields. Nursing also lends itself to writing, community service, and even political involvement.

You may decide to set your goals in relation to all three foci. That is, you might identify a clinical area, care setting, and functional category.

Setting Your Goals

The first step in setting personal career goals is a thorough self-assessment. Determine how your abilities and competencies correspond to your own expectations and to those of employers. Other factors to explore are your likes and dislikes and the situations or types of work you particularly enjoyed as a student. Consider the area in which you were most successful. Were there areas in which you or your instructor felt that you were an above-average student? Consider your health and personal characteristics in relation to types of work. Do you have physical restrictions? Do you prefer working independently or with others? How do you respond to close supervision or to freedom in the job setting? Do you prefer a work environment that is relatively predictable, or do you thrive in situations that change frequently? Do you work well with long-term goals and a few immediate reinforcements, or do you need to see results quickly? Another factor to consider is your own geographic mobility: would you be willing to move or travel as part of a job? Both your personal responsibilities and preferences operate in this arena.

As you plan ahead, examine many of the options offered by nursing. What types of jobs and opportunities are open to you? What education and personal abilities are needed in these areas? Are you interested? Does the education you have meet the educational requirements? Are avenues for additional education available to you? All of these considerations are important as you plan for the future. Career goals need to be both short- and long-term. They will help you to plan your future constructively. This does not mean that goals are static. Just as client goals must be realistic, personal, and flexible, so must your own goals.

Short-term goals encompass what you want to accomplish this month and this year. What do you want to do and what do you want to be in the immediate future? For example, you might decide that your short-term goal is to have 2 years of solid experience in a busy metropolitan hospital.

Long-term goals represent where you want to be in your profession 5 or more years from now. A long-term goal may be to work in a small, remote community in which you will have the opportunity to function autonomously.

COMMUNICATION IN ACTION

Planning for Short- and Long-Term Goals

John Wilson and Richard Martin were both in the final term of their bachelor's degree program. They were making plans about job applications. John said, "I am not sure what to do. I really want to work in public health, but a lot of people have been telling me that I have to have a couple of years of basic med-surg before even considering that and public health is more of a long-term goal. What do you think?" Richard replied, "I am not sure about that. My goal is intensive care, and a year of general med-surg seems good to me. I think I need to get my assessment skills and my organizational abilities firm before I take on intensive care. I have already begun applying with that in mind. However, I don't think you should just put your goal for public health aside. I remember my clinical instructor in public health told us that the necessary 2 years of med-surg was an old-fashioned myth." John responded, "Wow—I had not heard that perspective. Maybe I should check it out with the public health department before I make a decision. Thanks for the input."

Although both long- and short-term goals will be revised as your life evolves, they guide you in making day-to-day decisions more effectively. In today's world of rapid healthcare change, you may need to keep your goals somewhat broad and flexible. Be ready to consider alternative goals and a variety of pathways to one goal. These approaches will be of value as you enter a system in transition (Fig. 4.2).

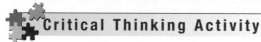

Critical Thinking Activity

Write out your short- and long-term professional goals, with a brief plan on how you can achieve these goals. Think critically about the obstacles you will need to overcome to reach these goals. How will you deal with the obstacles?

Maintaining and Enhancing Your Competence

Included in your goal setting should be an approach to maintaining and enhancing your competence. Every nurse has an obligation to society to maintain competence and continue practicing high-quality, safe care. Most state boards of nursing have identified a mechanism for identifying continued competence for ongoing practice. Some of the most common ways are through work as an RN, through reflective practice, through continuing education, and through self-directed study.

Practicing as an RN keeps you up-to-date and provides you the opportunity to learn new technology, to see new procedures, and to care for complex clients requiring critical thinking and decision-making skills. Most employers provide in-service education in regard to policies and procedures to enhance your competence. Maintaining and enhancing competence through practice requires that you focus your critical thinking on your own development as a nurse. You may develop the habit of reflective practice for this purpose. In reflective practice, you take the time to debrief after incidents and go back over the

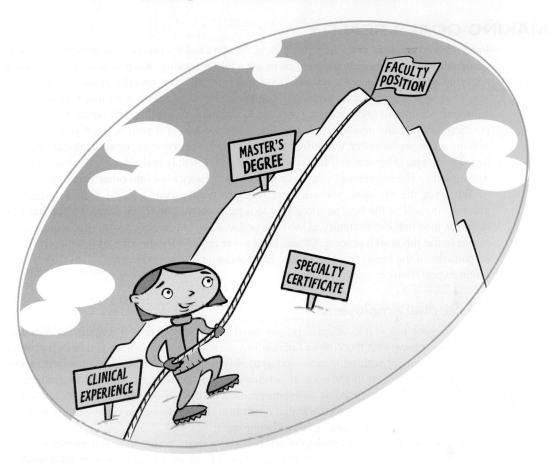

FIGURE 4.2 Clearly visualizing goals helps you to achieve them.

situation identifying what went well and what needed improvement. This may be done in a group or independently. Reflective practice is often enhanced by keeping a journal in which you write down your reflections (being sure to eliminate any personally identifiable health information regarding patients). Thus, you move your own practice forward improving your own competence. You may set goals for your own learning and professional development.

Continuing education may occur through many kinds of workshops and conferences, as well as by completing online or in-person classes. Computer instruction programs and examinations related to journal articles may be completed on your own time frame. Self-directed study may involve subscribing to and reading journals, participating in a journal club, or researching web information. Some nurses may want to advance through specialty or higher education. Any of these avenues may be appropriate, depending on the circumstances.

MAKING GOALS REALITY

Philosophic questions regarding goals must be resolved by practical approaches. As a new graduate, your first goal simply may be to get a job in nursing. Keep in mind that you are not applying only for an entry-level job. If you have identified a specific clinical area in which you wish to work, a specific employer you prefer, or a long-term goal that requires moving from one position to another, then you need to do those things that will obtain your preferred position, not just any position. Additionally, when applying for your first job you also may be making an impression that will affect later promotions or requests for educational opportunities. Those who interview you for an entry-level position may make decisions about future job assignments. The impression you make initially will carry over into other situations.

Whatever the situation, you are more likely to realize your goals if you are prepared to present yourself in the best possible way to a prospective employer. Many of you have held different jobs in the community as students and as adults. You may be familiar with and competent in the job search process. Others have never applied for the kind of job that truly could be considered the beginning of a career. Employers and prospective employees may hold different expectations in such a situation.

Identifying Potential Employers

To begin your job search effectively, you need to identify potential employers. You might begin your review with those more familiar to you, such as those where you have had clinical experiences during your education, and gradually move outward in an ever-widening circle to identify others. You might network with instructors, colleagues, and fellow graduates for opportunities. If you worked as an employee in a healthcare setting before graduation, you may be given preference in hiring at that institution. This is one reason for seeking healthcare employment during your nursing education process.

Job fairs for healthcare employers are becoming more common. Each employer participating sets up a booth or table to provide information on job openings in its agency. An individual looking for employment may explore a variety of employers, learning about job openings, benefits, and opportunities in a brief time without the difficulty of searching out each employer. The employer may see many potential employees in a focused period. Thus, job fairs benefit both employers and potential employees. Job fairs may be held in the community, attracting experienced healthcare workers as well as students and new graduates. Some colleges arrange job fairs on campus. Nursing programs or nursing student clubs also may arrange job fairs. When attending a job fair, prepare and dress as if you going to an interview (see below). Prospective employers begin to form their impression of you at the job fair.

A prominent source of potential jobs is the Internet. Many government job openings are posted online. An online search may reveal the names of nursing employers in your area as well as those at other locations of interest to you. If you do not have personal online access, use the computers at your local library. Using a search engine, look for "employment opportunities," "jobs," or "careers" combined with the term "nursing." Some online service providers have additional support services for a job search that might include career guidance (for a fee) or sample documents such as résumés and letters of application.

Major nursing journals have sections in the back pages devoted to advertisements. Some of these advertise nursing positions. Sometimes an entire issue is devoted to a specific geographic area. This provides the ability to do a quick overview of possible employers. Your nursing program may receive advertising magazines that are designed to present job opportunities for new graduates. These magazines provide a few articles about relevant job search topics, such as interviewing, as well as advertisements from healthcare agencies. These advertisements present information on the agency itself and how to make contact for an application.

Another source of potential jobs is the classified section of the local newspaper. There you are more likely to find single jobs in small facilities, as well as general recruitment announcements from larger facilities. However, just because an agency fails to advertise does not mean it will not be hiring any employees. Advertising is expensive and may not result in the desired outcome. Therefore, some healthcare agencies do not advertise and rely on those who independently seek them out as potential employers.

In areas of the country where jobs are very scarce for new graduates, unpaid nursing internships have been developed. These provide job experience to enhance the new graduate's skills and abilities and increase the potential for hiring.

Letter of Application

Writing a **letter of application** is an excellent way to approach many prospective employers (Display 4.2). This letter is often termed a **cover letter** because it is sent with your résumé. You can present yourself positively through a well-written letter. Some question the value of the cover letter; however, employment experts support the use of cover letters saying that an effective cover letter forges a connection with the employer and can set you apart from other applicants. The cover letter should package your résumé so that it will get more than just a glance. It provides the opportunity for you to reveal a bit of your personality and connects your experience to the position's requirements.

Before you write your letter, make sure you have information about the prospective employer. What kind of facility is this? What types of clients does it serve, and what special services does it offer? It makes a poor impression to write to a prospective employer stating that your goal is to work in pediatrics when that facility does not provide any pediatric services. Many agencies maintain a Web site with information regarding their mission, goals, and services. You might also obtain this information by calling the human resources department of the facility or by contacting a public information office. In a small agency, you may simply speak with a receptionist or secretary. If you call for information, be honest and straightforward in explaining that you are considering applying for employment and would like information about the agency before making that decision. The letter is sent to the nurse recruiter (if the agency has one) or to the human resources department along with your résumé. If you are not sure to whom to address your letter, check the agency's Web site or ask when you call to inquire about the agency itself.

Another part of your advance planning is identifying how you will focus your letter on your special qualifications and what you want to highlight. Focus on the skills or accomplishments related to the position you want. Your letter should be no more than one page in length, but should present all essential information. Introduce yourself and your purpose for writing in the first paragraph so that the reader immediately understands why you are writing. You may want to state briefly your reasons for applying for a position with this particular employer. The more specific the reasons, the better the impression you are likely to make.

DISPLAY 4.2   Letter of Application

Maribeth Wilson
3428 1st Ave. N.
Seattle, WA 98103
(206) 274-5978
E-mail: maribethw@email.com

May 20, 2010

Joyce Montgall, R.N.
Nurse Recruiter
Seattle General Medical Center
321 Heath Blvd.
Seattle, WA 98101

Dear Ms. Montgall:

Enclosed please find a copy of my résumé, along with my application to Seattle General Medical Center's New Graduate Residency Program. I will graduate from Shoreline Community College's associate degree nursing program on June 8, 2011. I expect to acquire my registered nurse license by the end of July. I am extremely interested in a medical-surgical nursing position within your upcoming residency program.

I believe that I would bring many strengths to a new graduate position. I have worked here at Seattle General as a nursing assistant for the past year, and my experience has given me an excellent foundation in understanding the philosophy and mission of the Medical Center. During this time I have been assigned to several different units, including 4 West and 4 Center, where new graduate positions are available. The nurses at Seattle General have been generous in their mentoring and have helped me to increase my understanding of the patients' conditions. They have been supportive as I developed increased problem-solving and decision-making skills. I am familiar with the documentation system and the policies of the institution.

Within my nursing student educational experience, I have had the privilege of working in a wide variety of healthcare institutions throughout the city. From these experiences I would bring an understanding of the community standards of care as well as a unique appreciation of the position of Seattle General in the healthcare community.

I hope that I will be selected for an interview and look forward to hearing from you. My phone number, e-mail address, and home address are at the top of this letter. I am available most afternoons. If I do not hear from you within the next 2 weeks, I will contact your office to ascertain the status of my application.

Sincerely,

Maribeth Wilson

Use the body of the letter to briefly highlight your qualifications for the position. This should not be a simple recitation of what is in your résumé, but should either present the information in a slightly different light or add pertinent detail that is not in the résumé. If you are responding to an advertisement, touch on each of the qualifications listed in the advertisement. You might include personal qualities that would make you an effective employee in the position, such as interest in learning and skill in teamwork. Relate your skills and abilities to the needs of this particular agency. If your healthcare experience is limited, point out skills you have gained from other jobs that would be useful in nursing. These might be interpersonal skills, management skills, or adaptability.

In the final paragraph, make a summary statement indicating why you want to work for this employer and ask for an appointment for an interview. Be sure to indicate the times you are available and how and where you can be contacted if the employer so wishes. It also is wise to indicate that you will contact the person to whom the letter is addressed to request an appointment. This allows you to maintain some initiative in the process. Thank the person for considering your application, and close.

Another point to remember is that the letter's appearance and its content both represent you. You will be judged on spelling, grammar, clarity, and neatness, in addition to content. Be cautious about relying on the spell-checking function on your computer. An incorrect word may pass the spell-check but be clearly seen as an error by the careful reader. Your letter of application should be written in standard business format on plain white or off-white business paper. Make it brief and clear. Ask a friend or family member to check your first draft if you have any questions about its correctness.

▶ *EXAMPLE*

Seeking Information Regarding a Potential Employer

Joseph Williams will be graduating from a basic nursing program in 3 months. He has decided he would be interested in applying to a hospital in the state capital. He wants to move to a larger community and be in an institution where research is being conducted, advanced technology is used, and nurses have a voice in the operation of the institution. Through a Web search using the name of the city and "hospitals," he obtains a list of hospitals. He saves the search for future access and begins linking to each of the hospitals. On the hospital sites, he reads the mission statement and any other general information about the hospital. He reviews the services that they describe and narrows his exploration to those that mention research. He notes that one hospital prominently displays that it has achieved designation as a Magnet hospital. He links to the human resources page to gather information about applying for a job in each institution that interests him. In some institutions, a link to a nurse recruiter is found prominently displayed, but in others, there is no indication of a specific nurse recruiter. He decides to start his personal contacts with the nurse recruiter at the Magnet hospital.

Critical Thinking Activity

Identify an area of the country and type of nursing position that interests you. Using the various Internet resources, learn about job availability, salaries, and working conditions for at least three employers in that area. Determine which of the three would be of most interest to you and provide a brief rationale for why you would choose that employer.

Preparing an Effective Résumé

A **résumé** is a brief overview of your qualifications for a position. Its purpose is to present you in the most positive light to be considered for the position in which you are interested and to provide the employer with a way to identify quickly whether you have the basic qualifications for a position. Résumés are used primarily to screen applicants for interviewing; therefore, you will want to make a good impression that will result in an interview. You will want to include your résumé with your initial letter. In addition, have copies of your résumé to take with you to any interview or appointment. You may want to leave a copy of your résumé with a unit manager at the end of an interview because your original résumé may be retained in the human resources office. Résumés may be posted online by job search sites. If posting online, check on the privacy policies of the site. Use care in what you place in an online résumé for your own safety. Often you will not include personally identifying information, but rather a code from the job site.

Appearance of Your Résumé

The appearance of your résumé is important because it initially presents your image to the prospective employer. You want its appearance to reflect a competent, professional image. It is not necessary to have a professionally produced résumé. Nursing employers, when asked, have indicated that it neither adds to nor detracts from their impression to read a résumé that has been produced by some professional printing method. The important point is that it be a somewhat formal, standard, informative document that is neat and without errors.

Your résumé should be on standard-sized (8.5″ × 11″), white or off-white, good-quality paper so that it is easy to handle, file, and read. A résumé that is individually printed (or reproduced well enough so that it appears to be) usually will be received more positively than an obvious photocopy. You will find it valuable to create a résumé and save it to a disk. In this way, you will be able to revise it easily, and you may even be able to tailor it to an individual job situation. In addition to the capabilities of standard word processing software (which usually include résumé templates), there are inexpensive software programs especially designed to facilitate the production of a well-organized and formatted résumé.

To achieve legibility, use sufficient margins (usually 1″), spacing, indentation, bullets, and even line separators to separate different sections and topics. You might want to underline or italicize related items or bold print or highlight important items to draw swift attention. A résumé looks better when the content is evenly balanced on a page. Dense paragraphs do not attract the reader, but lists and topics do. Use capital letters, bold font, and underlining to draw the reader's eye to what you want that individual to notice first, but be careful not to overdo this approach. When an employer is reviewing many such documents, anything that facilitates review and makes you stand out is an advantage. Often the use of bullets helps to break up the tedium of words. Ask individuals you trust to review the appearance of your résumé and identify those areas that first caught their attention. This helps you to evaluate its appearance.

If your résumé will be sent or posted online, consider how that will affect the appearance. Special fonts or nonstandard résumé programs may not transfer effectively into the online environment. A job site will provide directions for a posted résumé. If your résumé is to be sent as an attachment to an e-mail, then it should be composed in a common word processing program such as Microsoft Word or in rich text format (.rtf). You might check with the receiving human resources department as to its preference for format.

Traditionally, applicants have been advised to keep résumés to one page if possible although an online résumé may be longer than one page. To develop a one-page résumé, consider how you might most effectively present employment history. However, more important in today's market is that the information supports your candidacy for the position you are seeking and thus may be more than a single page.

Content of Your Résumé

The content of your résumé is critical. When you are beginning the preparation of a résumé, first list the information that you want to include in some way. Making such a list before beginning the process of actually formatting a résumé helps you to take an organized approach and not forget to include important information. If you will be submitting a résumé online, this process should include identifying specific key words that you want to include within the résumé. Often employers search online résumés using key words that pertain to the type of position they have available or specific skills and abilities that are needed in the position. If your résumé does not contain these key words, it will not be identified as relevant to the employer.

A standard résumé always begins with your name, address, and telephone number (including area code). If you will be moving, indicate the date the move will be effective and provide an alternate method of contacting you after that date. You may use the address of a permanently settled relative or friend. Employers are not permitted to ask about age, race, religion, marital status, and dependents (and in some jurisdictions, sexual orientation), and you do not need to include this information. An e-mail address is helpful to employers. However, if your e-mail address is an informal phrase, plan to set up a separate e-mail address for business use. This can be done for no cost through one of several Internet mail providers such as Gmail, Yahoo, or Hotmail. Use a simple derivation from your name that creates a professional impression. One final comment regarding content: be certain that it is accurate. You may be checked on what you say in your résumé so truthfulness is always the best bet.

Objective. Many résumés include a personal goal or objective. This is helpful to a recruiter or human resources department that considers many different occupations within the agency. The objective immediately alerts the reader to the type of position being sought. This may include both a short-term goal such as "employment as a beginning registered nurse" and a long-term goal such as "with eventual move to employment in coronary care." You may wish to write an objective that is tailored to a specific employer or job announcement. When you are more experienced, you may want to make your objective more specific to a particular department or role (see Display 4.4 for an example).

Some career advisors today are suggesting a statement of what you can provide for the employer is more effective than an objective that focuses on your own goals. It should show the employer how they can benefit from hiring you, how you can make a contribution. This statement should focus on what you can do rather than on what you want. This must be done very succinctly so as to quickly catch the attention of the individual reading the résumé. The remainder of the résumé should reinforce this first impression (see Display 4.5 for an example).

Credentials. Include information regarding your licensure and other credentials. Indicate the date your license will be effective and whether you have a temporary permit to work as a nurse. Your nursing license or permit number should be listed after you have received it. If you do not have a license at the time you are preparing your résumé, you may choose to include information about when you expect to have your license in your letter of application.

Education. Educational background should form a separate section and cover your nursing education and any specialized courses or postgraduate work you have completed. It is appropriate to note any college-level work. Do not include high school information. In each group of information, list the most recent items first.

Employment History. Work experience is of critical importance, and you should provide a meaningful employment history. If using a traditional format, for each job you held include employer, address (city and state are sufficient), dates employed, position, and duties. List the most recent employer first and follow with the remaining information in reverse chronological order. The prospective employer will be especially interested in a previous nursing assistant position or any other position that demonstrates your knowledge of or experience in some area of healthcare or the assumption of responsibility. Other positions also may be important if you are clearly able to identify skills used in those settings that are transferable to nursing.

If you have had only one or two part-time jobs during your educational program, it would be appropriate to include them in detail. However, if during your educational program you held 15 part-time jobs, for example, it is appropriate to list only significant ones that offered valuable experience.

Focus on accomplishments and use active verbs to describe skills. These give life to your résumé and create interest in the reader. See the accompanying display for a list of active verbs you might use in describing your skills and abilities (Display 4.3). If you were part of a team that accomplished a significant project or task, you might indicate that. However, be careful not to take personal credit for team accomplishments. If you are responding to a specific job announcement, be sure that your résumé reflects the education and skills that are noted.

In a position-focused résumé, you can emphasize the responsibilities you had within each position. See Display 4.4 for an example of a position-focused résumé. You might also highlight specific experiences in an area that especially relates to the position for which you are applying. For example, you might have had a senior leadership practicum on an orthopedic unit—this would be particularly relevant to an application for a nursing position in orthopedics. If you had a practicum in the facility or agency to which you are applying, indicate this in some way. Your familiarity with its policies and procedures will be a valuable asset. If you attended any special workshops, include those in a separate section. Information included in this part of the résumé can be used to demonstrate your ability to meet deadlines, produce good work, and relate to people in ambiguous situations. Use numbers when possible to describe achievements. For example, if you previously worked evenings in a long-term care facility as an LPN, you might state, "Supervised five nursing assistants" or "Administered all medications to 30 patients per shift." Be sure to include language proficiency if you are fluent in more than English. Computer literacy is also a valuable skill.

DISPLAY 4.3 Power Verbs for Résumés

- Use of verbs without subjects will be more concise and space conserving.
- Use of active, not passive, voice, such as "advanced to" rather than "was promoted to," "earned" rather than "was given," indicates a person who does things rather than receives them.
- Use of "-ed" or "-ing" as verb endings can both be effective.

Accompanied	Directed	Inspired	Processed
Achieved	Discovered	Installed	Procured
Acquired	Displayed	Instructed	Produced
Activated	Doubled	Insured	Progressed
Administered	Earned	Integrated	Promoted
Advanced to	Educated	Intensified	Prompted
Advised	Employed	Interviewed	Proposed
Analyzed	Enacted	Invented	Proved
Arranged	Encouraged	Led	Provided
Assembled	Engineered	Located	Reconciled
Assessed	Established	Maintained	Reduced
Assisted	Evaluated	Managed	Regulated
Balanced	Executed	Marketed	Related
Budgeted	Exhibited	Mastered	Reorganized
Clarified	Expanded	Mediated	Reported
Composed	Facilitated	Motivated	Represented
Conceived	Financed	Negotiated	Researched
Concluded	Formalized	Nominated	Satisfied
Conducted	Formed	Obtained	Secured
Constructed	Formulated	Officiated	Served
Consulted	Founded	Operated	Simplified
Controlled	Generated	Ordered	Solved
Converted	Governed	Organized	Structured
Coordinated	Graduated	Originated	Succeeded
Counseled	Headed	Overcame	Supervised
Created	Identified	Participated	Trained
Decided	Implemented	Perceived	Transferred
Delegated	Improved	Perfected	Transformed
Demonstrated	Improvised	Performed	Unified
Designed	Increased	Piloted	Verified
Detailed	Induced	Pioneered	Won
Determined	Influenced	Placed	Wrote
Developed	Informed	Planned	
Devised	Initiated	Prepared	
Diagnosed	Innovated	Presided	

You may choose a more skill-focused résumé and not include details of all your previous positions separately. For individuals who are older and have an extensive employment history, a résumé providing types of positions with a focus on related skills rather than a chronologic list of employers is often the most effective. List a position such as LPN and include respon-sibilities and skills for all employers followed by a simple list of employers. This keeps the résumé from becoming repetitive as the same information is presented for each employer. See Display 4.5 for an example of a skill-focused employment section.

 DISPLAY 4.4   Position-Focused Résumé of a Recent Graduate

Sarah Mitchell
5714 31st Ave. N.
Seattle, WA 98117
(206) 555-0000
E-mail: sarahmit@email.com

Objective

A beginning Registered Nurse position that will provide the opportunity for professional development and advancement toward critical care nursing.

Overall qualifications: Possesses a positive, energetic approach to working collaboratively with others, solving problems, and providing evidence-based, patient-centered nursing care.

Experience

2009–present   Seattle General Medical Center   Seattle, WA

Patient Care Technician, Medical-Surgical Units

• Provide basic care and ADLs with attention to psychosocial needs for acutely ill medical-surgical patients.
• Assist RN with procedures and carry out delegated duties.
• Work collaboratively with nursing team, assuring prompt response to patient needs.
• Effectively manage time to support seven patients on evening shift.
• Document care on computerized system, maintaining accuracy, and confidentiality.

2007–2009   Health Choice Urgent Care Center   Seattle, WA

Nursing Technician, Urgent Care Clinic

• Interviewed clients, took vital signs, initiated documentation, and prioritized care for urgently ill and injured adults and children.
• Under RN supervision, performed assessments, dressing changes, ECGs, nebulizer treatments, and hospital admission processes.
• Attended to psychosocial needs of family and others accompanying a sick or injured individual.
• 2005–2007 First United Bank Lynnwood, WA.

Bank Teller

• Maintained excellent customer service by following detailed bank policies and procedures.
• Utilized a variety of computerized systems to assure accurate and detailed documentation of all activities.
• Incorporated information from employee training classes into job skills to assure up-to-date function.

Education

2008–2011   Shoreline Community College   Seattle, WA

AAAS Nursing, to be Awarded June, 2011

DISPLAY 4.5   Skill Focused Résumé of a Recent Graduate

Joseph M. Sanchez
1298 Avenida Diaz
La Quinta, CA 92252
(619) 524-4321

Objective
An opportunity to provide excellent, customer-focused care using evidence-based practice and contributing to Main Medical Center's status as the premier hospital in the tristate region.

Skills/Accomplishments
• Work effectively in a multicultural environment.
• Communication skills: Earned award for communicating in a positive, supportive way with coworkers, clients, and families.
• Bilingual Spanish/English: Developed Spanish language instructions to assist clients.
• Collaborative/cooperative worker: Volunteered to work multiple shifts/floating positions in order to allow colleagues to meet important family needs.
• Excellent critical thinking and problem solving: Identified cost saving approaches to work processes.

Education>
College of the Desert, Palm Desert, CA
Management practicum, Desert Health Center 5-West: Working with RN preceptor, demonstrated RN level skills in managing care of a module of five acutely ill patients. Delegated care appropriately to nursing assistant. Facilitated interdisciplinary communication.
Associate in Science in Nursing, June 2011

Experience
Manor Care Center, Palm Desert, CA
Nursing Assistant, Certified: 2005–Present
• Maintained function and dignity of dependent elderly adults by providing direct care, strong interpersonal relationships, and effective collaboration with nursing and allied health.
• Earned promotion to position of mentor for new hires and team leader for a group of nursing assistants. Facilitated team performance to accomplish assigned responsibilities.
Northrup Corporation, Los Angeles, CA
Machinist: 1995–2005
• Performed precision skills with accuracy and attention to detail.
• Followed precise written protocols and procedures to ensure quality.
• Led a team in a program of total quality management within our department.

Awards
• College of the Desert Merit Scholar 2010
• Golden Acorn Award for Leadership in Parent Involvement, Cactus Valley Elementary School PTA, La Quinta, CA

Additional Experience. Volunteer or community work and awards and honors form two sections when you have these experiences. Choose the items you list under volunteer and community work carefully. Employers are interested in skills you would bring to the job that

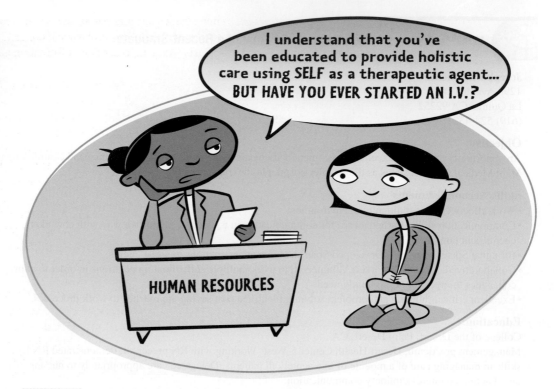

FIGURE 4.3 Employers are often interested in specific skills needed in their setting.

require decision making and the exercise of good judgment both in volunteer work and in past work experience (Fig. 4.3). In some instances, you may want to list briefly the skills or abilities gained from a particular volunteer activity just as you would for employment targeting the particular skills you think are important to the position for which you are applying. For example, you might use your volunteer experience to demonstrate past success in the skill of organization, managing or coordinating people and events, and effectively delegating responsibilities. It also might be used to highlight public relations skills: the ability to write, work within or control a budget, prioritize multiple tasks, or cope with deadlines. For some volunteer positions, you might focus on your ability to direct, coach, and teach others.

List awards, honors, and professional associations (such as the National Student Nurses' Association) that would demonstrate your competence, professional involvement, or leadership ability. This provides an opportunity to show responsibility in directing the activities of others, public speaking, and, perhaps, motivating people. You may omit this section if you feel that you have nothing pertinent to enter.

References. References are typed on a separate page and given to the prospective employer or copied onto an application form, if they are requested. Be selective in choosing the people you list as references. Consider people who know you, would be able to speak positively of you to a future employer, and would have credibility with the employer. Seek the person's permission before giving his or her name as a reference. When seeking permission to use someone as a work reference, you might outline what you would like the person to emphasize if contacted—for example: "If you are contacted, I would particularly like you to provide information about my work habits and effectiveness as an employee."

A primary reference should be an instructor from your basic educational program. This person would be able to affirm your ability in the nursing field. Some agencies request two instructor references, so be prepared for that. Another reference should be someone who has employed you and who can describe your work habits and effectiveness as an employee. If you have had any healthcare work experience, this would be the best work reference. Also look at the position in which you assumed the most responsibility. This should be reasonably recent (within the past 10 years). Again, some employers ask for two work references.

If the agency indicates the type of references they want, supply the names of references that comply with the agency's request. When types of references are not specified, include professional or work-related references only. Include full names with titles (if any), addresses, and telephone numbers, so that the employer will be able to contact the references easily.

Employers express differences of opinion about the value of a standardized letter of reference addressed "To Whom It May Concern." Some employers may consider this a useful initial presentation of your qualifications. Other employers want the reference to address the specific position needs or the qualifications outlined on a reference form. One advantage of the general letter is that you might be able to obtain this reference from a part-time faculty member or supervisor who may no longer be employed by the institution. If you do obtain this type of letter, be sure to preserve the original carefully (perhaps in a clear, plastic page protector) to show to a potential employer; you then would provide a good-quality photocopy for the employer to place in your file. Even when an employer accepts this as an initial reference, your references usually will be personally contacted as well.

Critical Thinking Activity

Create an effective résumé and at least two application/cover letters that present you as a positive addition to a nursing staff. Base these letters on two specific nursing positions you have learned about in a search of possible employers.

Completing an Application

Whether the application is online or completed in a print format, there are similarities. First, be sure that you fill in all the information requested. Do not simply write on the application form "see résumé" or leave the sections blank. Information often will be entered into a database, and the employer wants it in a standardized format. The failure to follow directions accurately is a poor reflection on your skills and abilities. If the application must be completed onsite, bring all needed information with you, including information about references and names, addresses, and dates for past employers. If it is an online application, you may need to complete it at one time and then submit it. Sometimes it is beneficial to print out the online form to be certain you have the information before starting it on the computer.

Successful Interviewing

The interview should be a two-way conversation in which you will gain as well as give information. Typically, employers have three major concerns for which they seek answers in the interview: they want to know whether you have the required knowledge and skills to do the job, whether you possess an attitude toward the job and the organization that is compatible with what they are seeking, and whether your personality and style will fit with the image the organization wishes to put forth. They are going to be interested in what you can do for them and, at this point, are often more interested in what you can do than in your opinions. They may be especially interested in your problem-solving and critical thinking skills. When planning for an employment interview, consider your appearance, your attitude and approach, and what the content of the interview will be.

Learning About Your Potential Employer

Once you know that you have gained an interview with a potential employer, learn as much about that specific position and the organization as you can. This can be done a number of ways. Review information you received when you were searching for organizations to which you would apply. Look again at information on its Web site if one exists. Be sure you have information regarding the organization's mission statement and other public pronouncements. Look especially for information on the various types of healthcare service the institution provides. If possible, contact current employees. Check local newspapers for information regarding the facility.

Preparing Your Questions for the Interviewer

Think through the situation before going to the interview and outline information that you want to obtain and questions that you want answered. It is helpful to write out your questions so that they are clearly stated, and so that you do not forget items while in the tense atmosphere that often exists in an interview situation; for example, "How and when will I learn of your decision?"

Time spent reflecting on your personal views in advance will be valuable for the interview. Remember that an interview is a chance to sell yourself to an employer, a chance to present yourself as a valuable addition to their nursing staff, and an opportunity to determine how you will fit into that work setting. A question such as "Please tell me about the educational opportunities that would be available to me," indicates an interest in learning.

Dressing for the Interview

The minute you walk in the door, people start making assumptions about you. How you dress plays a significant role in this aspect of job seeking. You need to make a conscious decision about the impression you want to create through your attire. Your personal appearance and demeanor may make a significant difference in whether you are offered a position.

Consider what you would like the interviewer's response to be and choose your attire with that in mind. This means that what you wear when applying for one type of job might be different when applying for another type of job. And you don't always know who you will be talking with—someone fairly conservative or someone with an informal approach. Being neat and well-groomed is always essential. In most instances, such as applying for a position at a hospital, you would wear business-like clothing, such as dress pants or skirt and shirt or blouse or sweater, or a suit or dress. If you were applying for a position in a walk-in healthcare clinic that offered services to persons who are uncomfortable in a traditional environment, it might be appropriate to wear more casual clothing, such as khaki trousers and a polo shirt with a collar. Never appear at a job site wearing leisure or sports clothing such as attire with a bare midriff, shorts, athletic attire, body piercing jewelry other than the earlobe, pants with holes in the legs, or flip-flops. Avoid the use of strong cologne or perfume. Most interviewers indicate that being more business-like in dress is never a mistake, while being too casual is a frequent mistake.

In all instances, your hair should be clean and neatly styled. Do not chew gum while in the interview. If you smoke, avoid smoking immediately before the interview so that the odor of smoke is not apparent on your clothes or person.

Today many people have tattoos and piercings. They can be limiting when seeking a job. It is advisable to remove jewelry from obvious pierced locations other than earrings (which should not be elaborate) and to wear clothing that covers tattoos. Jewelry should be conservative and limited in amount. You want the attention to be on you and what you have to say rather than focused on the jewelry you are wearing.

Things to Take With You

Take several copies of your résumé with you to the interview. You may want to refer to it or you may find it appropriate to leave a copy with someone. In addition, be prepared with the names, addresses, and telephone numbers of all references, as well as your Social Security card and photo identification. If you should be offered a position, you will need these last two items to complete employment forms. If you have received your nursing license, take that with you or in states with a paperless system, have your license number. Take along a black pen to fill out any forms, and a note pad with your questions listed and a place to make personal notes of important information obtained during the interview. You might want to purchase a special job interview hard-backed folder that will hold materials in a pocket on one side, has a notepad on the other, has a place for a pen, and will be a surface upon which you can write. You do not want to infringe on an interviewer's space by using that person's desk to take notes. Having all the information and supplies you need with you can increase your self-confidence if you have forms to fill out or if questions about statements on your résumé arise during the interview.

Arriving at the Interview

Plan to arrive at an interview early. This gives you time to check your appearance and focus your thoughts. If you carry a cell phone, turn it off before the interview. Having it ring in the middle of the interview is disrespectful to the interviewer.

Your manner during the interview is important also. It has been said that a first impression is made in the initial 10 seconds of contact. Although the employer expects an applicant to be nervous, he or she will be interested in whether your nervousness makes you unable to respond appropriately. Follow common rules of courtesy. Greet your interviewer with a smile and firm handshake and establish eye contact and maintain it throughout the interview. Making and maintaining eye contact communicates confidence and honesty—two important characteristics employers value. Wait to be asked to sit down before you take a chair. Do not put anything of yours on the interviewer's desk other than your résumé. Avoid any distracting mannerisms, such as chewing gum or fussing with your hair, face, or clothes. Nervousness often causes people to fidget, bounce their feet, or drum their fingers; be careful to avoid these behaviors. Sit up straight, as slouching communicates a message of disinterest. Be serious when appropriate, but do not forget to smile and be pleasant. The interviewer is also thinking of your impact on clients, visitors, and other staff members.

Anticipating Interview Questions

When you prepare your responses, try to anticipate possible questions from the interviewer. To do this, you must know the role of the person conducting the interview; for example, your first interview might be with a human resources department employee, not a nursing department representative. If you are successful at this stage, you might be recommended for an interview in the nursing department. Each might ask different types of questions.

Role-playing an interview situation with a friend or relative may help you to feel more confident in your responses. Another technique is to visualize the interview situation in your mind and mentally rehearse responses to questions.

An interview usually covers a wide variety of subjects. The interviewer may direct the flow of topics or may encourage you to bring up the ones that concern you during the process. Some interviewers focus on asking questions about your past experiences and your future plans. Others focus their questions on specific accomplishments and problems encountered in your past nursing experiences. Presenting hypothetical problems for you to consider and asking you to provide appropriate nursing responses is common. You may find it helpful to use your nursing process approach to any situation presented. Specifically state, "I would need to begin by assessing …" Talk about clearly identifying the problem (analysis of data) and planning for action. Don't neglect to indicate that you would evaluate the effectiveness of your actions. See Display 4.6 for a list of questions you might reflect on as you prepare.

In most instances, be sure to answer questions that are asked, rather than skirting them. However, if the interviewer asks a question that is illegal or inappropriate, such as a question regarding age or marital status, you might want to redirect the question to address what appears to be the concern of the interviewer. For example, in response to a question about your age, you might say, "Perhaps you believe that I appear to be young and inexperienced. I want to assure you that I have demonstrated my maturity and responsibility both in my nursing education and in my position with [name of employer]." In response to a question about marital status or children, you could reply, "Perhaps you are concerned about how long I plan to stay in my first position? I want to assure you that whatever my personal situation, professionally, I am looking for a position in an organization where I can be a long-term employee and plan for advancement within the organization." Avoid simple yes or no answers, but try to describe or explain to give a more complete picture of yourself.

Some interviews are conducted by a group of interviewers. This might include a person from nursing administration, a unit manager, and a staff development nurse. For an applicant to sit across the table from three to five individuals can be intimidating. You will need to look around the group, being sure to make eye contact with each individual. Make sure that you understand the role of each person present. You might actually write down individual names and roles on your notepad. This would allow you to direct a question to a specific individual or to use an individual's name when replying to a question. If you use a name, be sure to address

DISPLAY 4.6 Potential Interview Questions

Philosophy
- What is your philosophy of nursing?
- Is there a nursing theorist that you use as a basis for your nursing practice?
- What do you believe is the most central concept to support excellence in nursing?

Personal Goals and Planning
- Where do you see yourself in 1 year? 5 years? 10 years?
- Have you developed any professional goals? If so, would you share those with me?
- Why do you want to work here?
- What plans do you have for continuing education in nursing?
- What do you see as your weakest area in nursing?
- What do you see as your strengths in nursing?

Your Experiences
- What experience in your nursing education did you find the most rewarding? Why?
- What experience in your nursing education did you like the least? Why?
- In what kind of settings did you have an opportunity to work as a nursing student?
- What other job experiences have you had? What skill did you develop there that will be useful in nursing?

Problem Solving
- Identify a problem in patient care that you encountered as a student and explain how you solved that problem.
- Describe a difficult patient with whom you worked. Include why you found that patient difficult and how you managed the situation.
- Identify a situation in which you were involved in a conflict and describe how you handled that situation. If you had to do it over again, what would you do differently?
- Explain how you would use the nursing process in patient care.
- A problem may be presented to you for your solution. Plan ahead to approach it in a systematic manner.

Technical Skills
- What technical nursing skills do you feel comfortable performing?
- What skills will you require assistance with?
- What do you do when you encounter a technical skill you have not performed before?

The Employment Setting
- In what type of unit do you wish to work?
- Why do you want to work here?
- Why do you think we should hire you for this position?

them formally as "Mr.," "Ms." (if marital status of a woman is not known), "Miss," or "Mrs." rather than by first name. If they want you to use another form of address, they will let you know. While replying to the person who asks the question, glance at others as you make your point. Be sure that you do not ignore any individual, even if one of the interviewers does not seem to ask questions or to be as active in the process as the others. Interviews of this type are often longer than interviews with one person.

Some interviewers are less skilled than others; in these situations the questions may seem less focused and vaguer. You may sometimes feel at a loss as to exactly what is being asked. Before proceeding, seek clarification, but be careful that your manner of asking for clarification does not offend the interviewer. In this situation, you may have to take the initiative to be sure that you have an opportunity to present your strengths and skills. Don't hesitate to elaborate on questions to more effectively present yourself.

COMMUNICATION IN ACTION

Clarifying Questions in an Interview

Cheryl Layton, a new graduate, interviewed for a nursing position. She found that she did not understand many of the interviewer's questions and decided to use clarifying questions and statements throughout the interview. When there was a rather unclear question about communicating with others, she asked, "Would you give me an example of the type of situation you were thinking about?" Another clarifying approach she used was to state clearly what she perceived to be the central question before continuing: "Let me be sure I understand. You would like me to identify a situation in which I believe I responded effectively to a problem. Is that correct?" Still another clarifying response she used was, "If I understand correctly, your unit will be switching to computerized charting, and you are interested in my experience with computerized documentation. Is that right?" In this way, she indicated interest and attention to accuracy but did not challenge or offend the interviewer.

Almost all interviews provide an opportunity for the interviewee to ask questions before the interview is terminated. If you are asked to present questions, ask professional questions first. Make sure your questions are appropriate for the interviewer. In the human resources department, you might ask about the overall mission and philosophy of the organization, its organizational structure, and how authority and accountability are determined. You might also ask, "Do you have any questions about my résumé? Are there other details I can provide?" With a nursing interviewer, demonstrate that you are concerned about how nursing care is given and by whom, where responsibility and authority for nursing care decisions lie, the philosophy underlying care, the availability of continuing education, and where you would be expected to fit into the facility's overall picture. For example, you might ask, "Can you outline for me the responsibilities of this position?" or "What type of individuals do well in this type of position?"

Then be sure to cover such topics as hours, schedules, pay scales, and benefits. Recognize that the replies to these questions may be quite general when you have not yet been offered a specific position. Before you leave, be sure to ask when you can expect to know the results of your interview and how you can follow-up. State clearly that you are interested in the position and hope to be hired (if that is true). An important reason for not getting a position is the failure to clearly state that you want to work there.

If you are unfamiliar with the interview process, you might benefit from reading books on the topic. Reading several different books will give you a variety of viewpoints and might provide you with strategies that are comfortable for you.

COMMUNICATION IN ACTION

Replying Professionally to an Interview

Rosa Quintana had been interviewing for a position in a new graduate residency program in which she would really like to be a participant. The interviewer said, "Well that concludes my questions, do you have any questions for me?" Rosa responded, "I prepared some questions before I came. Some of those were already answered. However, I would like to hear more about the shared governance system you briefly mentioned on your Web site. Exactly what types of issues are addressed through shared governance and how might I, as a newly hired new graduate, participate in shared governance?" In this reply, Rosa demonstrated her preplanning and organization as well as her understanding of organizational function. After hearing the response to this question, Rosa then said, "Thank you so much for that information. It really confirms that I would really like to work here. I do hope to be chosen to enter this new graduate residency. What are the next steps I can take to learn about my status in the selection process?"

Telephone and Online Interviews

Because interviews are costly to an employer, telephone and online interviews may be conducted and an in-person interview only scheduled for individuals in whom the organization is interested in employing. Do not mistake these telephone or online interviews for unimportant or casual conversations. Plan for them in the same way that you would for an in-person interview. Prepare and have all your materials at hand. You will want to be professional and business-like in this context also. The one advantage is that you do not need to worry about your appearance.

Interviewing Errors

Several errors can occur during an interview that almost certainly will result in the position being offered to someone else. The first relates to making a negative comment about a former employer. If asked why you left a position identified on your résumé, be careful not to use this as a time to vent your frustrations about the employer or the employment situation. You may be labeled a troublemaker.

Bringing your personal problems to the interview may create a negative response. You may be asked why you would like this position. This is no time to talk about the economic necessity of having the job to repay your student loans, make your car payment, or even meet the monthly rent. Instead, focus on professional issues related to this employer.

Taking a friend or relative with you to the interview gives the impression that you are not an independent thinker. If you take children, they will be a distraction. Some interviewers will refuse to have children in the office. Arrange with a friend who also has children to exchange babysitting time or make other plans.

Do not take over the interview. Let the interviewer lead the interview. It is important to know when to talk and when to listen. When answering questions, be brief and concise; don't ramble. Also, watch your nonverbal responses.

Follow-up Strategies

Always follow up after your initial inquiry. If you were granted an interview, follow up with a letter. If you did not obtain an interview, you should continue to contact the potential employer at intervals to learn of other job opportunities and to indicate that you still seek a position.

When a new position opens, employers do not necessarily go back through previous employment files. They are more likely to interview a person who appears to be currently searching for a position than one who was searching several months previously. They will assume that you have found desirable employment.

After your interview, write a brief thank-you letter to the person who interviewed you. If a group interviewed you, direct the letter to the person who seemed to be in charge. In that letter, thank the individual for the time and attention to your questions and concerns. Restate any agreement you feel was reached. For example, write, "I understand that I am to call your office next week to learn whether I have been scheduled for an interview with the birth center unit manager." Close your letter with a positive comment about the organization. Even if you are not offered a job or do not choose to work at that facility, you are leaving a positive impression. You can never tell when that will be important to you in the future (Display 4.7).

DISPLAY 4.7 **Interview Follow-up Letter**

Maribeth Wilson
3428 1st Ave. N.
Seattle, WA 98103
(206) 274-5978
E-mail: maribethw@email.com

June 9, 2010

Joyce Montgall, R.N.
Nurse Recruiter
Seattle General Medical Center
321 Heath Blvd.
Seattle, WA 98101

Dear Ms. Montgall:

I want to thank you for meeting with me today to discuss your new nursing graduate residency program at Seattle General. I am particularly interested in the medical-surgical positions available on 4 West and 4 Center, although I am certainly willing to consider another unit.

I am confident that my educational background, clinical experience, and commitment to excellent patient care make me an ideal match with Seattle General. In addition, I feel very "at home" in the Seattle General environment, having worked there as a nursing assistant for the last year.

Again, I hope that you will consider me for one of the medical-surgical positions in the July 1 new graduate program. I am available to meet with any of the unit managers, which I understand is the next step in your hiring process. I can be contacted at the above telephone number or by e-mail. I do have an answering machine and would promptly return your call if I were not there to receive it. If I have not heard from you within 2 weeks, I will check with your office regarding the status of my application.

Thank you again for your time and consideration.

Sincerely,

Maribeth Wilson

Do not let this letter be your last contact with that potential employer. Call back as agreed. Even if you do not get a position at this time, you might ask that your application be kept on file because you are still interested in employment with that particular agency. You might then continue to call back every month or so to find out if any other positions are available.

▶ **EXAMPLE**

Following Up After an Interview

A student in her last term of a nursing program interviewed for a position in a new graduate residency program of a major medical center. She was disappointed when she called to follow up and was told that she had not been selected. The nurse recruiter assured her that she was a good candidate but that they had just had more applicants than they could place. After thanking the recruiter for notifying her, she asked if she could call back every couple of weeks to see if any new opportunities were available. She emphasized how much she would like to work at this medical center. She kept in contact with the recruiter as she widened her job search. Four weeks after she had been told that she was not selected, she called the nurse recruiter. The nurse recruiter told her, "I am so glad you called. One of the new graduates selected for the program has decided to move back to her hometown. We will have a place for you after all. Can you come in today or tomorrow to complete the paperwork?" Continuing her contact in a professional manner was a successful strategy.

Setting up your own record-keeping system often enhances managing a job search. Maintain a record of when you contacted an agency, in what manner (letter or telephone call), interviews—including the interviewer's name and the content of the interview—and dates and times of any follow-up letters or calls. Have a place to record your own notes or impressions. This will enable you to keep track of details when you manage an extensive job search. By keeping this type of record, you will not forget to call an agency to recheck on job availability, or mistakenly send an inquiry letter and résumé twice to the same agency.

Resignation

When you decide to leave a nursing position, it is important that you provide the employer with an appropriate amount of time to seek a replacement. The more responsible your position, the more time the employer will need. For a staff nursing position, strive to provide a month's notice, unless an urgent matter requires that less notice be given. Notice of resignation should be in a letter that is directed to the manager of your department. Copies should be sent to other supervisory people, such as the chief nursing officer.

The letter of resignation is important in concluding your relationship with the employer on a cordial and positive basis. The feelings left behind when you resign may influence letters of recommendation and future opportunities for employment with that agency. Give a reason for your resignation and the exact date when it will be effective. If you have accrued vacation or holiday time and want to take the time off or be paid for it, clearly state that. Comment about positive factors in the employment setting and acknowledge those who have provided special support or assistance in your growth (Display 4.8).

DISPLAY 4.8 Letter of Resignation

1546 Avenida Escuela
Palm Desert, CA 76321
February 14, 2011

Marvin Short, R.N., Unit Manager
Transitional Care Unit
Desert Hospital
509 Desert Highway
Palm Desert, CA 76320

Dear Marvin:

It is with mixed feelings that I am submitting my resignation to be effective March 23. I will be moving to Oregon and returning to school full time beginning spring quarter.

My 2 years here at Desert Hospital have been an excellent foundation for my future career. The nurses were supportive of me as a new graduate and have always encouraged me to think of my career as a lifetime opportunity for growth.

The last day I plan to work will be at the end of this pay period. My understanding is that my unused vacation and holiday pay will be included in my final paycheck.

Thank you again for all of your help.

Sincerely,

John Webster, R.N.
cc: Maria Gonzales, Vice President for Patient Care Services

If you are resigning because of problems in the work setting, you may find it wiser to address those in person, separate from your letter of resignation, and in a manner that will not affect future recommendations. However you address problems, do so in a clear, factual, unemotional way. Avoid attacking anyone personally and do not make broad, sweeping negative comments. Try to make any written statement a clear and reasonable presentation of your position as a professional. Remember that the nursing community is not large and a career path may bring you back to this agency or may bring these individuals to a place where you work. Try always to leave with appropriate professional relationships intact.

KEY CONCEPTS

- Developing a successful career pathway involves setting personal short- and long-term goals and developing a plan for maintaining and enhancing your own competence.
- Throughout the history of nursing, employment patterns have changed, moving from a focus on the home and the community in the first part of this century to a focus on acute care institutions.
- In today's healthcare world, the percentage of nurses employed in hospital inpatient settings, while still high, is diminishing as more outpatient, home care, long-term care, and community settings are established for the delivery of care.

- Competencies expected of the newly licensed RN can be categorized by frequency and by importance.
- Employers have expectations in eight basic areas: theoretic knowledge for safe practice and decision making; ability to use the nursing process; self-awareness; communication skills; understanding the importance of documentation; commitment to a work ethic; proficiency in specified technical skills; computer literacy; and speed of functioning.
- To obtain a nursing position, you will need to identify potential employers, develop a professional résumé, write appropriate letters to employers, and interview effectively using both in-person and online strategies.
- Successful interviewing involves learning about the organization, dressing appropriately, arriving a bit early, being self-confident, maintaining eye contact throughout the interview, and remaining attentive.

- To make the best impression, interview questions should be answered directly and clearly. The use of clarifying statements and questions may help to assure that you are providing needed data, while specific details rather than generalities in your response often are received more favorably. Approaching problem-solving questions using the nursing process provides a pattern for effective response.
- Following up after the interview has been completed includes sending a note of thanks to the key decision makers, and checking back to learn of decisions about the position, and maintaining contact with the institution if not selected if you still would like to be considered for a position there.
- When resigning from a position, communicating your plans to the head of the department with a sufficient time interval to allow the organization to find a replacement to fill your position leaves a professional impression and may result in a more positive reference.

RELEVANT WEB SITES

Web sites relevant to this chapter can be found at thePoint, accessed through *http://thePoint. lww.com/Ellis10e* and by entering the code found on the inside cover of your text.

REFERENCES

American Association of Colleges of Nursing. (2008). *The essentials of baccalaureate nursing education for professional nursing practice*. Washington, DC: Author.

American Health Care Association. (2008). *Projected number of nursing staff positions and vacancies in nursing facilities: 2008–2020*. Retrieved September 14, 2009, from http://www.ahcancal.org/research_data/staffing/Documents/ProjectedNH_Vacancy.pdf

Buerhaus, P. I., Auerbach, D. I., & Staiger, D. O. (2009). The recent surge in nurse employment: Causes and implications, *Health Affairs, 28*(4), w657–w668. Retrieved September 10, 2009, from http://content.healthaffairs.org/cgi/content/abstract/hlthaff.28.4.w657

National Council of State Boards of Nursing. (2009a). *The 2008 RN practice analysis: Linking the NCLEX-RN® examination to practice*. (Research Brief Vol. 36). Chicago: Author. Retrieved September 15, 2009, from https://www.ncsbn.org/2008_RN_Practice_Analysis.pdf

National Council of State Boards of Nursing. (2009b). *2010 NCLEX-RN test plan*. Chicago: Author. Retrieved June 26, 2010, from https://www.ncsbn.org/1287.htm

National Council of State Boards of Nursing. (2009c). *Report of findings from the post-entry competence study*. Chicago: Author. Retrieved September 12, 2009, from https://www.ncsbn.org/09_PostEntryCompetenceStudy_Vol38.pdf

National Council of State Boards of Nursing. (2010a). *The 2009 PN practice analysis: Linking the NCLEX-PN® examination to practice*. Chicago: Author. Retrieved November 30, 2010, from https://www.ncsbn.org/10_LPN_VN_PracticeAnalysis_Vol44_web.pdf

National Council of State Boards of Nursing. (2010b). *2011 NCLEX-PN test plan*. Chicago: Author. Retrieved November 30, 2010, from https://www.ncsbn.org/2011_PN_TestPlan.pdf

National League for Nursing. (1990). *Educational outcomes of associate degree nursing programs: Roles and competencies*. Publication No. 23-2348. New York: Author.

National League for Nursing. (2009). *Percentage of students enrolled in nursing programs by sex and program type, 2008–09*. Retrieved October 15, 2010, from http://www.nln.org/research/slides/pdf/AS0809_F19.pdf

National League for Nursing, (2010). *Outcomes and competencies for graduates of practical/vocational, diploma, associate degree, baccalaureate, master's, practice doctorate, and research doctorate programs in nursing*. Atlanta: Author.

U.S. Bureau of Health Professions. (2008). *The registered nurse population: Findings from the 2008 national sample survey*. Retrieved June 26, 2010, from http://bhpr.hrsa.gov/healthworkforce/rnsurvey/

U.S. Bureau of Labor Statistics. (2008). *Occupational outlook handbook: 2008–2009 edition*. Retrieved October 14, 2009, from http://www.bls.gov/oco/ocos083.htm

U.S. Bureau of Labor Statistics. (2010) *Occupational employment and wages for 2008* Retrieved October 15, 2010, from http://www.bls.gov/news.release/pdf/ocwage.pdf

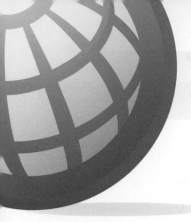

The World of Healthcare Employment

After completing this chapter, you should be able to:

1. Discuss the purpose of organizational mission and vision statements and statements of philosophy and analyze how these differ.
2. Discuss the concept of organizational structure and explore the relationships among organizational charts, chains of command, and channels of communication within the structure of organizations.
3. Delineate the characteristics of shared governance, and explain the advantages of a shared governance approach.
4. Discuss the development of the Magnet Recognition Program for hospitals and list the characteristics required to achieve this status.
5. Describe various patterns of nursing care delivery, and identify the major characteristics of each and a situation in which each would be employed appropriately.
6. Compare and contrast the characteristics of a grievance with those of a complaint.
7. Analyze the processes through which resolution is achieved in collective bargaining issues.
8. Discuss the history of collective bargaining as it applies to nursing.
9. Identify at least four professional concerns that should be addressed in a contract for nurses.
10. Discuss the concerns nurses have regarding membership in a collective bargaining group and the reasons for each of these concerns.
11. Outline the advantages and disadvantages of having the state nurses association serve as a bargaining agent for nurses.

KEY TERMS

Accountability	Chain of command
Agency shop	Channels of communication
Arbitration/arbitrator	Clinical ladders
Authoritative mandate	Collective bargaining
Authority	Concession bargaining
Bargain in good faith	Contract
Binding arbitration	Cross-training
Bureaucracy	Deadlocked
Case management	Functional method
Case method	Grievance/grievance process
Centralized/decentralized/matrix	Impasse

(key terms continues on page 156)

KEY TERMS (continued)

Injunction
Interest-based bargaining
Lockout
Mediation/mediator
Mission statement
Modular care
National Labor Relations Board (NLRB)
Negotiate/negotiation
Organizational chart
Organizational hierarchy
Partnership models
Policy
Primary care
Procedure

Protocols
Ratified
Reinstatement privilege
Shared governance
Span of control—broad, narrow
Standards of care
Statements of philosophy
Strike/strike breaking
Structure
Team nursing
Total patient care
Unfair labor practice
Union
Vision

As you seek employment as a professional nurse, you will most likely find an initial job in a healthcare organization. Organizations—formally constituted groups of people who have identified tasks and who work together to achieve a specific purpose defined by the organization—are the backbone of the American economy. We believe you will move from student to staff nurse more easily and function more effectively in any organization if you have some understanding of the structure and makeup of organizations. By gaining an understanding of the makeup of organizations, you will be best equipped to participate effectively in the activities of the workplace. This also will help you anticipate some of the difficulties that may occur and, thus, handle them with greater ease and adeptness.

This chapter begins with a brief discussion of the structure of organizations and some of the most common conditions of employment and then presents the most common avenues, including unions, through which employees participate in workplace decisions. Because we can only touch on these topics, you are encouraged to gain greater depth in this area by reading books devoted to this topic.

UNDERSTANDING ORGANIZATIONS

All organizations have structure and purpose. **Structure** refers to the way in which a group is formed, its chains of commands, lines of communication, and processes by which decisions are made. These comprise the formal working relationships and serve to identify who is accountable and responsible for the various jobs within the organization. The purpose identifies the goals of the organization—what it intends to accomplish. In other words, the structure outlines how individuals work together to reach the purpose.

Mission Statement and Philosophy

The purpose of an organization is often expressed in the form of a **mission statement**, which outlines what the organization plans to accomplish, including its goals and function. Sometimes, mission statements incorporate **statements of philosophy** (beliefs) and goals or

DISPLAY 5.1 Typical Hospital Mission Statement

Mission, Vision, Values, and Strategic Goals for Mercy Valley Hospital
Mission: To provide services resulting in the improved health of all individuals we serve.
Vision: To make available high-quality, high-tech, and high-touch healthcare to residents of the community.
Values:
- Patient centered
- Caring, compassion, and consideration
- Cooperation and collaboration
- Ongoing development and improvement
- Leadership
- Best care provider
- Best employer
- Best partner

objectives into a single statement; other times, the philosophy and goals are addressed in a statement separate from the mission statement. The mission of an organization may be combined with a **vision**, which is a broad conceptual view of what the organization desires to be and do. The mission statement is the responsibility of the board of directors or board of trustees. Input may be gathered from many sources and drafts are developed by top management with final approval by the board. Display 5.1 provides an example of a typical mission and vision statement for a hospital.

Mission and vision statements serve as a standard against which an organization's performance can be evaluated. A large research hospital might incorporate into its mission statement obligations for research, teaching, and the care of clients with complex problems. A smaller community hospital may reflect a goal of meeting the healthcare needs of citizens of the community in its mission statement. The hospital's ability to meet these goals would be reviewed as part of the overall evaluation of the organization.

Critical Thinking Activity

Based on your perception of the needs of the community in which you live, write a mission statement for a hospital in your community. How did you arrive at the decision to offer the services you outlined? What facts support this decision? What services did you not include? Examine your response for personal biases.

Organizational Structure

A central goal of most organizations is to seek an organizational structure that is efficient while providing maximum cost-effectiveness. The structure of an organization outlines the formal working relationships and identifies who is accountable and responsible for the various jobs required within the organization. Thus, it refers to the way it is put together to accomplish its goals. The structure determines the manner and extent to which roles, power, and responsibilities are delegated, controlled, and coordinated and how communication occurs between levels of management (BusinessDictionary.com, 2009). Size, age, services, technical components, and environment influence the structure of an organization.

The concept of organizational structure is credited to a German social scientist, Max Weber, who is known as the father of organizational theory. He highly valued **bureaucracy**— the administration of institutions through departments or subdivisions managed by sets of officials who followed an inflexible routine. Historically, hospitals have functioned in the bureaucratic mode, which also dominated both government and corporate life throughout the 20th century.

To continue operation, any organization must make enough money to meet its expenses and to improve and develop; some also seek to provide a profit return to investors. This is as true in healthcare as it is in retail businesses. As the values and priorities of our society change and as new technology becomes available, healthcare organizations also must make adaptations in their structure and function. Thus, today we encounter a healthcare system experiencing tremendous transformation (see Chapter 6).

Types of Structure

The power to make decisions is a key factor in the structure and function of any organization. Organizations may be described as having a centralized (or tall) or a decentralized (or flat) structure. When the structure is **centralized** the authority to make decisions is vested in a few individuals in the top layer of management. For example, in the patient services area of a hospital, major decisions may be made by the vice president of patient care and two or three associates (Fig. 5.1).

Conversely, when the decision making involves a number of individuals and individual employees are responsible for making decisions in areas in which they have expertise, the organization is said to operate in a **decentralized** manner. Major decision making is distributed, and decisions may be made by the individual closest to the action; a head nurse or unit manager may be responsible for more than one patient care unit. Currently, many organizations are going through a process of restructuring to embrace a transformational approach to decision making that places the responsibility for finding solutions to problems at the site where the activity occurs. Decentralized structures have the advantage of simplified communication patterns, which flow easily and directly from lower levels to higher levels. Later in this chapter, we discuss the concept of shared governance, which embraces a decentralized structure and function (Fig. 5.2).

Another type of organizational structure, the **matrix** structure, may be either flat or tall and also may be referred to as cross-functional. The unique characteristic of the matrix structure is that a second structure overlies the first, creating two directions for lines of authority, accountability, and communication. An organization will have an underlying structure (either tall or flat) that is a functional structure over which is imposed a project structure. In short, the individuals in the functional structure perform the duties of operating and maintaining the organization, and the individuals in the project structure oversee the application of various projects or special responsibilities. The relationship that exists among individuals in the project structure is outside the regular chain of command of the underlying structure. We typically see the matrix structure in large, multifaceted organizations. Individuals with special expertise or authority

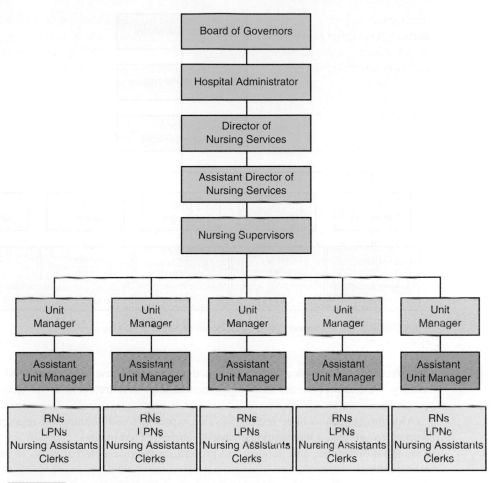

FIGURE 5.1 Centralized (tall) organizational structure of nursing service.

in an area serve as resource persons for several departments, all of which can benefit from the knowledge. For example, in Figure 5.3, three types of expertise (financial services, planning and marketing, and quality assurance) cross all aspects of this large hospital corporation, which include acute care, long-term care, and home care. Another example of a matrix-type relationship could be illustrated when a nurse with expertise in gerontologic nursing provides assistance, advice, and information to employees in each branch of this hospital organization.

ORGANIZATIONAL RELATIONSHIPS

When examining organizational function, it is important that you identify relationships among people and departments and realize where the authority and accountability are placed within that organization. When one has **authority**, it means that the individual has the power or the right to take action, give directions or commands, and make final decisions. **Accountability** refers to being obliged to answer for one's actions and sometimes, as when certain tasks are

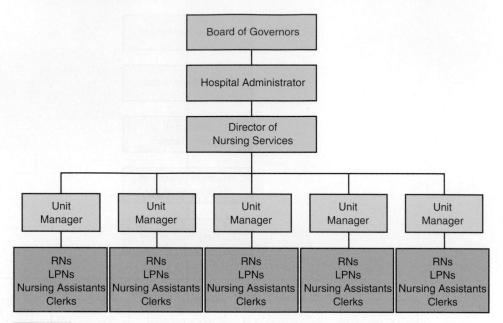

FIGURE 5.2 Decentralized (flat) organizational structure of nursing service.

delegated, for the actions of others. A synonym frequently used for accountability is responsibility. We discuss both authority and accountability in more detail in the section on shared governance.

Most organizations have several ways of expressing and defining the relationship of one worker to another. Organizational charts, chains of command, channels of communication, job descriptions, and policies and procedures provide different views of organizational relationships.

Organizational Chart

The structure of any large group comprises both a formal and an informal organization. The formal organization can be seen on an organizational chart. The **organizational chart** is a graphic, pictorial means of portraying roles and patterns of interaction among parts of a system. It identifies formal chains of command, communication channels, and the authority for decision making.

The organizational chart typically is represented on the page by boxes stacked in a pyramid formation. The greatest authority exists at the top of the chart (often a single box), and authority declines as you move toward the base (many boxes). Persons occupying jobs at the top of the organizational chart are considered administrators, executives, or management, and individuals with jobs closer to the base are considered employees or staff members. Located between these two levels is an area known as middle management, comprising those who coordinate and control activities of specified groups of workers.

The organizational chart may take one of several forms, reflecting the type of administration operating within that organization. One term used to describe these forms is **span**

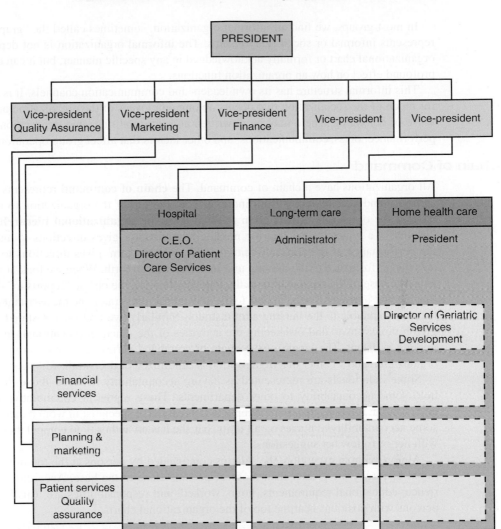

FIGURE 5.3 Matrix organizational structure of nursing service.

of control, which refers to the number of employees supervised by a manager. A **narrow** span of control exists when a manager has responsibility for only three to five subordinates. If, however, the organization operates with a **broad** span of control, it places authority and responsibility for decision making in the hands of fewer individuals, with each manager supervising a large number of employees. The larger the number of individuals to be supervised, the more difficult it is to control each worker through direct observation. If two organizations of equal size were to exist—one with a narrow span of control and the other with a broad span of control—the organization choosing to implement a narrow span of control would have more managers. One limitation of the organizational chart is the difficulty in keeping it current. Positions and people change frequently, and each change requires updating the chart.

In most groups, we find an informal organization, sometimes called the "grapevine," that represents informal or social relationships. The informal organization is not depicted on an organizational chart or formally acknowledged in any specific manner, but it can often have a profound effect on how an organization functions.

This informal structure has its own leaders and communication channels. It is responsible for much of the socialization that occurs among employees of the organization and creates a sense of belonging. There may be unwritten and informal rules and expectations regarding performance, dress, communications, and other factors that affect group operation.

Chain of Command

All organizations have a chain of command. The **chain of command** represents the path of authority and accountability from individuals at the top of the organization to those at the base of the organization. It is often referred to as the **organizational hierarchy**. Thus, in hospitals we typically find that the nursing administrator gives directions to and evaluates the performance of the assistant administrator, who, in turn, gives directions to and evaluates the performance of the nursing unit manager, and so forth. When we look at this process from the base of the organization to the top, we often use the phrase "reports to"—indicating that the unit manager is accountable to the assistant administrator and the assistant administrator is accountable to the nursing administrator. Similarly, we find the registered nurse (RN) giving directions to and overseeing the activities of the practical (vocational) nurse and the nursing assistant. The length of the chain of command varies depending on the size of the organization and whether that organization is centralized or decentralized.

Some individuals are represented as having accountability to those above them but also hold some accountability to other departments. These represent collaborative rather than authoritarian relationships. For example, a clinical nurse specialist in wound care might hold some accountability to nurses on all units, but she has no authority to compel them to consult with her or follow her suggestions.

Almost without exception, the salaries commanded by persons at the top of the organizational hierarchy are greater than those of persons close to the base. Accordingly, the experience, educational requirements, hours worked, and responsibilities are usually greater for persons with positions near the top of the organizational chart.

Channels of Communication

Channels of communication are, as the name implies, the patterns through which messages are delivered within an organization. The channels of communication usually reflect the chain of command; they run up and down the organizational chart, moving from one level of responsibility and authority to the next. Thus, the nurse manager communicates concerns and information to the assistant administrator, who either has the authority and responsibility to deal with the problem or relays the concern to the nursing administrator. The nursing assistant reports her concerns to the staff nurse, who either has the authority to deal with the issue or reports it to the head nurse or clinical manager. Some types of communication move along to individuals in parallel positions.

For nurse managers to report a concern directly to administrators rather than to assistant administrators to whom they report is referred to as "looping" the system. It is generally considered improper and inappropriate to skip or bypass any level in the communication system.

For example, if a staff nurse disagrees with a pharmacy technician who delivers medications to the unit and takes this problem directly to the nursing supervisor without first discussing it with the unit manager, this individual is looping the system. You can see how this would put the unit manager at a distinct disadvantage, should the supervisor ask about the incident.

COMMUNICATION IN ACTION

Missing Supplies

Mary Allioto had been working on a medical unit of a community hospital for 4 months. Over that period of time, she noted that one of the nursing assistants, Jane, often left with towels, washcloths, and other unit supplies in her backpack. Mary approached Jane as they were leaving one afternoon and said, "I've noticed that you often carry home towels and other unit supplies." Jane quickly replied, "Oh, these ones are becoming ragged and should not be used anymore." Further observation suggested that Jane continued to remove unit items. Mary decided she needed to report this to her unit manager. Talking with the manager in private, Mary explained, "On several occasions within the past 3 months I have noticed Jane leaving the hospital with unit supplies in her backpack. I asked her about it 2 weeks ago and she stated that the supplies were worn and should not be used with clients. I thought you should know about this." The unit manager thanked Mary and said, "I'll look into it."

Not all communications follow the formal pathways. New approaches to leadership and management have encouraged communication outside those lines if the result is accomplishing a desired action more efficiently. The informal structure of the organization mentioned earlier also functions outside the formal pathways, often communicating messages much more rapidly than within the formal structure.

▶ ## EXAMPLE

Informal Communication Networks

Betsy Archer had been working on a medical unit of a community hospital for about 7 months. During lunch, a colleague said, "I hear that our unit will be the first to start on the new computerized charting system." Betsy replied, "How do you know that? The newsletter said that the hospital has not even decided on a vendor for computerized charting. I thought we were going to get to evaluate systems before the final choice." Her colleague replied, "Oh, they didn't mean that people at our level would get to evaluate the systems. It's a done deal. My friend in technology says they are making plans for implementation right now and we are first! Jenny [the unit manager] will learn the news at today's manager's meeting."

Job Descriptions

Job descriptions form another important aspect of any organization. Job descriptions are written statements, usually found in policy manuals, that specify the duties and functions of the various jobs within the organization and the scope of authority, responsibility, and accountability involved in each position. Job descriptions should explain the role of each individual working for the company or organization, from the chief executive officer to the housekeeper.

Sometimes job descriptions are very detailed; other times they are more broadly stated. If broadly stated, policy and procedure manuals may help to specify a task or responsibility. Job descriptions provide the foundation for performance standards for each position and should provide the basis for evaluation. Job descriptions also may include competencies expected of employees and can provide the basis for competency-based orientation. Increasingly in today's healthcare environment more care is delegated by the RN to those with lesser educational preparation; therefore, it is critical that job descriptions provide sufficient description of the competencies of various workers, so that the document can be used to guide delegation activities (see Chapter 13 for more information on delegation).

Job descriptions also are important when cross-training is used in the organization. **Cross-training** requires that a person hired to perform functions of one position in the healthcare team be trained in the skills needed to perform those of another position. For example, a respiratory therapist might learn to perform basic patient care skills and, when not needed for respiratory therapy treatments, be available to answer call lights and respond to patient needs. Cross-training is viewed by some administrators as a method by which costs can be reduced by having an individual able to do more than one set of tasks within the organization. It can help manage peak times and provide for greater flexibility in scheduling. It also may be viewed as a method of job enrichment, giving an employee more control or more responsibility. Some persons enjoy the challenge of learning new skills and excel in the stimulation; others prefer to stay in the area they have chosen and know well (Reh, 2009). The effectiveness of cross-training between different disciplines has not been well documented. Certainly issues related to scope of practice, liability, and patient safety must be considered. Patients may express concerns if a care provider, wearing an identification badge stating he or she is a radiological technician, is functioning as a phlebotomist.

Cross-training of nurses between different specialties has become common, and many nurses welcome the employment flexibility this provides. It also allows nurses to move with greater comfort from one area of the hospital to another when patient census surges or drops in an area. Some nurses express concern over their ability to maintain a high level of expertise in multiple areas. As you enter into your first nursing position, check with your state board of nursing to learn what position your practice act has taken regarding cross-training.

Job descriptions also may describe **clinical ladders**. A clinical ladder differentiates and defines the skills and performance expected of nurses in terms of advancing levels. Typically, three or four levels of performance are defined, with each higher level having greater responsibility and authority than the previous one. A new graduate usually enters the system as a clinical nurse one (or similar title) and moves to clinical nurse two and then to clinical nurse three as that individual becomes more proficient. Salary increases typically accompany movement from one level to another, and the responsibility the individual is expected to assume also increases.

Sometimes additional formal education or continuing education is required for advancement. Through this process, the nurse is supported and encouraged to develop greater clinical expertise. The clinical ladder also serves as a mechanism for recognizing and rewarding nurses who wish to remain in direct care positions rather than seek administrative positions.

Policies, Protocols, Procedures, and Standards of Care

A **policy** may be defined as a designated plan or course of action to be taken in a specific situation. In organizations, the governing board holds the responsibility and authority for ensuring that appropriate policies are adopted and followed. The governing board usually delegates the development of policies to the chief administrative officer who usually delegates the responsibility for the development of policies for a specific department to individuals or groups in the department who will be most affected by the policy. The policy once developed is returned to the governing board for review, possible revision, and adoption.

Written copies of all policies usually are placed in a policy manual that is available in each department, or a current copy may be available online in the institution's computer network. Online policy manuals ensure that all departments refer to the most current policy and that the information is always available. Depending on the area in which you are employed, you will find varying reasons for referring to the policy manual in your role as a new employee. As you might anticipate, the need for special policies related to occurrences in an emergency department, a delivery room, or a critical care unit is greater than in a general medical or surgical unit in a hospital. When you are confronted with a new nonclinical problem to solve, always check your policy manual to see if it offers guidance; if you do not find help there, ask your manager.

Special unit policies are sometimes termed **protocols**. A protocol is a detailed "plan for carrying out a scientific study or a patient's treatment regimen" (Dictionary.com, 2009). For example, the protocol for dealing with a patient seen in the emergency department suffering from a dog bite determines the wound assessment instrument to be used, a reference to the procedure to be used for wound care, when tetanus immunization would be included in care, discharge criteria, and teaching needed. Protocols may be available online so that any unit confronted by an unusual situation has access to the protocol even when it is not commonly used.

Procedure manuals contain the written instructions describing the accepted method for satisfactorily performing a particular nursing activity (**procedure**), often describing it in a number of steps. Each unit or department should have a procedure manual. In the manual, you might find a procedure for changing the dressing on a central intravenous line, administering chemotherapy agents, and doing many other procedures, such as catheterizations. Procedures may also be available online.

Institutions are giving nurses more responsibility for developing institutional policies, protocols, and procedures and serving as representatives to various committees that monitor, review, and update these policies, protocols, and procedures. As hospitals move to broader spans of control and to greater involvement of all employees in decision making, grassroots participation in policy formation is becoming more common. The nature of a policy and the breadth of its scope will determine whether it needs further review within the organization.

Standards of care are authoritative statements that describe a common or acceptable level of client care or performance. Thus, standards of care define professional practice. In 1973 the American Nurses Association (ANA) first formulated general standards and guidelines for nursing practice, which were revised in 1991 and again in 2004. Additionally, standards for more than 20 areas of specialty practice have been developed. (The individual standards can be purchased from the ANA, or all may be purchased as a package.) They apply across the nation, are broad and general in nature, and have the purpose of establishing the best practice and eliminating as much variation as possible. Similarly, state practice acts contain language describing the standard of practice that applies to all nurses licensed in that state.

Each agency also may develop standards of care for patients with selected healthcare problems. These more detailed and specific standards may take the form of standard nursing care plans. Some standards are being incorporated into documents termed "care pathways," *critical pathways*, or *clinical pathways*. These are intended to serve as guides to direct the healthcare team in daily care. The individual standard organizes and sequences the care and describes the care required for a patient at specific times in the treatment. It involves a multidisciplinary approach and identifies both the care activities and the outcomes for each 24-hour period of hospitalization. These specific standards of care become the basis for evaluation of care, quality improvement within the organization, and cost analysis.

SHARED GOVERNANCE

In the realm of administrative structure, one of the more important changes in healthcare delivery has been the move to a pattern of shared governance within healthcare agencies. Governance establishes how the power and authority for decision making is structured within an organization.

Shared Governance Model

Shared governance may be viewed as a system in which nurses have organizational autonomy as reflected in control over their practice and have input into decision relating to patient care. It is a professional practice model in which both the nursing staff and the nursing management are involved in decision making, as opposed to the administrative decision area being controlled by management. Fundamental to the successful implementation of shared governance is the belief that staff nurses at every level within the organization should govern their practice and be involved in decisions that affect that practice; it enables staff nurses to assume greater levels of autonomy and control over their practice. It involves the concepts of equalitarianism, collegiality, and shared professional accountability. Thus, shared governance is more than a structure—it is also a way of thinking.

The concept of shared governance could be found in business and management literature in the 1950s when concepts of participative management and decentralization were popular. It made its way into healthcare and nursing by the late 1970s and 1980s (Swihart, 2006). It gained further status and recognition as an alternative to bureaucratic management during the 1990s when nurses became dissatisfied with the institutions in which they worked. A shared governance structure allows nursing staff to make major decisions within the organization and attempts to get the decision-making process as close to where the action occurs as possible, typically through the development of internal councils. Fundamental to shared governance is accountability. Although the terms accountability and responsibility are often used interchangeably, experts in the area of shared governance define responsibility as focusing on work, the competence of the worker, and the excellence of its application or the quality effort. Accountability on the other hand focuses on the effect of the work rather than the processes related to the work itself—the results of the work, the difference the work makes, whether the work mattered in relationship to expectations or the quality impact (Porter-O'Grady & Malloch, 2007).

Over the past 35 years, four structural models of shared governance have emerged: (1) councilor, (2) congressional, (3) administrative, and (4) unit-based. A councilor model is structured around specific committees and councils that have defined authority and functions within identified areas. The congressional model involves elected representatives who oversee the operations of a unit or department. The administrative model consists of committees or forums in which people communicate and share ideas and more closely resembles a traditional hierarchy. The unit-based model (which is the least frequently used) operates when members define their own basic accountabilities, and the structure may not affect the organization outside the unit (Swihart, 2006). The committees or councils result in staff actively participating in management and, as a consequence, gaining autonomy, control over the work environment, and greater job satisfaction. Often, councils report to a nursing executive board that serves as a coordinating and approval body. Within this framework, the nurse is held to greater accountability within the context of peer-defined and peer-operated parameters (Porter-O'Grady & Malloch, 2007).

Effect of Shared Governance on the Role of the Manager and Staff Nurse

In a shared governance model, the traditional role of the manager as one who hires, evaluates, promotes, and fires becomes a thing of the past. The nurse manager's role is changed to become one of facilitator, integrator, and coordinator of the processes that support the work of the staff nurses who have been empowered to control their own practice. Managers must learn to share authority over key areas such as scheduling. In some instances, it has required that they give up seats on various hospital committees to staff nurses. Managers are required to understand their own change style, decision-making style, and leadership style (Brooks, 2004). The inability of managers to make these changes has been a major impediment to the success of shared governance. Many managers have found their new and changing role difficult to accept.

The implementation of a shared governance structure requires that staff nurses understand that it is their right and professional obligation to participate in how decisions are made about nursing practice (Brooks, 2004). They need to participate in professional development sessions that increase nurses' understanding of the decision-making process, team building, group dynamics, leadership and budgeting, and how to participate in and conduct meetings.

Pros and Cons of a Shared Governance Model

The shared governance model has waxed and waned in hospitals over the past 25 years. Strong advocates for the empowerment, autonomy, and professional development of staff nurses encourage the implementation of shared governance. Because shared governance models were introduced to improve nurses' work environments, satisfaction, and retention (Anthony, 2004), their popularity has grown. Nurses engaged in evidence-based practice (see Chapter 16) believe the environment that most facilitates and nurtures critical thinking and autonomous decision making is that of shared governance in which engagement and participation are encouraged. Nurses involved in workplace advocacy, which endeavors to strengthen nursing's voice and ensure nurse involvement in workplace decisions, also see shared governance as an avenue by which to accomplish their goals. An entire nursing journal has been devoted to the topic, with many of the articles describing implementation of shared governance models.

Some question the continuance of shared governance models in today's healthcare system stating that shared governance is costly to an organization, and the cost-effectiveness of shared governance in terms of patient outcomes is dubious.

Systems for evaluating the effectiveness of shared governance are being implemented. Evidence that sorts actual costs of the various shared governance models is being collected. Information that examines the returns on the investment in terms of what is attained and in relationship to retention rates, nurse satisfaction, and vacancy is beginning to be gathered and analyzed.

Critical Thinking Activity

Interview nurses who work in a shared governance environment. Identify what they find satisfying about shared governance. How would they like to see it changed? If shared governance is not used in your area, contact your state nurses association and learn what information it has regarding shared governance. Analyze the information you receive, and make a list of the advantages you see in this form of governance; list disadvantages you identify with its implementation.

MAGNET HOSPITALS

Along with the concept of shared governance, within the past 20 years the hospital workplace has witnessed the development of the Magnet hospital concept. A Magnet hospital is described as one where nursing delivers excellent patient outcomes, where nurses have a high level of job satisfaction, and where there is a low staff nurse turnover rate and appropriate grievance resolution (Fagin, Maraldo, & Mason, 2008). In the early 1980s, the American Academy of Nursing recognized that acute care facilities, in particular, were having difficulty attracting and retaining RNs. They appointed a task force on hospital nursing practice to examine the situation. The task force determined that it was necessary to research the various factors involved in creating environments that would attract and retain professional nursing staff (McClure, 2005). Nurse researchers, sponsored by the ANA, conducted "reputational" studies to identify successful hospitals, and a body of literature developed from these studies.

Initially 41 hospitals were selected as Magnet hospitals. Gold standards were then identified. In 1991, the American Nurses Credentialing Center (ANCC) established a program through which hospitals could apply to be designated Magnet hospitals. Today, more than 100 healthcare organizations have been awarded Magnet designation for excellence in nursing practice (ANCC Magnet Recognition Program, 2010).

As the study of hospitals continued, characteristics emerged that resulted in the hospitals being considered a good place to work. In the initial study conducted by Kramer and Schmalenberg (2005), 14 forces of magnetism were identified. Over time, some of these became outdated; for others the operational definition changed. These forces were narrowed down to 10 items staff nurses identified as important to enabling them to give quality patient care, and eventually down to 8 (see Display 5.2). Note that many of the forces of magnetism relate to characteristics of hospitals discussed earlier in this chapter (ie, flat, decentralized organizational structures; shared governance; and nurse autonomy). Other concepts are

DISPLAY 5.2   Eight Essentials of Magnetism

- Support for education
- Clinically competent coworkers
- Autonomous nursing practice
- Positive RN–MD relationships
- Supportive nurse manager
- Control over nursing practice
- Adequate staffing
- Culture that values concern for the patient as paramount

Compiled from Kramer and Schmalenberg (2005).

tied to processes such as team building and participative leadership, which are discussed in Chapters 12 and 13. Magnet hospitals have been identified as having strong leadership, offering educational resources to employees, providing a work environment in which nurses can grow and challenge themselves, and allowing nurses to be involved in problem solving. A strong aspect of Magnet hospitals is a decrease in the turnover of staff, a factor that speaks to employee satisfaction.

Although Magnet recognition was initiated by nurses and is carried out through the ANCC, the Magnet effort involves all departments and disciplines within the institution. Excellent patient care is an interdisciplinary process, and participants in the process of gaining Magnet recognition experience feelings of pride and satisfaction.

PATTERNS OF NURSING CARE DELIVERY

The nursing department of any healthcare institution carries major responsibility for the quality of nursing care delivered. Throughout the years, the structure of the delivery of care has taken many forms, with the particular pattern of care in common use changing about every 20 years. Among the factors influencing the delivery pattern selected in each era were the types of patients served, the type of care provided, the cost of the care, the structure of the hospital, and the number and education level of potential employees. Perhaps a wider variety of patterns of care are being used today than at any other time in nursing's history. In the following section, we describe the typical implementation of several patterns of care delivery. However, remember that you might find a particular pattern of care practiced a little differently in different settings.

Case Method

The **case method** was the first system used for the delivery of nursing care in the United States (around the beginning of the 20th century) and should not be confused with the term case management practiced today (more discussion occurs later in this chapter). With the case method, the nurse worked with one patient (or case) only and was expected to meet all of that patient's needs. The nurse often lived in the patient's home and was expected to assume other household duties, such as cooking for the patient and family and light housekeeping, when not busy with the patient. While able to provide total care, the chief disadvantage was that nurses worked long hours and were poorly paid. Advancing technology and increasing costs made this type of care delivery impractical, but vestiges of its structure can be seen in today's home health nursing. However, the role of the RN in home healthcare is typically one of assessment, planning, skilled intervention, supervision of care provided by a home health aide, and evaluation of the client's progress.

Functional Method

The **functional method** of care delivery emerged during the Great Depression of the 1930s and allowed for the care of greater numbers of patients in hospitals and for the use of advancing technology. At the time, the industrial model of narrowly defined and frequently repeated tasks had revolutionized manufacturing, and this approach to work was being transferred to all types of work environments including nursing.

A head nurse assigned nursing tasks to various persons employed on the unit, according to the level of skills required for performance, the size of the unit, and available personnel. One nurse might take all temperatures and another would do all dressings, while yet another administered all medications, charted them, and provided a list of replacement needs to the head nurse. The head nurse gave a report to the next shift.

Although economical and efficient, this system of care delivery had the disadvantage of fragmenting care—no single individual was responsible for the planning of care. Patients were confused about who was caring for them, and communication among caregivers was lacking. Individual nurse–patient relationships were limited. Nursing care came to be viewed as a list of procedures and tasks. This pattern of care still may be used in long-term care facilities or subacute units, largely because of the educational preparation of the care providers.

Team Nursing

The concept of **team nursing** was introduced in the early 1950s, with the promise that it would result in more patient-centered care. It also was responsive to the nursing shortage that followed World War II (see Chapter 1) and the involvement of nurse aides and licensed practical (vocational) nurses (LPNs) in patient care. Each unit had two or more teams composed of variously educated care providers, for example, two nurse aides, an orderly, an LPN, and an RN. An experienced RN was the team leader. Team members worked together, each performing those tasks for which they were best prepared, thus providing high-quality and comprehensive care. The team leader made assignments, had overall responsibility for the care of patients on the unit, typically administered all medications, and gave a report to the team that followed on the next shift. An important part of this form of nursing was the team conference, during which members of the team met to communicate about the needs of their patients and to plan care. The conference provided each team member with the opportunity to participate in decision making. A disadvantage was that continuity of care might be threatened as the assignment of teams varied. Today, as we see more healthcare facilities decreasing the number of RNs and adding more unlicensed assistive personnel, team nursing has again become a prevalent method of care delivery (Fig. 5.4).

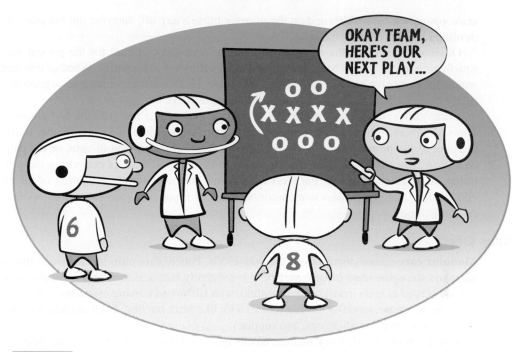

FIGURE 5.4 Team conference, planning, and communication are critical elements of team nursing.

Total Patient Care

During the late 1970s and early 1980s, many hospitals returned to **total patient care** in which an RN or LPN was assigned to all the care needs of a group of four to six patients, depending on patient acuity. This type of care focused on the total person (from which its name is derived), rather than on a collection of tasks or procedures, and returned a greater sense of control to nurses, gave them a greater sense of autonomy, and fostered a greater sense of involvement in the whole spectrum of care and patient outcomes.

This approach to care was costly because an individual with less training could satisfactorily complete many of the tasks performed by the RN and at a lesser cost. However, studies demonstrating the relationship between nurse–staffing levels and quality of care in hospitals would question this conclusion. Higher RN staffing was associated with less hospital-related mortality, failure to rescue, cardiac arrest, hospital-acquired pneumonia, and other adverse effects, as well as shorter stays (Nurse Staffing and Quality of Patient Care, 2007). This topic is discussed in greater detail in Chapter 10.

Primary Care Nursing

In a pattern of **primary care**, which came into popular application in the 1980s, one nurse was assigned the responsibility for the care of each patient from patient admission until that patient's discharge. The primary nurse was responsible for initiating and updating the nursing care plan, patient teaching, and discharge planning. An associate nurse worked with the same patient on other shifts and on the primary nurse's day off, carrying out the plan of care developed by the primary nurse.

Obvious benefits of this method included the continuity of care for the patient and job satisfaction for the nurses because they had more autonomy and control. Whether this method was more expensive has been the subject of debate. Healthcare administrators argued that the salary costs for RNs make this a more costly approach to care.

Under this system, every nurse was a primary nurse for a few patients and an associate nurse for others. Sometimes the nurse functioning in an associate role had difficulty following the plan of the primary nurse or disagreed with the established plan of care, or the patient's condition changed rapidly, requiring the plan to be changed without consulting the primary nurse. Another concern was the level of expertise and commitment required of all nurses and the fact that nurses who work autonomously with patients soon forget how to delegate responsibilities.

Modular Care

Modular care gained popularity in the mid-1980s. Patient care units were divided into modules, and the same team of care providers consistently was assigned to a particular module. An RN served as team leader of each module, with LPNs and nursing assistants making up the team. In this sense, modular nursing looked a lot like team nursing. Each module was stocked with its own linens, medications, and supplies.

This form of care delivery had the advantage of offering continuity of care, because the same team cared for the same group of patients each day. It also had the advantage of involving the RN in planning and coordinating care and resulted in more efficient communication because of the geographic closeness of the unit. The disadvantages center on the increased costs of stocking each unit and the fact that many hospitals, with long corridors and halls, do not lend themselves architecturally to a modular staffing pattern.

Partnership Models

In some areas of the country, there currently exists a trend toward **partnership models**, in which patient care is provided to a group of patients by an RN and an LPN or unlicensed nursing assistant. If an unlicensed care provider is involved, this individual does nonnursing tasks, and the RN provides the professional care, thus making it less expensive than some other models. When an LPN is employed, the patient care is shared, with the RN responsible for planning and directing the care. This form of care delivery may also be referred to as "care pairs." The difficulty of maintaining consistent partnerships among staff creates a major disadvantage.

Case Management

Case management, although not a system of care delivery in the sense that we have mentioned earlier, involves nurses in the role of managing patient care and bears mention here. Case management refers to a system in which the healthcare services are controlled and monitored carefully to ensure that policies are followed, that neither too much nor too little care is provided, and that costs are minimized. A key to case management is the identification of a critical pathway for care and treatment that includes specific timelines and protocols. The case manager typically follows the patient from the diagnostic phase through hospitalization, rehabilitation, and back to home care, ensuring that plans are made in advance and that the patient receives care that will achieve the most positive outcomes. The case manager may not provide direct care but is responsible for managing the patient's interaction with the entire healthcare system. For a more detailed discussion of case management, please refer to Chapter 6.

RNs are the healthcare professionals who most often act as case managers. In some settings, social workers also act as case managers. Case managers may be employed by third-party payers (such as insurance companies) or by healthcare agencies (such as hospitals or long-term care facilities). Case managers employed by a particular institution also might be involved in wellness programs (eg, blood pressure management, stress management, smoking cessation programs, and exercise classes).

Some objections to this form of care delivery come from physicians, who see the role of the case manager as an infringement on their historic rights of autonomy in decision making. Providers may also believe that the case manager is more concerned with cost factors than with what is best for the individual, arguing that quality is sacrificed to cost containment.

Critical Thinking Activity

Compare the various patterns of nursing care delivery with the pattern being used in a facility where you currently receive clinical experience. Analyze the pattern in current use and evaluate whether another pattern of care delivery would be more or less effective. Provide a rationale for your answer.

WORKPLACE ACTIVITIES THAT INVOLVE NEGOTIATION

Negotiation involves the exchange of ideas and values for the purpose of reaching a mutual decision regarding a particular situation. While it occurs on a day-to-day basis as we work with others, it often is also a part of the mediation process. The following section of this chapter discusses some of the major activities in healthcare environments when negotiation occurs.

Grievance Process

A **grievance** is a circumstance or action believed to be in violation of a contract (or of policies of an institution if a contract is not in place). The **grievance process** represents an established and orderly method to be used in the adjustment of grievances between parties. In this sense, it represents a problem-solving mechanism.

Grievances usually are related to interpretations of a contract or policies and procedures. They may occur as a result of a misunderstanding or difference of opinion about the contract or its language, or as a result of direct violations of policies or of the contract. Although either the management or an employee can file grievances, in most instances, it is an employee who initiates the case.

The grievance process spells out in writing a series of steps to be taken to resolve the area of dissension and a timeline for accomplishing those steps. If a contract exists, the steps to be used in mediating grievances are usually included in that document. If there is no formal contract, internal policies exist that outline grievance procedures. Perhaps you are aware of grievance processes from your student handbook, where the processes in place in an educational program are shared with students.

Initially, the employee and the immediate supervisor attempt to resolve the disagreement through an informal talk. If no resolution occurs, the discussion moves to the steps of the grievance process, involving others within the organization. The steps include providing notifications and responses in writing, adhering to strict timelines for action, and eventually involving people at higher levels within the organization (eg, representatives from the bargaining unit, a grievance chairperson, the human resources director, and administrative representatives). Perhaps the services of an arbitrator will be needed toward the end of the dispute. Failure of either side to comply with the timelines that are in effect regarding its own actions or responses ends the process. If an arbitrator is involved, that person's decision is usually binding.

It is important to differentiate between complaints and grievances (Fig. 5.5). Employees may have complaints that are not violations of the contract. For example, Nurse No. 1 may object that she was required to float from the postpartum unit to the nursery; she had been oriented to the nursery but preferred to work in the postpartum unit. Nurse No. 2 was required to float from a medical unit to a surgical unit to which she had not been oriented. If the contract in this hospital stipulates that no one would be floated to a unit to which he or she had not been oriented, Nurse No. 1 had a complaint, whereas Nurse No. 2 had a grievance.

The absence of grievances, once thought to be an indication of an effective, well-managed organization, may not be the best indicator of the organization's health. It is entirely possible that problems are not being addressed. By the same token, a high number of grievances may

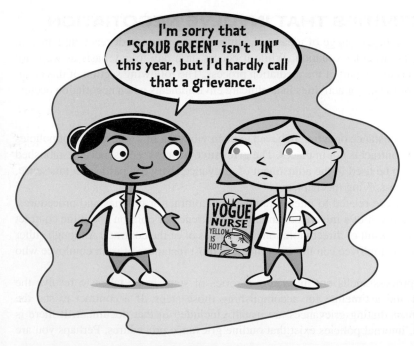

FIGURE 5.5 It is important to discriminate between complaints and grievances.

indicate problems within the organization. These problems also may relate to the language of the contract or the education of the employee regarding the conditions of employment. Another barometer of the health of an organization is the level at which the grievances are resolved. It is most desirable to settle most grievances at the informal level, without the involvement of an arbitrator.

Although most grievances are settled short of arbitration, they are still time and energy consuming. Grievances can best be avoided if everyone has a good understanding of the terms of employment and if sound personnel policies are developed and applied consistently and equitably. A part of the orientation of new employees to an organization should be spent reviewing and explaining these features. Open discussions between the employees and management to review mutual concerns and share information help reduce the number of grievances. Mutual respect is a critical element in any organization.

 ## Critical Thinking Activity

What are the reasons that grievance processes should be spelled out? How would you determine whether an issue is a grievance or a complaint? What resources are available to you as you search for the answer?

Collective Bargaining

Collective bargaining consists of a set of procedures by which employee representatives (typically a union) and employer representatives negotiate to obtain a signed agreement (contract) that spells out wages, hours, and conditions of employment that are acceptable to both. A key word in this definition is **negotiate**. The goal of negotiations is to obtain a signed agreement, which is a legal contract that spells out in writing the decisions that are reached.

Because of nursing's long history as a profession of dedication, altruism, and service, collective bargaining initially was a controversial issue within nursing. Some saw this process as detracting from the professional role of the nurse and ethically improper.

Today, however, nurses are vitally concerned about contracts, services, third-party payers, comparable worth, patients' rights and safety, shared governance, staffing ratios, and a host of issues that can be discussed at the bargaining table. Nurses believe that people who choose nursing as a career should have the opportunity to have some voice in patient care assignments, length of the workday and workweek, fringe benefits, and wages, without losing face with the public at large, members of the medical profession, or other colleagues. Additionally, at a time when nurses are campaigning for a safer practice environment free of mandatory overtime and other work issues, collective bargaining takes on a new countenance—an avenue by which to address these and other work concerns and gain control over practice.

History of Collective Bargaining

Interest in the rights of workers began to gain attention in the United States as early as the 1850s. The highlights of the history of collective bargaining are presented in Table 5.1. We summarize those activities in the following paragraphs.

Table 5.1 **History of Collective Bargaining**

EVENT	DATE	EFFECT(S)
Horace Greeley writes articles in *New York Tribune* columns regarding collective bargaining	1850	Impetus and interest generated in the issue of workers' rights
National Industrial Recovery Act	1933	Nation required to accept a 35–40 hour workweek and 30–40 cents per hour minimum wage, and prohibited child labor
NLRA (Wagner Act)	1935	Gave workers protection in their efforts to form unions and organize for better working conditions Created the NLRB
Taft-Hartley Act (Labor Management Relations Act)	1947	Excluded nonprofit hospitals from the legal obligation of bargaining with employees
Taft-Hartley Act amended	1974	Provided economic security programs for those employed in nonprofit hospitals, thus requiring hospitals to bargain with nurses for better salaries and working conditions Required 10-day written notice of intent to picket or strike

Under the administration of Franklin D. Roosevelt, who was elected president in 1932, several acts were passed related to the rights and privileges of the worker. These culminated in the establishment of the **National Labor Relations Board (NLRB)**, a quasi-judicial body that was to ensure proper enforcement of the conditions of the legislation.

The NLRB has the responsibility for administering the National Labor Relations Act (NLRA). In addition, it has two primary functions: to conduct secret ballot elections that will determine that the majority of employees of a unit desire the representation of a given union in collective bargaining procedures and to prevent and rectify unfair labor practices committed by employers or unions. It also has the responsibility for determining to which of the bargaining units established for healthcare workers various employees will be assigned. This is important to nurses because it enables them to have a separate unit and, therefore, to deal with issues important to their role in healthcare delivery.

Because the original NLRA used the term "labor organization," the language was interpreted to exclude nursing and several other professions, such as teaching and medicine that were organized through professional organizations. These early labor unions often were viewed negatively by the public—an image that was reinforced in movies, in newspapers, and on radio. Often portrayed as rowdy, aggressive, and hostile, unions did not seem to fit well in nursing. Although prevented from bargaining collectively in the 1947 amended Taft-Hartley Act, in 1974, additional amendments provided economic security programs for those employed in nonprofit hospitals and brought healthcare facilities and their employees under the jurisdiction of the NLRB. Nonprofit hospitals were legally required to bargain with nurses for better wages, hours, staffing conditions, and patient–nurse ratios, and for a voice in hospital governance. To ensure that the public would be protected from strikes or work stoppage, several amendments were attached to the NLRA passed in 1974, including the requirement of longer notification periods and provisions mandating participation in mediation.

Understanding the Basic Concepts of Collective Bargaining

Intelligent and effective bargaining begins with an awareness of the process itself. The information that follows is designed to provide a better understanding of the terms and processes involved in bargaining collectively to achieve an agreed-upon contract.

Bargaining and Negotiating. To negotiate means to bargain or confer with another party or parties to reach an agreement. It implies that there will be a discussion of the terms of the agreement and suggests that there will be give-and-take—that neither party will obtain all items asked for in the contract. Ideally, negotiations would proceed in a somewhat philosophic vein, moving toward reasonable compromises that would allow each side to achieve many of the conditions it requested, but this does not always occur.

A typical bargaining session has three phases. The early sessions include a formal exchange of proposals, during which each side may ask for more than it knows it can expect to receive and emphasizes its commitment to certain issues. The second phase gives the most attention to secondary issues. The third phase occurs as the deadline approaches, and primary issues are discussed realistically.

Several forms of bargaining have evolved. **Interest-based bargaining** represents a nontraditional style of bargaining in which the parties

- Focus on interests or what each side wants rather than proposals
- Agree on the criteria of acceptability that will be used to evaluate alternatives
- Generate several alternatives that are consistent with their interests
- Apply the agreed-upon acceptability criteria to the alternatives so generated in order to arrive at mutually acceptable contract provisions

Much of the success of the technique depends on mutual trust, openness, and a willingness to share information. But even where these are lacking, the technique, with its focus on interests and on developing alternatives, tends to make the parties more flexible and open to alternative solutions and thus increases the likelihood of agreement (Labor-Management Relations Glossary, n.d.).

Another variation sometimes seen is concession bargaining. **Concession bargaining** is a process in which there is an explicit exchange of reduced labor costs for improvements in job security. This occurs with increasing frequency. An example would be a shift in emphasis from one that asks for increases in salary to one that focuses on eliminating the practice of calling nurses and telling them not to report for work because the census has dropped (on such days, the nurses do not receive salary). These are issues of concern to nurses today.

Unions and Collective Action. A union is a legally authorized organization that has been empowered by its members to negotiate and enforce a contract. Therefore, in order to engage in collective bargaining, employees must choose a union that will represent them. This usually is done through an election. The major areas in which a union may bargain are the wages, hours, and working conditions of its members.

When a branch or part of a professional association assumes the role and responsibility of a union, as often occurs in nursing, the negotiating group may be known as a collective action division, although it is legally considered a union. A professional organization works under the same legal constraints as any other union. It provides legal counsel and representatives to assist with negotiations, may lobby on behalf of issues, or may participate in other activities that would further the economic welfare of nurses. It oversees the development of the contract, monitors adherence to the contract, and represents employees in any grievance process.

Contracts. The conclusion of the bargaining process should result in a signed contract that converts to writing the agreements that have been reached. A **contract** is "an agreement between two or more parties, especially one that is written and enforceable by law" (www.freedictionary.com). This signed contract is enforceable under law and cannot be changed by either party acting unilaterally.

Some would suggest that the contract is the most important product of the collective bargaining process because it is a legal agreement on all issues that have been discussed. It provides the foundation for further activities. Unlike the policies of an agency, which can be changed by management alone, the agreement of both management and employees is required for any change to be made in a contract. The contract remains in effect until breached or terminated. Most negotiated contracts define the period of time—usually 2 or 3 years—during which the established conditions are effective.

Before being put into effect, a contract must be **ratified**. This means that the members of the bargaining group must accept the terms of the contract. This is usually done by a vote of the membership. Factors to be considered in a contract will be discussed later in this chapter.

Rules Governing Labor Relations. When two parties agree to begin the negotiation process, it is understood that both will **bargain in good faith**. Bargaining in good faith is a poorly understood concept, but generally it means that the parties will meet at regular times to discuss (with the intent to resolve) any differences over wages, hours, and other employment conditions. Failure to carry out these activities could lead to an unfair labor practice.

An **unfair labor practice** is any action that interferes with the rights of employees or employers as described in the amended NLRA. It is not possible to discuss all of these in detail; however, some examples follow. An employer must not interfere with the employee's right to form a union or other organized bargaining group, join the group, or participate in the group's activities. The employer may not attempt to control a group, once organized, or to discriminate against its members regarding hiring or tenure. Most important, the employer must bargain collectively and in good faith with representatives of the employees.

Likewise, labor organizations have constraints placed on their activities. They, too, must bargain in good faith. They must not restrain or coerce employees in selecting a bargaining group to bargain collectively. They may not pressure an employer to discriminate against employees who do not belong to the labor organization.

One of the issues brought up in negotiations that usually results in a dispute is that of **agency shop**. When an agency shop clause is in effect, all employees in the unit pay dues or fees to the union to defray the costs of providing representation. There are several variations in provisions related to an agency shop. If, because of religious or philosophic beliefs, employees are unwilling to pay dues to the bargaining group, provisions may be made to pay the same sum to a nonprofit group, such as a charity or foundation. In some instances, those who are already members of the union are required to remain members for the life of the contract, although no one is required to become a member. In some states, laws referred to as "right to work laws" forbid the establishment of an agency shop. If you seek employment in an agency where nurses bargain collectively, it would be wise to explore the options available to you.

Settling Labor Disputes

When labor disputes arise, several actions can be taken to help resolve the differences. Initially, of course, the parties continue to negotiate and may agree to extend the negotiation period if progress in settling differences is being made. When the two parties negotiating cannot come to an agreement on an issue, they are considered to be at **impasse** or **deadlocked** on the issue.

Mediation and Arbitration. Perhaps the most commonly used method of seeking agreement between parties when negotiating has not been successful is through **mediation** and **arbitration**. A **mediator** is a third person who may join the bargainers to assist the parties in reconciling differences and arriving at a peaceful agreement. Although the mediator may join the parties at any point in the negotiations, due to the cost of mediation, most negotiations proceed until things are at an impasse. Mediation involves finding compromises, and the mediator assists with this. He or she must gain the respect of both parties and must remain neutral to the issues presented.

An **arbitrator** is technically defined as a person chosen by the agreement of both parties to decide a dispute between them. The primary difference between a mediator and an arbitrator is that the mediator assists the parties in reaching their own decision, whereas the arbitrator has the authority to actually make the decision for the parties if necessary. However, the terms mediator and arbitrator and mediation and arbitration often are used interchangeably; in fact, a mediator may also serve as an arbitrator (Fig. 5.6).

Arbitration may take several forms. It may be mediation arbitration, in which a third person joins the parties in the negotiation process before any serious disputes arise. This person's role is to act as a mediator, who attempts to keep the parties talking, suggests compromises, and helps establish priorities. If an agreement is not reached by a specified date, or if it appears that the issue is deadlocked, with neither party willing to compromise, the mediator then assumes the role of an arbitrator and makes a decision based on the information gained in the role of mediator.

Another form of arbitration is called **binding arbitration**. This means that both parties are obligated to abide by the decision of the arbitrator. Some people see this as the least desirable alternative in settling disputes because it may result in a decision that is not satisfactory to either side, but one by which both must abide. It has been suggested, in instances in which binding arbitration is used, that the parties spell out exactly which of the issues are to be decided by the arbitrator. Binding arbitration has the advantage of resolving deadlocked issues without a strike. It also encourages both parties, knowing that the arbitrator's decision may not please either side, to reach a compromise on their own.

One type of binding arbitration uses a final offer approach. Employer and employee bargaining representatives reach agreement on as many issues as possible. The deadlocked issues and a final position (final offer) from each side are then presented to the arbitrator, who is obligated to select only the most reasonable package. The arbitrator may not develop a third alternative, which would split the difference. The final offer approach encourages both sides to come up with a realistic package and serves to close the gap on issues, as each side seeks to maintain some control over the outcome of the deliberations.

One criticism of any type of arbitration is the expense involved. Arbitrators must be paid for their services. Arbitration is also criticized because it undermines voluntary collective bargaining and allows parties to avoid unpleasant confrontation with their own difficulties by

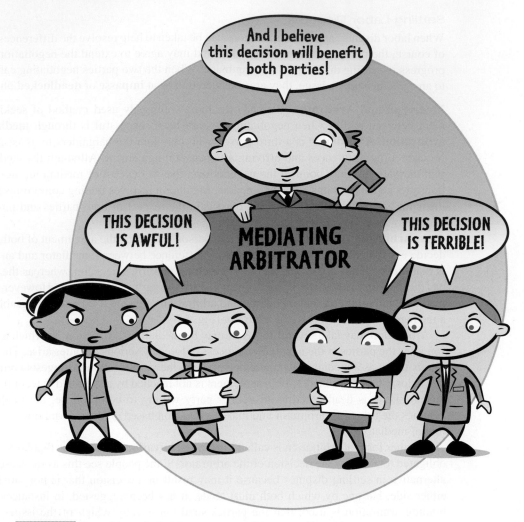

FIGURE 5.6 The arbitrator's decision may not really please either side.

shifting that responsibility to a public authority. However, it is useful in preventing the disruption of services.

Arbitration may be requested from the American Arbitration Association or from available state, public, and private mediation and conciliation services. The American Arbitration Association is a nonprofit, nonpartisan organization that, for a nominal fee, can provide a list of qualified arbitrators. Most states have available groups, such as the Public Employees Relations Commission, that also can provide a list of mediators and arbitrators.

Lockouts and Strikes. When the negotiation process breaks down, lockouts and strikes are likely to occur. A **lockout** occurs when an employer refuses to allow the employees to work. It is done to force employees to agree to the terms offered by the employer. The employer may close a place of business, or the employer may choose to remain open, discharge the workers, and use replacement workers. One readily can see how undesirable this would be in the healthcare system, but it has occurred in rare instances.

A **strike** occurs when workers refuse to continue to work until certain demands are met, thus imposing economic hardship and pressure on the employer. When the negotiation process breaks down, employees may use the strike to emphasize the need to improve their working conditions, salaries, and benefits. The most recent strikes by nurses, however, have been over issues related to patient care rather than those related to the economic status of the nurses. Striking places a serious economic hardship on employees and therefore is not undertaken lightly. Sometimes a strike is used to gain public attention to the labor dispute and to create public pressure for a settlement. This is only successful if the public agrees with the position of the striking workers.

At one time, nursing strikes were viewed by some as unprofessional and detrimental to the health of the community and, as indicated in Table 5.2 (see page 186), were forbidden by ANA policy until 1968. When strikes occurred, they drew major media attention, and it was feared that they would damage the image of nurses and nursing.

Some nurses view with great concern the issue of whether nurses should participate in strikes if negotiations break down. These nurses believe that the withholding of services from patients is unethical and unprofessional, and therefore, personally unacceptable. Others view the strike as a final method for bringing attention to the needs of the nurse as a citizen. Fortunately, as bargaining groups representing nurses become more knowledgeable and skilled in the process, strikes occur less frequently. Disagreements at the bargaining table are more commonly resolved through mediation and arbitration, much to the relief of many professionals.

Strikes in nursing are undertaken only with advance notice, to enable patients to be transferred to another facility and to make other plans for care of individuals in the community. Typically, arrangements are made with another hospital to admit patients during the strike, and all elective procedures are canceled. The striking nurses may also agree to provide staffing to critical care, labor and delivery, and emergency departments of the facility in which the strike occurs. Often the notification that nurses intend to strike on a certain date is sufficient incentive to move negotiations to the point of settlement.

In spite of efforts to avoid them, strikes do occur in nursing. When this happens, it is often an unpleasant experience for all. Those who choose to cross picket lines may be subjected to harassment and verbal abuse by their colleagues. Those striking for better working conditions and patient safety may feel betrayed by nurses who make the strike less effective. Nurses may feel pitted against one another as well as against the management (Williams, 2004).

Reinstatement Privilege. A reinstatement privilege is a guarantee offered to striking employees that they will be rehired after the strike as positions become available, provided that they have not engaged in any unfair labor practices during the strike and provided that the strike itself is lawful. The hospital may replace a striking nurse during the strike. If strikers agree unconditionally to return to work, the employer is not required to rehire a striking nurse at that time. However, recall lists are developed, and if the nurse cannot find regular and equivalent employment, he or she is privileged to recall and preference on jobs before new employees may be given employment. Nurses may lose their reinstatement privileges because of misconduct during a lawful strike. For example, strikers may not physically block other nurses and personnel from entering or leaving a hospital during a strike. Strikers may not threaten nonstriking employees and may not attack management representatives. These types of activities usually do not occur during strikes conducted by nurses, but are not outside the realm of possibility.

Other Methods of Influencing Settlement. There are a wide variety of methods by which solutions can be reached in the negotiating process. The following discussion briefly addresses the more formal and far-reaching of these activities.

One method of reaching solution is to employ an **authoritative mandate**, in which a president, secretary of labor, or other high-ranking or influential person encourages a peaceful settlement. This is usually employed when the situation becomes critical and when the continuance of a strike would cause problems for a great number of people.

Another technique is informational picketing, which involves employees carrying informational signs outside of the institution. Informational picketing is not designed to stop work, but rather to inform the public of the concerns under dispute and to create public pressure on behalf of the union and the employees; it happens frequently. Other methods of obtaining community support also may be employed. These include newspaper editorials, letters to the editor, and even paid advertisements. Rallies and marches may be used to draw public attention to the issues.

In some instances, an **injunction** may be requested. This may result in a court order that requires the party or parties involved to take a specific action or, more commonly, to refrain from taking a specific action. Employers may use this measure to forestall or end a strike. Unions may use this measure to stop a lockout.

In still other instances, an institution or company may be subjected to government seizure and operation. Government employees are then used to run the plant, firm, or industry in question. This is seldom seen in the healthcare industry, for obvious reasons. However, this option was used in Montana in 1991, when state employees decided to strike. The National Guard was called in to replace striking state patrolmen.

What to Look for in a Contract

The negotiation process should ultimately conclude in the development of a written contract that is signed by both union and management representatives.

A contract must meet certain specified criteria to be legally binding. It must result from mutually agreed-upon items arrived at through a "meeting of minds." Something of value must be given for a reciprocal promise, that is, professional duties for an agreed-upon sum. Contracts can be enforceable whether written or oral but are easier to work with when written. Written contracts are also considered formal contracts. Although each agreement will differ, most contracts have a fairly general format. Display 5.3 includes items included in that format.

Issues Negotiated in Contracts

Many have come to believe that the collective action of nurses provides one of the best avenues for achieving professional goals and exercising control over nursing practice. Provision 6 of the ANA Code (2001) states, "The nurse participates in establishing, maintaining, and improving healthcare environments, and conditions of employment conducive to the provision of quality healthcare and consistent with the values of the profession, through individual and collective action." As nurses are called on to assume greater responsibility for complicated

DISPLAY 5.3 **Items Typically Included in Contracts**

- A preamble stating the objectives of each party
- A statement recognizing the official bargaining groups
- A section dealing with financial remuneration, including wages and salaries, overtime rates, holiday pay, and shift differentials
- A section dealing with nonfinancial rewards, that is, fringe benefits such as retirement programs, types of insurance available, free parking, and other services provided by the employer
- A section dealing with seniority in respect to promotions, transfers, work schedules, and layoffs
- A section establishing guidelines for disciplinary problems
- A section describing grievance procedures
- A section that may explicitly state codes of conduct or professional standards

decisions and control over practice, collective bargaining through a professional organization may provide the means to implement the concept of collective action. Today, the terms and conditions of employment have taken on a prominence over wages and hours in contract negotiations. Common issues to be negotiated include the following:

- Provisions for shared governance
- Mandatory and voluntary overtime
- Acuity-based staffing systems
- Use of temporary nurses
- Protections from reassignments and other issues related to assignment of duties
- Provisions for orientation to the work environment and continuing education
- Whistleblower protection
- Health and safety provisions such as free vaccines and needle safety
- "Just cause" language provision for discipline and/or termination
- Provisions for nursing and interdisciplinary practice committees (Budd, Warino, & Patton, 2004)

The manner in which the bargaining is conducted greatly influences how it will be perceived. Nurses as a group need to develop the skills necessary to communicate to the public the importance of their role in healthcare delivery. They must be able to handle conflicts and work toward resolution while maintaining integrity and dignity. Nurses need to become enlightened and informed, and they need more than a superficial understanding of the process of collective bargaining.

It is important that, as a new graduate, you know whether there is a contract in effect in the institution in which you seek employment or in the community in which you plan to work. You should also be knowledgeable about the terms of the existing contract so that you might best fulfill your obligations and recognize and benefit from the provisions to which you are entitled. The organization to which you are applying for employment can provide you with a copy of the current contract. Contact state nurses associations for information regarding the organization that represents nurses in a particular hospital or facility. They can also provide a copy of any contracts that have been negotiated for which they represented the nurses.

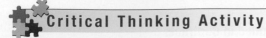

Critical Thinking Activity

As a new employee in a hospital, how will you find out whether there is a contract? Whom will you ask? How will you obtain a copy of the contract? What will you do if the contract includes language that you do not understand? What would you do if you were in total disagreement with some of the stipulations of the contract?

Issues Related to Collective Bargaining and Nursing

Four major issues of collective bargaining affect the nursing profession: the fact that some nurses see collective bargaining as unprofessional, the matter of which bargaining group will represent nursing when nurses participate in collective bargaining, the question of whether to join a union when one exists, and the issue of the role of the supervisor. These issues may take on greater or lesser importance depending on the area of the country involved, the length of time the nurses in that area have been participating in collective bargaining, and the group chosen to represent the nurses at the bargaining table. Additionally, as a staff nurse, you may, at some time, have to make a decision regarding whether to strike. In making this decision, you want to be well grounded in the issues at hand and knowledgeable about the arrangements that have been made for the continuance of services in emergency situations and in special hospital areas, such as labor and delivery.

Collective Action and Professionalism. In addition to the historic view of nursing as an all-serving, altruistic calling with strong religious influences, another factor that has hampered the strong development of unionization in nursing is the socialization of women and the fact that nursing is primarily a woman's profession. Although more men now enter nursing, currently fewer than 10% of the RNs in the United States are male. Early social beliefs that a woman's role should be submissive, supportive, and obedient were extremely compatible with the expectations that our society placed on nurses. The paternalism that has existed in the healthcare delivery system has also made the process of collective bargaining for nurses a slow one. The combination of the role of women and the role of the nurse under earlier paternalistic practices were once described by a nursing author as the nurse caring for the "hospital family," looking out for the needs of all (from patient to physician) and being responsible for keeping everyone happy (Ashley, 1976). The tendency to see the physician as the father figure in the healthcare system, the nurse as the corresponding mother figure, and the patients as the children has done little to promote the autonomy of nursing as a profession.

Today we see nurses involved in collective bargaining in greater numbers than ever before. Several of the factors responsible for this change include

- Legislated changes that allowed nurses to bargain collectively
- The rising cost of healthcare that resulted in the examination of all factors, including salaries that contributed to the cost
- Issues in the delivery of care such as patient–nurse ratios, workplace safety, and overtime that lent themselves to negotiation
- A new generation of nurses who approach the world of employment with different goals and attitudes than did the previous generations

Representation for Nurses. As collective bargaining has become accepted for nurses, the number of groups that seek to represent them at the bargaining table has constantly increased, with many groups now bargaining for nurses. Representation is determined by elections that are supervised by the NLRB. To become the certified collective bargaining representative of a group of employees, the organization seeking that role must receive 50% of the votes cast, plus one.

When nurses first began to organize, the ANA, through the state nurses associations, was the sole bargaining representative; this group still represents more nurses than all other organizations combined.

Activity of the ANA. Although nurses were not permitted to engage in collective bargaining activities until 1974, by 1931, the ANA publicly recognized its obligation regarding the general welfare of its members and developed within its organization a legislative policy addressing this concern. Some suggest that this effort was spurred by the fact that other groups—particularly the Service Employees International Union (SEIU), an affiliate of the American Federation of Labor/Congress of Industrial Organizations (AFL/CIO)—were actively working to organize healthcare workers. Other factors also were important. Before 1930, most nurses were employed in public health, visiting nurse, or private duty positions. Students, aides, and orderlies, under the direction of a head nurse, delivered much of the care in hospitals. As more care was delivered in the hospital setting, the number of nurses employed by these facilities grew. The existing working conditions affected more people.

In 1946 the ANA's House of Delegates approved a resolution that called upon the state nurses associations to work actively to secure the general and economic welfare of its members. The ANA has worked constantly since those early years to provide leadership and support to nurses as they negotiate salaries, working conditions, benefits, and governance opportunity. In 1966, they adopted the Resolution on National Salary Goal, which established a salary goal of not less than $6,500 per year for entry-level RNs. Lacking the right to bargain collectively for salaries, nurses sometimes used mass resignations as a method to change employment conditions.

The United American Nurses (UAN) was established in 1999 as an affiliate of both the ANA and the AFL-CIO. Six state bargaining groups (New York, New Jersey, Ohio, Montana, Oregon, and Washington) separated from the UAN in 2007 over issues of decision making and control and formed the National Federation of Nurses (NFN). In 2009 the UAN voted to join with the California Nurses Association and Massachusetts Nurses Association (groups that broke away from the ANA) to form the National Nurses United (NNU) as a national union. Both the UAN and the NFN assist state nurses associations to organize and to negotiate in regard to work hours, staffing levels, health and safety, and wage benefits and issues.

In 2000, the Commission on Workplace Advocacy was established by the ANA House of Delegates. Its purpose was to work through policy and legislative activities that affect nurses in all work environments, both those who participate in collective bargaining and those who do not.

Following on the heels of the establishment of the commission, a new membership category for Associate Organizational Members was created in 2003. The Center for American Nurses was established to deal with issues of workplace advocacy. The Center, which is independent of ANA, offers tools, services, and strategies designed to make nurses their own

Table 5.2   **ANA Activities Related to Collective Bargaining and Workplace Advocacy**

YEAR	ACTIVITY
1931	Developed within its organization a legislative policy addressing general welfare concerns of its members.
1945	Appointed a committee to study employment conditions.
1946	Established the ANA Economic Security Program as an outcome of the 1945 study. State nurses associations encouraged to act as exclusive bargaining agents for their memberships.
1947	Collective bargaining between nurses and hospital administrations implemented in several states with negotiated contracts in effect.
1949	ANA is certified as a labor organization.
1950	No-strike policy adopted officially by ANA due to the concern for the image of nursing.
1967	ANA identified as the bargaining agent for nurses in Veterans Administration hospitals.
1968	No-strike policy rescinded.
1991	ANA embarked on a Workplace Advocacy Initiative to improve the work environment of nurses.
1999	UAN established as an autonomous arm of ANA to carry out collective bargaining for nurses at the national level and to coordinate the work of state collective bargaining units.
2000	Commission on Workplace Advocacy established to address the needs of individual nurses in the workplace not represented by collective bargaining.
2003	The Center for American Nurses established as an outgrowth of the Commission on Workplace Advocacy. Created a new membership category for Associate Organization Members and addresses challenges and opportunities individual nonunion nurses face in their practice environments.
2009	NNU formed as a *super-union* by three founding organizations, UAN, Massachusetts Nurses Association, and CNA/NNOC.

best advocates in their practice environments. Table 5.2 summarizes the activities of ANA in relationship to collective bargaining and workplace advocacy.

Some would contend that it is not realistic for one group to work with the professionalism aspect of nursing as well as with the issues of wages, benefits, and working conditions. This has encouraged other organizations to compete for the right to represent nurses. As a result a large number of nurses are represented by the American Federation of Teachers, the Teamsters Union, the National Union of Hospital and Healthcare Employees, The Federation of Nurses and Health Professionals, United Food and Commercial Workers, or the SEIU. In some instances, as with the SEIU, the organization represents other workers employed in the organization. The SEIU organizes what are called "wall-to-wall" unions, in which all employees of all categories from housekeeping and maintenance to nurses and pharmacists belong to one bargaining unit. This may be favored by hospital administration, which often expresses frustration with the number of groups with whom negotiations must be carried out. However, when the SEIU is bargaining for all employees, it has the distinct disadvantage of diluting the ability of nurses to include professional issues in the negotiation process.

Nurses face a difficult decision when choosing which group can represent them best. In the past years, this decision has occupied perhaps more time and effort on the part of nurses than has the actual bargaining. Some contend that only RNs should bargain for RNs because nurses face different issues than other workers. Many believe that only nurses can effectively negotiate such items. These people contend that hospital administrations, fearing the power of labor unions, will bargain more constructively and positively with nurses themselves.

The state nurses association serves as a collective bargaining agent in many states. To do this, they must organize in such as way that the collective bargaining is separated in terms of finances and control from the other activities of the organization. Those who are members but not part of a collective bargaining unit pay lesser dues than those who are part of a collective bargaining unit. Only those who are part of bargaining units have a vote regarding collective bargaining issues.

Some nurses prefer two organizations—one to represent issues related to professionalism and another to negotiate salaries. This does require dues to two organizations. Although the dues for the state nurses association are reduced considerably if it does not serve as the bargaining agent for an individual's workplace, there remains an added cost when belonging to two organizations. Because of this, many who are represented by another union do not join their nurses association.

Critical Thinking Activity

If the collective bargaining agent in the hospital in which you worked was other than the state nurses association, would you belong to both organizations? What factors would you use to support your decision? Why are these factors important to you?

Decision to Join or Not to Join. Once nurses have gained an understanding of collective bargaining and have developed a personal philosophy about the professional role of the nurse, they are ready to make a decision regarding membership in the bargaining unit.

In working with students who are soon to embark on professional careers, we find that it is easier for them to decide whether to bargain collectively than it is to decide to part with the money that is required for membership. Many nurses want better working conditions and higher salaries, but are all too willing to let someone else fund these endeavors and work to achieve them.

It is in response to these concerns that many agency shop clauses have been added to contracts. Those who are members and are active in the negotiation process believe it is inappropriate for some to benefit from the labors of the bargaining process without having contributed, at least financially, to the effort. The presence of agency shop clauses may serve as either an asset or a deterrent to recruitment, depending on the applicant's viewpoint.

COMMUNICATION IN ACTION

Seeking Information Regarding a Union

Will Jones had just begun working at the medical center. He was given a copy of the contract for RNs during his orientation. He was also given the name of a union representative on his unit. During his first week there, he approached the representative and said, "Hi Carol, I was told you are the union representative for our unit. Do you have some time to talk with me at lunch? I would like to understand more about the process here." She replied, "Sure—let's plan to go down to the cafeteria at 11:30—first lunch. Does that work for you?" He said, "That is when I was scheduled for lunch too. Just so you know, I don't really know anything about the union, what its goals are, the issues here, or anything. I hope you can help me get that kind of information." Will had set the stage to become a knowledgeable participant in the bargaining process.

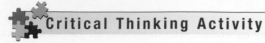

Critical Thinking Activity

Do you support the concept of nurses becoming members of a union? Why or why not? If so, do you believe all employees of an organization should be required to pay membership fees? Analyze your response to this question and provide the rationale to support your views.

Collective Bargaining and the Role of Supervisor. The question of whether nurses are considered supervisors because they direct the care of others first surfaced in 1994, when a nursing home argued before the Supreme Court that the LPNs in its employ were supervisors, directing the work of others, and, therefore, were not protected by the NLRA. The Supreme Court, in a 5 to 4 decision, ruled in favor of the nursing home ("Striking at bargaining," 1994).

This issue was again addressed in February 1996, when the NLRB ended nearly 2 years of deliberation by ruling that charge nurses at Alaska's Providence Medical Center could not be called supervisors simply because the role requires some direction of other workers. The board stated that the essence of the nurse's role was judgment and went on to explain that the authority that arises from professional knowledge is distinct from the authority of a front-line manager ("NLRB to the Supreme Court," 1996). The fact that the nurses did not have the authority to hire, evaluate, and terminate others was important in the court's decision. The issue continues to occur with surprising frequency.

Changes in the Number of Bargaining Units. Within hospitals, there are many different positions and job titles, ranging from professional staff through office staff to those responsible for hospital maintenance. In nursing alone, there are groups of RNs, LPNs, and nursing assistants. As these groups have been granted authority to organize into bargaining units, concern has been expressed about the number of unions with which any hospital administration must bargain at any given time. Some fairly elaborate estimates have been made regarding the amount of time demanded by the collective bargaining process.

When the NLRA was first passed in 1974, the NLRB specified that seven employee bargaining units would exist within the healthcare industry (Wilson, Hamilton, & Murphy, 1990, p. 37): RNs, physicians, other professional employees, technical employees, business office employees, clerical employees, and skilled maintenance employees. In 1984, the NLRB determined that bargaining units would be decided on a case-by-case basis. This resulted in reducing the number of bargaining units to three: all professionals, all nonprofessionals, and guards.

In 1989, the NLRB proposed a new rule that resulted in the establishment of eight collective bargaining units. At this time, it was also determined that the rule would apply to hospitals of all sizes. In response, the American Hospital Association (AHA) sought and obtained a permanent injunction against the rule. Subsequently, all-RN units were legally approved. The latest activity regarding this issue occurred in April 1991. The U.S. Supreme Court upheld the NLRB in its authority to define bargaining units for healthcare workers in acute care hospitals and allowed for all-RN bargaining units ("Supreme Court Okays," 1991). As might be expected, the AHA and the ANA occupied opposite points of view regarding this issue.

Changing Trends With Regard to Collective Bargaining

At one time, economic concerns and working conditions may have been the principal motivators for collective action. However, by the mid-1980s, subtle, and at times not so subtle, changes occurred throughout the United States regarding collective bargaining, unionism, and labor-management relations.

Some working in the area of contract management have reported a shift from the adversarial relationship that historically had existed between the employee and the employer (which focused on salaries, work hours, and the like) to one that placed greater emphasis on the quality of work life.

Thrust of Collective Bargaining in Nursing. The focus of collective bargaining issues changed during the 1990s. As nurses have become more comfortable and knowledgeable about the bargaining process, their energies have been directed toward many issues. Originally focusing on wages and benefits, today the major concerns of nurses also include staffing patterns, involvement in decisions affecting patient care, cross-training, the use of unlicensed assistive personnel, workplace safety and the rights of employees to know the hazards with a work environment, comparable worth, and discriminatory practices against employees (both male and female). This shift in emphasis reflects the general acceptance of the process of collective bargaining by nurses and the fact that significant headway has been made through this process regarding basic issues.

Elimination of Unions and Strike Breaking. A trend seen in healthcare institutions during the 1980s, and persisting in some areas today, is an effort toward eliminating unions. Although technically illegal when referring to methods used to eliminate an existing union, the movement has been expanded to include a wide range of legal activities that slow down collective bargaining or prevent a union from forming or functioning effectively. Pressured by rapidly escalating healthcare costs and influenced by the changing attitudes toward work, hospital administrators have hired consultants and law firms to assist and advise in discouraging and impeding organizational activities.

Another closely related approach involves mutual cooperation between management and the union without undermining the legitimate roles and rights of either. The union encourages wholehearted employee participation by its members while exercising flexibility on issues. With this approach, the union should have input into the managerial decision-making process through representation on committees at every level of the organization. Unions should be expected to be cooperative with management but not be co-opted. Management must be fair with the union, neither seeking to destroy the union nor meekly acquiescing to every union demand.

Strike breaking refers to efforts directed at causing employees on strike to cease the strike without having reached an agreement. In an effort to break a strike, employers hire temporary nurses at very high wages plus living stipends to entice them to come to work. Some temporary agencies specialize in providing nurses to work when the regular employees of the institution are on strike.

Impact of Shared Governance on Collective Bargaining. Although the greater involvement of staff nurses in healthcare agency decision making may have a significant impact on the collective bargaining process, the number of nurses represented by collective bargaining is increasing. When both collective bargaining and shared governance are present, there is a separation of those issues that are the purview of the union and those issues that can be decided within the shared governance structure. If there is a union, it has the responsibility and authority to negotiate those things that fall under wages, benefits, and working conditions, such as the use of agency nurses, work load, and policies regarding floating from one unit to another. The shared governance committees work with clinical standards. Each nurse has greater accountability for participation in decision making outside of the bargaining process and for implementing decisions that have been made.

Looking to the Future

As with many of the issues with which nursing wrestles, there are no easy answers to the matter of collective bargaining. Some view it as an absolute necessity; others find it unethical. And there are many who would prefer to play ostrich with regard to the entire concern, hoping it will not be necessary. Williams (2004) makes the following four recommendations regarding collective bargaining, all of which demonstrate opportunities for nursing leadership grounded in ethics:

- Because nurses are creative and powerful problem solvers, they should recognize the power that they have to observe, identify, and improve processes within the healthcare system.
- Nurses must recognize healthcare and hospital administrators as health professionals and be familiar and respectful of their ethical and professional obligations.
- Nursing curricula should provide graduates with a working understanding of all aspects of the ANA Code, especially provision six, which addresses collective action and advocacy.
- When selecting leaders and spokespersons for their groups, care should be taken to choose those who are able to listen, understand, and communicate the interests and problems identified by the other parties at the negotiating table. Powerful and creative leadership requires understanding both sides.

KEY CONCEPTS

- Mission statements provide information about critical elements of the organization. They explicitly outline the purpose of the organization and may also contain the philosophy and the vision or goals of the group. These statements serve as a benchmark against which an organization's performance may be evaluated.
- Organizations may be structured in a number of ways. Some are tall and centralized, where the authority to make decisions is vested in a few individuals. Others are flat and decentralized, with a number of individuals involved in decision making. Some have a matrix of functional roles.

- All organizations have chains of command, channels of communication, and spans of control that describe lines of authority and accountability. These can be depicted in organizational charts, which represent the formal organization and are a pictorial means of portraying roles and patterns of interaction among parts of a system.
- Written job descriptions outline the roles and responsibilities for all employees and are a necessary and vital part of any organization.
- Policies, protocols, and procedures guide the activities of the employees as they carry out their responsibilities.

- Shared governance, a form of practice model that involves decision making in which both nursing staff and management participate, results in a decentralized organization and often results in greater job satisfaction for nurses because they have more control over their practice.
- In the late 1980s, studies were conducted to determine what factors resulted in hospitals attracting and retaining RNs. Characteristics of these hospitals were identified, and the awarding of Magnet status to hospitals that achieve these goals has resulted. The process is carried out under the auspices of the ANCC.
- Patterns of nursing care delivery have varied over the years and include the case method, the functional method, team nursing, total patient care, modular care, and primary nursing.
- Case management provides an approach to the delivery of all patient care services (not just nursing) over an entire hospital stay or even throughout an entire healthcare concern. Nurses are involved in case management and may serve as case managers.
- Many workplace matters require negotiation. Major issues among these are grievances, collective bargaining contracts, and workplace safety issues.
- A grievance is an alleged violation of the provisions of the contract or institutional policies. Should a grievance arise, all steps must be followed as outlined in order for the grievance to be addressed effectively. Nurses need to distinguish between issues that are grievances and those that are simply complaints.

- Approaches to collective bargaining vary and include the historic adversarial approach, interest-based bargaining, and concession bargaining.
- Interest-based bargaining attempts to problem solve differences between labor and industry. Nurses can play a powerful leadership role in the process.
- The collective bargaining process culminates in a contract that places in writing the decisions reached at the bargaining table. Key aspects of a contract are the wages and benefits, issues of seniority and layoffs, grievance procedures, termination procedures, and working conditions (including professional involvement).
- One of the issues surrounding nurses and collective bargaining is related to which group should do the bargaining for nurses. Many believe this process is best conducted by a professional nursing organization; others believe they are served best by an organization that has collective bargaining as its only focus.
- Since 1974, nurses have bargained collectively for salaries, working conditions, and benefits. Collective bargaining may also negotiate for nurses' participation in committees focused on improving patient care and patient care standards and other issues of concern to nurses including staffing patterns, mandatory overtime, use of temporary nurses, workplace safety, and discriminatory practices.
- Trends regarding the collective bargaining process include constructive adversarialism, union busting, strike breaking, and changes in the number of bargaining units.

RELEVANT WEB SITES

Web sites relevant to this chapter can be found at thePoint✳ accessed through *http://thePoint. lww.com/Ellis10e* and by entering the code found on the inside cover of your text.

REFERENCES

American Nurses Association. (2001). *Code of ethics for nurses with interpretive statements.* Washington, DC: American Nurses Publishing.

ANCC Magnet Recognition Program. (2010). Retrieved July 29, 2010, from http://www.nursecredentialing.org/Magnet.aspx

Anthony, M. K. (2004). Shared governance models: The theory, practice, and evidence. *Online Journal of Issues in Nursing, 9*(1), Manuscript 4. Retrieved November 10, 2009, from www.nursingworld.org/MainMenuCategories/ ANAMarketplace/ANAPeriodicals/OJIN/TableofContents/Volume92004/No1Jan04/SharedGovernanceModels. aspx

Ashley, J. A. (1976). *Hospitals, paternalism and the role of the nurse.* New York: Teachers' College Press.

Brooks, B. A. (2004). Measuring the impact of shared governance. *Online Journal of Issues in Nursing, 9*(1), Manuscript 1a. Retrieved November 17, 2009, from www.nursingworld.org/MainMenuCategories/ ANAMarketplace/ANAPeriodicals/OJIN/TableofContents/Volume92004/No1Jan04/MeasuringtheImpact.aspx

Budd, K., Warino, L., & Patton, M. (2004, January 31). Traditional and non-traditional collective bargaining: Strategies to improve the patient care environment. *Online Journal of Issues in Nursing, 9*(1), Retrieved November 17, 2009, from www.nursingworld.org/MainMenuCategories/ANAMarketplace/ANAPeriodicals/ OJIN/TableofContents/Volume92004/No1Jan04/CollectiveBargainingStrategies.aspx

BusinessDictionary.com. (2009). *Organizational structure.* Retrieved November 17, 2009, from http://www.busi-nessdictionary.com/definition/organizational-structure.html

Dictionary.com. (2009). Protocol. Retrieved November 9, 2009, from http://dictionary.reference.com/browse/ protocol

Fagin, C., Maraldo, P., & Mason, D. (2008). What is magnet status and how's that whole thing going. *The Center for Nursing Advocacy.* Retrieved November 17, 2009, from http://www.nursingadvocacy.org/faq/magnet.html

Kramer, M., & Schmalenberg, C. E. (2005). Best quality patient care: A historical perspective on Magnet hospitals. *Nursing Administration, 29*(3), 275–287.

Labor-Management Relations Glossary. (n.d.). Retrieved November 29, 2009, from http://www.opm.gov/lmr/glos-sary/index.asp

McClure, M. L. (2005). Magnet hospitals: Insights and issues. *Nursing Administration, 29*(3), 198–201.

NLRB to the Supreme Court: Labor law protects nurses. (1996). *American Journal of Nursing, 96*(4), 67, 72.

Nurse Staffing and Quality of Patient Care, Structured Abstract. (2007, March). Agency for Healthcare Research and Quality. Rockville, MD. Retrieved November 23, 2009, from http://www.ahrq.gov/downloads/pub/evi-dence/pdf/nursestaff/nursestaff.pdf

Porter-O'Grady, T., & Malloch, K. (2007). *Managing for success in healthcare.* Philadelphia: Mosby Elsevier.

Reh, F. J. (2009). Cross training employees: Saves you money, makes them happy. Retrieved November 9, 2009, from http://management.about.com/cs/people/a/crosstrain.htm

Striking at bargaining rights, court says RNs are supervisors. (1994). *American Journal of Nursing, 94*(7), 67, 70–71.

Supreme Court Okays all-RN unit. (1991, June). *American Nurse, 33*(3), 1.

Swihart, D. (2006). *Shared governance: A practical approach to reshaping professional nursing practice.* Marblehead, MA: HCPro, Inc.

Williams, K. O. (2004). Ethics Column: Ethics and collective bargaining: Calls to action. *Online Journal of Issues in Nursing, 9(3).* Retrieved July 28, 2010, from http://www.nursingworld.org/MainMenuCategories/ ANAMarketplace/ANAPeriodicals/OJIN/Columns/Ethics/EthicsandCollectiveBargaining.aspx

Wilson, C. N., Hamilton, C. L., & Murphy, E. (1990). Union dynamics in nursing. *Journal of Nursing Administration, 20*(2), 35–39.

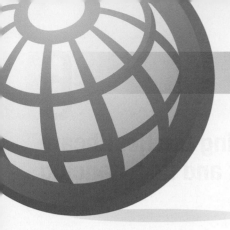

Understanding Healthcare in Today's Society

This unit provides you with a basic overview of the healthcare delivery system in the United States. Chapter 6 begins with the part of the system with which you are probably most familiar—those settings that employ nurses—and then expands to include some of those that are lesser known and understood. After gaining an understanding of the various players in the system, you should find it easier to analyze specific issues, such as access, finance, power, and control, which are also addressed.

A well-grounded understanding of the legal and ethical dimensions of practice provides the foundation for professional nursing. Chapter 7 initiates a discussion of the legal ramifications of practice. Concrete examples provide help in understanding specific legal issues of importance to consumers and healthcare providers. The chapter concludes with the role of the nurse as a witness.

Ethical and bioethical issues associated with healthcare constantly challenge us as professionals and as members of society. Each technologic advance brings additional questions and concerns to our attention. Chapters 8 and 9 explore these issues and their ramifications on nursing practice. A discussion of major questions posed by ethical and bioethical issues provides an understanding of the basis of ethical decision making and the factors that significantly affect it and outlines a framework for ethical decision making. Some of the specific problems you will encounter as you move into a professional role are explored in the hope that considering them before you become directly involved will help you to address them more comfortably.

Chapter 10, Safety Concerns in Healthcare, is devoted to issues related to safe patient care. Beginning with findings from the Institute of Medicine study conducted in 1999, the content expands to include a review of actions taken by other national organizations to increase patient safety. Areas of major concern are identified with discussion of strategies and tools to eliminate errors. The chapter concludes with a discussion of major areas in which nurses play a critical role in the prevention of adverse events.

The unit concludes with Chapter 11 and a discussion of nursing's role in the community. Wherever their individual practice settings, nurses have an impact on the health of their communities. Moving toward the goals of Healthy People 2020 will require a commitment from all those in the system. Included in this chapter is a discussion on complementary and alternative healthcare and how that affects the health of both individuals and communities.

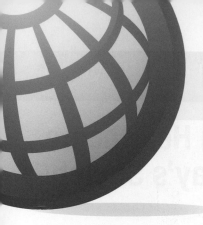

6

Understanding the Healthcare Environment and Its Financing

LEARNING OUTCOMES

After completing this chapter, you should be able to:

1. Explain the classification systems for healthcare organizations and the particular focus of each.
2. Differentiate the goals for client/resident care in acute care hospitals and long-term care facilities.
3. Describe the roles of the various healthcare providers, and analyze how these roles affect the relationships between providers.
4. Analyze how issues related to education, credentialing, and scope of practice of healthcare occupations affect individual providers and clients within the healthcare system.
5. Discuss the various mechanisms used for financing healthcare and managing costs in the healthcare system and how healthcare reform of 2010 may affect these.
6. Explain how quality in organizations and agencies that are delivering healthcare is measured and ensured.
7. Analyze the use of power by regulatory agencies, payers, providers, and consumers in the healthcare system.
8. Explain continuing concerns regarding the effective use of healthcare resources.
9. Describe how the nurse could use knowledge of the healthcare system and its financing when teaching clients and planning for continuity of care.

KEY TERMS

Access	Medicaid
Accreditation	Medicare
Capitation	Medigap insurance
Case management	Minimum data set (MDS)
Case mix	Point-of-service (POS) plan
Clinical pathway	Power
Comorbidity	Preferred provider organization (PPO)
Diagnosis-related groups (DRGs)	Primary care provider (PCP)
Entitlement	Prospective payment
Fee-for-service payment	Quality indicators (QI)
Independent practice association (IPO)	Resource utilization groups (RUGs)
Intensity measures	Skilled nursing facility (SNF)
Key indicators	Third-party payer
Managed care	Vertically integrated systems

Healthcare is an exciting and rewarding field but also a challenging one due to the issues that surround it. The entire healthcare system reverberates with change. The roles of nurses in this system constantly develop and expand. You can function more effectively within this system if you understand the various healthcare agencies and their services, the roles that nurses perform in those agencies, and the colleagues with whom you work. We will begin with an overview of healthcare agencies and then discuss the financing of healthcare.

CLASSIFICATION OF HEALTHCARE AGENCIES

The healthcare industry is so large, diverse, and complex that it is difficult to understand. Generally, agencies providing care are classified according to length of stay, ownership, or type of service. These classifications are somewhat arbitrary, and any agency may be placed in more than one classification. With the systemic changes that are occurring, one large entity may exist that includes multiple lengths of stay, types of service, and ownership patterns. Understanding these categories is useful because they are used to plan for services, to describe institutions, and to allocate funding and reimbursement. Your understanding also can be used to guide clients and families through what sometimes seems a maze of confusion in the healthcare system (Fig. 6.1).

Classification According to Length of Stay

One way of classifying inpatient agencies is according to the average *length of stay,* or how long patients remain in the facility. Ambulatory care, short stay, traditional acute care, and long-term care are terms that reflect the average length of stay in a facility. Table 6.1 outlines the various definitions of care according to length of stay.

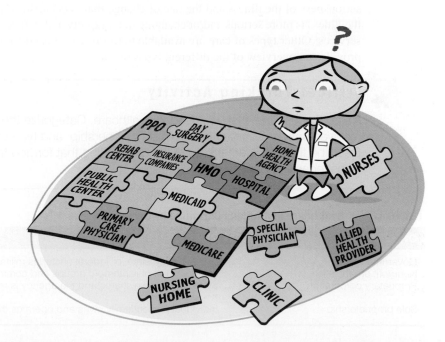

FIGURE 6.1 The many aspects of healthcare in the United States.

Table 6.1   **Healthcare Institutions Classified by Length of Stay**

LENGTH OF STAY	DESCRIPTION
In-and-out care	Contact with client is measured in minutes vs. hours. Typical examples are office visits, emergency department visits, and therapy sessions.
Short stay	Provides care to patients who suffer from acute conditions or require treatments that require <24 hours of care and monitoring. Diagnostic tests or minimally invasive surgery are examples.
Acute care	Traditionally occurs in hospitals where patients stay >24 hours but <30 days. Stays are shortened since the advent of managed care and DRGs.
Long-term care	Provides care to residents for the remainder of their lives; care also includes services to patients with limited recovery needs, functional losses, chronic disease, mental illness, or major rehabilitation, which may range from 30 to 90 days.

Classification According to Ownership

The second method of classifying healthcare agencies is according to ownership. Agencies may be classified as governmental (public) or proprietary (private profit-making) or nonprofit. Table 6.2 provides information about the various types of ownership. An important consideration is that all healthcare agencies, regardless of their ownership, need to have income sufficient to meet the costs of the care provided as well as to maintain and upgrade the equipment and physical facilities that support that care. No agency can continue to exist if it is not adequately funded.

Classification According to Type of Care

Healthcare agencies may also be classified according to *type of care* provided. Many agencies provide more than one type of care. The type of care is based on the acuity, which is the seriousness of the illness and the rate of change that is occurring. Higher acuity signifies that the illness is more serious and/or changing more rapidly and will demand a greater intensity of services. Other types of care are available to those whose need for services differs. Table 6.3 provides an overview of the different types of care.

Critical Thinking Activity

Recall the last time that you needed healthcare. Categorize the place where you received care in regard to length of stay, ownership, and type of care provided. Describe those characteristics of the care setting that formed the basis for your decisions regarding classification.

Table 6.2   **Healthcare Institutions Classified by Ownership**

OWNERSHIP	DESCRIPTION
Government	Local, county, state, or federal (includes military and veterans facilities).
Nonprofit organization	Religious and philanthropic groups and community organizations.
Proprietary corporation	Stockholders own shares and the agency is managed for the benefit of stockholders.
Sole proprietorship	Individual person/family owns and operates the agency.

Table 6.3 **Healthcare Institutions Classified by Type of Care**

TYPE OF CARE	DESCRIPTION
Acute care	Illness needing immediate hospitalization and provision of diagnostic tests, treatments, and/or monitoring that require the continuous availability of skilled nursing care. Goals are recovery from illness or injury and restoration to previous level of function.
Long-term acute care	Illness that has stabilized but still needs the ongoing provision of highly skilled care, such as ventilator support or care for major unhealed wounds. Goals are correction of the underlying problem and eventual move to a less skilled level of care.
Subacute care	Care provided after initial recovery from an acute illness needing inpatient care. Skilled care is needed but on a less frequent and intense basis. Goals are to restore function for discharge to home. It is usually provided in a separate unit in an acute care hospital.
Skilled nursing care	Care provided after initial recovery from an acute illness needing inpatient care or following subacute care. Skilled care is still needed, but on a less frequent and intense basis. Goals are to restore function for discharge to home. It is usually provided in a nursing home.
Custodial care	Care is needed because of functional deficits in the ADLs rather than due to the illness itself. Care may be provided in an assisted-living setting, an adult family home (board and care home), or a nursing home. The goals of care are maintenance of functioning and maximum wellness in the face of disability.
Hospice care	Care provided for the terminally ill in the last 6 months before expected death. Care may be provided in the home or an inpatient hospice. Goals are patient autonomy and relief of symptoms while supporting the patient toward a peaceful death and the family and others in their mourning processes.
Ambulatory care	Care for the person who can come to the healthcare agency, receive needed healthcare, and then be discharged to home. It may be a clinic or office. It may also be in hospital departments that provide skilled care for 24 hours or less. Goals are focused on treating a health problem and returning the person to an independent living situation.
Home care	Care providers visit the home to provide some types of care, teach the patient and family how to manage care in the home, and evaluate response to treatment. The goal is effective patient and family self-care.

UNDERSTANDING TODAY'S HOSPITAL

The modern hospital is often viewed as the hub or center of the healthcare delivery system and as central to the healthcare of a community, although more care is moving into community settings and the emphasis is on avoiding and limiting hospitalization. A primary characteristic of hospital care is its focus on the current problem, rapid assessment, stabilization or treatment, and then discharge.

In addition to supplying healthcare to clients, hospitals also provide education to a wide variety of healthcare workers and to the community. In many cases, they also serve as centers for research and research dissemination. Hospitals use their status and position in healthcare to enter into cooperative agreements and alliances with healthcare providers, insurance companies, and even other hospitals.

The Development of Hospitals in the United States

The history of hospitals in the United States can be traced back to the mid-1700s, when most cities built almshouses, also called poorhouses. Almshouses provided food and shelter for the homeless poor and served as homes for the aged, disabled, mentally ill, and orphaned. "Pest houses" also were built at this time to isolate people with contagious diseases, especially those diseases contracted aboard a ship. These facilities housed people suffering from cholera, smallpox, typhus, and yellow fever, and the more common communicable diseases such as scarlet fever. Pest houses opened and closed as needed.

Neither almshouses nor pest houses were institutions from which most individuals would want to seek or receive care. They were crowded and unsanitary, with insufficient heat and ventilation. Cross-infection was common, and mortality was high. Those with financial means were cared for in their homes.

The first hospital, founded in what was to become the United States, was started in Philadelphia in 1751, at the urging of Benjamin Franklin. Franklin believed that the public had a duty to provide care to the poor, friendless, sick, and insane. A bill passed that year authorizing the establishment of the Pennsylvania Hospital (Kalisch & Kalisch, 2004). The New York Hospital in New York City was established in 1773, primarily to prevent the spread of infectious diseases brought by sailors and immigrants. Massachusetts General Hospital in Boston opened its doors in 1816 and New Haven Hospital in Connecticut in 1826.

The early hospitals cared for people with acute illnesses and injuries but did not admit the mentally ill. Separate hospitals were established for this purpose. The first such facility was established as a department of the Pennsylvania Hospital in 1752. The second was founded in Williamsburg, Virginia, in 1773; the third, known as Friends Hospital, was located near Philadelphia in 1817. By 1840, eight hospitals to treat the mentally ill had been established (Kalisch & Kalisch, 2004). The cruel and inhumane treatment of patients in the early mental hospitals is legendary. Dorothea Dix campaigned vigorously for and brought about much reform in the area of mental health treatment. Although never educated as a nurse (she was a schoolteacher), Dix volunteered as a nurse during the Civil War and is included in the Nursing Hall of Fame because of her significant contributions to the profession.

The earliest hospitals left much to be desired. Most were housed in large buildings that had been converted from other uses. Often they were dirty, rank with infection, and poorly ventilated. Linens were used for several patients before being laundered, even though draining, suppurating wounds were common. The stench was overwhelming, and it is said that nurses used snuff to make working conditions more tolerable (Kalisch & Kalisch, 2004). Hospitals constructed during the early 19th century often followed a block plan in their design, and the buildings resembled large barns. Much of Florence Nightingale's writings on hospital design pushed for the use of a "pavilion" plan in which smaller units would be constructed to enable cross-ventilation and sunlight, would be equipped with smooth walls and floors to facilitate cleaning, and would separate patients from one another (Bostwick, 2008). In the 1850s, Massachusetts General Hospital constructed a facility divided into wards or pavilions, each one a separate building with high ceilings and good ventilation. The buildings were built of wood because it was believed they would need to be replaced after 20 years because of contamination (Kalisch & Kalisch, 2004, p. 21).

Factors Affecting the Development of Hospitals

Six major forces can be cited as influencing the growth of hospitals throughout the United States. Each played a unique role in the continued development of hospitals and patient care.

Advances in Medical Science

By the end of the colonial period, two medical schools had been established in the United States. Before that time, physicians learned their skills through an apprenticeship with a practicing physician. As medicine became more of a science, advances occurred. One of the most significant was the discovery of anesthesia and the rapid progress in surgery that followed. The germ theory also did much to improve the practice of medicine because it inspired the development of agents or techniques that would sterilize or serve as antiseptics and provided a rationale for cleanliness. The growth of hospitals in the United States was a direct result of such progress, which made hospitals safer and more desirable. The discovery of sulfa in the mid-1930s and antibiotics in the mid-1940s heralded even greater changes.

The Development of Medical Technology

The development of specialized medical technology was a natural successor to the advances in medical science. The first hospital laboratory opened in 1889, and x-rays were used in diagnosis in 1896. The electrocardiogram was invented in 1903 and the electroencephalogram in 1929 (Haglund & Dowling, 1993). Since those early days, new technology has continued to expand.

Changes in Medical Education

Advances in medical education also had a significant impact on the development of hospitals. *The Flexner Report*, a study of medical education, was completed in 1910, and it led to changes in the structure and content of curricula in medical schools. It also expanded the role of hospitals to include education and research and resulted in internships and residencies for medical students.

Growth of the Health Insurance Industry

The growth of the health insurance industry is another factor responsible for the development of hospitals. Although there were some antecedents, most sources indicate that the first hospital insurance plan was initiated at Baylor University Hospital in 1929 to serve the needs of schoolteachers in Dallas, Texas. Their approach formed the model for Blue Cross plans around the country. As health insurance grew more widespread, individuals more often could afford hospital care.

Greater Involvement of the Government

In early times, the government was involved in healthcare delivery primarily at a local level, building almshouses and facilities for the insane. The federal government built public health hospitals for seamen and military hospitals for members of the armed services. By 1935, the government was providing grants-in-aid to assist in the establishment of public health and other programs to furnish health assistance to citizens. The Hospital Survey and Construction Act of 1946 (also called the Hill-Burton Act) resulted in the construction of many hospitals and other health facilities. The initiation of **Medicare** (the federal health plan for those on Social Security and their dependents) and **Medicaid** (state health plans for certain low-income individuals paid through a combination of state and federal funds) in 1965 made another significant impact on the healthcare industry, because the legislation encouraged capital construction and the development of hospitals through the manner in which the system of reimbursement was structured. The passage of the Patient Protection and Affordable Health Care

Act of 2010 (healthcare reform) was another major step in the federal government's attempt to assure healthcare for all legal residents of the United States (see Chapter 15 for an overview of this legislation).

The Emergence of Professional Nursing

Another force that significantly influenced the growth of hospitals was the development of professional nursing. According to Haglund and Dowling (1993, p. 139), first, it "increased the efficiency of treatment, cleanliness, nutritious diets, and formal treatment routines" that resulted in patient recovery. Second, it resulted in considerate, skilled patient care that made hospitals acceptable to all people, not just the poor. The role of the nurse and nursing influences the healthcare delivery system more today than ever before.

Hospital Services for Patients and Families

The two terms used frequently to describe today's modern hospital services are "inpatient care" and "outpatient care." Individuals are termed inpatients when they have been admitted for the purpose of staying 24 hours or longer. The outpatient comes to the hospital for services, but is expected to stay less than 24 hours.

Inpatient units comprise what most people think of when they use the designation "acute care hospital" (see Table 6.1). Nurses work in all of these service departments, coordinating the nursing care for individual clients, managing the care environment, delegating and supervising care provided by others, and providing direct skilled care.

In addition to these usual acute care units, hospitals have developed transitional care and rehabilitation units that provide long-term care services, often closing some units and converting them to areas offering these other types of care. A transitional care or rehabilitation unit allows a hospital to discharge an individual from acute, inpatient care in a timely fashion because the next level of services is guaranteed to be available. Reimbursement for the transitional or rehabilitation care is based on long-term care guidelines, and the care must meet long-term care standards for skilled nursing care. Inpatient rehabilitation services may be provided only for a brief period of time, followed by outpatient rehabilitation services.

Outpatient care, also termed "ambulatory care," is care that is provided for a period of time expected to be less than 24 hours. The outpatient goes through an admission process, has a procedure performed or care delivered, is determined to be ready for home care, and is discharged. Many diagnostic and treatment procedures, surgeries, and emergency health needs are treated as outpatient care. When people must remain longer than 24 hours for observation and management, their status may remain as an outpatient and may not be converted to inpatient unless a continued stay is expected.

The distinction between the categories of inpatient and outpatient is important in regard to both billing and discharge to a nursing home. Both Medicare and Medicaid are billed differently for outpatient care than for inpatient care. Medicare payments for nursing home care after hospitalization require that the person be admitted as an inpatient with a minimum 3-day hospital stay. When these conditions are not met, Medicare payment is denied for a nursing home stay even if it meets the standards of being for recovery and return to home. Patients and their families may not understand this distinction and how it affects the bills they receive and their eligibility for some types of reimbursement. Nurses must understand that different rules

Table 6.4 **Hospitals Classified by Mix of Services**

TYPE	SERVICES
General or community hospital	Medical, surgical, obstetric, emergency, and diagnostic, plus laboratory services.
Tertiary care hospital	Referral centers for clients with complex or unusual health problems such as level 1 trauma, major burns, bone marrow transplant, and research-based oncology, in addition to standard care. Part of a large medical center associated with a university. Serves a wide geographic area
Specialty hospital	Offers only a particular type of care (ie, psychiatric, pediatric).

may apply and refer patients and families to appropriate resources for accurate information as they help patients to plan for needed care after discharge.

Hospitals may also be referred to by the mix of traditional inpatient services that are offered (Table 6.4). Not every hospital offers each of the services mentioned earlier, but more are becoming part of a corporate entity that provides all services. The terms most commonly used to describe the mix of services are the "general" or "community" hospital, the "tertiary care" hospital, and the "specialty" hospital.

Hospitals may offer other services that are not directed solely at client care. Day procedures and early discharge for inpatient care may present travel difficulties for individuals who live a long distance from a major care center. To facilitate care for these patients and their families, some hospitals have developed hotel-like services, often termed "hospitality units," where the patient scheduled for day surgery may plan to arrive the day before and stay overnight. A family member may also stay in the unit during the individual's hospitalization. After discharge, both the patient and the family member may stay one or more days before traveling home. The cost of staying in a hospitality unit is not covered by insurance, but it is much more convenient than staying in a hotel and typically the cost is less than in a hotel. Additionally, if an emergency occurs, the patient in a hospitality unit has care immediately available.

Hospitals as Educational Institutions

The education of healthcare providers is an important function of many hospitals. Although the number of hospital-based schools of nursing offering diplomas has decreased steadily, some are well supported and expect to continue operation. There are also hospital-based programs for respiratory therapy, dietetics, medical laboratory technology, and other health-related occupations.

Many hospitals serve as clinical laboratory sites for individuals who enrolled in colleges and universities that provide education for healthcare professionals. These individuals include students in nursing, laboratory sciences, nutrition, pharmacy, radiology and imaging, and other disciplines as well as medicine.

Graduate medical education includes all the residency programs for physicians preparing for independent practice. Residents receive a salary from the hospital and are responsible for providing services in return. Residents augment the services of primary physicians, who are often referred to as the attending or staff physicians. Residents often provide the majority of medical services for individuals who are part of the medically underserved in a community, consulting with the staff physician in charge as needed. Part of the funding for graduate medical education comes from the money made available through Medicare.

THE LONG-TERM CARE FACILITY

Long-term care refers to any of the different care settings that involve coordination of the entire multidisciplinary team to provide counseling, nursing care, rehabilitation, nutritional support, social services, and sometimes special education programs over months to years. Managing a positive living environment is as important as managing health problems for long-term care residents. Long-term care facilities include nursing homes, assisted-living centers, adult care homes (also called board and care homes), chronic disease hospitals, psychiatric hospitals, and group homes for those with developmental disabilities or chronic mental health problems. The majority of long-term care facilities are nursing homes that care primarily for the elderly.

Nursing Homes

The nursing home is the care facility most often associated with long-term care. Although nursing homes suffer from negative images of the past and not all meet appropriate standards for care, they do offer a far different environment than they did 20 years ago. Nursing homes in the United States provide care and a positive living environment for individuals who have the greatest number of deficits in activities of daily living (ADLs). ADLs include dressing, bathing, eating, toileting, and ambulating. Just as the acute care hospital, the nursing home is expanding services beyond those traditionally associated with nursing home care. A nursing home that provides skilled care in nursing, physical therapy, and speech therapy is termed a **skilled nursing facility (SNF)**.

History of the Nursing Home

Like acute care facilities, the nursing home had a rather harsh beginning. In the 19th century, almshouses sheltered the destitute elderly. These facilities attracted a strange mixture of residents, including those who needed asylum and detention, as well as the poor, the chronically disabled, and the mentally ill. According to the moral perspective that prevailed at the time, poverty and disability were viewed as indications of an undisciplined and wasteful life. A person who was housed in a "county poorhouse" often had no financial resources and no family to provide care and assistance and endured a certain social stigma. In time, these almshouses became the community dumping grounds for all of society's cast-offs. The early facilities for the country's dependent elderly offered the same grim surroundings as the early hospitals. They were unsanitary, overcrowded, and poorly ventilated. Residents were expected to work to assist with their keep if they were able. Individuals who provided care sought employment there usually as a last resort. Appropriations to manage these facilities were meager because most citizens did not identify with the institutions that housed the poor and the transient.

As the United States grew as a society, various groups became concerned about the conditions that existed in the almshouses. Eventually, patients were separated according to their condition, and the mentally and chronically ill were reassigned to different institutions. An increasing number of churches and fraternal organizations started homes to care for their elderly members. As a result of the Social Security Act of 1935, private (for-profit or proprietary) nursing homes emerged during that decade.

In the postwar period, the Hill-Burton Act of 1946, which supported hospital construction, was expanded to include voluntary (nonprofit) nursing homes, and some states also developed grant programs. Since 1950, government funding for nursing home care has increased steadily. Governmental regulation of nursing homes has become increasingly involved and complex.

As changes in funding occurred and as short-term acute care hospitals became increasingly specialized, the role of the nursing home changed. In the 1950s and 1960s, the deinstitutionalization movement, which saw large numbers of the elderly population with dementia discharged from mental hospitals, also affected nursing homes. Nursing homes began to assume the role of providing specialized care for the elderly. By the 1960s, this role was well established, but the nursing home industry was plagued by constant reports of substandard and negligent care and, in some instances, charges of absolute abuse of patients and misuse or embezzlement of their funds. This resulted in even greater scrutiny and regulation by the government.

Today, "nursing home" is a broad term that encompasses over 16,000 facilities ranging from special units in acute community hospitals to those that are a part of the campus of continuing care retirement centers (Centers for Disease Control and Prevention [CDC], 2009). The facilities are licensed by the state in which they operate, and each state has its own definitions and requirements; however, 87.6% are certified for payment by Medicare and/or Medicaid (CDC, 2009), and thus are subject to federal standards. The major reason for admission to a nursing home is functional dependence in terms of basic ADLs and cognitive impairment rather than medical diagnosis.

The Nursing Home Resident

Although most of the elderly live in community settings, many will spend their last years in a nursing home. Seventy one percent of the residents are women, reflecting the longer life span of women and the greater likelihood that a woman's spouse will precede her in death. The most recent data available from the National Nursing Home Survey (NNHS) indicate that over 98% are dependent in at least one ADL and more than half of all residents are dependent in all five ADLs. Typically, nursing home residents range in age from 65 to older than 100, with 45.2% aged 85 and older (CDC, 2009).

The number of individuals requiring nursing home care is expected to steadily increase, based on the increasing number of the elderly. According to the 2000 census, the number of people aged 80 to 84 increased by 26% from the 1990 census, those 90 to 94 increased by 45%, and those over 100 increased by 35% (U.S. Census Bureau, Statistical Abstract 2004–2005). While complete data from the 2010 census is not yet compiled, it is expected to show further increases in all categories of older adults. The CIA Factbook provides an estimate that 13.1% of the 2011 U.S. population is over 65 (CIA, 2011).

Health Services in Nursing Homes

The majority of residents in nursing homes remain there because of major deficits in self-care abilities and the need for ongoing care that is custodial in focus rather than treatment oriented. Maintenance of function, independence, autonomy, and rehabilitation are all goals for nursing home residents. Residents are concerned with the living environment and the healthcare environment.

Units designed for the cognitively impaired are free of restraints and barriers to mobility. Facility design and alarm systems prevent residents from wandering away. These units provide special approaches to care delivery that decrease stress and reduce the potential for hostile, angry outbursts. Reality orientation is used for those who might benefit from this therapy. Validation therapy and reminiscence also are planned to provide a supportive and rich environment. Staff development assists caregivers in responding appropriately to the special challenges of working with the cognitively impaired.

Some nursing homes have entire wings devoted to individuals receiving post-hospital convalescent care where the major goal is rehabilitation and return to independent living. These individuals are admitted with a specific planned stay of 14 to 30 days. During this time, the individual is aided in restoring functional abilities and planning for self or family care. Activities might include physical therapy for the person with a hip replacement or speech therapy after a stroke.

The level of autonomy expected of nurses employed in nursing homes where physicians visit monthly is often surprising to those who have always worked in acute care hospitals, where physicians visit patients daily and resident physicians are available when needed. In nursing homes, the individual may be a permanent resident and the nurse may be charged with managing both quality of life and quality of care. Additionally, nurses in these settings must manage care conducted by a variety of assistive personnel and work effectively with an interdisciplinary team.

Funding Nursing Home Care

The cost of nursing home care is a concern for many. The annual cost of nursing home care in a semiprivate room ranges from $44,553 in Texas to $189,891 in Alaska, with a national average of $66,850 (Genworth, 2009). Medicare pays for only a limited number of days for individuals who meet specific criteria regarding hospitalization and who need skilled care or rehabilitation rather than custodial care. Some individuals have long-term care insurance that will pay part of their costs. An increasing number of individuals are purchasing policies, which are available through a number of organizations. Personal financial resources are frequently exhausted by a prolonged nursing home stay. State-administered public assistance in the form of programs such as Medicaid and Medi-Cal (as it is called in California) pays for nursing home care when an individual's personal financial resources have fallen below a certain state-determined level. By 2007 Medicaid (including both federal and state portions) covered approximately 42% of all nursing home costs and Medicare covered another 17.5%, leaving 40.5% covered through personal resources including private long-term care insurance (CMS, 2008a). Payment for an individual resident may come from multiple sources with insurance paying a sum, personal resources (such as savings, Social Security, and/or pension) paying a portion, and Medicaid paying for the remainder. As the number of elderly individuals requiring nursing home care continues to rise, these costs create a serious budget concern in most states.

Regulation of Nursing Home Care

Nursing homes are among the most regulated of all healthcare facilities. Because the federal government pays for some of the care, federal regulations affect nursing homes across the country. Starting primarily with the Federal Budget Act of 1987, government regulations mandate specific assessment tools; planning processes; standards of care, including the use of restraints and psychoactive medications; documentation systems used; and evaluation tools. Data are collected according to a standardized minimum data set (MDS). State regulations may place additional requirements on nursing homes. Nursing homes are visited by a survey team that is responsible for ensuring adherence to regulatory standards. The results of nursing home surveys are public documents and must be displayed in each facility in a place accessible to the public and to residents who wish to review them. Nursing home survey results may be seen on the Medicare Web site at *www.medicare.gov/Nhcompare/Home.asp*.

Critical Thinking Activity

Use the Web site *www.medicare.gov/Nhcompare/Home.asp* to investigate a nursing home in your community. Find out its average length of stay, the types of services it offers, and its type of ownership. Analyze the quality of care provided as represented through the nursing home survey. Compare this facility with two other nursing homes in your geographic area.

Assisted-Living Facilities

The assisted-living facility provides care for those needing help with up to three ADLs. In an assisted-living arrangement, the resident can maintain maximum independence and use a shared decision-making model to decide when additional help or support is needed. Husbands and wives reside together and may often bring their own furniture and belongings to create a homelike atmosphere. Those who are able to perform any ADLs seek the less costly and more independent and flexible living found here. Assisted-living facilities have been much less regulated than nursing homes. As these facilities admit more impaired individuals, or as individuals living in them want to "age in place," concerns are being raised about the quality of care provided. Increasing regulation is expected. The Joint Commission provides a voluntary accrediting process for assisted-living centers.

Care in Assisted-Living Facilities

In an assisted-living facility, all instrumental ADLs such as shopping, cleaning, meal preparation, and laundry are provided. A resident is expected to have some mobility (even though it may require a walker or a cane) and to eat in a dining room except when the person is temporarily ill. Residents also are expected to manage their own medication and health needs, although they may be assisted with remembering to take medications. Assistance is provided with bathing, dressing, and other personal care as needed. Most care is provided by unlicensed assistive personnel. Licensed nurses may be employed in a supervisory capacity and may plan for care. One area of controversy is the level of assistance with medications and health needs that can be provided by unlicensed, unregulated personnel. Some states are authorizing delegation to appropriately trained assistive personnel of selected nursing tasks, such as giving oral medications, for residents of assisted living.

The level of disability that requires a move to a nursing home may vary based on the regulations governing assisted living. In some jurisdictions, there is very little regulation, and decisions are made by the agency as to whom it can continue to care for. This sometimes creates difficulties when residents require skilled care and the facility does not have the resources to provide that level of care. For some individuals, the transitions from independent living to assisted living and from assisted living to nursing home care are smooth ones, thus avoiding the transition or relocation stress that affects their well-being. This is particularly true when multiple levels of care are available in the same retirement living setting. (See the discussion of continuing care retirement communities below.) For others, this change triggers serious stress and is one of the reasons for pressure to allow residents to remain in assisted-living settings even when very incapacitated.

Board and care homes, sometimes termed *adult family homes*, that provide assisted living and some services similar to nursing homes are licensed in some states. These individual residences usually house six or fewer adults needing care and assistance. Originally planned as care in private homes that would be operated by the owner or resident, many now are commercial operations with a paid staff. The costs are usually less than for a nursing home. One concern is the difficulty of regulating these small residences where there are no professional caregivers.

Funding Assisted Living

Assisted living is not supported with Medicare funds and therefore does not have to meet the stringent regulatory standards of federal legislation. Public assistance, in the form of Medicaid, Medi-Cal, or other programs, may provide some support for assisted living when the alternative would be expensive nursing home care for which the state would be responsible; however, this is not true in all jurisdictions. Most assisted living is paid for by the individual or family.

Retirement Communities

Retirement communities, which continue to grow, may be self-contained towns, retirement villages, retirement subdivisions, retirement residences, or continuing care retirement communities. The basic retirement complex is designed to provide the environment for self-care and may support independence longer than would a regular house or apartment. Home care services are provided to those in retirement communities in the same way that they are provided to those in regular homes or apartments.

Continuing care retirement communities provide a variety of levels of independent and dependent living and care to residents based on each resident's needs. Most residents enter the community to reside in a retirement apartment or home and then move within the community to an assisted-living section and from there to a convalescent or nursing home center if that becomes necessary. Services such as occupational therapy, physical therapy, and dental care also may be available as home care or for those in the convalescent center. The aim is for people to reside in the setting that provides maximum autonomy and independence while ensuring that needs are met. A major limiting factor is the cost of such communities to the individual residents.

Rehabilitation Centers

Rehabilitation centers typically focus on a specific healthcare problem; for example, there are centers for those with spinal cord injuries and other centers focusing on head injuries or cerebral vascular accidents. Although many of these agencies prefer nurses who have taken advanced courses in rehabilitation nursing, many employ nurses with different backgrounds, such as those who have worked in a nursing home focused on rehabilitation principles.

Other Long-Term Care Facilities

Some of the other long-term care facilities available are the group homes for the developmentally disabled and for those with chronic psychiatric illnesses. These smaller residences, most with 12 or fewer residents, strive to create a home-like atmosphere in which individuals can function at their highest capacity. They are often hampered by the lack of stable funding and the difficulty of hiring qualified care providers because of the low wages typically offered.

AMBULATORY CARE SETTINGS

Ambulatory care has long been provided in offices, clinics, and the day-procedure units of hospitals. Some ambulatory care is provided in settings where people work and go to school. Providing care where people routinely spend their days rather than requiring them to go to a different site for healthcare often results in a more effective use of healthcare services. Some ambulatory care settings rely heavily on the skills of registered nurses (RNs) to provide assessment and teaching, while others focus on medical care provided by physicians, nurse practitioners, and physician assistants, with medical assistants for routine tasks.

Healthcare Provider Offices

One of the major changes in healthcare has been the decrease in the number of solo practice offices and the growth of group and organizational practices. Many medical practices are owned by health systems that also own hospitals. Within a private-physician practice setting, there may be several general practice physicians and many specialists. Advanced practice nurses (APNs) and physician assistants also are working in many of these group practice settings. Other RNs in these settings may have responsibility for triage, assessment, teaching, and providing direct care. Nursing roles in ambulatory care are expanding as the need for the cost-effective use of physician time is modifying practice patterns.

Walk-In Clinics

Walk-in clinics treat clients with emergent conditions that do not require the high-technology resources of the emergency room. Walk-in clinics may be referred to as immediate care facilities, urgent care centers, or emergent care centers and are usually open during extended hours that include evenings and weekends, in addition to the traditional Monday through Friday office hours. Some operate within retail pharmacies. Walk-in clinics have grown in popularity as people find it increasingly difficult to gain access to traditional healthcare settings because of their personal time constraints.

Many walk-in clinics have gradually added services such as sports physical examinations for school-age children, pelvic examinations and Pap tests for women, and routine immunizations. Some are beginning to act as primary care providers, advertising the willingness of staff doctors to become family doctors. Walk-in clinics have relatively small nursing staffs, often employing only one RN during a shift; therefore, each nurse must have a wide variety of skills and be able to function with a high degree of autonomy. Some settings do not use RNs in direct care; they are hired in these settings only to supervise other clinic staff members and may oversee more than one facility. Licensed practical nurses (LPNs) may be employed in ambulatory care to collect data, carry out specific treatments, and give medications.

COMMUNITY AGENCIES

Agencies providing care in the community include public health agencies, home care agencies, and hospice care.

Public Health Agencies

Public health departments are operated as agencies of the government. In general, the focus of health departments has been on broad community issues, communicable diseases, and infant and child health. Public health nurses originally did a great deal of individual family visiting, but today fewer funds are available for visits. As a result, public health nurses now focus on individuals who are at high risk and whose health affects the entire community, such as those with tuberculosis. Public health nurses responsible for community health issues are required to have a baccalaureate degree in nursing; however, some agencies operate a variety of clinics (such as immunization clinics) in which RNs with an associate degree or diploma provide teaching and direct care services. With severe cutbacks in state and local funding, many programs traditionally operated by public health agencies are being eliminated.

Home Care Agencies

Home care agencies, such as the traditional visiting nurse services and the proprietary home healthcare companies, provide a broad spectrum of care that may include nursing care, personal care assistance, minor housekeeping, physical therapy, occupational therapy, speech/language therapy, and respiratory therapy for individuals in their homes. Teaching family and caregivers is a large part of the home care professional's responsibility. The focus of home care agencies is broad. It ranges from providing short-term visits for clients who need assistance after a hospital stay or acute illness to assisting clients who will need ongoing home care for years, such as those requiring dialysis or ventilator support in the home. People with these conditions may require nursing care for 8- to 12-hour shifts in the home or episodic visits that last from 15 to 60 minutes.

Hospice Care

The goal of hospice care is to assist the terminally ill individual to maintain the highest possible quality of life until death. Hospice care may be provided in the home with care providers visiting as needed. Some hospices provide services to individuals living in assisted-living or nursing home settings. There are inpatient hospice units for those who do not have a family and friends to act as home caregivers or for whom this would be too great a task. Multidisciplinary teams may include physicians, nurses, clergy, occupational and physical therapists, home health aides, social workers, and volunteers who work with both the hospice patient and the family or other caregivers. Nurses provide special skills in symptom management for physical problems, such as pain, nausea, anorexia, and constipation and psychosocial support for end-of-life events and issues. Nurses are usually responsible for the management and coordination of hospice care.

Community Mental Health Centers

Community mental health centers were established to allow individuals with psychiatric problems to remain in their communities. Services may include individual counseling and therapy, group or family counseling, evaluation, and referral. For those who must be hospitalized, the community mental health center provides follow-up care that facilitates early discharge. These centers usually employ a variety of mental health workers including psychiatrists, clinical psychologists, social workers, marriage and family counselors, psychiatric nurses, and community workers.

Many psychiatric care providers hoped that psychiatric clients who remained in their communities on an outpatient basis, with family and community ties intact, would have more successful treatment outcomes. Another hoped-for advantage of community mental health centers was that people would seek help more readily when it was available in the community. Unfortunately, community mental health centers have not been funded adequately to meet the many and varied needs of individuals with mental health problems. Mentally ill clients often are eligible for care only when they become acutely ill and not for care that can maintain their health. Some people are not eligible for help because of the complex rules and regulations governing funding. Others do not continue with prescribed treatment and experience a relapse; legal constraints do not allow involuntary treatment. Although recognition of the rights of the mentally ill has been important, there also is a concern that society expects mentally ill people to make rational decisions about their own best interests when, in fact, they are not mentally capable of understanding the consequences of their actions. The entire area of community mental health has many challenges.

Critical Thinking Activity

Identify an agency in your community that offers home healthcare. Investigate the services offered by this agency. Compare these with the list of possible services offered by home care agencies mentioned in this chapter. If the lists do not match, analyze the factors in your community that may be responsible for the difference.

Adult Day Centers

Adult day centers provide care for adults who cannot safely be alone throughout the day. Transported daily to the center by a family member or a van operated by the center, clients receive a variety of social and health services that enable them to continue to live in their own home or a family member's home. Various maintenance and rehabilitative services usually are available, including exercise classes, medication education and supervision, recreational activities, mental healthcare, and an opportunity to interact with other people. Some centers provide "drop-in" or intermittent services for clients who need only one aspect of the program. Other centers provide care each day for clients who need continuing supervision while family members are at work or school. The nursing role in these settings may vary considerably. Some settings have APRNs who plan care and work with families. Others have RNs who provide medication supervision, assessment for ongoing health problems, and who may lead groups in reminiscence, reality orientation, or validation therapy. LPNs may be hired to give medications and carry out specific treatments.

Ambulatory Care Dialysis Centers

A dialysis center provides an environment where the individual, who has complex dialysis needs or who does not have a family care provider or a home dialysis assistant, can go two to three times a week for dialysis. Nurses in dialysis centers must have high-level skills, because clients with renal failure who need in-center dialysis usually have the most complex problems and coexisting illnesses. Both LPNs and RNs may be employed in these centers.

COLLEAGUES IN HEALTHCARE

Hundreds of types of healthcare workers have been identified in the United States, each of which meets the needs of our society in some way. It is not within the scope of this book to discuss each of these occupations individually. Table 6.5 provides a list of the more common healthcare occupations and a web reference for information regarding education and credentialing. The discussion below focuses on some of the issues related to the healthcare professions.

Roles of Healthcare Workers

Although the major health occupations provide academic education with legal licensure and a defined scope of practice, many of the allied health workers have much less defined roles,

Table 6.5   Common Health Occupations and Certification Organizations

Dentistry	
American Dental Association (*www.ada.org*)	Doctor of dental surgery (DDS) dentist
	Registered dental hygienist (RDH)
	Dental assistant
Diagnostic Imaging Technology	
American Society of Radiologic Technicians (*www.asrt.org*)	Radiologic technologist
Society of Diagnostic Medical Sonography (*www.sdms.org*)	Sonography technologist
Nuclear Medicine Technology Certification Board (NMTCB) (*www.mntcb.org*)	Nuclear medicine technologist
Nutrition	
American Dietetic Association (*www.eatright.org*)	Registered dietitian
	Dietetic technician registered
Occupational Therapy	
American Occupational Therapy Association (*www.aota.org/*)	Occupational therapist registered
	Occupational therapy assistant
Optometry/Vision Care	
American Optometric Association (*www.aoanet.org*)	Doctor of optometry
	Certified paraoptometric (CPO)–certified paraoptometric assistant (CPOA)
	Certified paraoptometric technician (CPOT)
Pharmacy	
American Pharmacists Association (*www.aphanet.org*)	Registered pharmacist
	Pharmacy assistant
Physical Therapy	
American Physical Therapy Association (*www.apta.org*)	Registered physical therapist (PT)
	Physical therapist assistant (PTA)
Physician	
American Medical Association (*www.ama-assn.org/*)	Medical doctor (MD)
American Osteopathic Association (*http://www.osteopathic.org*)	Doctor of osteopathic (DO) medicine
Podiatry	
American Podiatric Medicine Association (*www.apma.org*)	Doctor of podiatric medicine (DPM)
Respiratory Therapy	
American Association for Respiratory Care (*www.aarc.org/*)	Respiratory therapist (RT)
Speech, Language, and Hearing Therapy	
American Speech, Language, and Hearing Association (*www.asha.org*)	Speech/language pathologist (CCC-SLP)
	Speech/language pathology assistant (SLPA)
	Audiologist (CCC-A)

Organization Web sites provide an overview of the profession and educational requirements.

which creates concerns about how education or training is provided and how the role is regulated. For some, regulations and requirements may differ from state to state. National organizations that provide **accreditation** for allied health educational programs serve to provide standardization of some occupations (Display 6.1).

Even within professions, increasing specialization has sometimes created conflict over expertise and territory (Fig. 6.2). Pressure from insurers has mandated a decreased use of specialty physicians and mandated that more care be delivered by family practice physicians. In some states, clinical psychologists may obtain authority to prescribe medications, a treatment modality formerly limited to physicians and certain APRNs. This eliminates the need for referral to another mental healthcare provider solely for the prescription of medications to treat psychiatric conditions. When nurse anesthetists can be reimbursed independently, more facilities hire those nurse specialists, which decreases the demand for anesthesiologists. Those with greater education argue that the patient loses when the provider has a lesser background. The education, regulation, and use of all healthcare workers will continue to be an issue in the coming years.

Access to Primary Healthcare

The healthcare provider contacted initially by clients who seek healthcare is considered a **primary care provider (PCP)**, who furnishes entry into the healthcare system. Today the federal government considers family practice specialists, pediatricians, internal medicine specialists, obstetricians, physician assistants, and nurse practitioners to be PCPs. The PCP is the mainstay of basic care for most individuals.

All states require licensure of physicians, nurse practitioners, and other providers who are authorized to treat illness and prescribe drugs. The cornerstone of many managed healthcare plans is an emphasis on the primary healthcare provider as the gatekeeper for the system. The primary provider implements health maintenance activities that prevent the need for more expensive care as well as provides care for common health problems. In order to assure coordinated care, the concept of the *medical home* is being emphasized. This is the primary care setting where all care can be coordinated. Because fewer physicians are choosing primary care fields of practice, the availability of adequate numbers of PCPs has been identified as a concern with the expansion of health plans to over 40 million uninsured in the United States through healthcare reform. Nurse practitioners and physician's assistants may fill this gap.

Lack of access to primary care has been one of the healthcare problems for individuals without health insurance, the unemployed, those residing in rural areas and in economically

DISPLAY 6.1 Approaches to Financing Healthcare

- Personal payment
- Charitable care
- Health insurance plans
- HMOs
- State-administered health plans
- Federal government programs

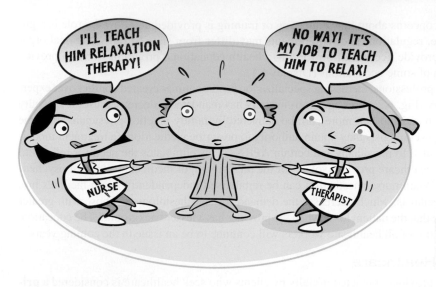

FIGURE 6.2 Overlapping roles and unclear boundaries between healthcare occupations can lead to conflict.

disadvantaged areas in large cities, and those on welfare programs. Often it has resulted in delaying care until the problem is more complex and requires greater resources to resolve. In urban areas, the lack of access to primary care has often resulted in the inappropriate use of emergency room services for routine illnesses.

Interdisciplinary Teamwork

As the healthcare system grows more complex, it is clear that it is impossible for one individual, educated to a specific role, to manage all aspects of care. This has led to an increasing emphasis on collaborative work that will provide the benefits available through the expertise of different professions. Multidisciplinary teamwork has always been part of hospice care—physicians, nurses, social workers, therapists, home health aides, and pastoral staff all bring their unique insights into the client's care. The current regulations for long-term care require that there be interdisciplinary collaboration in planning for resident care.

Healthcare Worker Supply

The shortage of RNs that was very acute as recently as 2008 was alleviated during the economic downturn (Buerhaus, Auerbach, & Staiger, 2009). A variety of factors have created this short-term change including fewer people seeking healthcare because of lack of health insurance due to job loss and people putting off elective healthcare due to an uncertain economic situation. Current RN employees have moved from part-time to full-time status, postponed retirement, and been willing to work overtime. In response to actual changes and uncertainty about the future, many hospitals have greatly decreased hiring, especially the hiring of new graduates who need costly orientation. Other employment settings have also stopped recruiting. This change is allowing nurse employers to look at issues other than recruitment and focus on other issues related to quality nursing care (Fig. 6.3).

According to the Bureau of Labor statistics, the long-term expectation is that the employment market for nurses will grow 22% between 2008 and 2018. The biggest growth is expected

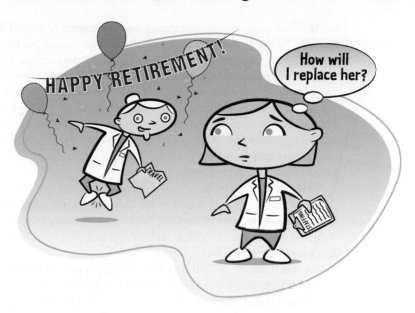

FIGURE 6.3 The aging of the nursing workforce will affect the supply of nurses.

to occur in ambulatory care, with hospitals showing the least growth (BLS, 2010). The challenge will be to sustain the nursing workforce and nursing school enrollments in the face of this temporary downturn in employment. If these falter, the future supply will be in serious jeopardy.

Nurses are not the only healthcare workers in short supply. There are predicted shortages in almost all areas of healthcare over the next 15 years. As the population ages and more people enter the system due to the expansion of healthcare insurance coverage, the shortages are likely to persist.

PAYING FOR HEALTHCARE

Throughout the world, the concern over healthcare has everyone's attention. In most of the industrialized world, healthcare is seen as a right, or an **entitlement**, of every citizen. Based on this right, healthcare in most industrialized countries is operated by government systems that provide universal healthcare coverage. In some countries such as Sweden (see *www.sweden.se/eng/Home/Society/Health-care/*) and the Netherlands (see *www.minbuza.nl/en/You_and_the_Netherlands/Living_in_the_Netherlands/Health_care*), there is strong centralization of financing and control. In other countries such as Canada (see *www.canadian-healthcare.org*) and Germany (see *www.civitas.org.uk/pubs/bb3Germany.php*), systems are controlled regionally through provincial authority. These governmental systems are successful in accomplishing overall health outcomes such as low maternal–infant mortality, high immunization rates, and reduction of preventable deaths. The problems found in these systems are related to the high cost of providing healthcare and subsequent attempts to control those costs. The delay before receiving care may be long, and some care, especially care that is very costly such as dialysis, may be limited. Because of these situations, private medical care that is paid for by individuals also may be available to those with sufficient income.

In developing nations, healthcare may be limited or almost nonexistent. Some care may be paid for by the government and some by private means, but there are not enough individual or institutional providers to meet the needs of the population. The available resources may not meet the standards that those in more affluent countries have come to expect. Hospitals may lack adequate safe water and sanitation. Ordinary supplies such as dressing materials and sterile needles may be unavailable. Drugs may be in short supply, and diagnostic and laboratory testing may be nonexistent. Healthcare outcomes in these countries tend to be poor, especially regarding infant and child mortality. The World Health Organization is most active in these developing nations, trying to improve health outcomes through immunization, sanitation, and other public health programs.

In the United States there has been no mechanism to build a coordinated healthcare system. Much of the complexity found in the U.S. healthcare system relates to the variety of mechanisms for funding and controlling healthcare. Although the United States has ready access to the most sophisticated medical technology and expertise, deficiencies are seen in some of the key measures of population health.

As noted above, in 2010 the U.S. Congress passed the Patient Protection and Affordable Care Act commonly referred to as the Healthcare Reform. This act set up a process through which the United States would move toward healthcare coverage for all by requiring everyone to be enrolled in some type of health plan. The various health plans described below will continue to exist, but enrollment will change. The provisions of this act are set to go into effect over a period of years beginning in 2010. Changes mandated by this act will be identified as part of the discussion below. The Republican Party has announced a goal to reduce or repeal the Health Care Reform Act. Therefore, you will need to watch legislative developments carefully to learn what provisions are in place.

Financing Healthcare for Individuals

Currently, there are many different approaches to financing healthcare for individuals in the United States. Personal payment, charitable care, insurance plans, health maintenance organizations (HMOs), and a variety of government programs are all forms of healthcare financing. Agencies such as insurance companies and government programs that pay providers for health services provided to individuals are termed **third-party payers**. Increasingly, decisions about an individual's healthcare are made by a combination of the patient-consumer, the provider, and the payer, rather than by any one of them alone.

Under healthcare reform these options will remain. Individuals will have access to one or more health plan options through employers, subsidies for low-income individuals, expansion of the rules for Medicaid, and the use of insurance pools for high-risk individuals. All will be mandated to participate by 2019.

Personal Payment

Today most individuals still pay for healthcare but often in indirect ways that make them less aware of the specific costs. Health insurance premiums may be deducted from a paycheck, or an employer may pay premiums directly, considering them part of employee compensation. Most health insurance plans require the subscriber to pay a deductible (a portion of the bill), which may be computed for each service or may be an aggregate for the year. The size of the deductible that is the individual's responsibility is increasing in many insurance plans, giving people greater incentive to use services wisely. The Healthcare Reform bill will continue to allow co-pays and deductibles to be part of insurance plans, but it does limit the co-pays for those on Medicare beginning in 2011.

Charitable Care

Charitable care has played a significant role in the history of healthcare. The earliest hospitals were religious institutions that provided healthcare as a form of ministry and as a charitable service. Some large charitable groups, such as the Shriners Hospitals for Children, still provide a great deal of care for people who are unable to pay. Although these hospitals do collect insurance and payment from those who can afford care, they also raise money for the purpose of providing high-level care to children in need.

Hospitals constructed with the use of Hill-Burton funds made available in 1946 accepted an obligation to provide some charitable care in their communities. As these obligations expired, concern about what was happening in emergency care led to legislation that requires hospitals to provide emergency care regardless of an individual's ability to pay.

Historically, some money for charitable care was raised through donations. As insurance became more widespread, hospitals often supported charitable care by charging paying clients more than the cost of their care and using the excess income to offset the costs of charitable care. However, as negotiations for lower healthcare costs for managed care continue and regulations have limited Medicare reimbursement, hospitals are experiencing a decreased ability to provide charitable care without severe financial difficulties. (Medicare is discussed more fully later in this chapter.)

Individual physicians also have provided forms of charitable care. Only rarely did people directly ask physicians for charitable care; rather, the physician sometimes did not pursue the payment of a bill that could not be paid by a family. Physicians and other care providers also have provided charitable care by volunteering their time at free clinics.

To meet the needs of society, free clinics have been established throughout the country and now number more than 1,200. The National Association of Free Clinics (NAFC), founded in 2001, serves as an advocate for the issues and concerns of free clinics, their volunteer and paid staff, and their patients. Free clinics are becoming PCPs for those without other access to care (NAFC, 2010).

Charitable care is expected to continue to be a part of financing of healthcare. There will always be some individuals who fall outside of the system due to immigration status or other such issues. Additionally, individuals with very high healthcare costs may continue to need help with the deductibles and co-pays that can mount during a prolonged or high-cost illness.

Health Insurance Plans

Starting in the 1930s through the 1970s, insurance companies gradually began to pay a larger share of medical fees. The basic framework of insurance coverage is that of shared risk of having high-cost healthcare needs. Individuals pay for coverage whether or not they incur healthcare costs; when an insured individual requires healthcare, the insurance pays for that care. Thus the individual has a stable healthcare cost without the risk of incurring costs that are difficult to meet from ordinary income, and the insurance company stays financially solvent because more money is coming in than is going out.

Historically, health insurance was for hospital care and related services only. Outpatient visits, immunizations, costs of drugs, and other such benefits were not covered by insurance policies. One disadvantage of this system was that consumers had no incentive to reduce their use of services; they paid the same regardless of their needs or use of the system. People sought to have care delivered on an inpatient basis to obtain reimbursement. Another disadvantage was that individuals often neglected preventive healthcare that had to be paid for out-of-pocket. Health insurance policies now cover many preventive services, outpatient costs, and some prescription costs.

At the heart of the process of setting insurance rates and specifying coverage are identifying what will be covered, determining the risk (probability) of health services being needed for different groups of individuals, and projecting the costs of care. It has been found that the more heterogeneous the group, the more likely that the average cost for those in the plan will mirror the population average, thereby keeping insurance costs reasonable for all. Limitations on coverage that eliminate individuals with high probability of needing services (such as the elderly diabetic) protect insurance companies from the risk of excessive costs. When high-risk individuals are excluded from insurance, it lessens the cost for low-risk subscribers within the plan, but leaves those who are most in need of assistance without the benefit of insurance.

Most insurance companies are private profit-making companies owned by stockholders. They provide service to policyholders in return for insurance payments and create profit for stockholders in the company.

Nonprofit insurance companies are established within different legal regulations from profit-making companies. They are owned collectively by those who hold insurance policies. All profits from the company are theoretically used to enhance benefits or to decrease the cost of the insurance. Additionally, the nonprofit companies have certain advantages in terms of taxes. The "Blues" (Blue Cross and Blue Shield companies) originally were established as not-for-profit organizations.

Legal regulations place restrictions on the rate setting, investments, and general management of nonprofit companies that do not apply to private profit-making companies. This has limited their ability to grow in size and compete for some types of business. In some areas of the country, Blue Cross and Blue Shield companies have asked regulatory authorities for permission to convert from nonprofit to profit-making status and to sell stock in the company (and have changed their names in the process). In some states, courts have required that these corporations provide remuneration to their communities in return for this change in status. In other states, these changes have occurred without public input. In still others, the change was blocked.

One of the major controversies in the 2010 healthcare reform act was the requirement that all individuals be covered by an insurance company plan unless they are enrolled in a government plan such as Medicaid, Veterans' Administration (VA), or Medicare. This mandate provides private companies with a very large source of new subscribers.

As the cost of healthcare has increased, insurance premiums have increased greatly. An additional public concern has been that health insurance has been unobtainable for individuals with existing health problems and often economically beyond the means of those who are not insured as part of an employee group. The new law requires access to insurance for all individuals with preexisting illnesses through high-risk pools. These will continue until the

Medicaid standards are widened and new state-run insurance exchanges have been developed. Subsidies are being enacted for those who meet low income standards, and Medicaid requirements are being changed. Dependent young adults up through the age of 26 will have access to insurance through their parents' insurance.

Although insurance companies originally focused on paying for healthcare, they now are involved in establishing standards for care, evaluating care, and negotiating charges. They are active participants in all areas of healthcare and, because of the economic power they wield, have great influence. Insurance companies determine whom they will pay and what procedures they will reimburse. Thus, insurance companies can and do limit healthcare choices.

All insurance plans have written rules regarding notification, acceptable providers, and precisely when and how reimbursement will occur. Sometimes these rules result in a denial of payment. Many people have expressed concern about the process of reviewing and denying insurance claims (Fig. 6.4). Realistically, the foremost goal of most health insurance plans is to return a profit to investors. Providing good healthcare to an individual is a means to that end and not the focus of effort.

Federal legislation, the Health Insurance Portability and Accountability Act (HIPAA), was passed in 1996. Title 1 of the act focuses on measures that assist in maintaining healthcare insurance coverage for those who change or lose their jobs (see *http://aspe.hhs.gov/admnsimp/ pl104191.htm*, for the full text of the act). The Centers for Medicare & Medicaid Services (CMS) maintains a Web site (*http://cms.hhs.gov/hipaa*) with consumer information regarding the protections provided by this federal legislation to allow people to maintain coverage when they change jobs. This legislation also has provided tax incentives for those purchasing

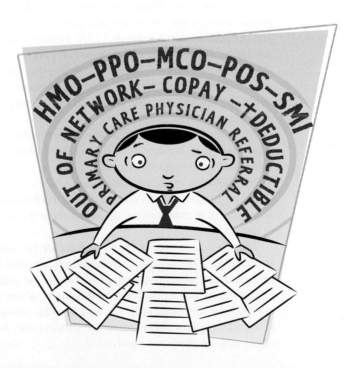

FIGURE 6.4 Healthcare insurance plans are complex and often confusing to the ordinary consumer.

long-term care insurance. The HIPAA legislation had additional provisions regarding the privacy of patient health records, which will be discussed in Chapter 8.

Managed Care Organizations

Managed care refers to any system for "financing and organizing the delivery of healthcare in which costs are contained by controlling the provision of services" (Taber's, 2005). The concept of managed care has broadened since its beginning, and now it includes many types of health plans.

A managed care plan may be controlled by the payer (eg, an insurance company), include both payers and providers, or be a business entity that serves only as a go-between. HMOs (discussed below) always have acted as managed care systems. Many of the current health plans referred to as HMOs are in reality managed care systems that do not focus on health maintenance.

In some cases, a group of primary healthcare providers, termed an **independent practice association**, may contract with a managed care organization to provide services for a preset fee per individual in the program. Managed care organizations also may directly provide healthcare and therefore employ many healthcare workers, including nurses. In some managed care organizations, clients have a choice of care providers; in others they do not. Managed care plans that allow an individual the option of going outside of the plan for services that the plan does not or will not provide are called **point-of-service plans**. Usually the subscriber is eligible for some reimbursement of costs for these outside services, but by a greatly reduced amount.

In a managed care system, someone, usually the primary physician, is assigned to the role of gatekeeper. This person monitors and restricts the use of services by the client. The physician sees the client first and then determines whether referral or diagnostic services are needed. In some managed care systems, the primary physician has decision-making authority. However, in many managed care systems, the actual gatekeeper is a plan manager, who must be consulted regarding the use of services. A written request may be required before the client receives permission for a referral. This may result in delay or denial of needed care and is one source of consumer dissatisfaction with some managed care plans.

Many managed care decisions about individual clients are made based on a set of predetermined protocols for treatment. The original protocols were developed by physicians, based on broad statistical patterns. Thus the protocol may not be responsive to individual differences. These protocols often are administered by plan employees who are not healthcare providers. Some physicians express dismay over a mechanism that allows a nonphysician who has never seen a client to make critical decisions about the care needed and to deny any individualization of the plan.

Managed care usually requires that care be authorized or approved for payment before it is provided. Clients identify the required approval of any type of care as a major problem. A managed care plan may not approve or pay for care that it considers nonessential. If a healthcare provider and a plan consultant disagree about which type of treatment is appropriate, the client often feels caught in the middle. This situation frequently occurs in emergency care. Even when approval is granted, the process may have been long and frustrating for both the client and the physician involved.

Some plans require that an individual travels to a designated hospital when an emergency is not life threatening. Thus, a consumer may be denied payment if he or she goes to the closest hospital as may occur when the consumer is away from home.

Managed care controls extend to such matters as the medications that can be prescribed. A managed care company may have a specific formulary or list of drugs that are allowed to be prescribed. The company usually negotiates for drug purchases at lower prices than paid by the general public. For many conditions, there are clear therapeutic equivalents, and medication restrictions are not a concern. For the person with a chronic health condition who has been stabilized on specific medications, however, moving into a managed care plan can pose a real threat to health maintenance if the plan will not approve the client's current drugs.

People on Medicare also have the option of joining managed care plans under an option termed "Medicare Advantage." Under such circumstances, the person joins the plan and pays a monthly fee similar to the cost of a supplemental health insurance (Medigap) policy (see below). The government makes a single payment for each individual Medicare recipient directly to the plan and the plan provides all care. The amount per individual was calculated as an average of the expenses incurred by Medicare recipients for all costs. Most Medicare Advantage plans have co-payment fees for services and assess charges for prescriptions.

Health Maintenance Organizations

The first managed care organizations were HMOs that originated as an alternative to traditional insurance plans and were nonprofit in nature. Although traditional insurance plans paid for care when subscribers were ill, HMOs were the first to provide payment for care aimed at preventing illness. HMOs provided well-child care, prenatal care, immunizations, gynecologic examinations, and other preventive services when insurance companies did not.

Because the HMO receives the same income (except for modest co-payments) whether a client requires extensive care or very little care, there is a built-in incentive to emphasize preventive care and avoid costly hospitalization. A flat charge per month covers routine preventive healthcare; care for illness; hospitalization and, in some instances, prescription costs; outpatient care; and other services. HMO-enrolled individuals are often responsible for a co-payment. These co-payments support part of the cost of care and give the consumer an incentive to use services wisely. The line between HMOs and traditional insurance plans has blurred as all health plans pay for preventive care services and the term HMO has become synonymous with managed care plan.

State-Administered Health Plans

States may operate a variety of healthcare resources for their residents. All states manage some type of workers' compensation plans for those injured on the job. This plan may be managed as a state monopoly or contracted to private insurance companies. Employers are required to pay premiums based on statistical information about covered injuries and hazards in various job categories.

Some states administer health insurance plans on a wider basis. Hawaii ensures universal healthcare coverage for its residents. Minnesota was a leader in attempting to provide health services for all its residents. The state of Washington developed an insurance plan called the Basic Health Plan for working individuals who earn too much money to be eligible for tax-supported healthcare, but who do not have incomes high enough to afford regular insurance.

Unfortunately state plans that rely on tax subsidies face decreased revenue while incurring increased costs. They cannot accommodate all who are eligible and long waiting lists may result. In many states this has become a crisis (Kaiser Family Foundation, 2010). As healthcare reform is established, these state plans may be expanded and modified with federal subsidies for costs.

Most states support state mental hospitals and public health services. Additional public health services may be supplied through county and city governments. Hospitals designed to provide care for those who are indigent may be operated by the city (such as New York City hospitals) or by the county (such as Cook County Hospital in Chicago).

Federal Government Programs

The federal government in the United States is deeply involved in healthcare financing. Federal programs cover the elderly, the poor, federal workers, the military, the veterans, and Native Americans and Native Alaskans, some through special programs and some through Medicare and Medicaid. Some individuals express concern about government involvement in the U.S. healthcare system. When all of these programs and agencies are considered together, it is clear that, for good or ill, the federal government already controls many aspects of healthcare.

Medicare. In 1965, after years of effort and testimony by many health-related groups (including the American Nurses Association [ANA]), and with widespread public support, an amendment to the Social Security Act was passed. Title XVIII of the act, which was termed Medicare, provided payment for hospitalization (Part A) and insurance that could be purchased to meet physicians' fees and outpatient costs (Part B) for people over age 65 and certain others who were receiving Social Security payments. In 2004, Medicare Part D, which covers prescription drugs, was approved, and it took effect in 2006 (see below).

Participation in Medicare Part A is automatic for those on Social Security, whereas participation in Medicare Part B is optional and a premium is deducted from the Social Security check to pay for Part B. Medicare Part A pays only for acute hospitalization and a limited amount of rehabilitative care that may occur in a nursing home. Medicare does not pay for any long-term or custodial care in a nursing home. Part B reimburses for physician care and outpatient services based on a fixed schedule of payments. Medicare is administered through CMS, which uses contracted insurance companies termed *Medicare carriers* or *Medicare intermediaries* to process claims (*www.cms.gov*). Payments from Medicare do not cover the entire cost of the care provided. The amount authorized is determined by CMS. Medicare then pays a fixed percentage of that authorized amount. The individual pays the remaining percentage. If the provider charges more than the authorized amount, that portion of the fee is not recoverable from either Medicare or the patient. Many individuals who receive Medicare also pay for supplemental insurance to cover the part of the healthcare bill for which Medicare Parts A and B do not pay. This is commonly referred to as **"Medigap" insurance** and is available from many different insurance companies, such as Blue Cross and Blue Shield.

The premium for Part D prescription coverage may be added to the premium for the Medigap policy or Medicare Advantage contract or may be a separate Part D policy. The cost of prescriptions under Part D is subsidized by Medicare. Plans differ in cost and have different benefits and requirements, such as co-pays, deductibles, coverage of different generic and brand name drugs, and additional coverage in the "gap" or "doughnut hole" (that area of costs between $2,600 and $3,600 for which no reimbursement is provided) that is built into the general plan. The Health Care Reform act has scheduled changes to reduce this gap in coverage. Each plan is free to establish its own formulary of drugs that are covered and may change that formulary once a month. Participants must investigate each plan to determine whether the drugs they currently take are covered. If new drugs are prescribed, the provider will need to check on the plan to learn what therapeutic equivalent drugs may be covered by that particular plan. Participants may change plans once each year. Individuals who belong to Medicare managed care plans have their Part D integrated into that plan. These drug plans have significantly increased the cost of Medicare. Details are available on the CMS Web site at *www.medicare. gov/medicarereform/drugbenefit.asp.*

The complexity of filing claims with Medicare and with an insurance company designed to supplement Medicare coverage (the Medigap policy) is problematic for many people because the insurance company will not pay until Medicare has determined coverage and paid its share. If there are many different health claims, the sending and receiving of the various claims requires careful record keeping. Even when claims are filed by the provider, they may be denied payment if they do not conform to specific rules and regulations. Often elderly people accept an initial denial of payment for the claim as the final decision and do not pursue the matter further. There is a high rate of reconsideration when denials are appealed. Therefore, it is often wise to encourage clients to appeal a denial of payment.

Medicaid. Title IX of the Social Security Act, which was termed Medicaid, provides funds for healthcare for those dependent on public assistance and certain other low-income individuals. Costs for Medicaid are shared between the federal government and each state. Very-low-income individuals who are eligible for Medicare may be covered by Medicaid in the same way that those who can pay are covered by Medigap policies. This often is referred to as being "dual-eligible." Each state is responsible for administering Medicaid: The state determines eligibility and level of coverage. Payments from the federal government to the states are administered by CMS. Benefits vary greatly among states. California's plan, called Medi-Cal, historically has been one of the most comprehensive plans. As healthcare costs rise and state budgets are severely impacted by decreased tax revenue, there has been great pressure to cut this program. To avoid federal control, a few states have not participated in the Medicaid program. Some states, such as Oregon, have requested waivers from the usual regulations of CMS governing Medicaid to allow experimentation with different plans that might help to control costs.

In 1999 the federal government provided a mechanism for states to enlarge their Medicaid programs, so they could enroll children from low-income families who did not qualify for Medicaid and who would otherwise be without healthcare coverage. This State Children's Health Insurance Plan (SCHIP) represented the first time that the United States has supported healthcare as a right for all children. Not all states agreed to participate in the plan because it required their financial contribution and provides for some federal control of the program.

Problems Facing Medicare and Medicaid. Medicare and Medicaid are important healthcare resources, but they have not been without problems. Costs have been higher and have been rising faster than anticipated at their inception. There has been a great deal of publicity about instances of abuse and even fraud, associated with these two programs.

The Medicare bill contains many provisions that have made a significant impact on nursing. The definition of skilled nursing care in the original bill was narrow and excluded many important aspects of care necessary to maintaining the health of clients. Through later efforts and testimony, nursing organizations were instrumental in convincing legislators to recognize that the definition of skilled nursing care was critical. As a result, a Senate subcommittee asked the ANA to study skilled nursing care, to provide background data for the Senate. Amendments to the Medicare/Medicaid Act of 1972 encouraged the study of alternative ways of providing healthcare to contain costs. These alternatives included the use of nurses in expanded roles and the use of managed care.

Amendments to the Medicare/Medicaid Act were responsible for mandating review and evaluation of healthcare. This was done in the interests of cost containment. Institutions must review records of Medicare/Medicaid clients and compare them with specific criteria for care. Many insurance companies have followed this pattern and required review and evaluation of care of their clients.

In 1982 and again in 1993 Congress revised Medicare to prevent serious financial deficits in the system that escalating costs could create. The healthcare reform bill contains some modifications of Medicare, but there is still concern that increased demand by an aging population will undermine the financial stability of Medicare and that further cuts in Medicare spending are being proposed.

The growing number of the elderly; the rising costs of medications, supplies, and wages; and the widespread use of costly, highly technical diagnostic tools and therapies all have contributed to escalating healthcare costs. With the baby boom generation moving into retirement years, further strain will be placed on the financial resources of the system. Despite these concerns, Medicare and Medicaid have provided healthcare dollars and services to many people who would otherwise have done without.

Critical Thinking Activity

What changes are occurring in the healthcare systems in your community? Are some hospitals growing or merging? Are some facilities changing their focus? Have any healthcare providers had economic difficulties or even closed? Have new providers established facilities? Analyze how these changes may affect nursing practice.

Military Healthcare. TRICARE is "the health care program serving active duty service members, National Guard and Reserve members, retirees, their families, survivors and certain former spouses worldwide" (TRICARE, 2010). This program has many different options as well as a pharmacy plan. While care is available in military facilities, most participants receive care in the private sector with TRICARE acting as the health plan.

Other Federal Healthcare Programs. The U.S. Department of Health and Human Services (DHHS) provides direct healthcare services through the Indian Health Service (IHS), which operates hospitals, health centers, school health centers, health stations, and urban Indian health centers and provides payments to community providers where no IHS facilities are present (DHHS, 2008). Most other healthcare provided through the DHHS is through payments to community clinics and other support for meeting the needs of low-income and disadvantaged individuals.

The Department of Veterans' Affairs operates many clinics, hospitals, and nursing homes for veterans. These are found across the country. For those who are eligible for care from the VA, benefits are comprehensive. The VA is engaged in a major effort to improve services to veterans. Information on the VA's services is available at *www.va.gov*.

Patterns of Payment

Understanding the various methods of paying for healthcare services can help you understand what is happening in the organizations and agencies involved in the healthcare system. The following discussion covers those most commonly used methods of paying for healthcare services.

Fee-For-Service Payment

Fee-for-service payment means that each time a service is provided a fee is generated and then billed to the care recipient. The more services provided, the more fees charged. This was the traditional method of charging for healthcare in the United States. Initially, private individuals paid almost all fees. When insurance companies began assisting with payment, the bill was sent to the insurance company and to the client. The insurance company then paid the amount established in the policy (eg, 80%), and the client was required to pay the rest.

As costs rose, insurance companies began setting a standard for reimbursement. Under this system, if a policy stated that a company reimbursed at 80%, this meant 80% of a fee that the insurance company determined was reasonable. If the provider charged more than what was considered reasonable, the client was responsible for the excess, in addition to 20% of the "reasonable" fee. Insurance companies usually set these fees based on statistical analysis of prevailing fees in a geographic area. In a time of rapid inflation, providers complained that there was often a serious discrepancy between the fee used for calculating benefits and the actual fees being charged. This standard fee still provided for paying a fee for each service rendered.

Prospective Payment

A **prospective payment** is a fixed reimbursement amount for all the care required for a particular surgical procedure, an illness, or an acuity category. This reimbursement amount is determined in advance of the provision of service. The predetermined amount is paid without regard to actual services required or the costs of those services in individual situations. Thus, the same payment is made whether the person is healthy and has an uncomplicated hospital stay or whether the person is in poor health and has complications that increase the cost of care or the length of the hospital stay.

Prospective payment is designed to provide an incentive for providers to control costs. Prospective payment has accomplished this as hospitals began to monitor the use of high-cost testing and pharmaceutical products and to limit the length of stay. Another advantage to payers in a prospective payment system (PPS) is that costs are predictable. The system transfers the burden of risk (the probability that an individual may require extraordinary services) from the payer to the provider. Several specific types of prospective payment have particular significance for nurses. These are DRGs and resource utilization groups (RUGs).

Diagnosis-Related Groups. The first major change in the method of payment for healthcare services began October 1, 1983, when the federal government stopped using a fee-for-service reimbursement system for Medicare and introduced a PPS using **diagnosis-related groups (DRGs)** to determine the payment for each Medicare client admitted to the hospital. This change was designed to stop the spiraling costs of Medicare and to correct inequities that made the costs of care in one facility very different from those in another facility.

The method of determining the rates to be paid in the Medicare PPS—the creation of DRGs—resulted from a computerized analysis of costs that had been billed for hospitalized individuals in the past and a determination of an average length of stay. This analysis led to the formation of categories of medical diagnoses that require similar treatment and for which costs are similar. Each category (or DRG) has a name and number; for example, DRG 236 is "fracture of the hip and pelvis." In addition, a decision was made to increase the payment for care when another illness or condition is present. This second condition is termed a **comorbidity**. Thus, a person with heart failure whose basic DRG is "fractured hip" is designated "fractured hip with congestive heart failure." A hospital receives greater reimbursement for providing service to this person because care is more complex and costs are higher. Hospitals also receive additional amounts for cases that are determined to be "outliers." An outlier is a case in which the client's length of stay significantly exceeds the average. The number of days needed to qualify a case as an outlier is predetermined. For example, the average length of stay for DRG 236, "fractured hip and pelvis," is 6.2 days, but the stay must reach 29 days for the case to be considered an outlier. Pressure is placed on all providers to ensure that the patient is discharged within the average length of stay on which payment is based.

Most hospital costs are included in the DRG reimbursement. The actual DRG reimbursement amount is recalculated each year by CMS through a complex formula that considers the area of the country in which care was provided (eg, Northwest, Southeast), the urbanization of the area (eg, rural, suburban), and the type of care required. Some hospital costs still are reimbursed separately. In the past, the separate reimbursements included costs for medical education of resident physicians and research conducted by the hospital. These were reimbursed because the federal government supports the need for research and medical education and also acknowledges that the resident physicians provide care to Medicare and Medicaid recipients.

Most of the controversy surrounding the implementation of DRGs has not been concerned with the incentives for cost control or the prospective reimbursement system itself, but rather how the payment amounts are determined and how the system is being administered. Hospitals with a large population of extra-high-risk clients (eg, the very elderly or the poor) have expressed concern that discharging a client for convalescence in a home with a caring family, good food, and a clean environment is much different from discharging a client to an impoverished environment. Many believe the individual situation should be considered when determining regulations for length of stay. The proponents of shortened stays point out that shortened stays are effective cost-containment measures. They argue further that a client's lack of a support system is a social problem and that hospitalization cannot be used to solve social problems. Alterations and modifications of the system will continue, but the basic prospective plan is not expected to change.

Resource Utilization Groups. Resource utilization groups (RUGs) are the categories used to determine prospective payment for nursing home clients. Each RUG represents a group of residents who require a similar amount of care and would have a similar cost of daily care. Unlike the hospital prospective payment, which is a flat amount for the entire hospital stay, the prospective payment for nursing home care is a fixed daily rate. This daily rate must include all the services, including medications and treatments, that a resident needs. The actual daily rate of reimbursement to the nursing home is the average of the RUGs for all residents. This is often referred to as the **case mix**.

The basis for determining to which RUG a nursing home resident will be assigned for reimbursement purposes is the comprehensive **minimum data set (MDS)** prepared by the RN. This assessment must be transmitted electronically to the appropriate center for review and payment categorization. If the assessments are not completed accurately or are not submitted in a timely manner, the resident automatically is assigned to the lowest reimbursement RUG category. The facility is then unable to recover the difference between the lowest RUG and the actual RUG to which the resident is eventually assigned. Reassessments are required at specified intervals and are used to reassign the resident to a RUG.

The nursing home industry is lobbying for changes in the reimbursement plan because it believes that low reimbursement is undermining its ability to provide appropriate care. The costs of compliance are high, the reimbursements are low, and there are restrictions on such items as the provision of therapy services. Many nursing homes have reduced staff, changed practice patterns, and made other adjustments to adapt to the effect of RUGs. One unintended result of the move to PPS for the nursing home has been the refusal of nursing homes to admit high-cost residents. For example, an individual with an extensive wound that requires intensive wound care with expensive products might cost more per day for care than that the highest RUG category allows. In the past, it was possible to bill separately for the expensive dressings and topical agents used. When this is not possible, the facility may refuse to admit the patient. This actually may increase costs for the payer, because patients remain in the high-cost hospital if no long-term care facility will admit them.

In addition to Medicare and Medicaid, many states are adopting systems similar to DRGs, and some private insurance carriers are now using these basic concepts in their cost-control efforts through prospective payment. These prospective payments are often the result of negotiations between healthcare agencies and the insurance companies. Although the specific amounts and the totals of what is included may differ, some of the same concerns regarding the adequacy of payments remain.

Capitation

Capitation is yet another way of determining payment within the healthcare system. In a capitated system, a fee is paid to a provider organization for each person (each "head," thus the term) signed up for the plan whether that person uses any healthcare services. Global capitation refers to the inclusion of all services, both inpatient and outpatient, including physician costs in the capitated amount. Capitation may also be limited and only include outpatient and physician costs.

Capitation shifts an even greater share of the risk of providing costly healthcare from the third-party payer to the provider organization. Providers in a capitated system have an incentive to guide individuals to low-cost outpatient services or other care environments rather than to the acute care hospital. A goal of this payment system is to encourage preventive services that may make high-cost interventions unnecessary. Thus, in a capitated system you may find that services such as mammograms, immunizations, stop-smoking clinics, and back-injury classes do not have any co-payments attached, or the co-payments may be quite low. HMOs were the original capitated systems.

A criticism of a capitated system is that when the provider is at risk for providing care, there may be an unconscious (or even deliberate) attempt to deny medically necessary care to keep costs down. In some capitated systems, consumers have complained that they were unable to obtain services they believed were medically necessary.

COST CONTROL IN HEALTHCARE

Because healthcare costs continue to rise, cost control is a major focus of today's healthcare system. Many factors contribute to the rising costs of health, and many strategies have been used to attempt to limit the rate of increase.

Understanding Increasing Costs

Many factors contribute to the rising costs of healthcare (Display 6.2).

High Technology and New Facilities

One important factor in cost increase is the price of new, more sophisticated technology. The rising cost of technology affects every area of the healthcare field, from the cardiac care unit to the laboratory. Companies that manufacture health-related devices and drugs reportedly have some of the highest profits in any industry. These companies justify their profits as appropriate relative to the risk and cost involved in research and development. However, some critics believe these companies take advantage of the public's dependence on their products. For example, recent evidence indicates that the drug companies spend as much on advertising as they do on research. For those health insurance plans and HMOs providing prescription

DISPLAY 6.2   Contributing Factors in Rising Healthcare Costs

- Price of new technology
- Construction of new facilities
- Higher survival rates, leading to greater need for costly intensive or long-term care
- Growing population of the elderly adults requiring healthcare
- Rise in salaries for healthcare workers
- High costs of drugs and health-related equipment

coverage, the costs of prescription drugs are cited as a key reason for premium increases. The public has expressed concern that drug companies sell identical drugs in other countries for far less money than what they charge consumers in the United States. Drug companies contend that high costs in the United States are essential to support continued drug research, which is very costly. One of the realities contributing to this situation is that other countries place price controls on drugs, and the United States does not.

An increasing population needs a greater number of facilities, and the construction of new care facilities also contributes to rising costs. In addition, existing facilities often require modifications. More space is needed for new technologies both at the bedside and in many hospital departments. Electronic healthcare records require space and infrastructure of wiring and servers as well as the computers and software. More offices and conference rooms are needed. The regulations governing hospital construction also have become more stringent, requiring more fire-safety and infection-control measures and protection against environmental hazards. These factors combine to make the per-bed cost of new hospital construction or hospital remodeling increasingly expensive. Additionally, decreases in the length of hospital stay and the move to outpatient services have left many hospital beds unused on a fluctuating basis. Unoccupied hospital beds create a major drain on organizations, because large sums of capital investment are tied up and not returning any income.

Changing Patient Profile

The average length of hospital stay for standard diagnoses has decreased steadily. The typical client in today's hospital is discharged rapidly to convalesce at home or in a long-term care facility, leaving behind only the acutely ill. Many clients who would have died quickly in the earlier years live through a crisis but require long and intensive care. All of these factors make the acuity level of a client today much greater. This in turn requires more intensive observation and care and the use of more specialized equipment.

The population of the United States as a whole is growing older, and, statistically, the elderly have an increased incidence of all chronic illnesses. A greater percentage of that population requires healthcare on a regular basis and may depend on medications, treatments, and therapies for continued functioning.

Uninsured Individuals

Health plans in the United States are primarily linked to employment, except for those eligible for Medicare and Medicaid, because the cost of independent plans is prohibitive. Major incentives to pass the health reform act were to provide a mechanism for more individuals to be able to purchase insurance, to subsidize those unable to afford insurance, and to reduce the effect of uncompensated care on healthcare providers. Another concern has been the effect on businesses of their having to provide health care benefits to employees, which are provided by government plans for their competitors in other countries.

Many healthcare providers have struggled with the financial problem of uncompensated care. Uncompensated care is a particular concern for hospitals. Individuals arrive at emergency rooms, and laws require that they be assessed before they leave. If an acute problem is found, they must be treated. If the patient has no insurance and is not able to pay privately (which is the common case for those without insurance), the provider is never compensated for the care given. For hospitals with trauma centers and busy emergency rooms, these cases may be ones that require extensive resources lasting over months. Uncompensated care may threaten the viability of these institutions. The provisions of the healthcare reform act are expected to decrease the demand for uncompensated care. However, there will continue to be those not covered by the provisions of healthcare reform, and thus uncompensated care will not disappear altogether.

Other Factors Affecting Costs

Salaries for healthcare workers are part of the cost equation. In the mid-1900s the salaries of healthcare workers (except for physicians) were far below those of the general society. To remedy this, for a time, salaries of healthcare workers rose more rapidly than the general inflation rate. Physicians also had an increase in income greater than the relative inflation rate, until the mid-1990s, when changes in the system began to affect income levels for physicians.

Lack of competition in the healthcare field is one factor that may contribute to higher costs. Although physicians continue to be primary gatekeepers in the system, the advent of other PCPs, such as nurse practitioners, nurse midwives, and physician assistants, offers alternative and less costly care for many routine problems and normal life processes such as respiratory infections, pregnancy, and well-child care. However, there is opposition to allowing these practitioners to operate in collaborative rather than dependent or subsidiary roles.

Critical Thinking Activity

Choose a patient you currently care for. Make a list of all the therapies, medications, diagnostic tests, and surgeries or procedures that this patient has received. Research the cost of these therapies and the daily rate for hospital care in your area for 1 day. Research the DRG reimbursement for that diagnostic group. Compare the reimbursement with the costs being incurred for this individual patient. Identify ways that nurses could reduce the costs involved in this patient's care.

Strategies for Cost Control

As healthcare costs continue to rise, third-party payers have used several methods to control costs, including changing patterns of payment and controlling the actions of providers. These strategies are often referred to as *cost containment* actions.

Limiting Hospital Costs

With the changes in payment, hospitals have developed many mechanisms to limit costs. Because federal regulations limit the reimbursement to hospitals, physicians are asked to judge carefully the necessity of diagnostic studies and costly procedures for hospitalized patients. Physicians sometimes are asked to consult with a pharmacist before prescribing certain high-cost drugs to determine whether a low-cost therapeutic alternative exists. There is great pressure on physicians to discharge patients by the average length of stay to ensure that costs remain within the established prospective payment amount. Physician practices are monitored, and they have even been threatened with denial of hospital privileges if their patients consistently stay beyond the expected length of stay. Many physicians are upset about these cost-containment measures because they may interfere with the physician's independent decision making about what care is needed and when.

To add new high-cost equipment or additional client care facilities, a healthcare institution may be required to apply for a certificate of need from the state. This establishes that there will not be unnecessary duplication of services in an area and that a need for them exists. For example, if every hospital purchased magnetic resonance imaging equipment that was used to only one-fourth or one-third of its capacity, the cost per use would have to be higher to cover the investment and maintenance costs than if the device were used to capacity.

In many states, nonprofit hospitals must apply for rate increases. In their applications, they must document all the factors contributing to the need for an increase. Hearings are held, and permission for rate increases is given only when the evidence indicates that all possible economies are being observed. Private profit-making hospitals are not held to these rules.

Preferred Provider Contracts

In an attempt to contain costs, third-party payers such as insurance companies, HMOs, and managed care organizations sometimes negotiate with providers of healthcare to supply certain kinds of care at an agreed-upon, usually lower, price. The third-party payers then provide incentives for clients to use these preferred providers. These incentives may include the waiver of all or part of co-payments by the insured or coverage of additional conditions or situations.

Preferred provider organizations (PPOs) include hospitals, nursing homes, corporations employing care providers, or groups of care providers who have cooperated to negotiate more successfully with third-party payers for these special contracts. The advantage to the provider is the ensured number of clients and the guaranteed income that in a time of competition in healthcare may be significant. Each PPO operates independently without government regulation. Therefore, the exact structure and contractual arrangements are independently determined.

Case Management

Case management is a technique used to efficiently move an individual requiring major health services through the system resulting in more effective use of services and reduced cost. According to the Case Management Society of America (CMSA), case management is

> a collaborative process which assesses, plans, implements, coordinates, monitors, and evaluates options and services to meet an individual's health needs through communication and available resources to promote quality cost-effective outcomes (CMSA, 2010).

Case managers typically are assigned to high-risk clients, such as those with chronic illnesses or major traumas, who will require rehabilitation. In some settings, the case manager specializes in a particular group of high-risk clients, such as those with diabetes, and is referred to as a *disease manager*.

The case manager is an experienced health professional with knowledge of available resources who oversees or monitors a case to ensure that necessary care is instituted promptly and is provided in the most cost-effective setting. Nurses have often assumed the role of case manager. In this role, the nurse monitors the care as it is provided, ensuring that appropriate referrals are made, changes in the plan of care are instituted appropriately, and the care follows established standards. Because of their understanding of the whole person, both physiologically and psychosocially, and their understanding of how the system works, nurses are particularly well suited to this role. The CMSA provides a system for certifying professional case managers.

Case managers may work as internal case managers where they operate within only one part of the system (eg, managing cases from admission through discharge in a nursing home or hospital) or they may manage cases across all phases of care from outpatient through hospitalization, rehabilitation, and back to outpatient-external case managers. At their best, case management systems ensure that delays in patient transfer or breaks in communication do not occur and that costs are minimized through efficiency. Case managers often act as advocates for clients in the system. Physicians sometimes object to what they see as the interference of the case manager in a decision-making process that previously included only the client and the physician.

Vertically Integrated Healthcare Systems

Organizations contracting to provide managed care are expanding their own control through the development of **vertically integrated systems**, that is, those that provide every level of healthcare service. A vertically integrated system may have contracted physicians, laboratories, a hospital, a subacute facility, a rehabilitation facility, and a home care agency. This allows the contracting organization to offer managed care corporations a package that provides care at all levels for each enrolled member of the managed care plan for a capitated fee. The contracting organization then has an incentive to control costs by decreasing the use of high-cost services and more effectively using low-cost alternatives. It is also in a better position to negotiate with the managed care system about reimbursement. This merging of systems is resulting in the closure of hospitals in many communities.

Using Acuity Measures to Determine Costs

Healthcare providers who negotiate contracts and plan care need accurate data regarding the specific cost of each service. One way of trying to understand and control these costs is through the development of acuity measures. Acuity in this context refers to the severity of illness and the rapidity of change in the client, and thus the intensity of medical and nursing care and other therapies required.

There are various ways of measuring acuity in both acute and long-term care settings. Most systems use categories that reflect the different types of care needed. Each category is assigned a numerical value (eg, a scale of 1 to 4). All applicable category values are summed and compared with a standard. For example, an acuity measuring system might have one category reflecting the need for assistance in personal hygiene. As a person needs more assistance, more points are assigned. Another category might reflect the amount of time needed for monitoring vital signs: The more time required, the more points assigned. Each category is assigned an appropriate number of points, and the total is computed. The points identified for an individual client are then compared with a standard, and the client is assigned an acuity level. Clients with the fewest points are level 1 and require the least care. Those with the most points are level 4 and require the most care. Each system in use has its own scale for determining acuity. Acuity values are sometimes called **intensity measures** because they reflect the intensity of care needed.

In some settings, acuity levels or intensity measures are used as a mechanism for determining the staffing needs of a client care unit. Acuity levels also are used as a means of billing for the level of nursing care needed and are reflected in a variable, rather than flat, charge for the nursing portion of a client's room charge. It also has been suggested that prospective reimbursement might be based on acuity level rather than on medical diagnosis because acuity levels reflect the real impact on resources more accurately than do medical diagnoses. The RUGs developed for prospective reimbursement in long-term care are essentially an acuity measure based on the nursing assessment.

Increasing the Availability of Mid-Level Providers

Because physicians are the most costly healthcare providers, increasing the use of nonphysician PCPs, such as nurse practitioners and physician assistants, is being used to decrease healthcare costs. These are referred to as mid-level providers. The use of nonphysician providers relies on the ability to obtain reimbursement for the care these individuals deliver. The report The Future of Nursing (IOM, 2010) emphasized the importance of allowing APRNs to practice to their fullest scope of practice in all settings nationwide to meet the needs of the public for care.

One attempt to increase the availability of nonphysician care has been the movement to obtain legislation requiring that government agencies and third-party payers make payments directly to nonphysician providers of primary care service rather than requiring that payment always be made to a physician, who employed the nonphysician provider. Progress has been made in regard to third-party reimbursement for nurses in primary care. However, this continues to be a problem and a major thrust of political pressure by nurses.

Changing Fee Structures

In addition to reducing payments through PPSs, the federal government has sought to control costs for Medicare and Medicaid by establishing higher deductibles (the portions that individual clients must pay) and by limiting the fees that the government will pay. Because the elderly and the poor are often unable to pay these deductible amounts, they become liabilities for healthcare providers, who cover these costs by collecting higher fees from those who do pay their bills. Hospitals, physicians, and pharmacies argue that as more limits have been imposed, the limited reimbursement no longer covers the actual costs of care. This jeopardizes the entire system. Medicaid costs also have been contained by tightening eligibility requirements, which shuts more people out of the healthcare system. Healthcare reform relies on expanding eligibility for Medicaid to cover the working poor. Many employer plans are requiring more cost sharing by employees both to reduce the cost to the employer and as an incentive for the employee to use healthcare wisely. Fee structures have historically rewarded procedures and medications with higher reimbursement than teaching or addressing psychosocial needs. Changing fee structures to support actions that promote health and avoid exacerbations of chronic illness has been proposed as one possible source of cost containment.

Controlling Fraud and Abuse

As Medicare and Medicaid have become a larger part of the financing for the healthcare system, fraud has become a larger problem with individual cases responsible for millions in fraudulent payments (Rashbaum & Wilson, 2010). HIPAA created a federal Healthcare

Fraud and Abuse Control Program that coordinates federal, state, and local law enforcement activities in fighting healthcare fraud and abuse. Information on preventing Medicare fraud is available at the Medicare Web site (*www.medicare.gov/*) under Help and Support.

Other Cost-Containment Measures

In medical facilities, personnel now are asked to be more cost conscious. Nursing personnel must be aware of the tremendous cost of any complication or prolonged length of stay. Preventing complications and getting clients ready for early discharge have become a major focus of care. Care pathways specify care and identify outcomes for each day of hospitalization, with the goal of ensuring that resources are used wisely. Cost consciousness involves such ordinary measures as being conservative with telephone use, canceling meal trays when clients are discharged, and using expensive supplies with care.

Efforts at reducing costs affect the entire healthcare environment, the decision-making processes, power structures, the kinds of care provided, and the ways that individual healthcare providers practice. Concerns about cost continue to exert pressure for change in the system.

Critical Thinking Activity

What cost-control measures have you seen in places where you have had clinical practice? Analyze the effects of these cost-control measures on client care.

ACCESS TO HEALTHCARE

Access to healthcare refers to the individual's ability to obtain and use needed services. Access can be an economic, a geographic, or a sociocultural issue. Creating access requires a broad approach that encompasses access to health providers and hospitalization as well as addressing other factors that affect health. In addition to providing a family with a prescription, for example, a provider must determine whether there is a way to fill that prescription. Prescribing a special diet requires learning whether that the individual has the necessary knowledge and resources to follow that diet.

Economic Access

The problem of economic access to healthcare was discussed from a system perspective when the various methods of paying for healthcare were presented. Economic access is often dependent on having a health plan or being eligible for one of the government programs. Some of the decisions made for purposes of cost containment may have unforeseen consequences in terms of economic access. Although giving people an incentive to use services wisely is the stated goal of raising deductibles and co-payments, the result for lower-income families may be the delay or avoidance of timely care. Many of the provisions of the healthcare reform were for the purpose of increasing economic access to healthcare.

Some groups, such as minorities and the elderly, that experience disparities in healthcare access, are heavily affected by the coexistence of poverty in these groups. Even those eligible for Medicaid-financed care may not be able to find a PCP willing to care for them. The low reimbursement rates and the need to cope with the complex governmental system lead many private providers to opt out of such care.

Geographic Access

Geographic access to healthcare is a special concern for those in rural areas. As changes occur in the healthcare system, small rural hospitals have found themselves unable to compete or to manage financially, leading to the closure of some of those hospitals. When a rural hospital closes, area residents lose emergency room care, hospital access, and diagnostic services. The need to travel to receive healthcare especially affects the elderly and poor.

Communities without hospitals find it more difficult to recruit physicians and other PCPs. Historically, most healthcare providers have preferred not to work in areas where hospitals are not available to provide diagnostic and treatment services; consequently, rural communities find it difficult to recruit healthcare providers. Many medical schools, with the support of both federal and state funds, developed programs to encourage medical students and residents to consider family practice as a specialty and to practice in a rural location. Although successful in increasing the number of physicians entering rural practice, in some states that number couldn't make up for the number of physicians leaving rural practice.

Geographic access may be a concern for those in urban areas as well. Economically depressed areas of large cities have fewer healthcare providers, forcing the residents of those areas to travel long distances, often using inconvenient public transportation, to receive healthcare.

Nurse practitioners have a long history of moving into underserved areas both rural and urban. Significant support for the education of nurse practitioners and for removing barriers to their reimbursement was part of the healthcare reform legislation and the recommendations of the report on The Future of Nursing (IOM, 2010). As more individuals have economic access, the demand for PCPs is expected to increase. Nurse practitioners are expected to be major players in providing primary care.

Access to healthcare is affected by whether all services are available in one location. Some organizations now offer all health services in one geographic location. A single healthcare site allows an individual to see a primary provider and a specialist and have diagnostic tests and procedures in one trip to one location. This makes efficient use of the client's time, increases the likelihood that the client will follow through with recommended procedures, and simplifies communication between providers.

Sociocultural Access

Sociocultural differences affect access. When individuals feel uncomfortable in a setting because of their socioeconomic status or because their cultural background and beliefs are not respected, they are reluctant to use the services provided. Making care culturally accessible may mean having available in the care setting translation services, materials in multiple languages, and care providers who understand and are sensitive to cultural differences.

EVALUATION AND ACCREDITATION OF HEALTHCARE AGENCIES

A variety of standards and processes to enforce those standards have been established to evaluate healthcare. Meeting the standards of a state governmental agency is termed approval or *certification*. Meeting the standards of a nongovernment agency is usually designated as *accreditation*. Healthcare institutions are often both certified by a government body and accredited by a nongovernment agency. In some instances, government bodies accept accreditation as the equivalent of government standards and do not require an additional approval process. Approval by a specific organization may be required for an agency to receive some types of third-party payment. Therefore, accreditation is important for the agencies involved. Most evaluation processes involve evaluating client outcomes as well as the structure of the organization and the processes used to provide care.

Government Approval

Approval may take the form of state licensing, which usually focuses on maintaining minimum standards to safeguard public health. For some agencies, this meets their needs. Additional approval is required for reimbursement under federal programs and health plans.

Medicare/Medicaid Certification

Those agencies that seek Medicare or Medicaid funding must meet specific federal standards (termed the "conditions of participation" [COP]) and be Medicare certified in addition to meeting the basic state standards for operation. For Medicare or Medicaid to reimburse nursing home care, the state inspection must include Medicare/Medicaid standards, which relate to many aspects of care. By designating those to whom payment will be given, Medicare effectively exerts control. Because the costs of private care are so high, most people choose to receive care where it can be reimbursed, making other choices when the care is not reimbursed.

Healthcare institutions and agencies may seek accreditation from nongovernment bodies that set standards for high quality and provide guidelines to assist in developing policies and procedures. Medicare and Medicaid have granted several of these nongovernment agencies what is called "deemed status." This means that the standards of the agency are considered equal to or exceeding the Medicare standard. Therefore, a healthcare agency that has been accredited by the voluntary process from an agency discussed below may be deemed as meeting the standards set by Medicare and Medicaid and not required to pursue an additional Medicare certification process.

The Joint Commission

Hospitals, nursing homes, and related organizations may seek accreditation from The Joint Commission. This nonprofit, voluntary organization was established in 1951 by the American College of Surgeons, the American College of Physicians, the American Medical Association, and the Canadian Medical Association (Joint Commission, n.d.) to set standards for hospital care. Today's organization has a board of directors with members from many healthcare and public occupations. The standards of the organization are comprehensive and involve evaluating the structural aspects of institutions, the processes used within that agency to deliver and monitor care, and the outcomes of care provided. It has deemed status for federal programs. In the past, assisted-living settings have not had a standard accreditation and, in many states, little regulation. The Joint Commission now provides accreditation for a wide variety of healthcare facilities including home care, ambulatory care, and assisted living.

During visits to facilities referred to as *surveys* (done approximately every 3 years), the Joint Commission investigates all aspects of an organization, including the physical plant, the entire delivery of care process, and the evaluation and quality improvement plans being used. It has the power to demand change to maintain accreditation status. In most instances, however, problems that are not of serious danger to patients are noted for remediation and the facility is asked to report on the changes made.

DNV Accreditation

In September 2008, DNV (Det Norske Veritas) Accreditation became the first alternative to Joint Commission accreditation for hospitals. This nonprofit organization has been in existence for many years, working with manufacturing and other industries on developing effective quality improvement processes and managing risk. The expansion into health care follows their same model of operation. The surveys are done annually. Those institutions that meet the Medicare/Medicaid COP are accredited but are then guided toward improvement to meet the international ISO 9001 standard, which reflects continuous quality improvement and customer satisfaction. DNV does not provide consulting nor does it provide prescriptive processes for institutions. They state that their focus is to help organizations develop their own best practices by focusing on outcomes. While at this writing, only 120 hospitals in the United States are accredited by DNV. This may change as organizations examine their options for accreditation (Information from DNV, n.d.).

Community Health Accreditation Program

The Community Health Accreditation Program (CHAP) was established to provide a voluntary accreditation system for community-based health services including home health agencies, hospices, and home medical equipment providers (*www.chapinc.org*). This is a peer-reviewed process governed entirely by community health agencies with public representation. Medicare and Medicaid do not require a separate Medicare certification for an organization that has CHAP accreditation.

National Committee for Quality Assurance

The National Committee for Quality Assurance (NCQA) reviews and evaluates health plans and provides recognition of plans that meet standards of excellence. NCQA has established a set of statistical measures called the Healthcare Effectiveness Data and Information Set (HEDIS) and is a tool used by more than 90 percent of America's health plans to measure performance on important dimensions of care and service. This information is available from its Web site, *www.ncqa.org*. These data provide a standard set of information that both employers and consumers can use to compare and evaluate health plans.

Quality Improvement Organizations (QIO)

The first systematic evaluation of healthcare services was established through the Professional Standards Review Organization set up by Medicare and Medicaid in the 1980s. These efforts have continued to expand through quality improvement organizations (QIOs). "QIOs are private, mostly not-for-profit organizations, which are staffed by professionals, mostly doctors and other healthcare professionals, who are trained to review medical care and help beneficiaries with complaints about the quality of care and to implement improvements in the quality of care available throughout the spectrum of care" (CMS, 2008b).

Areas of concern in terms of quality improvement are patient safety, care coordination or transitions, clinical treatment advancement, and preventive care methods. QIOs also work to promote best practice models and serve as a resource in the areas of health information technology and electronic health records. Consumers may appeal decisions made by healthcare providers to their state QIO (CMS, 2008c).

Outcome Measures for Evaluation

Outcome measures refer to actual health results in the clients and communities served. Outcomes now are measured in relationship to hospitals, long-term care facilities, and the population as a whole. Some outcomes have been designated **key indicators**, also termed **quality indicators (QIs)**, which are specific, measurable aspects of healthcare that show the effectiveness of the system as a whole. Some of the outcome measures are based on the outcomes identified by Healthy People 2020 (DHHS, 2009).

Hospital Healthcare Outcomes

The federal government compiles statistics related to hospital healthcare outcomes. These include infection rates and morbidity and mortality rates associated with specific hospitals and procedures. In 1995, the federal government began releasing these figures to the public. These government statistics may be helpful in evaluating some aspects of care. One result of outcome studies has been the recommendation that only hospitals that perform a specified number of highly technical surgeries (eg, cardiac surgeries) each year should offer those procedures. Hospitals that perform fewer procedures per year have higher complication and mortality rates.

The Agency for Health Care Research and Quality (AHRQ) has identified a set of items that could be used as indicators of quality of care and community access to care. It identified three groups of QIs: prevention QIs, inpatient QIs, and patient safety QIs. Since their beginning in the early 1990s, these QIs have been refined through the use of extensive data banks maintained by the HHS (AHRQ, n.d.).

The prevention QIs are "a set of measures that can be used with hospital inpatient discharge data to identify 'ambulatory care sensitive conditions' (ACSCs) in adult populations. ACSCs are conditions for which good outpatient care can potentially prevent the need for hospitalization, or for which early intervention can prevent complications or more severe disease" (AHRQ, 2006a). The inpatient QIs are "a set of measures that can be used with hospital inpatient discharge data to provide a perspective on quality" (AHRQ, 2006b).

The patient safety indicators are adverse outcomes for hospitalized patients that reflect an adverse event that is preventable such as falls and nosocomial (originating in the healthcare system) infections (AHRQ, 2006c). Programs to facilitate the collection and aggregation of data in relationship to these QIs are now available on-line. Safety is discussed in detail in Chapter 10.

Many healthcare agencies are constructing their documentation systems to collect data that demonstrate performance in relationship to these QIs. This is enlarging the purpose of documentation from a focus on the individual client to a focus that includes system concerns.

Institutional Outcomes Measurement

Individual institutions are establishing ways to measure the outcomes of the care they provide. Outcomes here refers to data such as the number of clients admitted with a fractured hip who had uncomplicated recoveries leading to effective rehabilitation and the number of clients who had complications or did not recover. Knowledge of outcomes is essential for planning and for effective marketing. Often data have been collected but are scattered among many different records, making retrieval difficult. Because data only become valuable for planning when they are organized in a useful framework for analysis, healthcare agencies have moved rapidly to the computerization of data and the implementation of standardized protocols for data collection.

One of the standardized tools hospitals use to monitor outcomes is called the **clinical pathway**. This is also referred to as a critical path, a care map, or an anticipated recovery path. The clinical pathway describes the optimum progression through the system of the individual with a particular health problem. By establishing the desired outcome for day 2 of the postoperative client with a fractured hip, it is possible to determine when an individual client is not meeting the desired outcome. The advantage for the client is that care can be modified immediately to address the problem. The advantage for the system is the ability to aggregate data across all clients and examine what is working well and what needs to be changed.

Long-Term Care Quality Measures

Quality measures (QMs) are used in long-term care as part of the regulatory process. QMs differ from QIs. "Measures are values that are based upon sufficiently credible data to allow the user to make an informed, appropriate decision regarding the process under consideration based upon the data alone, without further investigation" (CHSRA, 2010). CMS has identified 14 QMs for long-term care residents (CMS, 2010). These QMs serve as the focus for the state surveyors. Long-term care facilities track these indicators themselves and use them as a focus of improvement.

Home Care Quality Indicators

The home care quality indicators provide tools for measuring quality in home care (Rosati, 2009). They are based on assessments using the MDS for home care. These indicators can be monitored to evaluate the performance of a home care agency. Examples of indicators are "prevalence of weight loss in individuals who are not palliative care clients" and "prevalence of decrease in ability to dress one's upper body." One area of concern in comparing agencies based on these indicators is that the population served by the agency affects the outcomes of care. Those agencies caring for a greater percentage of the poor and the disadvantaged face challenges in meeting the same outcome standards.

National Health Indicators

In 1992, DHHS and the Public Health Service published *Healthy People 2000, National Health Promotion and Disease Prevention Objectives*. The purpose of this document was to establish national goals to serve as a focus for health promotion and disease prevention activities by individuals, organizations, and the federal government. The Healthy People program has continued to guide federal efforts through Healthy People 2010 and now through goals and objectives for Healthy People 2020 (DHHS, 2009).

POWER IN THE HEALTHCARE SYSTEM

Part of trying to understand any system involves examining some of the unique sources of power and authority within it. If we define **power** as the capability of doing or accomplishing something, then understanding how power is distributed and used in the healthcare system can help us to function more effectively. Sources of power unique to the healthcare system are the authority to decide who may enter and leave the system, who may practice in it, and how funding is controlled. An understanding of power in the healthcare system provides a foundation for nurses to accomplish their goals for patients and their families. Without this understanding, nurses may find themselves without power and thus unable to accomplish desired goals.

Regulatory Power

The primary regulatory agencies in healthcare are government bodies as discussed above. Through regulation, these agencies have a profound effect on how institutions operate. The accrediting bodies (eg, The Joint Commission, CHAP, and NCQA) all have power to stimulate change in the system. If you have the opportunity to be in an institution when accreditation visitors are present, you will note that every aspect of the physical plant, the policies and procedures, and the competence of staff are examined. Preparing for an accreditation visit stimulates the agency to self-evaluate and correct any deficiencies.

Third-Party Payer Power

Because they represent the financial interests of large groups of people and control payments for services, third-party payers have the power to demand changes in the healthcare system. When they were first established, these agencies did not see their role in healthcare as anything beyond a financial relationship. As healthcare costs rose, these agencies began looking for ways of controlling costs to maintain their competitive place in the insurance market and have set increasingly rigid criteria for payment for services. The standard rates set for payment for procedures tend to place some restraints on charges (although actual fees often are slightly ahead of payment schedules). By determining whom they will pay for services, insurance companies reduce the choices available to those who carry insurance, and subscribers usually must select from the choices available if they wish to be reimbursed. Third-party payers therefore exert a more powerful influence over institutions and care providers than do individual subscribers.

Physician Power

Physicians historically had almost unlimited power within the healthcare system. They determined who entered the system and when. They decided whether and when other services and personnel would be used, and they determined when clients would leave the system. As other agencies and professionals in the healthcare system have obtained some power and independence, the overall power of the physician has diminished.

As a group, physicians have opposed changes that would disperse power in the system, arguing that they are the most educated and knowledgeable of all healthcare providers and that their professional judgment should be accepted. Those favoring increased distribution of power have argued that more competition, more choice for consumers, and input from a greater variety of healthcare providers and from consumers will make the system more balanced and more responsive. Despite changes, physicians remain powerful in the healthcare system.

Consumer Power

The sources of power previously discussed present problems because the client is excluded. Clearly, the client is involved in only the most basic aspect of entry into the system: determining that he or she needs care. The client cannot enter any institution without the express approval of a physician. The client may have no control over who can become a PCP, and, with the advent of HMOs and PPOs, may have limited choice in selecting providers. Funding usually is controlled by third-party payers, and the client is often powerless to determine who will be paid, how much will be paid, and when payments will be made.

Consumers do have rights in the healthcare system. These are stated in different ways by different institutions and groups, but all revolve around the recognition of the healthcare consumer as an individual with the ability and right to be self-determining. As a general rule, consumers are not aware of their rights, and even when they are aware, they may be reluctant to take advantage of them. Consumers are in a particularly vulnerable position in the healthcare system. Because they put their lives in the hands of those in the system, they are often reluctant to complain or request changes for fear of offending those on whom they depend. In addition, when consumers try to exert power in the system, they may meet with resistance. Consumers are most often effective in exerting power in the system by working in groups and through established committees and agencies.

The 2008 edition of the American Hospital Association's document "The Patient Care Partnership: Understanding Expectations, Rights, and Responsibilities" provides a framework for viewing the rights of individuals with the hospital system. This document, which emphasizes that responsibilities accompany rights, is further discussed in Chapter 8.

Nurse Power

Historically nurses have had limited power in the healthcare system, a situation that has its roots in many of the traditional aspects of nursing discussed in Chapter 1. Change may not occur as rapidly as desired, and nurses often are frustrated because of their inability to influence the system. Many new graduates are especially distressed to learn that, as individuals, they cannot affect the system. Somehow they expect that if they speak with a voice of reason and act in the best interest of their clients, others will respond positively. But this may not happen. Nevertheless, things are changing in nursing. Nursing organizations are working to provide nurses with a voice at higher decision-making levels in healthcare. By understanding the political realities and the ways in which decisions are made, and by working together to speak with a united voice, nurses can increase their power in the system (see Chapter 15). Nursing education programs increasingly try to educate nurses to act as client advocates and agents of change (see Chapters 2 and 13). Collective bargaining and shared governance have provided nurses with mechanisms for demanding recognition of the importance of their role within the system (see Chapter 5).

There are a variety of implications for nurses in the current cost-control environment. The availability and accuracy of documents that reflect the acuity level and multiple problems of a client when records are audited for compliance is essential (determination of acuity level is discussed earlier in this chapter).

Critical Thinking Activity

Nurses are actively seeking power in the healthcare system. Consider the roles of nurses in the facilities with which you are familiar. How might nurses in these settings increase their power?

IMPLICATIONS FOR NURSES

Nurses have continuing interest and concern in the direction in which healthcare moves. They are most concerned about client well-being in the midst of a powerful system. As pressures to change increase, nurses continue to speak out for consumers. Who will help consumers cope with their health problems and those of their families? Who will assist them in negotiating the various parts of the healthcare system? Will the individual identities and unique needs of consumers be addressed, or will each person be treated as the mythical "standard client"? Nurses in home health agencies and long-term care facilities are caring for clients with complex nursing needs. A major concern is whether the reimbursement system provides adequate funds for quality nursing care to be delivered.

Another important concern of nurses is whether that aspect of healthcare that we call nursing, with its focus on the individual, will be maintained. Will the pressures for demonstrating cost-effectiveness result in a loss of caring because it is not always quantifiable? Will the system recognize the critical thinking skills and abilities of nurses as well as their technical skills? Will many educated and skilled nurses be replaced by unlicensed assistive personnel? The future poses many as yet unanswered questions.

There are ongoing concerns in the healthcare system relating to the actual use of healthcare services by the public and to the structure of the system itself. The impetus for change in many ways continues to grow. Several states already have instituted efforts to create a more coordinated healthcare system for their citizens. With the passage of the health reform bill in 2010, major changes in the system are expected. No one can predict all the details of the future system with certainty, but we have tried to point out the major changes now occurring and the directions in which the new healthcare system is moving. Nurses need to remain knowledgeable and involved in the political processes involved as changes are proposed in the healthcare system.

Critical Thinking Activity

Identify clients you have encountered from a variety of social, cultural, and economic backgrounds. Given these clients' needs and backgrounds, what type of practitioner would best meet their needs for primary care? What barriers might they meet in trying to gain access to primary care? What might you do to assist these individuals?

KEY CONCEPTS

- The various types of healthcare services are differentiated by the needs of the client being served and range from specific specialized services to skilled care to custodial care.
- Many different types of agencies provide healthcare services, including long-term care settings, acute care hospitals, ambulatory care centers, home care agencies, and healthcare businesses. There are a wide variety of nursing roles in these different settings. Healthcare agencies are classified according to length of stay, mix of services provided, and ownership of the agency.
- Acute care is centered in the work of the traditional hospital, which has become a hub for healthcare in most communities.
- Long-term care facilities provide many types of care. Nursing homes provide care for those without the ability to manage ADLs and who need ongoing care. Assisted-living centers provide supportive services to those who can manage most of their own ADLs. Rehabilitation centers assist the individual in returning to the maximum level of independence possible.
- Ambulatory care settings provide care on an outpatient basis. This care may range from simple office calls for common illnesses and health promotion activities such as immunizations to the performance of ambulatory surgery.
- Home health agencies offer a wide variety of care services that may include traditional public health services, high-intensity skilled care in the home, and rehabilitation services. Home care agencies offer services within the home that assist individuals in avoiding institutional care settings when they are unable to complete their own ADLs.
- Changes in the healthcare delivery system are creating many problems that affect healthcare workers. Among these are issues related to primary care, accreditation of health professional education programs, and the future of health professional education and licensure.
- The financing of healthcare is complex and involves personal payment, insurance companies, HMOs, preferred providers, and governmental systems, each of which operates differently.
- Through control of financing, third-party payers exert control over all aspects of healthcare.
- Cost increases have created stress in the healthcare system. Understanding the basis of these increases is essential for planning to contain costs.
- Mechanisms for controlling costs and improving patterns of care have been instituted. These have included changing methods of payment, controlling healthcare providers, and managing care. The federal government has played a major role in the development and implementation of these mechanisms.
- Access to healthcare must be considered in terms of economic, geographic, and sociocultural access. A major concern in the system is those who do not have access.
- Quality of care is maintained by a wide variety of mechanisms. Institutions and agencies providing care receive oversight in the form of governmental approval and accreditation by certifying organizations.
- Quality is evaluated through peer review and the use of outcome measures, including key indicators and individual patient outcome standards.
- Power is exerted in the healthcare system by those who control finances, those who control access, and those with special knowledge. Traditionally, nurses and consumers have experienced little power in the system. Both are working to gain recognition and to affect more significantly the way the system functions.
- There are many implications for nurses in the financing and control of healthcare, including cost control, the well-being of the client, the effective use of healthcare resources, and changing the healthcare system.

RELEVANT WEB SITES

Web sites relevant to this chapter can be found at The **thePoint** ✲ accessed through *http://thePoint. lww.com/Ellis10e* and by entering the code found on the inside cover of your text.

REFERENCES

Agency for Healthcare Research and Quality. (n.d.). *Quality indicators*. Retrieved December 2, 2010, from http:// www.qualityindicators.ahrq.gov/

Agency for Healthcare Research and Quality. (2006a). *Prevention quality indicators*. Retrieved June 5, 2010, from http://www.qualityindicators.ahrq.gov/downloads/pqi/2006-Feb-PreventionQualityIndicators.pdf

Agency for Healthcare Research and Quality. (2006b). *Inpatient quality indicators (QIs)*. Rockville, MD: Agency for Healthcare Research and Quality. Retrieved June 5, 2010, from http://www.qualityindicators.ahrq.gov/ downloads/iqi/2006-Feb-InpatientQualityIndicators.pdf

Agency for Healthcare Research and Quality. (2006c). *Patient safety indicators*. Retrieved June 6, 2010, from http:// www.qualityindicators.ahrq.gov/downloads/psi/2006-Feb-PatientSafetyIndicators.pdf

Bostwick, M. (2008). *Florence Nightingale: The making of an icon*. New York: Farrar, Straus and Giroux.

Buerhaus, P. I., Auerbach, D. I., & Staiger, D. O. (2009). The recent surge in nurse employment: Causes and implications, *Health Affairs, 28*(4), w657–w668. (Published online 12 June 2009) doi: 10.1377/hlthaff.28.4.w657, Retrieved March 25, 2010.

Bureau of Labor Statistics (BLS), U.S. Department of Labor. (2010). *Occupational outlook handbook, 2010–11 edition, registered nurses*, Retrieved March 25, 2010, from http://www.bls.gov/oco/ocos083.htm

Case Management Society of America. (2010). *Who we are*. Retrieved June 17, 2010, from www.cmsa.org

Centers for Disease Control and Prevention, National Center for Health Statistics. (2009). *National nursing home survey: 2004 summary*. Retrieved December 27, 2009, from http://www.cdc.gov/nchs/fastats/nursingh.htm

Center for Health Systems Research and Analysis. (2010). *Quality indicators vs. quality measures*. Retrieved June 5, 2010, from http://www.chsra.wisc.edu/chsra/projects/completed/quality/definitions.htm

Centers for Medicare and Medicaid Services. (2008a). *National health expenditure data,* Table 13 Nursing home expenditures. Retrieved October 11, 2009, from http://www.cms.hhs.gov/NationalHealthExpendData/downloads/proj2008.pdf

Centers for Medicare and Medicaid Services. (2008b). *Statement of work for QIOs*. Retrieved May 25, 2010, from http://www.cms.gov/QualityImprovementOrgs

Centers for Medicare and Medicaid Services. (2008c). *Quality of care concerns: What can your quality improvement organization address?* CMS publication 11362. Retrieved May 25, 2010, from http://www.medicare.gov/ Publications/Pubs/pdf/11362.pdf

Centers for Medicare and Medicaid Services. (2010). *Quality measures*. Retrieved June 6, 2010, from http://www. cms.gov/NursingHomeQualityInits/10_NHQIQualityMeasures.asp#TopOfPage

CIA. (2011). The World Factbook: North America, United States, Population, Retrieved April 7, 2011, from https:// www.cia.gov/library/publications/the-world-factbook/geos/us.html.

Department of Health and Human Services. (2000). *Healthy people 2010*, Washington, DC: U.S. Government Printing Office. Retrieved June 18, 2010, from www.healthypeople.gov

Department of Health and Human Services. (2008). *Statement of the Indian Health Service*. Retrieved June 5, 2010, from http://www.hhs.gov/asl/testify/2008/06/t20080626g.html

Department of Health and Human Services. (2009). *Healthy people 2020*. Retrieved December 2, 2010, from http:// www.healthypeople.gov

DNV. (n.d.). *Simply better accreditation: Making healthcare healthier*. Retrieved November 25, 2010, from http:// dnvaccreditation.com

Genworth Financial. (2009). *Genworth 2009 cost of care survey*. Retrieved October 13, 2009, from http://www. genworth.com/content/genworth/us/en/products/long_term_care/long_term_care/cost_of_care.html

Haglund, C. L., & Dowling, W. L. (1993). The hospital. In S. J. Williams & P. R. Torrens, *Introduction to health service* (4th ed., pp. 135–176). New York: Delmar Publishers, Inc.

Health Insurance Portability and Accountability Act of 1996. Retrieved June 18, 2010, from http://aspe.hhs.gov/ admnsimp/pl104191.htm

Institute of Medicine. (2010). *The future of nursing: Leading change, advancing health*. Retrieved December 3, 2010, from http://www.iom.edu/Reports/2010/The-Future-of-Nursing-Leading-Change-Advancing-Health.aspx

Joint Commission. (n.d.). *The Joint Commission history*. Retrieved December 3, 2010, from http://www.jointcom-mission.org/assets/1/18/Joint_Commission_History.pdf

Kaiser Family Foundation. (2010). *State health policy*. Retrieved June 16, 2010, from http://www.kff.org/statepolicy/

Kalisch, P. A., & Kalisch, B. J. (2004). *American nursing: A history* (4th ed.). Philadelphia: Lippincott Williams & Wilkins.

National Association of Free Clinics. (2010). *What is the NAFC?* Retrieved June 17, 2010, from http://www.freeclinics.us/index.php

Rashbaum, W. K. & Wilson, M. (2010). 44 Charged in huge Medicare fraud scheme. *New York Times*, City Room, October 13, 2010. Retrieved December 3, 2010, from http://cityroom.blogs.nytimes.com/2010/10/13/44-charged-in-huge-medicare-fraud-scheme/

Rosati, R. J. (2009). The history of quality measurement in home health care. *Clinical Geriatric Medicine, 25*(1), 121–134, vii–viii.

Taber's cyclopedic medical dictionary. (20th ed.). (2005). Philadelphia: F.A. Davis Co.

TRICARE. (2010). *What is TRICARE*. Retrieved June 5, 2010, from http://www.tricare.mil/Transparency/

U.S. Census Bureau. (2004). *U.S. interim projections by age, sex, race, and Hispanic origin*. Retrieved June 10, 2010, from www.census.gov/ipc/www/usinterimproj/

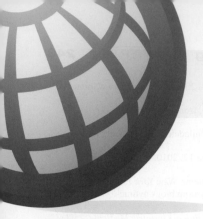

7

Legal Responsibilities for Practice

LEARNING OUTCOMES

After completing this chapter, you should be able to:

1. Differentiate the three general sources of law and explain how they apply to nursing.
2. Explain the role of institutional policies and protocols in legal decision making.
3. Identify nursing actions that violate criminal law and discuss how such violations may be avoided.
4. Explain liability in relationship to nursing practice, including situations in which liability is shared by employers or supervisors.
5. Analyze the benefits to individual nurses of purchasing professional liability insurance.
6. Explain the nurse's role in supporting patient rights through informed consent and advance directives.
7. Identify specific issues that can constitute malpractice and discuss the nurse's responsibility in relationship to them.
8. Identify factors that contribute to a suit being instituted against a healthcare professional, and explain how an individual nurse might prevent legal suits.
9. Explain the various phases of a legal action.
10. Differentiate the possible roles of a nurse when testifying for a legal proceeding.

KEY TERMS

Advance directive
Civil law
Commmown law
Competence
Constitutional law
Criminal law
Directive to physicians
Durable power of attorney for healthcare
Emancipated minors
Enacted law
Ethics
Expert witness
False imprisonment
Gross negligence
Healthcare proxy
Informed consent

Judicial law (decisional or case law)
Lawsuit
Liability
Living will
Malpractice
Mature minor
Misdemeanor
Negligence
Privileged communication
Protected health information (PHI)
Prudent professional
Reckless endangerment
Regulatory law (administrative or executive law)
Statutory law
Substitutionary decision maker
Tort

Every newspaper contains reports of sensational cases being considered in our courts and legal arenas. Concerns about lawsuits and liability are voiced in every business. Healthcare remains at the forefront of professions where legal issues constitute a major area of concern. The prudent nurse considers legal issues before a crisis arises and uses sound information to help guide action in situations where questions occur. This chapter provides basic information you will need in that process.

Examples and situations relating to legal issues discussed throughout this chapter are given to help you understand the application of the specific concepts. Many more factors are considered in arriving at an actual legal decision than can be presented in a paragraph or two. It is the interaction of multiple factors that makes it impossible to provide absolute predictions regarding legal outcomes in different situations; that is, data may be interpreted differently by judges and juries, resulting in different outcomes, even though cases may appear similar.

UNDERSTANDING THE SCOPE OF THE LAW

Legal issues are those that are decided by law. Law may be defined as "the principles and regulations established in a community by some authority and applicable to its people, whether in the form of legislation or of custom and policies recognized and enforced by judicial decision" (Dictionary.com, 2009). Laws are put in place to preserve public welfare and manage certain relationships (such as contracts) within the society. **Ethics** deal with "values relating to human conduct, with respect to the rightness and wrongness of certain actions and to the goodness and badness of the motives and ends of such actions" (Dictionary.com, 2009). Legal and ethical issues are often discussed together because they go hand in hand, with one supporting the other. In this chapter, we focus on how the law affects nursing practice. Ethics are discussed in more detail in Chapters 8 and 9.

SOURCES OF LAW

If nurses know the source of law, then they know how it can be challenged and changed, and how powerful it can be. There are three general sources of law: *statutory law*, *regulatory* (also known as administrative) *law*, and *common law*. All are relevant to nursing practice (Fig. 7.1).

Statutory Law

A statute is a written rule or formal regulation established by a government legislative authority, such as the Congress, the state legislature, or the city council. A violation of a statute is legally punishable. Statutory law is published in codes that are broken down into specific rules. In the United States, **statutory law** includes constitutional law and enacted law. All laws fall in a hierarchy of authority, with constitutional law having the greatest authority, and the enacted law the next. Regulatory law, which is discussed later, has less authority than statutory law.

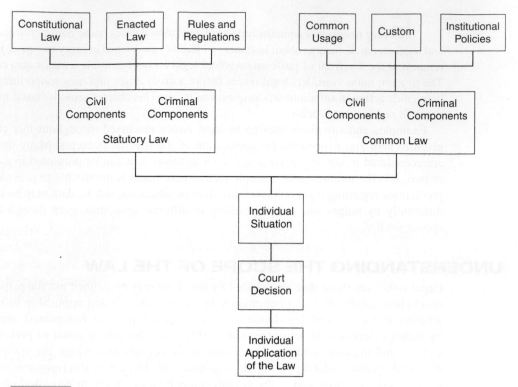

FIGURE 7.1 Civil law and criminal law both may affect a nursing situation.

Constitutional Law

Constitutional law is established by the federal government and based on the US Constitution. The Constitution was developed by the Constitutional Convention of 1787, approved by the Continental Congress, and then ratified by all the states. It establishes the general organization of the federal government and specifies the federal power and limitations to that power. The powers that are not specifically given to the federal government in the Constitution are retained by the states. The Constitution can be amended (ie, changed), with the amendments having the same status as the original provisions. Amendments to the US Constitution require similar passage and ratification by the states.

In addition, each state has its own constitution that acts as the highest law for that state. Many other nations, such as Great Britain, do not have a constitution or equivalent document. In those countries, the enacted law is the highest level of law.

Enacted Law

Enacted law includes all bills passed by legislative bodies, whether at the local, state or province, or national level. Enacted laws of the US federal government all carry the designation USC (United States Code) in their official title. The federal Social Security Act (42 USC 401) is an example of federally enacted law. Enacted laws of states or other governing bodies carry a title and number designation specific to each individual state. Nurse practice acts in the various states are examples of enacted laws at the state level.

Regulatory Law

Regulatory law (also referred to as executive or administrative law) includes the rules and regulations established by government agencies to carry out enacted laws. These appear as carefully written rules that apply to everyone. At the federal level, the Center for Medicare & Medicaid Services writes regulations governing the payment of Medicare and Medicaid funds that are authorized through legislation. At the state level, the board of nursing (or its equivalent) is authorized through enacted laws to establish and enforce rules and regulations that govern the practice of nursing in that state. The rules and regulations protect the safety of the public by defining standards for nursing education and practice (see Chapter 3). Rules and regulations of administrative bodies, often referred to as the "Administrative Code," can be enforced in court.

Common Law

Common law derives from common usage, custom, and judicial law (judicial decisions or court rulings). It is based on the English common law. Because it is based on occurrences of events, common law is less clear and exact than statutory law; it is composed of many actions and documents that are not specific written rules that apply to everyone. Common law is fluid and changes over time. In general, statutory law and regulatory law carry more weight in court than does common law.

Judicial Law

Judicial law (also referred to as decisional or case law) is derived from decrees or judgments from the courts. Judicial decisions or rulings in court cases apply statutory, regulatory, and common law to specific situations. These decisions then become precedents for interpretations of all types of law in other cases. A court also has the power to examine the same or a similar issue in a subsequent case and make a different decision, thus creating a new precedent. Court rulings are binding within the jurisdiction of the particular court that determines them but are used in a more general way (as guidelines) in other jurisdictions. In any specific situation, the final determination of the application of all types of law is the decision of the court in that case, although in most instances a decision may be appealed to higher courts.

Common Usage and Custom

As the term seems to imply, courts are empowered through the concept of common law to examine the common usage and custom in a community for patterns that reflect the community's standards for behavior. Common usage and custom are not usually written down and specific. However, written documents can be used to support common usage and custom in specific cases. For example, when examining standards of professional practice in a court case, the court may examine documents that specify standards of professional practice as reflecting common usage. These documents may be changed by the organization writing the standard and thus are not fixed.

The issue of safe medication practice illustrates how common usage applies to nursing. Neither statutes nor regulations are written about how to safely give medications. If a patient is harmed by receiving an inappropriate medication, the issue of whether the standard of practice was violated by the individual nurse might be considered in light of the standards of safe medication practice used in the healthcare facility and whether those standards were followed.

OTHER FACTORS AFFECTING LEGAL DECISIONS

In addition to the sources of law discussed above, several other factors can affect how laws are interpreted and enforced. These factors also play an important role in our legal system.

Administrative Rulings

An administrative ruling, also referred to as an advisory opinion, made by a state board or by an attorney general provides a guideline based on an interpretation of the enacted and regulatory law relative to a specific situation. It is not considered a final legal decision and different boards and attorneys general might vary in their opinions. The validity of an opinion stands until the issue is brought before a court and the court rules on the situation and provides a final decision. The court decision may or may not support the advisory ruling.

Rights and Responsibilities in Healthcare

Rights and responsibilities have both legal and ethical aspects. In the United States, basic rights are specified in the first 10 amendments to the US Constitution and are part of statutory law. This section of the Constitution is called the Bill of Rights and is an example of one of the limitations placed on the federal government. These rights protect the individual from government interference in basic areas of life. From these primary rights, other rights are deduced. For example, although the right to privacy is not specifically discussed in the Bill of Rights, the right to be secure in one's own home against unreasonable search and seizure is guaranteed. This basic right has led to court decisions supporting the right to privacy in some situations.

In some countries, rights may be part of the statutory law and thus carry less weight than a constitution does. Some countries have no counterpart to the rights found in the United States that are guaranteed through the constitution.

Some of the rights of which we commonly speak are not legally supported but are based on ethical values. For example, we often speak of a "right to healthcare." There is no legal basis for this right in the United States, but many people believe an ethical basis exists. In some countries, such as Canada and Great Britain, healthcare is a right supported by the law. In these countries, healthcare for all has been established through legislation and administrative rules and regulations.

In the United States, patient rights within the healthcare system continue to receive considerable attention by both government and consumer bodies. The federal **Health Insurance Portability and Accountability Act (HIPAA)** of 1996 contains a significant section regarding the privacy of **protected health information** . (**PHI**) refers to individually identifiable data about a person's health or healthcare. This act made privacy in regard to healthcare a legally supported right at the federal level. Based on this, all healthcare agencies and health plans are required to provide training for all employees in regard to the privacy rules and the procedures that ensure compliance. There are significant monetary penalties for breaches of privacy. Many facilities have adopted employment policies that include dismissal for certain types of breaches of patient confidentiality.

Recent attention has been directed to the patient's right to pain management. While managing pain has always been a healthcare goal, most providers did not think of it in terms of the patient's right to pain relief. The Joint Commission has added requirements to accreditation standards requiring that agencies have comprehensive plans for effectively managing pain and demonstrating that those plans are used. Human Rights Watch in its monograph (2009) regarding access to pain treatment has identified pain treatment as worldwide right of all human beings.

Responsibilities often accompany rights. If a right is guaranteed, the government and designated others have legally mandated responsibilities to ensure that the right is upheld. In the matter of the right to privacy of medical records, for example, all healthcare workers have legally mandated responsibilities to ensure that privacy is upheld.

Institutional Policies, Protocols, and Procedures

Institutional **policies** provide guidance in the proper actions to be taken in specific situations, identify the individuals responsible for taking action, and may establish specific timelines for action. Established agency policies may be considered the **standard of practice** for that agency and, therefore, common usage (common law) by the court and may become important as a basis for legal decisions. Policies may protect the institution and its employees from legal difficulties if they are based on current practice and sound legal advice. Standards of practice for nursing are often described in documents titled "Care Pathways," "Critical Pathways," or "Guidelines."

Members of the healthcare agency's staff who have expertise in the practice area under consideration usually develop the specific policy. An attorney also may be consulted to ensure that policies conform to legal requirements. Many larger institutions employ a risk manager who is frequently a nurse attorney. Final approval of policies often rests with the board of trustees, directors, or commissioners, who have ultimate responsibility for the financial and legal management of the organization.

Healthcare agency policies are changed in response to new situations and new expectations in society. Usually, there is an established route for the change or expansion of a policy. Nurses may be in a position to recognize the need for such a change as they use and compare a policy with the latest professional information.

Protocols, as the term is used in the healthcare environment, provide a list of actions for managing a specific problem that may involve the use of more than one procedure. For example, a protocol on the care of a central venous catheter might include frequency of tubing change, the type of fluid used for flushing, the frequency of dressing change, the type of dressing materials to be used, and other aspects of care. Protocols for nursing often include aspects of care that might be part of the medical orders for patient care. Therefore, they are usually developed with consultation between nursing and physician representatives and may be approved by the medical practice committee as well as by a nursing committee before implementation.

Specific institutional **procedures** outline the steps in a particular task. In the example of the central venous catheter, a procedure would be the list of steps to be taken when flushing the catheter to maintain patency. A procedure for nursing would be developed by the relevant nursing committee or sometimes by a clinical nurse specialist.

The purpose of policies, protocols, and procedures is to ensure that there is consistent, sound practice in an institution. Just as policies must be updated, so should protocols and procedures (see Chapter 5).

COMMUNICATION IN ACTION

Making Changes in a Procedure

Stan Wilson, a registered nurse (RN), was reading a nursing journal. He was surprised to learn that, according to an article, the procedure they were using at his hospital for intravenous (IV) site care was specifically not recommended. In fact, that practice was identified as showing an increased incidence of site inflammation. The next day he took the journal with him to work. He said to his coworkers, "Look at this article during your break if you can. It has some information that has made me concerned about our current IV site care procedure. I am going to show this to our manager Nancy and ask if we can start a study process to figure what really is best to do." He contacted the manager and asked for a time to sit down and talk with her about a concern. When they sat down to talk later in the day, he introduced the subject: "Nancy, I just read this article about IV site care. This is a peer-reviewed journal, and the article quotes some impressive research. According to the information here, our IV site care procedure does not meet current standards. Some specific concerns are our cleaning procedure and the ointment we are using at the site. Would you read this article? Then we can talk about the possibility of referring this issue to our evidence-based practice committee."

CLASSIFICATION OF LAWS

Law is divided into civil and criminal components. Both statutory law and common law may be subdivided in this way.

Criminal Law

Criminal law addresses the general welfare of the public. A violation of criminal law is called a crime, and it is prosecuted by the government. On conviction, a crime may be punishable by imprisonment, parole conditions, a loss of privilege (such as a license), a fine, or any combination of these. The punishment is intended to discipline the violator and deter further such actions by this person as well as discourage others from committing the crime. A crime may be classified as either a **misdemeanor** or as a **felony**. A misdemeanor is a lesser infraction of the law and is punishable by a fine or an imprisonment of less than a year. A felony represents a more serious violation of the law and carries heavier fines and longer periods of imprisonment, and, in the most serious of cases, perhaps even death (Guido, 2009.)

Civil Law

Civil law regulates conduct between private individuals or businesses and is enforced through the courts as damages or monetary compensation (Guido, 2009). Private individuals or groups may bring a legal action (a **lawsuit**) to court for breach (or breaking) of civil law. The judgment of the court results in a plan to correct the wrong and may award a monetary payment to the wronged party. Nurses may find themselves involved with both civil and criminal laws, either separately or within the same situation.

CRIMINAL LAW AND NURSING

It is costly to the state to undertake criminal prosecution; therefore, even when they are discovered, some violations of criminal law are not prosecuted in court. Knowing this, some nurses make the error of believing that "minor" violations are acceptable. Criminal action could result in the loss of a job and a license to practice nursing even when not prosecuted in court.

An example relates to laws regulating the distribution and use of controlled substances such as opioids. Violation of these laws is a crime. Thus, altering or changing narcotic records is a crime even if no diversion of drugs occurred. Falsification of a narcotic record may not result in criminal prosecution because of the cost to the state, but it usually would result in loss of a job and reporting to the licensing authority for disciplinary action.

Errors that result in serious injury or death of a patient are investigated and may be prosecuted and tried by the criminal courts. These legal actions may be based on such charges as **gross negligence**, **reckless endangerment**, or **criminal negligence**. (See discussion of negligence below.) A license to practice nursing may be temporarily withdrawn while such charges are investigated and tried. If the individual is found innocent, the license may be restored. If the individual is convicted of the crime, however, the nursing license may be revoked, in addition to sentencing and other penalties.

Nurses who commit felonies, such as theft, abuse, or deliberate harm, in which a patient is a victim are usually charged under both criminal laws and the laws regulating nursing practice. Nurses who commit felonies outside of the care setting can be prosecuted under criminal law and under the law regulating nursing practice if the felony reflects on their fitness to practice nursing. For example, an individual prosecuted for selling narcotics usually will have action taken under the Nurse Practice Act as well.

CIVIL LAW AND NURSING

Civil law relates to legal disputes between private parties. Malpractice actions brought in healthcare situations involve civil law.

Torts

"A **tort** is a civil wrong committed against a person or the person's property" (Guido, 2009, p. 92). The result may be physical harm, psychological harm, harm to livelihood, or some other less tangible value, such as harm to reputation. The action that causes a civil wrong may be either intentional or unintentional.

An intentional tort is one in which the outcome was planned, although the person involved may not have believed that the intended outcome would be harmful to the other person. For example, preventing a patient from leaving against medical advice may be based on concern for the patient, but it interferes with liberty and causes psychological harm and to do so is an intentional tort.

An unintentional tort is an action causing harm to another person or property that was not intended to happen. The most common cause of an unintentional tort is negligence.

Negligence

Negligence is a general term that refers to "conduct lacking in due care" (Guido, 2009, p. 92). If harm is caused by negligence, it is termed an unintentional tort and damages may be recovered. Experts differ on what should be termed the *essential characteristics* of negligence. For our purposes, we will identify four main characteristics and indicate common variations.

1. Harm: Harm must have occurred to an individual. Injury (which is the basis of harm) and damages (which include the consequences to the person of the injury) are considered separate characteristics by some.
2. Duty: The negligent person must have been in a situation where he or she had a responsibility or duty toward the person harmed.
3. Breach of Duty: The person must be found to have failed to fulfill his or her responsibility. This might include either doing what should not have been done (commission of an inappropriate action) or failing to do what should have been done (omission of a necessary or appropriate action). This is also referred to as failing to act as a reasonably prudent person. A reasonably prudent person in this context means someone who demonstrates careful and thoughtful action. Some authorities emphasize that this includes the responsibility to foresee possible results of a situation and act appropriately, also referred to as foreseeability. Foreseeability is identified by some experts as a separate characteristic.
4. Causation: The harm or injury must be shown to have been caused by the breach of duty.

Gross negligence or **reckless endangerment** includes the same four elements that are present in simple negligence as defined above, but the person's behavior is defined as "failure to use even the slightest amount of care in a way that shows recklessness or willful disregard for the safety of others" ('Lectric Law Library, 2006). There have been instances of nurses being charged with gross negligence under criminal law for serious errors resulting in the death of a patient; however, those charges were not sustained (Lyon, 1998). This degree of inappropriate behavior is very difficult for an individual to prove. This distinction becomes important in the discussion of charitable care and responding to community emergencies below.

Malpractice

Malpractice is a term used to identify professional negligence—liability resulting from improper practice based on standards of care required by the profession for which the person has been educated (Guido, 2009). Therefore, malpractice is a term used to describe negligence by nurses in the performance of their duties. The professional person must have had a professional duty toward the person receiving the care. For example, the nurse was performing the professional activities of a nurse for the person needing the care (in either a paid or volunteer capacity). Additionally, the harm that occurred to this person or to the property must be based on a failure to act as a **prudent professional** and in accordance with professional standards in the situation (Fig. 7.2). This is a higher standard than is required of the general public; it demands appropriate professional judgment and action (Guido, 2009) (Display 7.1).

DISPLAY 7.1   Essential Elements of Malpractice

- **Harm** to an individual
- **Duty** of a professional toward an individual
- **Breach of duty** by the professional
- **Cause of harm** is the breach of duty

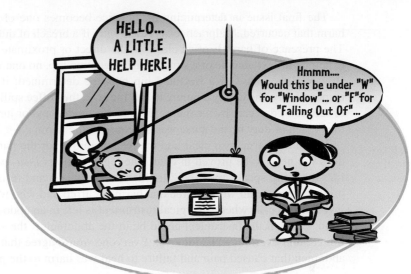

FIGURE 7.2 A reasonably prudent nurse uses common sense as well as nursing theory.

Just as all parts of the situation are clear in some general negligence situations and not in others, the same can be said of professional duty. The nurse who is assigned to care for a patient in a hospital clearly has a duty to that patient. In some situations, duties overlap and more than one nurse might have a duty toward the same patient, for example, the assigned nurse, another nurse on the unit, and a unit manager. Whether a particular nurse had a professional duty to a patient might be in dispute. In general, all nurses within a facility are considered to have a duty toward all patients and even toward visitors, in case of emergency, and are expected to act on behalf of the institution in that regard. For example, if a visitor falls, any nurse present is expected to respond, institute action, and summon help. Again, the court would decide whether a duty was present if any legal action occurred.

Critical Thinking Activity

You have taken a new position as a home health nurse. One of your patients is an elderly woman who has a leg ulcer and a long history of diabetes. Your role is to assess the patient in relationship to her diabetic management and wound care and teach as needed. While you are in the home, her husband tells you that he has been having pain in his knee and asks if you would examine it and tell him whether it is all right to use a heating pad on it, and whether he should take ibuprofen or some Tylenol. Do you have a duty to help him? Why or why not? What will your response be? What legal issues are involved in this situation? If you advise him and your advice turns out to be incorrect, what legal action could he take?

A breach of duty, as mentioned earlier, is a failure to act as a prudent professional, that is, according to the **standard of care** for the profession in a particular situation (Guido, 2009). The various sources of standards of nursing care were discussed above.

The final issue in determining malpractice becomes one of identifying the cause of the harm that occurred. Malpractice is present only if a breach of duty was the cause of the harm. The presence of harm is often clear but the direct or proximate cause may not be clear. For example, if the outcome of a situation is a fractured hip, no one will dispute that this is harm. However, the cause of a fractured hip must be determined; it might be the person's own responsibility, the family's failure to call for help, the coffee spilled on the floor by the visitor, or failure of due care by the nurse. Ultimately, a judge and/or jury must often decide whether the breach of duty by the nurse was the cause of the harm.

When the harm is so clear and the responsibility for the harm so straightforward that it does not need to be proved in court, the legal term *res ipsa loquitur* is used. This is Latin for "the thing speaks for itself." In this case, the harm and responsibility do not need to be proved, because all would agree that harm occurred and who was responsible. This may be invoked in a case where a surgical instrument is left in an abdomen and causes harm. There is no way that the instrument could be in the abdomen if the surgical team had not placed it there and overlooked its removal. Everyone would agree that a surgical instrument in the abdomen that caused pain and failure to heal was harm to the person.

LIABILITY

A **liability** is an obligation or debt that can be enforced by law. A person found guilty of any tort (whether intentional or unintentional) is considered legally liable, or legally responsible, for the outcome. The person legally liable usually is required to pay for damages to the other person. These may include actual costs of care, legal services, loss of earnings (present and future), and compensation for emotional and physical stress suffered. Although liability is legally determined by a court, an individual who believes that he or she would be held legally liable if a court were consulted may agree to pay damages (or that individual's insurance company may agree to pay) without actually going to court. Damages may be paid even when the person denies negligence, because a court case would cost more than paying damages.

Personal Liability

As an educated professional, you are always legally responsible or liable for your actions. Thus, if a physician or supervisor asks you to do something that is contrary to your best professional judgment and says, "I'll take responsibility," that person is acting unwisely. The physician or supervisor giving the directions may be liable also if harm results, but that would not remove your personal liability.

▶ *E X A M P L E*

Personal Liability

The RN who gives medications on a large medical unit at night notes that an order for dopamine is considerably larger than the usual dose. She looks up the medication in a reference book and finds that she is correct about the dosage: The ordered dose is several times the usual dose. The nurse then calls the supervisor and explains the situation and suggests that the physician be called (in this facility, night calls to physicians must be approved by the supervisor).

E X A M P L E (continued)

The supervisor double-checks the order with the RN and then states, "Dr. Jones is an outstanding physician. I am sure he has a good reason for ordering this dose. Go ahead and give the medication as ordered. I'll take responsibility. I don't believe it is worth bothering him at night." The RN then gives the medication, and the patient suffers a serious reaction.

The RN could be held liable for giving the incorrect amount of medication. She had the knowledge and judgment to recognize that the dose was much larger than usual, and she failed to check with the physician. A statement by the supervisor does not remove the nurse's personal responsibility for her own actions. Because even a competent physician might make an error, the nurse had a responsibility to clarify the order. The supervisor and the physician could be held liable in addition to the nurse, but this does not excuse the nurse from responsibility.

Although each person is legally responsible for his or her own actions, the example above illustrates that there are also situations in which a person or organization may be held liable for actions taken by others.

COMMUNICATION IN ACTION

Clarifying Your Actions

In the above situation, the RN might have responded differently and protected both herself and her supervisor. After being reassured that the supervisor would take responsibility for administering what appeared to be an excessive dose of the medication, the prudent nurse might reply, "I know you mean to be reassuring, but if the dosage is wrong I will be liable because I am the nurse administering the drug. I think it is best to call Dr. Jones and clarify the order. He has the same goal that we do: the safety and well-being of the patient. I will be glad to make the call now."

Employer Liability

In many instances, an employer can be held responsible for torts committed by an employee. This is called the doctrine of *respondeat superior* (Latin for "let the master respond"). The law holds the employer responsible for hiring qualified persons, establishing an appropriate environment for correct functioning, maintaining correct policies and procedures, and providing supervision or direction as needed to avoid errors or harm. Therefore, if a nurse, as an employee of a hospital, is guilty of malpractice, the hospital also may be named in the suit. The employer's liability may exist even if the employer appears to have taken precautions to prevent error.

It is important to understand that this doctrine does not remove any responsibility from the individual nurse, but it extends responsibility to the employer in addition to the nurse. If, for example, a hospital has a procedure that does not conform to good nursing practice as you know it, and you follow that procedure, you will still be liable for any resulting harm. You are expected to use your education and experience to make sound judgments regarding your work.

▶ *EXAMPLE*

Employer Responsibility for a Staff Nurse

A nurse working in a long-term care facility is responsible for planning and coordinating the care of a severely debilitated resident. This elderly man is totally dependent for all activities of daily living due to a recent stroke. He is not eating and drinking adequately. He faints and strikes his head. Upon assessment, he is discovered to have very low blood pressure and a rapid weak pulse. He is sent to the local hospital, where he is admitted for head injury and dehydration secondary to inadequate fluid intake. An investigation reveals that no assessment of his fluid or nutritional status had been recorded, nor was there any written plan to ensure that nutritional and fluid needs were met.

Both the nurse and the long-term care facility in this situation might be found liable for harm that resulted from the fall. The nurse had a personal, professional responsibility to accurately assess the resident and to institute care to meet his basic needs. And, the facility had a responsibility to guarantee that policies, procedures, and protocols were in place to ensure appropriate assessment and care and that the employees followed through on them.

Supervisory Liability

In the role of a clinical leader, charge nurse, unit manager, supervisor, or any other role that involves delegation, supervision, or direction of other people, the nurse is potentially liable for the actions of others. The supervising nurse is responsible for exercising good judgment in a supervisory role, including making appropriate decisions about assignments and delegation of tasks. If an error occurs and the supervising nurse is shown to have exercised sound judgment in all decisions made in that capacity, the supervising nurse may not be held liable for the error of a subordinate. If poor judgment was used in assigning an inadequately prepared person to an important task or if oversight was inadequate, the supervisory nurse might be liable for the resulting harm. The extent of the subordinate's responsibility would depend on his or her level of education and training. People with limited education or training might not be liable for some errors; the more education subordinates have, the more likely they will be liable (see Chapter 13 for more discussion of delegation).

▶ *EXAMPLE*

Supervisory Responsibility for an Educated Staff Member

Two sudden admissions to the coronary care unit (CCU) create a situation in which additional help is needed to care for the patients in the unit. A "float" nurse is sent to the CCU to assist. The charge nurse assumes that the temporary float nurse has education or experience in coronary care which she does not. The temporary float nurse does not volunteer this information.

The temporary nurse is assigned by the charge nurse to the complete care of two patients. Because of the float nurse's inability to accurately interpret the monitors, a potentially life-threatening problem is not identified until the patient "arrests." Resuscitation efforts are successful, but the patient suffers some brain damage.

In this scenario, both the charge nurse, who assigned the inadequately prepared nurse to total care, and the temporary nurse could be found liable: the charge nurse for incorrectly assigning the nurse, and the temporary nurse for not recognizing and communicating her own limitations. The educational preparation of the temporary nurse gave her the background to understand that she did not possess the expertise needed in this situation. If the situation were changed so that the temporary nurse was reviewed for expertise in coronary care and found to have that expertise, then the charge nurse might not be liable for the error of the temporary nurse. The supervisory function of ascertaining level of preparation and ability to meet the standards of the job would have been carried out.

▶ **EXAMPLE**

Supervisory Responsibility for a Staff Member with Limited Education

An RN is working on a unit that assigns a nursing assistant to work with each RN. One evening, the regular nursing assistant is absent due to illness. A new nursing assistant is assigned to work with the RN. During the evening, the RN asks the nursing assistant to monitor the new postoperative patient. The RN lists for the nursing assistant the items that are to be checked: vital signs, hourly urine output, pain, and condition of the dressing. Each hour, the RN stops the nursing assistant, asks if the patient is doing okay, and receives an affirmative reply. When the RN stops to chart, he reviews the past 4 hours of flow sheet information listed by the nursing assistant. He sees that the urine output has been only 15 ml/hour for the past 4 hours. When he questions the nursing assistant, he learns that the nursing assistant had no idea what information needed to be reported immediately. The RN completes an assessment and calls the physician. The patient is found to have developed renal failure.

The RN might be found negligent in this case for assigning the nursing assistant to monitor a critical postoperative patient without proper direction or supervision. The nursing assistant might not be found negligent because she had no basis for recognizing the seriousness of the situation or her own lack of ability to meet the responsibilities involved in this assessment.

Limits on a Patient's Claim to Negligence

Several situations may be viewed by the court as a valid defense to a patient's claim that negligence has occurred. *Contributory negligence* is based on the concept that the patient contributed to the injury by not acting prudently in that circumstance. For example, the patient may not have followed instructions, may have provided false information that led to improper treatment, or may not have followed warnings about the side effects of medications. In five states or territories (Alabama, District of Columbia, Maryland, North Carolina, and Virginia), contributory negligence prevents the individual from receiving any compensation for injury (Guido, 2009).

All other states incorporate the use of comparative negligence. If this is used, the court would determine what percentage of the injury resulted from the patient's negligence and what part rested with the nurse, and reduce the damage award accordingly (Guido, 2009).

Charitable Immunity

Charitable immunity refers to a situation in which an individual or an organization is held to a lesser standard of care because of the provision of charitable care. This lesser standard is that the person must be guilty of gross negligence (discussed above) in order to be liable. Thus, they are protected from liability for ordinary negligence.

Institutional Charitable Immunity

Historically, charitable immunity covered all the work of some hospitals and churches. Charitable immunity was granted if all the income for the institution was derived from charitable giving. Some laws even provided specific dollar amounts of liability limitation for charitable organizations. This type of immunity for institutions is rapidly disappearing because there are few major hospitals that do not provide both compensated care and uncompensated care. There is also a strong public interest in holding all organizations accountable for the actions of those who work under their auspices.

Charitable Immunity for Volunteers in Health Settings

In 1997, the federal government enacted the Volunteer Protection Act. This law provides for immunity from charges of simple negligence and only allows charges for gross negligence for volunteers in health clinics and other settings. This is an especially important protection for health professionals who choose to volunteer. State laws protecting volunteers may provide more protection but cannot limit the protection provided under federal law. This has been done to encourage health professionals to volunteer their services where they are greatly needed. If you choose to volunteer your services as a nurse, you should investigate the protections afforded in your state.

Charitable immunity does not mean that a person cannot sue a volunteer care provider; however, it makes it much less likely that they could win and, therefore, less likely that an attorney would help them to pursue such a case. Legislation in some states requires that the clinic inform clients in writing that by accepting free care they are agreeing to the limited liability of the care providers.

Good Samaritan Laws

Another type of charitable immunity is found in laws that relate to people responding to emergencies. These are often referred to as Good Samaritan laws. These laws are meant to encourage anyone to render assistance in an emergency situation without fear of liability for simple negligence. Liability is only for gross negligence. The nurse rendering aid in an emergency must behave as a reasonably prudent nurse in that situation. Thus, the standard is higher than for the nonprofessional person. For example, a person on the street might bend an injured person's neck in an effort to help the person, but a nurse might be found to be reckless for doing that because the nurse has more formal education regarding proper actions in accidents. However, in this scenario, the nurse is not expected to perform as if he or she were operating in a healthcare setting. The physical situation and the psychological situation are both considered when determining what is a reasonably prudent nursing action. An additional aspect of the professional responsibility is to not abandon the person until care can be turned over to another competent person. So the professional may relinquish responsibility to emergency services personnel who arrive on the scene, but not to a simple bystander. In reality, healthcare professionals have not been sued for rendering aid in emergency situations.

Each nurse must make an individual decision about rendering emergency aid in a specific situation unless the law mandates that people respond to emergencies. Vermont (Title 12, Chapter 23; SS 519, 1968) and Minnesota (Minn. Stat. Sec. 604A.0 1 [2003]) both require that a person encountering an emergency render assistance unless it would put themselves in danger.

The automatic external defibrillator (AED) is now being placed in public settings throughout the nation for the treatment of cardiac arrest victims. In 2002, the federal government passed the Community Access to Emergency Devices Act (Community AED Act), which provided grants for the purpose of placing AEDs in public locations and training individuals in their use, thus further expanding the presence of AEDs. The liability of those who use the devices became an immediate concern after their use was implemented. All 50 states have now enacted laws relative to the liability of those who use these devices. These laws again protect individuals from charges of simple negligence (National Conference of State Legislatures, 2006).

The decision to render aid involves ethical as well as legal considerations. If the profession of nursing is a public trust and nurses are truly involved in the business of caring, then failure to aid an individual who is in serious danger is an ethical violation of that trust. Professional liability insurance does provide coverage when assisting in this way, which may make a nurse feel more comfortable about rendering emergency aid.

LIABILITY INSURANCE

Liability insurance transfers the legal and any settlement costs related to a suit from the individual to an insurance company, which spreads the risks to a large group of policy holders. The expectation is that most individuals will not be sued and that the pool of premiums collected from policy holders, therefore, will adequately cover the costs of those who are sued, the administrative costs of managing the policies, and the profit for the insurance company. Individuals benefit by transferring risk from themselves to the insurance company for the cost of the insurance policy.

A liability insurance crisis exists in the United States. The cost of liability insurance for primary healthcare providers (such as physicians and nurse practitioners) has escalated at an extraordinary rate. Some of the factors that have caused this are the large judgments that have been made, the number of suits that have been brought, the large fees that attorneys receive, and the high profits of insurance companies. Nurses in independent advanced practice have been especially affected by the increase in premiums, because their incomes have traditionally been moderate and they cannot charge fees sufficient to cover insurance costs that may equal those of physicians. Nurses who are not employed in advanced roles are able to obtain malpractice insurance for a modest cost.

Some states have initiated legislation that allows for awards to cover actual losses and costs of care, while limiting awards for pain and suffering and other nontangible factors. Sometimes this legislation has been accompanied by restrictions on insurance company rates. Laws in some states are being amended to restrict the monetary liability of any party according to the percentage of responsibility. Liability laws continue to be a major concern for nurses, because nurses are being named in an increasing number of suits, although the total number is still low.

Institutional and Individual Insurance

Many hospitals and other institutional employers carry liability insurance that covers both the institution and its employees. Some hospitals may limit the coverage that their policies provide for individual employees in an effort to hold down costs. When healthcare institutions merge, are bought out, or go bankrupt, liability insurance coverage might be changed or dropped. Some institutions choose to self-insure part of their liability requirements and usually maintain a Self-Insurance Trust with funds to pay claims. If such an institution goes bankrupt, there may be no funds left to pay liability claims and pending claims may revert to individuals named in the suits.

Even if an employer carries liability insurance, it is usually advisable for the individual professional to carry an independent policy. If a legal action is instituted against you, your individual liability insurance policy provides an independent attorney who is focused on your welfare. An independent policy provides coverage in voluntary activities as well as on the job. It moves with you as you transfer from one employer to another. If the institution has charitable immunity and nurses are paid employees, the policy supports the individual nurse who may be sued when the institution is protected from a lawsuit. Many nursing liability policies also provide coverage for legal expenses incurred in defending your license in a disciplinary proceeding. Some policies may provide for personal liability in your home (for such things as a person tripping on a rug and being injured) as well as professional liability.

Keep in mind that insurance is not the only source of payment for a judgment in a legal action. Judgments may be levied against most tangible assets, including houses, cars, and savings; judgments also may be levied against future earnings. Married nurses who reside in community property states should realize that one half of the assets of a couple may be vulnerable to a judgment. Community property states at this time include Arizona, California, Idaho, Louisiana, Nevada, New Mexico, Texas, Washington, and Wisconsin. These factors combine to support the need for the individual professional to carry liability insurance that will provide an attorney and protection in the case of any judgment.

Analyzing Liability Insurance Coverage

Individual liability insurance for RNs is available from a variety of insurance companies (directly through their agents) and through professional organizations that offer coverage as a service to members. When investigating individual liability insurance, ask the agent or company the questions in Display 7.2. Of particular importance is the difference between a *claims occurred* and a *claims made* policy. A *claims occurred* policy is safer because if you subsequently drop the policy, it will still be in effect for any incident that occurred while you were covered. If a *claims made* policy was chosen, then the coverage for any claim ends when the policy premium is no longer being paid. Because the time limit on liability claims is substantial, you would have to continue to hold the policy and pay the premiums even if you were no longer employed in healthcare (Brooke, 2006b). Because the cost of nursing professional liability insurance is so low, any difference in cost between the two types of policies would be slight.

The questions in Display 7.2 can help you to compare policies from different insurance carriers. When coverage appears equal, you might ask how long a company has been in business and how long it has been providing nursing liability insurance. You want to be insured with a reliable, stable company.

DISPLAY 7.2   Questions to Ask Regarding Liability Insurance

1. In what situations would I, as an individual, be covered?
2. In what situations would I not be covered?
3. How is my coverage affected by my actions? For example, if I failed to follow hospital policy, would I still be covered?
4. What are the monetary limits of the policy?
5. Does the policy provide me with an attorney?
6. Does the insurance cover incidents that occurred while the policy was in force, regardless of when the claim is brought (claims-occurred insurance coverage), or does it cover incidents only if I am currently insured (claims-brought insurance coverage)?

Additional Questions Regarding an Individual Liability Policy
7. Is it renewable at my option? What factors affect renewability?
8. What is the cost compared with other policies?

Additional Questions Regarding an Institutional Liability Policy
9. Does the policy provide me with a personal attorney, or will the same attorney be working for the hospital?
10. At what point would the hospital no longer be responsible and would I become personally responsible?
11. How would my job be affected if a lawsuit was filed or payment awarded based on an action against me? (Check institutional policy as well as the insurance company policy.)
12. Does the insurance company have the right to seek restitution from me if it pays a claim based on my actions?

The nurse employee should investigate just as carefully liability insurance coverage carried by the hospital. Questions 1 through 8 in Display 7.2 apply to individual insurance policies. For an institutional policy, ask the questions 1 to 6 and 9 to 12.

 Critical Thinking Activity

You are accepting a position in a clinic. When might you ask about professional liability insurance coverage? Formulate specific questions. Identify the person who would be the best source of this information. How will you proceed if this person does not have the information you seek? If the interviewer tells you that the clinic is well covered by liability insurance, will you purchase personal malpractice insurance? Why or why not?

LEGAL ISSUES COMMON IN NURSING

Some legal issues recur frequently in nursing practice. It is wise for the nurse to understand these particular issues as they relate to individual practice.

Duty to Report or Seek Medical Care for a Patient

A nurse who cares for a patient has a legal duty to ensure that the patient receives safe and competent care. This duty requires that the nurse maintain an appropriate standard of care and take action to obtain an appropriate standard of care from other professionals when necessary. For example, if a nurse assesses a patient and determines that the attention of a physician is essential but fails to make every effort to obtain that attention, the nurse has breached a duty to the patient. *Failure to rescue* is shorthand for failure to prevent a clinically important deterioration, such as death or permanent disability, from a complication of an underlying illness or medical care (Agency for Health Research and Quality [AHRQ, 2009]) and is considered a nursing sensitive outcome. Reductions in *failure to rescue* rates are associated with low patient to nurse ratios. Monitoring patients to identify deterioration and intervening to assure care are critical RN functions.

▶ EXAMPLE

Failure to Seek Medical Care for a Patient

The RN is caring for a postoperative patient during the night. The patient's blood pressure begins to drop, and the pulse begins to rise. The nurse's assessment indicates that the patient may be bleeding internally. The nurse institutes a plan for close nursing monitoring and calls the surgeon to describe the situation. The surgeon gives a telephone order to increase the IV fluid rate and states that she will see the patient in the morning. The patient's condition continues to deteriorate, but the nurse does nothing further to ensure that a physician examines the patient.

If the outcome is unfavorable, the nurse can be found to have breached a duty to the patient. The patient relies on the nurse to provide appropriate care and to identify when a physician is needed. The nurse could have made more telephone calls to the surgeon and, failing the success of that, could have followed the facility's procedure for asking another physician (such as the emergency department physician) to see the patient.

The nurse has a duty to continue all efforts to obtain appropriate medical care for the patient. If the nurse had followed all procedures, sought another physician, and continued efforts when initial attempts were unsuccessful, the nurse would not have breached a duty. The nurse cannot guarantee a physician's care but can guarantee that the patient will not be left without an advocate.

Nursing Responsibility for Medical Orders

The nurse has a responsibility to critically examine medical orders that are written for a patient. Although the nurse is not responsible for the medical order itself, the nurse's education provides a background to identify obvious discrepancies or problems. In one reported case (Anonymous, 1997), two doctors left conflicting orders, which the charge nurse then transcribed. The court ruled that the nurse had a duty to understand the patient's plan of care and to communicate with the doctors who had written the conflicting orders. While this case happened some time ago, courts of today are likely to expect this level of critical thinking by the nurse.

Another area of important nursing responsibility is in relationship to telephone orders. The Joint Commission discourages these whenever possible, encouraging instead written orders that are faxed or communicated in writing in some other way (such as a secure online connection). However, there are situations when telephone orders are essential to timely care. In these instances, there should be clear guidelines as to how orders are documented and verified. The preferred method is for the nurse to speak directly to the prescriber, write down the order as received, and then read it back to the prescriber for verification. The prescriber must then review and sign the order as soon as practical. When it is entered into a computer system by the nurse, there is some method for the physician to verify the order at the next visit.

In some states, it is legal for the nurse to take a verbal order from the *agent* or spokesperson of the prescriber. This agent may be the nurse or medical assistant in the office. When receiving an order through an agent, the nurse should verify and document the identity and position of the agent, verify that the order did come from the prescriber (not at the discretion of the agent), and then follow the same procedure for verifying and documenting the order (Brooke, 2006a).

COMMUNICATION IN ACTION

Obtaining a Telephone Order

Evan Wilson was an RN on a medical unit. He called Dr. Marie Steven regarding the needs of a patient Esther Moran. The nurse in Dr. Steven's office answered the phone. Evan stated, "Hello, this is Evan Wilson, an RN on 4W at Mercy Hospital. I am caring for Dr. Steven's patient Esther Moran, who was admitted this morning for management of her heart failure. She is complaining of indigestion and has asked for an antacid, which Dr. Steven has directed her to use while at home. I would like to speak with Dr. Steven about this." The nurse replied, "Dr. Steven is with a patient now, but I am familiar with Mrs. Moran and I am sure that Dr. Steven would order the antacid. Go ahead and give it to her. I will talk with Dr. Steven and get her O.K. as soon as she is available." Evan replied, "I appreciate your interest in facilitating care for Mrs. Moran, but I can only accept an order that the physician has initiated after assessing the situation. It will be fine if you call me back after talking with Dr. Steven. If needed, Dr. Steven can call me on my cell phone for additional information. Thanks for your help."

Confidentiality and Right to Privacy

Confidentiality and the right to privacy with respect to one's personal life are basic concerns in our society. All information regarding a patient belongs to that patient. This right has been inferred from interpretation of the federal constitution but is explicitly stated in some state laws. HIPAA demands major efforts of all healthcare providers in regard to protecting patient privacy. In theory, the rights identified in HIPAA should protect a patient's privacy. Healthcare agencies are required to provide patients with a document on the agency's privacy policies. These policies are often multipage documents that may include a variety of ways in which an individual's health information is used and many patients do not read them carefully. Policies usually indicate that information will be used for business operations. Because third-party payers (such as insurance companies and health maintenance organizations) will not reimburse for care if they do not receive records documenting diagnoses and care provided, patients often must sign statements giving approval for all needed information to be sent to their insurance company. They may be unaware of exactly what information is sent or who may see it.

When computerized records are transmitted to insurance companies, they no longer contain only a brief statement of diagnosis and treatment; they may also contain detailed accounts of interactions between a patient and a mental health professional, health information of a sensitive nature, and genetic information that could be used inappropriately. Because increased use of computerized records can result in easier retrieval and cross-referencing of records from many sources, the general public, healthcare providers, and government officials are becoming more concerned about potential invasions of privacy. Safeguards must be built into all computerized medical record systems that prevent unauthorized access and the tracking of those who do access the system.

A nurse who gives out information without authorization from the patient or from the legally responsible guardian can be held liable for any harm that results. If you have question about who the legally responsible guardian of a patient is, be sure to consult with your administrative authority. If there is not a court-appointed legal guardian, then specific state laws identify who becomes the responsible guardian when the person is unable to give personal consent. The hospital administration should be able to ascertain the correct guardian.

Only those professional persons involved in the patient's care who have a need to know about the patient are allowed routine access to the record. A physician, nurse, or any other employee who is not involved in the patient's care or who does not have an administrative responsibility relative to that care is not allowed routine access. Persons not involved in care may be allowed access to the record only by specific written authorization of the patient or by court order. Be cautious about what information you share verbally and with whom.

Medical records professionals state that it is not uncommon for attorneys, family members, media representatives, or law enforcement officials to request access to patient records or specific patient information without having express consent from the patient or a legal court order to view the records or be given information. Those unfamiliar with laws regarding privacy sometimes reveal information inappropriately. If you are ever approached for patient information by someone who purports to have authority, your best course of action is to refer that individual to appropriate administrative personnel, who can determine the validity of the request.

▶ EXAMPLE

Breach of Confidentiality

A nurse in a small community hospital checks the computer to see if her neighbor was admitted after seeing the aid car at his house the night before. She learns he was admitted after a fall and determines that she will visit after work and offer help when he returns home. Even though her intent was to help, viewing this record was a breach of confidentiality. When records of access are reviewed, her accessing a record of a patient to whom she was not assigned would be flagged. She could be disciplined or even discharged for this breach.

Another concern is that many healthcare agencies are using fax machines to send patient information to one another and even between departments within an institution. Faxes have a legitimate purpose in that continuity of care is enhanced when information is shared. When you send a document via fax machine, it is difficult to ensure that confidentiality is maintained. Facilities must keep fax machines in areas not accessible to the public. Some facilities have a policy requiring that you call ahead and designate a specific person to be present to receive the fax. The cover page often states that this is confidential material and should not be read by anyone other than the designated recipient. If your facility or agency has no policy regarding the safeguarding of faxed information, you would be wise to raise the concern.

Other areas of concern are the Internet and e-mail. Through these avenues, a healthcare provider may consult with other professionals to provide the best diagnostic and treatment services to the patient. However, some online computer communications are not private. Those with the necessary skill may intercept and read any e-mail or Internet message. Therefore, the identity of patients must be protected in any such communication. Some online documents are shared through encryption and password protection within a protected computer system that may be accessed from remote locations.

In a world where social networking such as Facebook and Myspace and electronic communication such as Twitter and text messages have become common, healthcare providers may inadvertently breach privacy by comments made in an electronic posting or message. The safest approach is that no references of any kind regarding any patient should be made on an online site or in a message. Additionally, care should be taken to not disclose information regarding the healthcare facility itself. Once sent, messages and postings cannot be withdrawn and may be widely distributed without your consent or knowledge. When you are seeking employment, having made comments about patients even in general terms or about potential employers may be considered as showing poor professional judgment.

Defamation of Character

Any time that shared information is detrimental to a person's reputation, the person sharing the information may be liable for defamation of character. Written defamation is called libel. Oral defamation is called slander. Defamation of character involves communication that is malicious and false. Sometimes such comments are made in the heat of anger. Occasionally, statements written in a patient's chart are libelous. Severely critical opinions may be stated as fact. An example of such a statement might be, "The patient is lying," or "The patient is rude and domineering." Patients may charge that comments in the chart adversely affected their care by prejudicing other staff against them. The astute nurse will chart only objective information regarding patients and give opinion in professional terms, well documented with fact.

COMMUNICATION IN ACTION

Accurate and Responsible Documentation

William Whittier was caring for a patient who was brought in by an ambulance after being found unconscious on the sidewalk. There was considerable side discussion among the staff about whether the patient was intoxicated. In his documentation, William notes, "Skin red, flushed, and warm. Strong breath odor that resembles alcohol. Patient responds only to shaking and loud verbal stimulation." Later, when the patient has become more responsive and awake, he documents, "Patient states, 'Boy, am I hung-over! What happened?'" This provided factual information for the reader without making potentially libelous accusations.

Libel and slander may also be charged when written comments or verbal statements are made regarding another healthcare provider. Thoughtless or angry comments that impugn the abilities of a physician or that might cause a patient to lose trust in a physician can be slander. In conversations, the prudent nurse carefully considers any comments about other healthcare providers before making them. There are accepted mechanisms for confidentially reporting inappropriate care or errors; be sure to use them and do not make critical statements to uninvolved third parties. In many states, licensed professionals are required to report poor practice or illegal acts on the part of other professionals. Criticism reported without malice and in good faith, through the appropriate channels, is usually protected from legal action for defamation. If you have such a concern, you should investigate the appropriate channels to be used in your setting.

Privileged Communication

Privileged communication refers to information that is shared by an individual client with certain professionals but that does not need to be revealed, even in a court of law. This professional is said to possess "privilege"—that is, has the privilege of not revealing information. All states consider certain types of communication (between client and attorney, between patient and doctor, or between an individual and a member of the clergy) privileged. Not all states recognize the nurse–patient relationship as one in which privileged communication takes place; even those states that recognize nurse–patient communication as potentially privileged do not consider *all* communication between patients and nurses to be privileged. Privilege is a limited concept reserved for information given in confidence to the nurse within the nurse–patient professional relationship. Only a court can determine whether privilege exists in any specific case. If a court does not determine information is privileged, then you are legally obligated to testify about the communication.

Informed Consent

Every person has the right to either consent (agree) to or to refuse healthcare treatment. The law requires that a person give voluntary and **informed consent**. Voluntary means that no coercion exists. Informed means that a person clearly understands the choices being offered.

Consent for Medical Treatment

Consent for medical treatment is the responsibility of the medical provider (eg, physician, dentist, nurse practitioner). Informed consent contains information on

- The nature of the decision/procedure
- Reasonable alternatives to the proposed intervention
- The relevant risks, benefits, and uncertainties related to each alternative
- Assessment of patient understanding (University of Washington School of Medicine, 2009)

Consent (the acceptance of the intervention by the patient) may be either verbal or written and indicates a patient has decided to go ahead with the procedure based on a clear understanding of the options. Written consent usually is preferred in healthcare to ensure that a record of consent exists, although a signature alone does not prove that the consent was informed. A blanket consent for "any procedures deemed necessary" usually is not considered adequate consent for specific procedures. The form should state the specific proposed medical procedure or test.

Courts do not accept the patient's medical condition alone as a valid reason for withholding complete and accurate information when seeking consent. Currently, there are no clear guidelines as to what constitutes complete information. What constitutes adequate information about various alternative approaches to treatment often is unclear. Courts have generally supported the idea that commonly accepted alternatives and usual risks need to be disclosed, but that marginal or unusual treatments and rare or unexpected risks do not have to be discussed.

The law places the responsibility for obtaining consent for medical treatment on the provider who will perform the procedure. It is the responsibility of the provider to provide appropriate, accurate, complete, and correct information, and the provider is liable if the patient charges that appropriate information was not given. A nurse may present a form for a patient to sign, and the nurse may sign the form as a witness to the signature. This does not transfer the legal responsibility for informed consent for medical care to the nurse. If the patient does not seem well informed, the nurse should notify the provider so that further information can be given to the patient. Although the nurse would not be liable legally for the lack of informed consent, the nurse has ethical obligations to assist the patient in exercising his or her rights and to assist the provider in providing appropriate care.

Consent for Nursing Measures

Nurses must obtain a patient's consent for nursing measures undertaken. This does not mean that exhaustive explanations need to be given in each situation, because courts have held that patients can be expected to have some understanding of usual care. Consent for nursing measures may be verbal or implied. The nurse may ask, "Are you ready to ambulate now?" The patient answers, "Certainly," providing verbal consent. Alternatively, the nurse may state, "I have the injection the doctor ordered for you. Will you please turn over?" If the patient turns over, this is implied consent.

Similarly, consent for care should be requested in emergency situations, such as those mentioned earlier in the discussion of Good Samaritan policies, if the injured is able to give that consent. A simple statement such as, "I am a registered nurse. Do you want my help?" is sufficient.

The nurse should remember that the patient is free to refuse any aspect of care offered. Like the physician, the nurse is responsible for making sure that the patient is informed before making a decision. Good nursing care requires that you use all means at your disposal to help the patient comprehend the value of proposed care. For example, the postoperative patient needs to understand that getting into a chair is part of the plan of care, not a convenience for the nurse or simply a change to prevent boredom. Thus, a patient's refusal of care is accepted only after the patient has been given complete information. The nurse would then carefully document this situation.

Competence to Give Consent

A person's ability to make judgments based on rational understanding is termed **competence**. Dementia, developmental disabilities, head injuries, strokes, medications, and illnesses creating loss of consciousness are common causes of an inability to make judgments. Determining competence is a complex issue. The patient's illness, age, or condition alone does not determine competence. Legal competence is ultimately determined by the court. The general tendency of the courts has been to encourage whatever decision-making ability an individual has and to restrict personal decision making as little as possible.

When a person is determined legally to be incompetent, a legal guardian is appointed and consent is obtained from the legal guardian. A legal guardian is constrained from making some types of decisions. For example, if the healthcare action could be identified as injurious to the individual involved, a court may need to be consulted regarding consent for that specific action. An example would be the decision about discontinuation of dialysis for an incompetent individual. If a person left a living will or a detailed document naming a durable power of attorney for healthcare that included wishes regarding end-of-life issues, the guardian might be allowed to decide to end dialysis. When such an individual leaves no clear indication regarding personal wishes or never had the capacity to make such decisions, the healthcare providers might insist on getting a court decision before accepting the consent of the guardian to terminate the dialysis.

Healthcare providers often encounter clients for whom no legal determination of competence has been made but who do not seem able to make an informed decision; examples include the very confused elderly person, the inebriated person, and the unconscious person. There are usually institutional guidelines to follow in determining that a person cannot give his or her own consent. The guidelines may require examination by a physician and documentation of the patient's condition. More than one physician may be required to examine the patient.

This patient may not have a legally designated guardian or substitute decision maker. The law in each state specifies who is allowed to give consent in such situations. Frequently, this is the spouse, parent, children, or siblings. Your facility policy should contain directions to guide you in obtaining legal consent; if it does not, consult a supervisor for a decision. In situations where there are several persons in the category, such as children of an elderly person, agreement regarding decisions is needed before proceeding. Determining who is able to give legal consent in such a situation is not a nurse's responsibility.

Competence may change from day to day, as a person's physical illness changes. The person who has had major surgery and is receiving large doses of narcotics for pain may not be able to reason clearly. Forty-eight hours later, this same individual may be perfectly alert and capable of considering complex issues. An individual may be competent to make some decisions, such as "I don't like rice and I won't eat it!" but incompetent to make others, for example, decisions regarding financial matters. These differences in competence require care providers to adjust their own planning to incorporate patient self-determination whenever possible, even when the person is legally incompetent. If a person truly is not capable of making decisions, the nurse should attempt to present necessary nursing actions in a way that elicits cooperation and avoids confrontation over decisions. For example, rather than asking the cognitively impaired person if she wants to take her medications, the prudent nurse simply states, "Here are your medications. It is time to take them."

Withdrawing Consent

Consent may be withdrawn after it is given. People have the right to change their minds. Therefore, if after one IV infusion a patient decides not to have a second one started, that is the patient's right. As a nurse, you have an obligation to notify the physician if the patient refuses a medical procedure or treatment.

When individuals are participating in any type of research protocol for care, they are free to withdraw from the research study at any time. When caring for individuals who are part of a research process, you have obligations to protect the patient's right to make decisions, even if they are contrary to the interests of the researcher. You would have an obligation to inform the researcher of the patient's decision.

Consent and Minors

The parent or legal guardian usually provides consent for care of a minor. You also should obtain the minor's consent when he or she is able to give it. Increasingly, courts are emphasizing that minors be allowed a voice when it concerns matters that they are capable of understanding. This is especially true for the adolescent, but this consideration should be given to any child who is 7 years of age or older. Often courts do not seek consent from minors, but rather an indication that they understand the purpose of the care. For adolescents, the court may ask that negotiation with minors occur. When minors refuse care and legal guardians have authorized that care, do not proceed until legal clarification is given. Consult your nursing supervisor. This may be an issue for an ethics committee as well as for legal representation.

Minors who live apart from their parents and are financially independent, or who are married, are termed **emancipated minors**. In most (but not all) states, emancipated minors can give consent to their own treatment. Some states have specific laws relating to the **mature minor**, allowing sexually active minors to give personal consent (without also obtaining parental consent) for treatment of sexually transmitted disease or for obtaining birth control information and supplies (see Chapter 9). Be sure of the law in your state if you practice in an area where this is a concern. Most institutions have developed policies to guide employees in making correct decisions in this and other areas dealing with consent.

Advance Directives

Advance directives are legal documents stating the wishes of individuals regarding healthcare in situations in which they are no longer capable of giving personal informed consent. These documents are completed in advance of the situation in which they might be needed, and they direct the actions of others. There are several types of advance directives, such as a living will and a durable power of attorney for healthcare.

The Living Will

A **living will** or **directive to physicians** provides information on preferences regarding end-of-life issues such as types of care to provide and whether to use various resuscitation measures. The basis of a living will is an if–then plan. Most commonly, they declare that if "I am terminally ill and not expected to recover," then "I want this care given and do not want that care given." The if condition may also include the fact that the person is in a persistent vegetative state and not expected to recover function and capacity. The condition stated as the if must be diagnosed by a physician. Many states require that two physicians must agree that the person is terminally ill or in a persistent vegetative state. Even when this is not the law, healthcare agencies often require this as a policy. The determination of the patient's condition must be documented in the legal record by the physician. Although living wills or directives were originally advisory for families and physicians as they made decisions, some states have now passed laws requiring that these documents be honored. If the physician does not agree with the decision of the patient, then the physician in that state is obligated to withdraw from care and refer the case to another physician.

DISPLAY 7.3   Five Wishes for End-of-Life Care

• Which person do you want to make healthcare decisions for you when you can't make them?
• What kind of medical treatment do you want or don't want?
• How comfortable you want to be?
• How you want people to treat you?
• What you want your loved ones to know?

Aging With Dignity: *www.agingwithdignity.org/5wishes.html*

If the living will requests that no resuscitation or limited resuscitation efforts be undertaken, the physician must write orders limiting resuscitation in the record. However, remember that living wills may also request that all possible resuscitation efforts be made.

Living wills or directives to the physician may address other aspects of care in addition to resuscitation efforts. For example, they may indicate whether the individual wants to be tube fed if he or she is in a persistent vegetative state, whether surgery should be used in certain instances, or whether IV fluids or ventilator support should be used. Some advance directives are several pages long, as the person addresses many different possible concerns. For more discussion and an example of a living will, see Chapter 9.

Aging With Dignity, an organization in Florida, has developed and disseminated, in conjunction with the Robert Woods Johnson Foundation, an advance directive document called the "Five Wishes." This document addresses not only life-sustaining therapies that are desired or not desired but also other aspects of end-of-life care, such as the desire for people, for touch, for music, and so forth. The five wishes that form the structure of the document are listed in Display 7.3. The Five Wishes document is an accepted legal advance directive in the majority of states. The Five Wishes Web site lists states that accept this as a legal document. In other states, the Five Wishes document may be used as an addendum to the legally accepted advance directive document to inform healthcare providers of personal wishes for end-of-life care.

Durable Power of Attorney for Healthcare

A **durable power of attorney for healthcare (DPOA-Healthcare)** is a document that legally designates a **substitutionary decision maker**, should the person be incapacitated. This document may also be referred to as designating a **healthcare proxy**. This document provides individuals with the opportunity to identify a preferred legal decision maker if they are incapacitated. A standard power of attorney that addresses financial interests is in effect only as long as the person remains competent; however, the DPOA for healthcare is activated only when the person becomes incapacitated. It may be combined with a living will that contains specific advance directives, such as those discussed above, thus providing directions for that substitutionary decision maker regarding preferences.

If an individual has designated a substitutionary decision maker for healthcare, this supersedes all general legal designations for decision makers. In a society where there are many different family constellations and relationships, durable powers of attorney for healthcare are an important personal decision. For example, individuals who live in life partnerships other than marriage must have a durable power of attorney for healthcare to provide that life partner with decision-making ability for emergencies or critical situations. For the adult with no living parents or spouse and multiple siblings, the designation of one person as a decision maker may diminish family conflict and facilitate the provision of the care the individual wishes. An individual may wish to designate a trusted friend as a substitutionary decision maker rather than simply accepting the law that would designate a family member to assume the role.

Physician Orders for Life-Sustaining Treatments

Limitations on resuscitation in the event of a cardiac or respiratory arrest may take many forms. These orders are generally referred to as Physician Orders for Life-Sustaining Treatments (POLST). The most comprehensive is the order that reads "Do not resuscitate" (DNR) or "No Code," meaning that no resuscitation efforts of any kind are to be made and the patient be allowed to die naturally. There would be no cardiopulmonary resuscitation (CPR), no resuscitative drugs, and no mechanical ventilation. This is often the choice of the person who has a life-threatening disease such as terminal cancer and for whom resuscitation would only serve to prolong illness and discomfort. In some instances, the person may request a limited resuscitation effort, such as CPR and medications but no mechanical ventilation. Facilities may have a variety of ways to designate these limitations on resuscitative efforts and to communicate these directions to those providing care. An important understanding for nurses is that in the absence of a written order from a physician, other care providers are obligated to initiate resuscitation if an arrest occurs.

In an attempt to "effectively communicate the wishes of seriously ill patients to have or to limit medical treatment as they move from one care setting to another," the POLST organization at the Oregon Health Sciences University developed a set of standardized orders regarding CPR, medical interventions, antibiotics, artificially administered nutrition, and a summary (POLST, 2009). See the POLST Web site for examples of this form and for specific information in relationship to the use of similar forms in individual states.

An advance directive (or living will) provides information that the physician can use as a basis for deciding when an order limiting life-sustaining treatment is appropriate. In many states, there are laws that designate under what circumstances a physician may write an order limiting treatment in the absence of an advance directive. If the patient has not completed an advance directive and is not expected to recover, the physician may determine that resuscitation would be futile. Futile means that it would not add appreciably to life or have the potential for success. Laws or policies usually require the agreement of two physicians that resuscitation would be futile. After this medical determination, then the person who legally is the substitutionary decision maker is consulted, provided information regarding the patient's condition, and asked to consent to the physician's DNR order. This entire process must be documented in the patient's record.

All care providers must understand that a DNR order does not limit other types of care that will be provided. Treatment of wounds to promote healing, pain management, resolution of other physical problems (such as nausea or constipation), antibiotic administration to control treatable infections, and oxygen to ease breathing are all examples of care that will still be appropriate. Even radiation therapy might be determined appropriate to reduce tumor growth and increase comfort. This type of care is referred to as palliative treatment: therapy designed to relieve or reduce the intensity of painful symptoms but which is not designed to cure a condition.

In some instances, an order may be written that specifies "comfort care only." This order again occurs after consultation with the patient as able and family as appropriate. When this order is written, treatment of infections and other problems may not be initiated unless they would increase comfort. The focus becomes maximum comfort in the face of impending death. The patient for whom comfort care only is ordered should receive the same concerted focus on end-of-life care that would occur in a hospice setting.

Nurses sometimes find themselves in situations in which they believe that the patient's condition is futile and that a DNR or comfort-care-only order would be appropriate, but the physician has not made this determination or, having made this determination, has not consulted with the family and written a DNR order. In other instances, family insists on continuing all care options including resuscitation and ventilator support. Such situations can be difficult for nurses because they have no decision-making authority, and yet they are the ones who legally must carry out the resuscitation. Much depends on the nurse–physician working relationships, care provider–family relationships, and the ability to discuss difficult issues together. Some care facilities encourage care conferences where these matters can be raised for discussion. Nurses can be effective advocates for increased communication and discussion of these difficult issues.

Patient Self-Determination Act

In 1990, the US Congress passed the **Patient Self-Determination Act (PSDA)**. This Act took effect in 1992 and required that on admission to any healthcare service (hospital, long-term care center, or home care agency), patients be given an opportunity to determine what lifesaving or life-prolonging actions they want carried out. Much of the impetus for this legislation was the belief that many individuals were having their lives prolonged in situations in which they would have preferred this not be done. The Act requires the agency to provide adequate information for the individual to make an informed decision regarding these important matters. As a result of this legislation, agencies reviewed and revised policies and protocols regarding consent. In many agencies, a nurse has the responsibility to provide the education and obtain a signature on a document indicating preferences. Some difficulties arise in this process when the person giving the information does not clearly understand that the decision about resuscitation is not based on the current situation but upon the if condition of a patient becoming terminally ill and not being expected to survive, then what does the patient want to happen. Patients may become concerned that they will be abandoned if an untoward event happens.

Information regarding the results of the PSDA is being analyzed by several government agencies to determine whether there has been a change in practice. Some have suggested that the manner in which self-determination and the possible alternatives are explained greatly influences patient choices; one suggestion has been that these matters first be discussed in the healthcare provider's office, before admission. When this is possible, it allows for more time to consider alternatives and consult with significant others. The final decision is then made away from the pressure of the healthcare environment. See Chapter 10 for a further discussion of planning for end-of-life issues.

Emergency Care

Care in emergencies has many legal repercussions; therefore, the judgment that an emergency exists is important. Certain actions may be legal in emergencies and not legal in nonemergency situations. In emergencies, the standard procedures for obtaining consent may be impossible to follow. Further, in emergencies, personnel must sometimes take on responsibilities that they would not undertake in a nonemergency situation. Critical thinking on the part of all healthcare professionals is essential when differentiating an emergency from a nonemergency.

Most facilities that provide emergency care have policies and procedures designed to ensure adequate support for claiming that an emergency exists. Thus, the policy will often state that at least two physicians in the emergency department must examine the patient and concur that the emergency requires immediate action, without waiting for consent. This ensures maximum legal protection for the physician and the institution.

Consent in Emergencies

If a true emergency exists, consent for care is considered to be implied. The law holds that if a reasonable person were aware that the situation was life threatening, he or she would give consent for care. An exception to this is made if the person has explicitly rejected such care in advance; an example is a Jehovah's Witness carrying a card stating his personal religion and that he does not wish to receive blood or blood products. This is one reason why emergency department nurses should check a patient's wallet for identification and information related to care. Checking a patient's wallet should be done with another person, and a careful inventory of contents documented and signed by both. There should be little concern about liability in taking emergency action if this is completed.

Standards of Practice and Emergencies

Standards of practice in emergencies differ from those in nonemergency situations. In hospital emergencies, the nurse sometimes may be in the position of identifying an emergency and whether a needed action is one that only a physician usually performs. The hospital is expected to have a policy and protocol, which the nurse would follow, to verify and document the situation fully. This usually involves consultation with a supervisory nurse and verification of the emergency situation, as well as attempts to obtain medical assistance. Again, critical thinking by the nurse is essential to determine whether a true emergency exists. Review the information on scope of practice in Chapter 3 to help you with decision making in regard to emergency actions.

When life or limb is truly in danger, the courts have held that a nurse can do those things immediately necessary, even if they usually are considered medical functions, provided the nurse has the essential expertise to perform the actions safely and correctly. The matter of having essential expertise is crucial; this is why all members of an emergency response team must learn all aspects of the code procedure. If, for any reason, the physician were unable to respond to the code, a nurse who was prepared with this essential expertise would assume the role of the leader of the code team.

▶ *EXAMPLE*

Nursing Action in a Hospital Emergency

In an orthopedic unit, it is common to care for patients with new casts. A young man with a newly applied long-leg cast is admitted through the emergency department at 6 PM. The nurse assigned to this patient's care carefully makes all the appropriate observations throughout the evening and documents his findings. The nurse notes that the leg is beginning to swell and that the edges of the cast are beginning to cut into the skin. The nurse institutes nursing actions of increasing the elevation of the leg and

(display continues on page 274)

applying ice packs to limit swelling. At that time, the nurse notifies the supervisor that a problem is developing and that he thinks the physician should be notified. The supervisor agrees and the nurse begins trying to contact the physician. The nurse continues to make observations, noting increasing swelling, color changes in the exposed toes, and loss of sensation. The physician cannot be reached, and no other physician is immediately available.

The nurse follows the hospital procedure for seeking medical attention and for determining when an emergency exists. In consultation with the supervisor, it is decided that an emergency exists and that the cast needs to be cut open to relieve the pressure. Deciding to cut a cast open and cutting the cast are considered medical responsibilities in this hospital.

The nurse has been taught how and when to use a cast cutter in emergency situations. Thus, the nurse possesses the essential expertise. The nurse, with the supervisor's approval, cuts open the cast and secures the cast halves in place with an elastic bandage. From there, all observations are made, consultations carried out, physician notification attempted, and the final actions taken are documented carefully in the patient's record. Hospital policy was followed throughout the situation to ensure that all necessary steps had been taken.

Although the action in this example went beyond usual nursing practice, it would not be considered a violation of either the nursing or the medical practice acts, because an emergency existed and the results of inaction would have been serious. Additionally, the nurse had the expertise and was prepared to carry out the necessary action safely. This emergency care usually is limited to specific technical procedures that the nurse has learned.

Protocols and Emergencies

Most healthcare agencies have established protocols for nursing action in a variety of emergency or even urgent situations. These provide directions for nursing action that would usually be a physician's order. For example, if the patient's blood pressure drops precipitously, the protocol might indicate that the nurse would start an IV infusion with a specified fluid to maintain circulating volume and to provide IV access for emergency drugs. The administration of oxygen to a person suffering acute respiratory distress is another situation frequently covered by a protocol. When emergencies occur, nurses are protected from a charge of practicing outside the scope of the RN by following the protocol that was approved by the medical staff.

Noninstitutional Emergency Care

In many states, official emergency personnel must render all possible aid, including all resuscitative measures, when they are called to an emergency situation. This has sometimes resulted in the resuscitation of a terminally ill person who had previously stated that resuscitation was not desired. As more individuals receive terminal care in their homes, this has become an increasing concern.

Legislation allowing for patient self-determination regarding emergency responders has now been passed in most states. The law usually stipulates the precise circumstances under which an individual may provide an advance directive regarding emergency procedures, and how that directive must be documented so that emergency personnel can honor it. For example, the individual may be required to wear a specific armband and the DNR order may be posted on the door of the refrigerator or other prominent position in the home. All emergency responders must be aware of their responsibilities regarding advance directives.

Fraud

Fraud is deliberate deception for the purpose of personal gain and is usually prosecuted as a crime. However, it may also serve as the basis of a civil suit. Situations of fraud in nursing are not common. One example would be trying to obtain a better position by giving incorrect information to a prospective employer. By deliberately stating (falsely) that they have completed a nurse practitioner program to obtain a position for which they would otherwise be ineligible, individuals are defrauding the employer. This may be prosecuted as a crime, because they are placing members of the community in danger of receiving substandard care. Individuals also may commit fraud by trying to cover up a nursing error to avoid legal action. Courts tend to be harsher in decisions regarding fraud than in cases involving simple malpractice, because fraud represents a deliberate attempt to mislead others for one's own gain and could result in harm to those assigned to that individual's care.

Assault and Battery

Assault is saying or doing something to make a person genuinely afraid that he or she will be touched without consent. Battery involves touching a person when that individual has not consented to the action. Neither of these terms implies that harm was done; harm may or may not occur. For an assault to occur, the person must be afraid of what might happen because the individual appears to have the power to carry out the threat. "If you don't take this medication, I will have to put you in restraints" is an example of an assault. For battery to occur, the touching must occur without consent. Remember that consent may be implied rather than specifically stated. Therefore, if the patient extends an arm for an injection, he cannot later charge battery, saying that he was not asked. But if the patient agreed because of a threat (assault), the touching still would be considered battery because the consent was not freely given.

Assault and battery are crimes under the law. However, most of these cases in healthcare are instituted as civil suits by the injured party, rather than as criminal cases by government authorities.

Assault and battery are most commonly treated as criminal cases when they involve suspected abuse of a patient. Most of us in healthcare are shocked and dismayed to learn of instances in which care providers were abusive. Individuals who have difficulty with impulse control and anger may become frustrated with a patient and threaten, push, shove, or otherwise harm the individual. Another situation is when a confused patient hits or pinches a nurse. While a nurse has a right to a safe work environment, that is not justification for hitting a confused patient in response (Brooke, 2006c). Most jurisdictions have laws requiring that anyone who knows of abuse to an individual, whether a child, a developmentally delayed adult, or an elderly person, report that abuse to the proper authorities. Within an institution, there should be policies and procedures for this type of reporting. Appropriate authorities must conduct a careful investigation to ensure protection of the rights of the person accused and the person harmed.

False Imprisonment

Making a person stay in a place against his wishes is **false imprisonment**. The person may be forced to stay either by physical or by verbal means. It is easy to understand why restraining a patient or confining a patient to a locked room could constitute false imprisonment if proper procedures were not first carried out. Again, false imprisonment is a crime, but when it occurs in healthcare, it is most often the basis of a civil suit rather than a criminal case.

The law is less clear about keeping a patient confined by nonphysical means. Removing patients' clothing for the express purpose of preventing them from leaving could make a nurse liable for false imprisonment. Threatening to keep people confined with statements such as, "If you don't stay in your bed, I'll sedate you" can also constitute false imprisonment. If people need to be confined for their own safety or well-being, it is best to help them understand and agree to that course of action.

Any time patients pose a danger to themselves or others, the law requires that the least restrictive means available be used to protect patients and others. Healthcare providers are obligated to document the behavior of concern, problem-solve alternative actions, and then try those alternative actions before resorting to any type of restraint. Documentation of this entire process is essential. Nurses who determine the need for restraints must obtain a physician's order as soon as possible. Be sure to follow the policies of the facility.

In a conventional care setting, you cannot restrain or confine responsible adults against their wishes. All persons have the right to make decisions for themselves, regardless of the consequences. The patient with a severe heart condition who defies orders and walks to the bathroom has that right. You protect yourself by recording your efforts to teach the patient the need for restrictions and by reporting the patient's behavior to your supervisor and the physician.

In the same context, the patient cannot be forced to remain in a hospital. The patient has the right to leave a healthcare institution regardless of medical advice to the contrary. While this might not be in the best interests of the person's health, the patient has the right to decide to leave against medical advice. Again, document your efforts in the record and follow applicable policies to protect the facility, the physician, and yourself from liability.

False imprisonment suits are a special concern in the care of the psychiatric patient. Particular laws relate to this situation. In the psychiatric setting, you may have patients who have voluntarily sought admission. The same restrictions on restraint or confinement that apply to patients in the general care setting apply to these patients. Other patients in the psychiatric setting may have been committed involuntarily according to the laws of the state. Specific measures may be used to confine the involuntarily committed patient. Laws in terms of situation, type of restraint allowed, and the length of time restraining may be used often define these measures. If you work in a psychiatric setting, review specific policies regarding restraint to protect patients and to assist staff in functioning within the legal limits.

FACTORS THAT CONTRIBUTE TO MALPRACTICE CLAIMS

A suit usually does not always follow the poor results or harm that may on occasion occur in the course of nursing practice. An understanding of the factors that enter into whether a suit is instituted may be helpful to you.

Consequences of the Error

When an error results in serious consequences, such as prolonged hospitalization, disability, or even death, individuals are likely to institute legal action. The aim may be to cover costs such as needed care, lost wages, and other costs associated with the error. There also may be a wish to have the individual or organization pay for the pain and suffering experienced. For example, the person who was severely burned by a cautery used incorrectly in surgery would experience lost productivity and wages due to time off for care and healing. Additionally, the person would experience severe pain and suffering and might have permanent scarring. That person might seek compensation for these nonmonetary losses. In other situations, when no one seems to take responsibility for the error or people do not seem to care or feel regret for what happened, there may be a wish to punish those involved. Punitive damages may be awarded when the court determines that the injury reflects not just a single incident but a pattern of unsafe care.

Social Factors

Much is being written about changes in the public's attitudes toward healthcare personnel. Healthcare is big business, and patients complain increasingly of not being accepted and respected as individuals. In general, patients are more willing to bring suit against someone who is part of a large, impersonal system.

Health costs are high, and some people think hospitals and physicians have the ability to pay large settlements, whether directly or through insurance. If a patient's own income is lessened or disrupted by an illness, he or she might bring suit as a solution to economic difficulties. Increased public awareness of the size of monetary judgments that have been awarded also may be an economic incentive to initiating a suit.

Suit-Prone Patients

Some people are more likely to bring suit, for real or imagined errors. If these people are recognized as being suit-prone patients, it is possible for you to protect yourself through increased vigilance regarding care and thorough record keeping. Although it is important to guard against stereotyping, the following general descriptions may help you to avoid problems. Suit-prone patients usually are identified by overt behavior in which they are persistent faultfinders and critics of personnel and of all aspects of care. They may be uncooperative in following a plan of care and sensitive to any perceived slight.

Persons who exhibit hostile attitudes may extend their hostile feelings to the nurses and other healthcare persons with whom they have contact. The nurse who becomes defensive when faced with hostility only widens the breach in the nurse–patient relationship. It is necessary to pay careful attention to those principles of care learned in psychosocial nursing that deal with how to help the hostile patient. Assisting patients in solving their own problems and offering support are the best forms of protection for the nurse.

Another type of patient who appears more suit prone is the very dependent person who uses projection to deal with anxiety and fear. These individuals tend to ascribe fault or blame for all events to others and are unable to accept personal responsibility for their own welfare. Again, meeting these patients' needs with a carefully considered plan of care is the answer.

A common error is to withdraw and become defensive when confronting a suit-prone patient; this reaction occurs partly because a situation is unpleasant and partly because a staff member feels personally threatened by the patient's behavior. This reaction increases the likelihood of a suit if a poor outcome occurs.

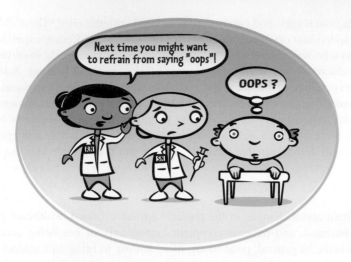

FIGURE 7.3 Certain things can be done to prevent malpractice suits.

Another incorrect nursing response to the suit-prone patient is to become more directive and authoritarian. This tends to increase the patient's feeling of separation and distance from the staff and again increases the likelihood of a suit.

When staff members are helped to view the patient as a troubled person who manifests his or her problems in this manner, sometimes they find it easier to be objective. The patient is in need of all the skill that the thoughtful nurse can bring to the emotional problems. The entire health team needs to develop a careful and consistent approach, which provides security and stability to the patient and family. The suit-prone patient does not always end up suing; much depends on the response of healthcare personnel.

Suit-Prone Nurses

Nurses may also be suit prone. Nurses who are insensitive to the patient's complaints, who do not identify and meet the patient's emotional needs, or who fail to recognize and accept the limits of their own practice may contribute to suits instituted not only against the nurse but also against the employer and the physician. The nurse's self-awareness is critical in preventing suits (Fig. 7.3).

Staff members may contribute to a patient's distrust of care through complaining about working conditions, telling patients about problems occurring on the unit, and disparaging other healthcare providers. There is a distinction between informing a patient that you must meet someone else's needs, and therefore will not return for a specified period of time, and giving the patient the impression that you do not have time to attend to his or her needs.

PREVENTING MALPRACTICE CLAIMS

A variety of things can be done to prevent malpractice claims from ever happening. Many of these actions are ones that you can take as an individual, while others require the involvement of the entire healthcare team.

Maintaining Excellent Standards of Care

The most significant thing you can do to prevent malpractice claims is to maintain a high standard of care. To do this, work at improving your own nursing practice and also the general climate for nursing practice where you work. You can do this in many ways. An important aspect of high-standard care is excellence in communication with patients and families. Therapeutic communication skills including listening, clarifying, and problem solving are especially critical.

COMMUNICATION IN ACTION

Talking with an Upset Family

Mr. Jenkins had been at the desk every hour demanding something for his very ill wife. Sometimes it was pain medication and at other times it was something such as a glass of water. He has said, "You people need to take better care of Mildred! If I weren't here, who knows what would happen to her?" Jennifer Tompkins approached Mr. Jenkins in his wife's room. "You seem really concerned about your wife's care," she said. "I would like to talk with both of you about it and see if together we can make some plans that help you both in this very difficult situation you are facing here."

Self-Awareness

Identify your own strengths and weaknesses in practice. When you identify a weakness, seek a means of growth. This may include education, directed experience, or discussion with colleagues. Be ready to acknowledge your limitations to supervisors, and do not accept responsibilities for which you are not prepared. For example, the nurse who has not worked in pediatrics for 10 years and accepts an assignment to a pediatric unit without orientation and education is setting the stage for an error to occur. The standard of care does not change for an inexperienced nurse. As a professional, do not accept a position if you cannot meet the criterion of being a reasonably prudent nurse in that setting. In instances of true emergency (eg, disaster or flood), courts may be more lenient, but "we need you here today" does not constitute an emergency.

Adapting Proposed Assignments

As discussed previously, nurses may find themselves assigned to units where they have little or no experience with the types of patient problems they will encounter. It is reasonable to be assigned to assist an overworked nurse in a special area if you can assume duties that are within your own competence and allow the specialized nurse to assume the specialized duties. It is not reasonable or safe for you to be expected to assume the specialized duties. Thus, if you were not prepared for coronary care, you might go to that unit, monitor the IV lines, take vital signs, and make observations to report to the experienced coronary care nurse; the experienced nurse then would be able to check the monitors, administer the specialized medications, and make decisions. Note that this does fragment the patient's care, and it would not be appropriate as a permanent solution but could alleviate a temporary problem in a safe manner.

Following Policies, Procedures, and Protocols

It is your responsibility to be aware of the policies, procedures, and protocols of the institution that employs you. If they are sound, they can be an adequate defense against a claim, providing they were carefully followed. In all circumstances, avoid shortcuts and "work arounds."

For example, the medication procedure may involve checking all medications against a medication administration record (MAR). If you do this and there is an error in the MAR, you might not be liable for the resulting medication error because you followed all appropriate procedures and acted responsibly. The liability would rest with the person who made the error in transcribing the medication from the physician's orders to the MAR. If, however, you had not followed the procedure in checking, you might also be liable because you did not do your part in preventing error. As discussed previously, policies are often designed to provide legal direction.

Changing Policies, Procedures, and Protocols

As nursing evolves, changes are needed in policies, procedures, and protocols. Part of your responsibility as a professional is to work toward keeping these up to date. Are there written policies to deal with emergency situations? Statements such as, "Oh, we've always done it this way" are not adequate substitutes for clearly written, officially accepted policies. Often facilities that are reluctant to make changes based on the suggestions of individual nurses are much more receptive to new ideas when the legal implications of outmoded practice are noted. References such as the guidelines produced by the Agency for Healthcare Research and Quality and articles with research results may provide strong support for needed changes in practice. See the discussion of evidence-based practice in Chapter 16.

Effective Documentation

Nurses' records are unique in the healthcare setting. They cover the entire period of hospitalization or long-term care, 24 hours a day, in a sequential pattern. Your record can be the crucial factor in avoiding litigation. Documentation in the record of observations made, decisions reached, and actions taken and the evaluation of the patient's response are considered much more solid evidence than verbal testimony, which depends on one's memory.

Because each case is determined by the facts as well as by the applicable law, clear documentation of all relevant data is important. For legal purposes, observations and actions that are not recorded may be assumed not to have occurred. Documentation needs to be factual, legible, and clearly understandable. Only use approved abbreviations. Make sure narrative notes have clear statements and correct errors according to the policy of the facility. In paper records, liquid erasing fluid, erasures, and heavy crossing out may be interpreted as attempted fraud in record keeping. In computerized charting, there are usually approved methods of making corrections after an entry has been made. Be sure to follow those processes carefully. Avoid any statement that implies negligence on the part of any healthcare provider. Nurses should be aware that their notes protect not only themselves but often other members of the healthcare team and the facility.

Properly kept records also may protect you from becoming liable for the error of another, by demonstrating that you did everything in your power to prevent harm, including consulting with others. These records might include a complete log of telephone calls to a physician and consultation with any relevant supervisor. Documentation should support that you followed all relevant policies and procedures when an emergency occurred. Although it is easy to become impatient with the time required by paper work and record keeping, complete and clear documentation is often the basis of a successful defense against a claim of malpractice.

One concern about problem-oriented records and charting "by exception" is that these formats may provide less-detailed information and may be less helpful in defense against litigation. This does not have to be the case. You can use any system of charting and record keeping to create appropriate and adequate documentation of care. If you identify something that needs to be recorded and cannot find a provision within your system to make that recording, you can be sure that others have experienced the same difficulty. You might begin making inquiries toward establishing a clear mechanism for the record keeping that concerns you. When nurses serve on committees to review and plan charting procedures, it is wise for them to seek consultation with the attorney for the facility. This helps to ensure that the plan for record keeping is legally sound as well as professionally useful.

ELEMENTS OF A LEGAL ACTION

An individual begins legal action by consulting an attorney and bringing suit against all of those who might have been responsible for the problem. Once the suit has been filed, the next step in legal action is the process of discovery. From there, it may be dropped, settled out of court, or settled by trial.

Discovery

In a civil lawsuit (one between parties for the recovery of damages), a lengthy discovery process commences. Discovery involves gathering information through documents (such as previous medical records and results of mental and physical examinations), interrogatories (written questions answered under oath), and depositions (verbal questions answered under oath and recorded by a court reporter) (Brooke, 2006d). Testimony refers to an individual's verbal or written account of a situation.

A deposition is a formal proceeding in which each attorney has an opportunity to question a witness outside of court, and a sworn verbatim record is made by a court reporter. On occasion, the deposition may be videotaped. Depositions in healthcare cases often are held in attorneys' offices or in the healthcare facility for the convenience of the witnesses. Sometimes depositions are taken to preserve the testimony of a witness for trial and are used in place of live testimony at trial. Most depositions in which you would participate, however, would be depositions for discovery purposes. The same guidelines that apply to testifying in court apply to giving a deposition (see below).

Settlement Out of Court

Often cases are settled before trial because of information obtained during the discovery process. The person bringing suit may be persuaded that no malpractice occurred or that it cannot be proved and may drop the suit. On the other hand, the persons or institutions being sued (or their insurance companies) may determine that it is in their best interests to avoid a trial and agree to pay damages; often this is done without admitting that malpractice occurred. A settlement may require that no party to the settlement reveals its terms to others. Often the cost in time and money to defend a malpractice case exceeds the cost of a settlement. However, any settlement must be reported to the National Practitioner Data Bank. This has made many healthcare professionals reluctant to settle a legal action for reasons of finances and convenience; however, the insurance company may have the authority to settle the case (Brooke, 2006d). Consult the policy at your facility to determine whether you would have a voice in determining any settlement.

Trials

A trial is a legal proceeding that takes place in a courtroom and is presided over by a judge. Some trials are settled before the judge (or panel of judges) alone, and others also have a jury present. In most instances, a trial is a public hearing, and anyone can attend and listen to the proceedings. The various witnesses may appear in person or, when agreed to by both sides, a deposition may be accepted in place of in-person testimony. The judge has full authority over all that takes place in the courtroom.

The plaintiff is the individual bringing suit. The defendants are all those being named in the suit. Each side presents its witnesses, who are examined (questioned) by the attorney. The attorney for the other side then is able to cross-examine (question) that witness about any of the information presented. The final decision is made by a vote of the jury meeting privately or by the judge, who considers all the information and makes a ruling. Monetary awards may be made at the time of the decision or may be established by further deliberation.

THE NURSE AS WITNESS

In the course of your practice as an RN, a time may come when you are asked to serve as a witness in a legal proceeding. Several kinds of cases may involve the nurse as a witness to fact or as an expert witness. When you become involved in any legal action, be sure that you understand both your rights and your obligations in regard to legal action. Always consult an attorney before talking to anyone about a matter in which you have been asked to testify, especially a malpractice action (Display 7.4).

The Nurse as Witness to Fact

A **witness to fact** is an individual who has firsthand knowledge of the specific situation that forms the basis of the legal action. A witness to fact (also referred to as a lay witness) testifies to the exact situation and circumstances of the event or events in question. For example, as a nurse, you might be asked to testify as a witness to fact when a person was injured in an automobile accident and you or your organization were involved in the care of that person. Your testimony in such a case might be on behalf of the injured person, to help describe the injuries and the care received for those injuries.

DISPLAY 7.4 Guidelines for Testifying

- Listen carefully to the entire question before answering and pause to let your attorney object if appropriate.
- Answer only the questions asked and frame your answer in your mind before beginning to speak.
- Do not volunteer additional information.
- Admit if you do not remember.
- Refer to your written documentation to support your answers.
- Be brief and direct.
- Do not use medical or technical terminology unless essential—then explain your terms.
- Explain when a simple yes or no would be misleading.
- Note differences between hypothetical cases presented and the one under consideration.

Another situation involving the nurse as a witness to fact is one in which a patient brings a lawsuit against persons or organizations who have provided healthcare that the patient believes was below the standard of the community. Medical malpractice is alleged in such a situation. For example, the nurse may have to give evidence regarding medical record notes or care given to the patient in the days before the alleged malpractice occurred. Sometimes a nurse is asked to provide information regarding the usual practices of the unit staff.

In both of these situations, the nurse's concern is with the specific factual details of a particular case. Nurses will testify only to what they have observed or done, not to hearsay or opinion. When nurses are asked to testify as to the facts of a situation, they sometimes believe that because they have done nothing wrong they do not need legal counsel. The law is complex, and you could jeopardize the position of an institution for which you work, or even jeopardize yourself and your professional future, with unwise statements. The person who is bringing suit may alter or amend the original complaint to involve new defendants, including you. If you have liability insurance, advise your insurance company of your role as a witness and an attorney will be assigned to talk with you. If you are covered by an employer's policy, consult with the appropriate administrative representative immediately to obtain legal counsel. This attorney should assist you in understanding the questions in the case, your role, and how you can protect yourself in the situation. However, they cannot tell you what to say, that would be illegal (Fig. 7.4).

Every witness is required to swear (take an oath) or affirm to tell the entire truth. Failure to tell the entire truth is perjury, which is a crime. As a witness, you are expected to answer the questions asked of you to the best of your ability; however, you do not have to provide an answer that would incriminate yourself, nor do you have to answer a question for which you do not remember or know the answer. It is perfectly permissible to state, "I do not remember" or "I do not know" if you do not.

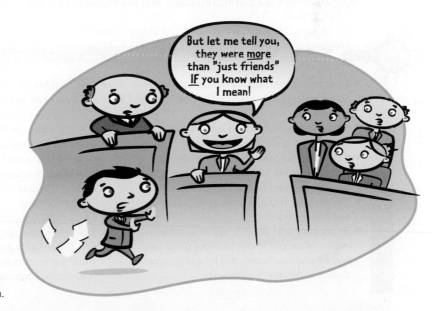

FIGURE 7.4 When testifying in court, you should answer only the questions asked. Do not introduce other information.

It is helpful to use words and terms that can be understood by those who are not familiar with medical terminology, or to explain medical terminology when its use is essential. Be brief and direct when answering questions. Answer the question asked of you. In clinical practice, nurses often use rephrasing techniques to gain information from clients. This is not appropriate when giving testimony. Do not volunteer additional information that has not been asked for by the attorney. You may open up entire areas of inquiry that would not be considered without your comments. However, be cautious about simply answering "yes" or "no." In some instances, an explanation is essential; a simple answer may sound as if you did not perform appropriately. It is the attorney's job to ask the questions to bring out the facts to which he or she wants you to testify. The opposing attorney will have an opportunity during cross-examination to ask you additional questions that the attorney believes are necessary for the facts of the case.

The Nurse as Expert Witness

A nurse also may be involved in a lawsuit as an expert witness. An **expert witness**, under Rule 702 of the Federal Rules of Evidence (accepted in the federal courts and many state courts), is defined as "a witness qualified as an expert by knowledge, skill, experience, training, or education who may testify in the form of an opinion or otherwise." An expert nurse witness may have long experience in a particular area of practice, be certified in the area, possess higher education in the area being considered, or have other evidence of special expertise. For example, in a case involving a patient's care in a critical care unit, the expert nurse witness may be certified in critical care, have a master's degree with a focus in critical care, and have worked in high-intensity critical care for 20 years.

The purpose of testimony as an expert witness is to provide information and opinion that can be used by the judge or jury to understand complex areas of care and make a decision. A nurse may provide a professional opinion, related to his or her area of expertise, on the appropriate care for a given situation. The expert witness may review the record and give an opinion as to what that record states and the meaning of the data found there.

KEY CONCEPTS

- Law includes those rules of conduct or action recognized as binding or enforced by government.
- Statutory law includes all written laws and government codes.
- Constitutional law, which has the greatest authority in any jurisdiction, is found in the US Constitution and in state constitutions.
- Enacted law includes those laws passed by legislative bodies.
- Regulatory law, also referred to as administrative or executive law, includes those rules and regulations established by administrative bodies within the government.

- Common law includes judicial law, also referred to as case law, and common usage or custom.
- Civil law encompasses those laws regulating private conduct between individuals.
- Criminal law regulates actions having to do with the safety of the community as a whole.
- Violations of criminal law are considered crimes, whereas violations of civil law are considered torts.
- Legal rights are derived from constitutional guarantees and carry with them responsibilities. Other rights are ethically determined and, while not supportable by law, do govern the behavior of healthcare professionals.

- Malpractice actions brought against healthcare workers involve civil law. Nurses may be involved in cases related to intentional torts, negligence, or malpractice.
- Individuals who are negligent or have committed malpractice are legally liable for the effects of that action. This means there is an obligation to the individual wronged.
- Liability may be focused on the individual, supervisor, or employer.
- Liability insurance may be purchased that transfers the cost of being sued and the cost of any settlement from the individual to a large group.
- A number of legal issues recur in nursing. Among these are the duty to report or seek medical care for a patient, protection of the patient's confidentiality and right to privacy, defamation of character, privileged information, issues related to informed consent, medication administration, and issues related to different types of emergency care.
- Many legal issues surround consent for care by the patient or by a substitutionary decision maker. These include the provision of advance directives (orders to the physician), such as living wills, durable power of attorney for healthcare, and physician orders for life-sustaining treatments.
- Nurses can be involved in criminal cases related to fraud, assault and battery, and false imprisonment. In some cases, however, a civil suit may be brought against a nurse for these issues and they may not be prosecuted as crimes.
- Many factors contribute to malpractice claims. These include seriousness of the error, social factors, characteristics of suit-prone patients, and characteristics of suit-prone nurses.
- A nurse can do many things to prevent malpractice claims. Being aware of your own practice; accepting only those assignments for which you are prepared; following policies, protocols, and procedures; and properly documenting care are among the most important.
- A legal action may include a process of discovery, dropping the action, settlement out of court, or a trial.
- Nurses may be called as witnesses in trials because of personal knowledge of the case (witness to fact) or because of their expertise in a particular area (expert witness). You must understand both your rights and your obligations regarding legal action before giving a deposition or testimony.

RELEVANT WEB SITES

Web sites relevant to this chapter can be found at the**Point** accessed through *http://thePoint.lww.com/Ellis10e* and by entering the code found on the inside cover of your text.

REFERENCES

Agency for Health Research and Quality. (2009). *Glossary, "F."* Retrieved October 21, 2009 from http://www.psnet.ahrq.gov/glossary.aspx#F

Anonymous. (1997). Court case: A failure to communicate. *Nursing 97, 27*(2), 32.

Brooke, P. S. (2006a). Legal Questions: Telephone orders: Risky chain of command. *Nursing, 36*(2), 67.

Brooke, P. S. (2006b). Legal Questions: Occurrence versus claims-made policy. *Nursing, 36*(3), 12.

Brooke, P. S. (2006c). Legal Questions: Slapping a patient: Strike one, you're out. *Nursing, 36*(7), 29.

Brooke, P. S. (2006d). So you've been named in a lawsuit. *Nursing, 36*(7), 44–48.

Dictionary.com. (2009). *"Law" and "Ethics."* Retrieved July 29, 2010, from http://dictionary.reference.com

Guido, G. W. (2009). *Legal and ethical issues in nursing* (5th ed.). Upper Saddle River, NJ: Prentice Hall.

Human Rights Watch. (2009). *"Please, do not make us suffer any more...": Access to Pain Treatment as a Human Right*. Retrieved October 22, 2009, from http://www.hrw.org/en/

'Lectric Law Library. (2006). *Gross negligence*. Retrieved October 25, 2009, from www.lectlaw.com/def/g020.htm

Lyon, C. (1998). Could you go to jail for a mistake? *Nurseweek 98, 5*. Retrieved November 16, 2009, from http://www.nurseweek.com/features/98-5/crime.html

National Conference of State Legislatures. (2006). *State laws on heart attacks, cardiac arrest & defibrillators*. Retrieved October 25, 2009, from www.ncsl.org/programs/health/aed.htm

Physician Orders for Life-Sustaining Treatments. (2009). *POLST*. Retrieved October 21, 2009, from www.ohsu.edu/ethics/polst

University of Washington School of Medicine. (2009). Informed consent. In *Ethics in Medicine*, Retrieved November 16, 2009, from http://depts.washington.edu/bioethx/topics/consent.html

Vermont Statutes. (1969). *Title 12, Chapter 23*; SS 519 (1968).

8

Ethical Concerns in Nursing Practice

LEARNING OUTCOMES

After completing this chapter, you should be able to:

1. Discuss the concepts of ethics and morality and how they are applied in the healthcare field.
2. Describe four ethical theories that may be used to guide ethical decision making and give an example of each applied to a nursing situation.
3. Explain the ways in which personal religious and philosophic viewpoints, the Codes for Nurses, and documents addressing patients' rights are used as a basis for ethical decision making.
4. Analyze ways sociocultural and occupational factors affect ethical decision making for nurses.
5. Outline a framework for ethical decision making.
6. Discuss how ethical standards are associated with commitment to the patient, personal excellence, and the nursing as a profession.
7. Analyze how ethics affect specific work situations, particularly your obligations related to a chemically impaired nursing colleague.
8. Discuss the importance of recognizing and adhering to boundaries with clients.

KEY TERMS

Autonomy	Morals
Beneficence	Moral distress
Boundary violations	Nonmaleficence
Chemically impaired professional	Paternalism
Code of ethics	Right
Cultural relativism	Standard of best interest
Deontology	Theory of social justice
Distributive justice	Utilitarianism
Ethical dilemma	Values
Ethics	Values clarification
Fidelity	Values conflict
Futile	Veracity
Justice	Whistleblowing

Have you ever overheard a physician discussing with a patient's family whether to start an elderly comatose patient on a series of antibiotics to treat pneumonia? Or have you been present at a nurses' conference at which attendees discussed an order to stop enteral therapy on a patient who has shown no response to stimuli? Or perhaps you have observed a staff nurse leaving the unit after completing the shift with a pocket full of pens, Band-Aids, or tape. These are examples of situations that involve moral and ethical judgments—judgments as to what is right, what is wrong, and what one ought to do in a given situation.

Bennis (2009, p. 2) points out that "organizational decisions inevitably have a moral dimension." This is especially true for nursing and healthcare organizations where situations that call for judgments requiring serious consideration of what is right or best for our clients, their families, and the community are impossible to escape. Although some of these decisions can be based on clinical knowledge, many will require additional expertise in the realm of ethical and moral decision making.

Fortunately, there are guiding principles to assist us in the process. As you work at the process of applying critical thinking to your ethical nursing decisions, look seriously at the assumptions that have been made. Assumptions often are based on ethical and moral values. All of these are good reasons why we need knowledge of ethics, morality, and the process of ethical decision making.

It is not possible in this text to explore the topic of ethics in depth; however, we provide an overview of the topic in this chapter. To assist you in understanding some of the terminology used in the discussion of ethics (and as a point of reference), we have provided a list of definitions in Table 8.1. We also discuss some of the approaches to ethical decision making and give examples of its application in healthcare. Some direct application to your performance as a nurse and to personal decision making is provided. As you read about ethical issues and conflicts, and discuss them in your classroom or with a classmate, respect others by listening carefully to what they have to say and honestly attempting to understand their positions and their accompanying values and beliefs. Only by considering all aspects of an issue can we seek and find understanding for ourselves.

Table 8.1   Terminology Related to Ethics

TERM	DEFINITION
Absolutism	View that there is only one correct moral principle or code for which there are no exceptions
Altruism	Behavior motivated by concern for the well-being of others and that is intended to benefit others
Amoral	State or quality of being indifferent to morality
Categorical imperative	From Immanuel Kant's ethics, the view that for an act to be moral, it must be able to be applied to everyone
Cultural relativism	View that there is enormous variety in the mores and morals of people in different cultures and times, and no single cultural position is correct
Descriptive ethics	Focuses on what people actually do in given situations
Ethics	Specific area of study of morality that concentrates on human conduct and human values (from the Greek ethos, meaning character, habitual uses, customs)
Ethical/moral egoism	When one considers only his or her own good or self-interest
Ethical/moral nihilism	View that no universally valid or true moral principles exist
Ethical/moral objectivism	View that universally valid and true moral principles exist
Ethical/moral relativism	View that no universally valid or true moral principles exist but, rather, that all moral principles are valid relative to culture or individual choice

TERM	DEFINITION
Ethical/moral skepticism	View that we cannot know whether there are universally valid moral principles
Ethics of care	Focuses on those traits valued in intimate personal relationships, such as compassion, love, sympathy, and trust
Hedonism	View that good can be defined as that which is pleasurable
Metaethics	Deals with the extent to which moral judgments are reasonable or justifiable
Moral	Generally accepted as dealing with what is good and what is bad, what is right and what is wrong
Moral agent	Person capable of making distinctions between what is right and what is wrong
Moral philosophy	Branch of philosophy that examines beliefs and assumptions about the nature of certain human values
Moral thought	Individual cognitive evaluation of right and wrong, good and bad
Naturalism	View of moral judgment that regards ethics as dependent on human nature and psychology
Normative ethics	Examines individual rights and obligations as well as common good
Philosophy	Intense and critical examination of beliefs and assumptions (from the Greek words *phila*, meaning love or friendship, and *sophia*, meaning wisdom)
Practical ethics	Use of ethical theory and analysis to examine commonly occurring moral problems
Situational ethics	View that one's actions are governed entirely by the situation rather than by principles or rules
Subjectivism	View that moral principles are applicable to the agent alone, that what is right for one might not be right for another
Virtue ethics	Places emphasis on the agents or people who make choices and take actions

UNDERSTANDING THE CONCEPT OF ETHICS

Since the time of Socrates and the Golden Age of Greece, philosophers have attempted to provide a logical approach to the questions of human conduct that arise in our lives. Why do we act the way we do? What constitutes good and evil, ethical and unethical? What are the factors that result in various cultures embracing different values? How are we to be guided in our decision making? How will the ethics of care affect our professional performance?

When we talk about **morals**, we are referring to the basic standards for what we consider right and wrong that typically are based on religious beliefs, social influences (including education), group norms, culture, and life experiences. If we are of good moral character, we would not steal from a neighbor or cheat on an examination. This word, derived from the Latin *mores*, means custom or habit.

In the formal sense, **ethics** is a branch of philosophy (the study of beliefs and assumptions) referred to as moral philosophy. The word *ethics* is derived from the Greek term *ethos*, which means customs, habitual usage, conduct, and character. Ethics offers a formal process for answering the question about what one ought to do in a given situation. Understanding some of the basic ethical principles and guidelines assists us in making logical and appropriate decisions. It helps us identify the motives for action and define relationships between human beings.

As we work at sorting out those behaviors that we typically describe as good, right, desirable, honorable, fitting, or proper (or the direct opposite), we also are dealing with values. Perceptions are based on values, and each of us (and each society) has a differing set of values. Generally speaking, **values** are important and enduring beliefs or ideals shared by the members of a culture about what is good or desirable and what is not that exert major influence on the behavior of an individual and serve as broad guidelines in all situations (Business Dictionary, 2010). Values are most commonly derived from societal norms, religion, and family orientation, and they provide the framework for making decisions about the actions we take every day. For example, if you were born in the United States, you may have been raised to believe it is unethical to restrict women's right to vote. Those in another society may have been raised to believe that this is the ethical (and logical) way to structure public life.

We all have been in a situation in which we experienced a **values conflict**. This occurs when we must choose between two things, both of which are important to us. For example, if you are a new mother, you probably value caring for your child on a full-time basis; however, if you also must help provide support for the family and your values support the concept that this is your responsibility, leaving your child to go to work results in a values conflict.

Most of the time we don't think about our values—we just accept them. We are most likely to think about them when we have a difficult decision to make, when something goes wrong, or when we find ourselves in a conflict because of differing values. In nursing, we work with a diverse patient population and therefore are exposed to a variety of values and ethical standards. The need to give conscientious care to all patients often forces us to examine the principles in which we believe.

The process of becoming more conscious of and naming what one values or considers worthy is known as **values clarification**, which Videbeck (2010) outlines as a three-step process: (a) choosing the value that feels right, (b) prizing the value or cherishing it (making it one's own), and (c) acting on the value. We examine what we believe is good, bad, beautiful, worthy, meaningful, and so forth and explore the process of determining our personal values. This increases our self-awareness or understanding of ourselves and assists us in making choices. It facilitates decision making, because we have a better grasp of our own value systems.

Having a good understanding of yourself will be helpful when you are faced with an **ethical dilemma**. If you spend a few minutes checking definitions of an ethical dilemma on your computer, you will find a variety of definitions. Some would suggest that it involves choosing between two unfavorable alternatives; others would say it requires choosing from among two or more morally accepted courses of action when one choice prevents selecting the other. We define ethical dilemma broadly: any situation in which guiding moral principles cannot determine which course of action is right or wrong. Examples abound: who should receive a needed heart transplant—a young 34-year-old male with a wife and two children or a 78-year-old gentleman who also has diabetes? Should assisted suicide be an alternative for an individual experiencing great pain and suffering from terminal stages of cancer when the focus of healthcare is to save lives? Should abortion be an alternative for a 14-year-old impregnated as the result of rape?

Ethical dilemmas usually have no perfect solution, and those making decisions may find themselves in direct conflict with another. Should you experience such a situation, be constructive (rather than destructive) in the methods you choose to work toward resolving the differences. Listen carefully without interrupting and be willing to hear what others have to say. Seek clarification using gentle questioning. Respect cultural differences and be attentive to body language. Explain the context of your point of view and try to picture the other person's perspective of what you are saying.

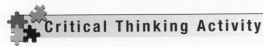

Critical Thinking Activity

Identify situations you might confront in nursing in which your personal religious or philosophic values would be involved. What would be the consequences of following the dictates of your value system? Do conflicts exist between your value system and actions required by the situation? If so, how will you recognize the differences and how will you deal with them? Are there any other alternatives? What might they be?

BASIC ETHICAL CONCEPTS

The most frequently addressed ethical concepts include autonomy, beneficence and nonmaleficence, justice, fidelity, and veracity. Let's examine each one.

Autonomy

Autonomy involves the right of self-determination or choice, independence, and freedom. It comes from the Latin *auto*, meaning "self," and *nomy*, which means "control." Many consider autonomy to include respect for the individual with the expectation that each individual will be treated as unique and equal to other individuals. Other words often associated with autonomy include dignity, inherent worth, self-reliance, individualism, and power.

In today's healthcare delivery system, it is important to respect patients' rights to make decisions about and for themselves, even when we do not agree with those decisions (rights are discussed later in this chapter). This is closely tied to informed consent because it requires that clients be provided clear and sufficient information to make good decisions for themselves. Even when the information is provided, you may have difficulty accepting the client's decision, for example, the decision of a new mother, who is a Jehovah's Witness and whose life is in danger because of blood loss, to refuse to have a blood transfusion.

As with most other rights, there may be restrictions on the right to choose—autonomy does not mean that individuals can do anything they want. When one person's autonomy interferes with another individual's rights, health, or well-being, limitations may be imposed. For example, should an individual have the right to choose a certain expensive treatment if that choice would unjustly deny money to another person for another treatment; should an expensive bone marrow transplant be administered when the physician does not believe a positive outcome is realistic? Does the autonomy of a patient with a highly communicable disease take precedence over the right of the community not to be exposed to the disease? And if rights are to be limited, who defines and enforces those limitations?

For some individuals, autonomy may be less important than values related to the family and community. Is this acceptable? Who decides how much autonomy is enough? Once again, we must consider the idea that autonomy is predominantly a Western value. Many cultures have deeply held values about the family, rather than the individual, as decision maker. So what happens when the family decision is not what health providers think is best for the patient?

COMMUNICATION IN ACTION

Exercising Autonomy

Joan Wagner often studied with a group of classmates as they prepared for examinations. An examination on medications and dosages was scheduled, and Joan believed she would profit most from studying independently because study sessions often strayed from the content being studied. Additionally her time was very limited the evening study was planned. As the group discussed study plans, Joan said, "I really appreciate the opportunity to study with you, but I believe I need to approach this material individually. I need to be sure I can independently master some of the areas related to dosage. Perhaps we can study together later for the content of our next unit." In addressing her own needs, Joan expressed autonomy.

Beneficence and Nonmaleficence

Beneficence comes from the word beneficent, meaning doing or producing good, especially performing acts of kindness and charity (Merriam-Webster Online Dictionary, 2010). The concept of beneficence extends from promoting good to **nonmaleficence** (the prevention of intentional harm). As far back as Hippocrates, physicians were entreated to do no harm. Florence Nightingale stated that the patient should be no worse for having been nursed. The *Code for Nurses with Interpretive Statements* (ANA, 2001) addresses this issue when it clearly delineates the steps to be taken to remove harm or evil. Some examples include reporting unethical practices of a colleague to appropriate authorities or expressing concern to the individual who is engaged in practices that result in substandard practice.

In healthcare, we recognize that sometimes we unintentionally do harm to individuals. For example, the discomfort associated with debridement of wounds, adverse drug reactions, and the side effects of such treatments as irradiation and chemotherapy for cancer are certainly harmful to the individuals who experience them. In many cases, given the alternatives, a patient will opt to have the treatment (eg, chemotherapy) in spite of the adverse effects. The ethical mandate is that we refrain from intentionally inflicting harm. Sometimes, it is difficult to accept that a side effect of a particular treatment might result in harm to a patient. Concern for the possible, although rare, reaction to vaccination for pertussis (whooping cough) is but one example.

Even more problematic is the continued use of medical therapies when they are **futile**, that is, do not have the potential for creating a positive outcome but clearly have the potential for adverse outcomes. Additional chemotherapy in the patient with terminal cancer may fall into this category. Deciding when a treatment is medically futile is a physician's decision, but there are many areas of gray in which one physician might identify a treatment as futile and another suggest that there is at least some possibility of effectiveness. Futility is discussed in greater detail later in this chapter. *Good* is a general term of approval or commendation, and may be defined as that which is "of a favorable character or tendency" (Merriam-Webster Online Dictionary, 2010). Thus, we tend to think of it as that which promotes life, development, and fulfillment. We view it as good when a friend makes a quick recovery from surgery, when a child graduates from high school or college, or when aging parents are able to take that long-awaited trip they have been planning for years.

It is sometimes difficult to decide who will determine what is good for a specific person in a specific situation. In most instances, we expect that people will make their own decisions about what is good for them (autonomy). But who decides for the infant regarding procedures such as immunizations that inflict some degree of pain and a low risk of side effects, but have long-lasting benefits? Who decides for the individual who is unconscious or mentally incompetent?

Another problem centers on how we identify what is good. There are often competing values that challenge our concept of "good." Is the ongoing support of life good if that life is filled with pain? If giving good care to one patient means that lesser care will be given to another (a situation encountered more frequently in today's healthcare environment), how can we defend such an action? What if giving good care means violating good nursing economics (ie, cost containment)? There are no simple answers, and the answers are not the same for everyone.

The issue of sanctity of life is of major concern in the healthcare arena. Some would argue that all life is good. Others would adamantly assert that life is not good when the quality of life is greatly diminished; this latter belief has led to serious discussions regarding euthanasia and assisted suicide, supported the establishment of such groups as the Hemlock Society, and at the time of the publication, has resulted in a few states legally permitting assisted suicide. Many people, particularly physicians, believe that the principles of respect for the patient and relief from suffering that are the basis for approving assisted suicide, fail to do justice to the internal values, professional integrity, and norms of medicine (Boyd, 2006).

Another example of a situation in which quality-of-life issues emerge can be seen in an instance in which parents are advised at a prenatal check up that the fetus has a life-compromising condition such as meningomyelocele. The parents must weigh the quality of the life and the complications inherent in the meningomyelocele in relationship to beliefs in the sanctity of all life when making decisions about terminating the pregnancy. Surrounding all issues regarding the sanctity of life are religious views and values that look upon all life as sacred. Certainly arguments regarding the sanctity of life play a major role in discussions regarding abortion, whether supported by religious beliefs or personal value systems. The sanctity of life also affects our personal beliefs about capital punishment.

Closely aligned to the issue of sanctity of life is the concept of medical futility mentioned briefly earlier in the chapter. Medical futility is a term applied to situations in which interventions are judged to have no medical benefit or in which the chance for success is low (Medical Dictionary, 2010). This concept is often applied to cardiopulmonary resuscitation and to "do not resuscitate" orders but also relates to situations in which a patient exists in a persistent vegetative state (see Chapter 9). The issue is further complicated by the fact that no set definition of the concept exists and that personal values affect the determination of futility. Should the decision regarding futility of treatment be different based on age, cost, or the ability to pay? Thus, it can be said that although the topics of the sanctity of life and medical futility are widely discussed, there exists little consensus about them. As a nurse, you will often encounter difficult situations in the care of your patients in which opposing values play against one another. Understanding your own values, which may change over time, is important in these situations.

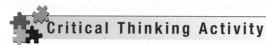

A Case of Unwashed Hands

You entered the women's lounge and noticed a fellow worker also there. After using the toilet, that individual walked to the door to leave the area without first washing her hands. You said, "Hey, Judy! You must have a lot on your mind this morning. You were heading out without washing your hands before returning to work. I know you know how important proper hand washing is and would want to be reminded." Preventing harm through speaking up reflects an ethical value.

Critical Thinking Activity

Identify ways in which the concept of beneficence has shaped medical and nursing care provided to patients. Do you believe this is a concept that will have the same impact in years to come? What assumptions are you making? Are your data accurate? What are the implications for the future?

Justice

Justice, sometimes referred to as fairness, refers to the quality of being just or fair; conformity to truth, fact, or sound reason; or treating like cases similarly (equity) and looks at the concepts of moral rightness in action or attitude (The Free Dictionary, 2010). We must ask, "How is fairness defined?" Does fairness mean that people should always be treated the same? In terms of access to healthcare, is it "just" for one person to receive more resources than another receives? If so, what makes it just, and how does that relate to the distribution of scarce medical resources? Does age make a difference in what we consider just? Should it? Does justice imply that the government should provide the resources or services individuals are unable to provide for themselves? Can we measure fairness in any objective sense? What should occur when one person's rights interfere with the rights of another? These issues are discussed in greater detail in Chapter 9.

The object of **distributive justice** is to distribute rewards and punishments to everyone according to his/her merits or demerits (Legal-dictionary, 2010). The expectation is that all individuals have an equal opportunity to access scarce resources and healthcare organizations and health plans will provide to individual recipients the care and service each is due. This has been a major issue in the United States as congress struggles to establish healthcare for all (see Chapter 6). Several criteria have been used to define the just distribution of limited medical resources: need, equity, societal contribution, ability to pay, effort, and merit. The use of these criteria is controversial. Need involves known medical need, not elective procedures. Equity addresses trying to distribute equally to all in need. Contribution considers what an individual might be expected to give to society at a future date. (This approach has met with concern over labeling those who are disabled or unable to contribute as less worthy and thus can be discriminated against.) Ability to pay is self-explanatory, but to deny needed health services because an individual cannot pay contradicts the concepts of charitableness that exist in our society. Patient effort deals with a patient's compliance or noncompliance with medical advice. For example, should a patient who refuses to quit smoking be eligible for a heart transplant? Merit (the good to be received) addresses the potential that exists for benefit from the additional investment of limited health resources, for example, the investment of federal dollars in cancer treatment. Who will decide about the future potential for a current investment? These six criteria have not always provided a strong basis for decision making, and the ethical issues related to allocation of scarce resources promise to become more complex in the coming years as people live longer and technology provides more alternatives.

Fidelity

Fidelity refers to the obligation to be faithful to the agreements, commitments, and responsibilities that one has made to oneself and others, both implicitly and explicitly. Fidelity is the foundation of the concept of accountability that we hear about so often in nursing today. What are the responsibilities of healthcare personnel to individuals, employers, the government, society, and each other? When these responsibilities conflict, which should take priority? In reality, which do take priority? Are nurses obligated to provide care to all patients? Under what circumstances, if any, might this be challenged? What are the nurse's promises to society? Would it also cover areas such as competence? Abiding by institutional policies? Operating within the profession's code of ethics?

Chaffee (2006) illustrates the conflict nurses may experience with this concept in a discussion of situations in which duties clash—as in a disaster where there is a clash between obligations to one's family (particularly if small children or elderly adults are involved) and to a professional obligation to report to work. She points out that the American Nurses Association's (ANA) *Code of Ethics for Nurses with Interpretive Statements* (2001) offers conflicting guidance: on the one hand stating that the nurse's primary commitment is to the patient and on the other that the nurse owes the same duties to self as to others. Chaffee suggests the following be considered when deciding whether to report for work in the event of a disaster: the nurse's safety, the prioritization of relationships of responsibility, the nurse's expertise, the benefits to be gained over the risks, consideration of the harm that would occur if the nurse fails to report for work, and consideration of the good that would come from reporting versus the good that would come from not reporting for work.

Another situation that often challenges us in healthcare is that of confidentiality. Is maintaining confidentiality a moral/ethical issue as well as a legal issue related to fidelity? Are there any instances when it is acceptable to violate the principle of confidentiality? If you are working with an impaired colleague, is it appropriate and ethical to violate a confidential situation in the interest of patient well-being? We discuss this issue in detail later in the chapter.

Veracity

Veracity refers to telling the truth or not intentionally deceiving or misleading patients. From childhood, we are all admonished to tell the truth and to avoid lying. When we are children, this seems straightforward. As we become adults, we see more instances in which the choices are less clear. For example, do you tell the truth (veracity) when you know the truth will cause harm to an individual (beneficence vs. nonmaleficence)? Do you tell a lie when it would make someone less anxious and afraid? You might see this as beneficence (doing good), but then you have abandoned the principle of veracity. Failing to be honest is considered by some as leading to a slippery slope, because when we conceal the truth from a patient, it suggests to all others involved (eg, family members, friends, nursing assistants, housekeeping staff) that health practitioners lie. This deception is later remembered, and the concept that one cannot rely on health professionals pervades. In other words, it diminishes one's esteem and reliability and erodes trust, which is an essential element of the nurse–patient relationship. Lying also diminishes oneself. Lying can change your concept of yourself as an honest person and may adversely affect future behavior if practice in lying makes it easier to lie in the future. Not all societies value telling the truth to the ill person. In some societies, such as Japan, the patient is to be protected from bad news or information that would provoke anxiety. Therefore, to lie and provide false reassurance may be considered doing good (beneficence) and avoiding harm (nonmaleficence). When health professionals relate to families with a different view of truth telling to the ill person, their values may come in conflict.

COMMUNICATION IN ACTION

To Tell or Not to Tell

You assessed your patient every hour because of elevated blood pressure. The fourth time you checked it during your shift, you noted that the reading was 195/105, more elevated than previously. The patient asked you, "How was the reading this time?" You replied, "This time I got a reading higher than before. I am going to check it again in 15 minutes and, in the meantime, notify your physician of my findings. I will return in just a few minutes." The choice of the nurse was to tell the truth to the patient even if it caused anxiety. The nurse also knew that the patient's anxiety may have been increased by feeling that information was being denied to him or by the uncertainty of not knowing. He may be reassured that action was being taken.

ETHICAL THEORIES

It is not our intent to delve with any depth into the writings of early philosophers. However, because ethical theories are mentioned frequently in the literature that deals with bioethical issues, some background information follows.

An ethical theory is a moral principle or a set of ethical concepts and moral principles that can be used to assess what is morally right or morally wrong in a given situation. Over the years, many people have called on the theories of philosophers to guide in decision making. The most widely used theories are presented in Table 8.2. You are encouraged to consider various ethical approaches and discuss with your classmates when each might be used appropriately.

An application of **utilitarianism** (or consequentialism) as seen in the healthcare industry would be the justification of capitation in the managed care organization (MCO). Because the MCO pays a certain amount of money per member per month to a contracted provider, the MCO would argue that it has provided the greatest good for the greatest number of members. In public life, it would be illustrated by the public health department fully funding immunizations and providing only limited funding for episodic care of illness. Preventing communicable disease will benefit many more people in the community than will caring for individual illnesses.

An example of **deontology** might be applied to a situation in which all persons involved in a research study have a complete understanding (informed consent) of the study and its purposes. The participant is treated as a moral being with freedom of decision making and

Table 8.2   **Major Ethical Theories and Theorists**

TITLE OF THEORY (OTHER NAMES)	THEORIST ASSOCIATED WITH WORK	BASIC PRINCIPLES OF THEORY
Natural Law (objectivism)	St. Thomas Aquinas (1225–1274)	Actions are morally right when they are in accord with our nature and end as human beings. Good should be promoted, evil avoided, and ethics grounded in our concern for human good.
Deontology (formalistic system, the principal system of ethics, or duty-based ethics)	Immanuel Kant (1724–1804)	Ethical decision making is based on moral rules and unchanging principles (or motivations that are derived from universal values), considered separately from the consequences. The fundamental principle is called the categorical imperative, unconditional commands that must be applied similarly in all situations without exception.
Utilitarianism (often referred to as teleology, consequentialism or situation ethics, although there are some differences)	Jeremy Bentham (1748–1832) and John Stuart Mill (1806–1873)	An act is right when it is useful in bringing about a desirable or good end. A second principle allows the end to justify the means. Fits well into Western society's values regarding work ethic and the behavioristic approach to education, philosophy, and life. Applicable to research.
Social Equity and Justice	John Rawls (1921–2002)	Sets forth principles of justice developed in 1971. Allows social and economic positions to be to everyone's advantage and open to all. Introduces a "veil of ignorance" whereby persons making choices would not have any specific information regarding those involved, thus choosing the alternative that supported the most disadvantaged person. Supports justice and equal rights for everyone.
Ideal Observer	Raymond W. Firth (1901–2002)	Requires that decisions be made from a dispassionate, disinterested, and consistent viewpoint with full information about the situation and the consequences available.

not simply a means to an end. The individual participant who has a bad result might be immediately dropped from the study because the well-being of the individual participant is considered more important than the study itself.

In applying Rawls' (1971) **theory of social justice**, one could not ethically justify using income inequalities or the ability to pay to determine a patient's eligibility for access to healthcare. According to social justice, the most disadvantaged person should receive the preferential benefit.

 Critical Thinking Activity

Of the ethical theories provided in this chapter, select the one that is of greatest interest to you and describe the aspects of the theory that make it most attractive. Examine factors that bring you to this point of view. What are your biases? What are the consequences of supporting this ethical theory on your professional practice? Which of the theories do you believe is most critical in the heathcare arena?

APPLYING BASIC CONCEPTS

The basic ethical concepts discussed so far have many applications to the way we live our daily lives and how we interact with others, as well as how we perform as professional nurses. A major application of these concepts is seen in how we view the rights of an individual, a concept tied to the concept of autonomy.

Rights

The discussion of ethical concepts is founded on the belief that people are entitled to certain rights or privileges. Typically, we think of a **right** as a just claim or entitlement, or as something that is owed to an individual on a legal, moral, or ethical basis. Most rights are based on the concept of autonomy of the individual. In common usage, this is often extended to include privileges, concessions, and freedoms. Rights are associated with many different areas of our lives. We tend to think of ourselves as having civil and political rights such as the right to assembly, to vote, to own property, and to speak freely. We have economic, social, and cultural rights, such as the right to healthcare, the right to education, and the right to work. Rights form the basis of most professional codes and legal judgments (see Chapter 7 for more discussion of rights as used in the legal sense). Legal rights include the right to due process and trial. And we have personal rights, such as the right of an individual to self-determination and privacy. Problems occur when one individual's rights come in conflict with the values of others. For example, if a patient is admitted to a hospital and refuses treatment, and there is a strong indication that with treatment the patient could recover, should the physicians and nurses respect the patient's right to self-determination? The conflict of rights provides us with many challenges and dilemmas. Although it is not within the confines of this text to discuss all of the circumstances, consider some of the major areas in which you may deal with rights in your role as a nurse.

Right to Self-Determination

Federal legislation has been passed to ensure that individual rights are respected. The Patient Self-Determination Act, also known as the Danforth amendment, is discussed in Chapters 7 and 9. This act was created because of our society's fundamental belief in the individual's right to decide. However, this act does little to recognize cultural diversity and sensibility to groups such as Chinese Americans, who have a unique set of values and well-defined role relationships, in which the role of family in making healthcare decisions is strongly valued.

Rights and Cultural Relativism

Although the concept of rights is almost taken for granted in our Western culture, there are some who suggest that the validity of all moral judgments is culturally relative. **Cultural relativism** is the principle that what an individual believes and does make sense in terms of his or her own culture. Cultural relativism embraces the notion that groups and individuals hold different sets of values that must be respected. The principle was made popular by anthropologists who wanted to compare and contrast a wide range of cultures in a systematic and even-handed manner. It gained greater popularity when the Commission of Human Rights of the United Nations began preparing the Universal Declaration of Human Rights. The Commission struggled to formulate a statement of human rights that would take into account the individual as a member of a social group of which he or she was a part.

Those of us raised in the Western culture have difficulty imagining the prospect of performing as a suicide bomber, as witnessed in news broadcasts from the Middle East where such behaviors are viewed as heroic by some groups. This is also an interesting concept to consider in relationship to practices such as female circumcision, often referred to in the west as female genital mutilation. Although it is appalling to Western cultures, in some non-Western cultures, concerns about virginity, ability to attract a husband, the husband's sexual pleasure, and religious beliefs dictate that female children be circumcised. Western countries have acted to make this practice illegal, indicating that it is outside the bounds of what can be accepted as simply a cultural difference.

Rights of the Unborn

There are many times when we grapple with whose rights should be respected. The most obvious example of this situation occurs when we consider the rights of the unborn to life versus the right of the mother to make choices regarding her own body. This issue is one that has continued to divide members of our society and is often an issue brought forth when candidates run for election or when appointments are made to the Supreme Court. The concern becomes even more contradictory, paradoxical, and convoluted when we consider that some states will permit a late-term abortion; however, in that same state, if an automobile accident occurs in which a pregnant woman is killed (thus also killing the fetus she is carrying), the offending driver can be charged with two cases of manslaughter—both the mother and the unborn child.

Right to Privacy and Right of Confidentiality

An area receiving much attention today is that of the rights of the patient to privacy and the confidentiality of medical information. Privacy may be thought of as the right to be left alone or free from intrusion. It also includes the right to select desired care based on personal values and beliefs and to have control over how sensitive information is shared.

Confidentiality deals with not sharing information. This has surfaced as a major concern, because sensitive health records are now computerized and can be e-mailed, telecommunicated, faxed, or copied to various individuals or groups who may have an interest in the information. This information, which could include individually identifiable health data, might be readily available to anyone who walks by a fax machine or logs on to a computer. People are concerned that exposure to personal health information, especially that related to genetic tests or communicable illnesses such as sexually transmitted diseases or HIV, could result in loss of or denial of health insurance, or could result in embarrassment or discrimination in the work environment.

In 1996, Congress passed legislation in the Health Insurance Portability and Accountability Act. It required that steps be taken or legislation passed to ensure the privacy of individually identifiable health information.

The ANA has been concerned about this issue for some time and continues to work with other national groups on the issue of privacy and confidentiality. Table 8.3 identifies some of the activities in which the ANA has been involved related to this issue.

The ANA Code of Ethics for Nurses with Interpretive Statements (2001) and the International Council of Nurses Code of Ethics for Nurses (2006) both address the issue of patient confidentiality. As a student and future nurse, remain ever mindful of your responsibility to maintain patient privacy and confidentiality in all matters.

Table 8.3 **ANA Activities Regarding Patient Privacy**

DATE	ANA GROUP	ACTIVITY
1994	House of Delegates	Approved a policy called "Privacy & Confidentiality" related to electronic data
1998	Board of Directors	Endorsed the "Core Principles of Telehealth" intended to regulate technology used to provide long-distance care and patient data
1999	ANA membership	Developed position statement on privacy and confidentiality
2006	Board of Directors	Revised and accepted updated position statement on patient privacy

The Standard of Best Interest

When a decision must be made about a patient's healthcare and the patient is unable to make an informed decision, the decision may be made based on the **standard of best interest**. As the name implies, it is based on what the healthcare providers or family believes is best for that individual, taking into account tangible factors such as how the patient may be harmed, how the patient may benefit, and any physical and fiscal risks. This is an application of the concepts of beneficence and nonmaleficence. Such decisions may be based on the individual's expressed wishes and preferences as noted in verbal statements or by written documents such as living wills if they are available. Healthcare professionals strive to avoid unilateral decisions made by a healthcare provider. Unilateral decisions often imply that the decision maker knows what is best for the patient. This is referred to as **paternalism**, or the deliberate treatment of people in a fatherly manner, especially by caring for them but not allowing them to have rights or responsibilities. In instances where parents have denied their children lifesaving care, the courts have, on occasion, overturned the parent's decision on the best-interest standard.

Ethics and Financial Compensation

Another issue receiving attention, discussion, and review is the practice of rewarding physicians (monetarily or not) for limiting care as was first seen in the advent of diagnosis-related groups under Medicare that established limits for payment for services. Recently, health maintenance organizations have come under fire for rewarding physicians who maintain lower costs of care or for penalizing those who do not. The impact this might have on nurses who are involved in the care of clients perceived to be receiving less than adequate treatment and the nurse's obligation to serve as an advocate for the patient are yet to be determined. It certainly emphasizes the importance of all nurses understanding ethics and ethical principles.

FACTORS THAT INFLUENCE ETHICAL DECISION MAKING

Ethical decisions are not made in a vacuum. Many factors influence us as we seek appropriate answers to the dilemmas that we face with new problems and new realities of today challenging yesterday's answers.

In determining their own bases for making ethical decisions, some individuals rely on formal philosophic or religious beliefs that define matters in relation to what is believed to be the truth or good or evil. Others make decisions based on personal life experiences or on the experiences of those close to them. Still others rely on professional codes of ethics to give guidance on ethical issues. In reality, ethical decision making often involves a combination of all of these factors.

In studying ethical issues, it is important for you to understand the many forces that are operating simultaneously in our society. These forces are not independent or mutually exclusive, but act and react with one another in a constantly changing milieu, causing evolutionary changes in all segments of society (Fig. 8.1). The following is a discussion of some of the factors that affect ethical decision making in the healthcare environment.

Codes for Nurses

Through their professional organizations, nurses have developed some common guidelines to use in making ethical decisions. They are contained in the ANA's code for nurses, the International Council of Nurses (ICN) code for nurses, and the National Association for Practical Nurse Education and Service's (NAPNES) Standards of Practice for licensed practical/vocational nurses. Each attempts to outline the nurse's responsibilities to the patient and to the profession of nursing.

The ANA code is unique among professional codes because it addresses specific issues and does not confine itself to matters of etiquette or broad general statements. Although identifying the need for a code of ethics as early as 1896, it was not until 1950 that a **code of ethics** was adopted after accepting tentative codes in the 1920s, 1930s, and 1940s. This code has been revised several times since then. Early versions stated that a nurse had an obligation to carry out a physician's orders; later versions, however, stress the nurse's obligation to the patient. This includes protecting the patient from incompetent, unethical,

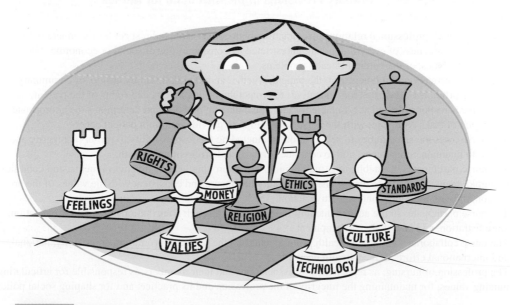

FIGURE 8.1 Decisions made in relation to one aspect of an ethical situation will affect all other aspects of the problem.

or illegal practice. The nine primary provisions of the code for nurses without explanatory provisions are presented in Display 8.1. You can view the entire code, including the preface, by visiting the ANA Web site, *http://nursingworld.org* and searching for "Code of Ethics for Nurses."

The ICN first adopted a code in 1953, and the code has been revised and reaffirmed several times since then. The most recent revisions occurred in 2005. The preamble of this code addresses the general responsibilities of the nursing profession. Four sections follow, dealing with the more specific concerns of people, practice, the profession, and coworkers. In addition, the ICN provides suggestions for use of its code and a chart to assist nurses in translating the standards into action. The four elements of the ICN code are presented in Display 8.2. The full document is available at the ICN Web site, *www.icn.ch/ethics.htm.*

Critical Thinking Activity

Compare and contrast the value statements found in the ANA Code of Ethics for Nurses with Interpretive Statements and the ICN Code of Ethics for Nurses. What topics are included in each? Which are not? What does the inclusion of similar topics signify to the profession of nursing? How do you account for topics that are not included in both?

DISPLAY 8.1   Primary Provisions of the ANA Code for Nurses

1. The nurse, in all professional relationships, practices with compassion and respect for the inherent dignity, worth, and uniqueness of every individual, unrestricted by considerations of social or economic status, personal attributes, or the nature of health problems.
2. The nurse's primary commitment is to the patient, whether an individual, family, group, or community.
3. The nurse promotes, advocates for, and strives to protect the health, safety, and rights of the patient.
4. The nurse is responsible and accountable for individual nursing practice and determines the appropriate delegation of tasks consistent with the nurse's obligation to provide optimum patient care.
5. The nurse owes the same duties to self as to others, including the responsibility to preserve integrity and safety, to maintain competence, and to continue personal and professional growth.
6. The nurse participates in establishing, maintaining, and improving healthcare environments, and conditions of employment conducive to the provision of quality healthcare and consistent with the values of the profession, through individual and collective action.
7. The nurse participates in the advancement of the profession through contributions to practice, education, administration, and knowledge development.
8. The nurse collaborates with other health professionals and the public in promoting community, national, and international efforts to meet health needs.
9. The profession of nursing, as represented by associations and their members, is responsible for articulating nursing values, for maintaining the integrity of the profession and its practice, and for shaping social policy.

Source: Reprinted with permission from American Nurses Association. (2001). *Code of Ethics for Nurses with Interpretive Statements.* American Nurses Publishing, American Nurses Association, Washington, DC.

DISPLAY 8.2 ICN Code for Nurses—Elements of the Code (2006)

Nurses and People

The nurse's primary responsibility is to people requiring nursing care.

In providing care, the nurse promotes an environment in which the human rights, values, customs, and spiritual beliefs of the individual, family, and community are respected.

The nurse ensures that the individual receives sufficient information on which to base consent for care and related treatment.

The nurse holds in confidence personal information and uses judgment in sharing this information.

The nurse shares with society the responsibility for initiating and supporting action to meet the health and social needs of the public, in particular those of vulnerable populations.

The nurse also shares responsibility to sustain and protect the natural environment from depletion, pollution, degradation, and destruction.

Nurses and Practice

The nurse carries personal responsibility and accountability for nursing practice and for maintaining competence by continual learning.

The nurse maintains a standard of personal health such that the ability to provide care is not compromised.

The nurse uses judgment regarding individual competence when accepting and delegating responsibility.

The nurse at all times maintains standards of personal conduct that reflect well on the profession and enhance public confidence.

The nurse, in providing care, ensures that the use of technology and scientific advances are compatible with the safety, dignity, and rights of people.

Nurses and the Profession

The nurse assumes the major role in determining and implementing acceptable standards of clinical nursing practice, management, research, and education.

The nurse is active in developing a core of research-based professional knowledge.

The nurse, acting through the professional organization, participates in creating and maintaining equitable social and economic working conditions in nursing.

Nurses and Coworkers

The nurse sustains a cooperative relationship with coworkers in nursing and other fields.

The nurse takes appropriate action to safeguard individuals, families, and communities when their care is endangered by a coworker or any other person.

Copyright © 2006 by ICN-International Council of Nurses, 3, Place Jean-Marteau, CH-1201 Geneva (Switzerland).

Since 1941, NAPNES has set standards for nursing practice of LPNs; they were last published in 2007. These standards also incorporate moral, ethical, and legal components to guide the practice of the practical nurse. The standards can be viewed online by visiting *http://www. napnes.org/about/standards/standards_read_only.pdf.*

The Patient's Rights

The patient's rights, as discussed earlier, are another consideration in decision making. Ideally, we have always recognized them in some way. As early as 1959, the National League for Nursing formulated a statement regarding patient rights. For many years, however, healthcare professionals assumed that they knew what was best for patients and made many decisions without consulting or considering the rights of the patient. For example, a patient with a specific disease was not offered information about possible treatment alternatives, even when valid alternatives did exist. The patient's physician decided which treatment method was preferable, and that was the only one presented to the patient. This is another example of paternalism, discussed earlier in this chapter.

As the health consumer movement became more active, greater attention was paid to the rights of the patient. Today, patients may expect to be informed of all alternatives for treatment and often want to participate in choosing a type of treatment, weighing the possible benefits and risks of the treatment methods presented. For example, a patient with a diagnosis of ovarian cancer may want to be involved in the decision whether to first start treatment with chemotherapy or surgery. Many research their health problems on the Internet and come to the physician with questions about specific therapies and approaches to treatment. The law also has supported the right to informed decision making.

In 1973, the American Hospital Association (AHA) published *A Patient's Bill of Rights* (AHA, 1992), which outlined the rights of the hospital patient and served as a basis for making decisions about hospitalized patients. Some criticized this document, saying it is rather innocuous because it simply reminded patients of their rights (such as privacy, confidentiality, and informed consent) but said nothing of hospitals that fail to act in accordance with these rights. The AHA revised this document in 1992 to speak more forcefully to the hospital's responsibility for providing medically indicated care and services and to emphasize the collaborative nature of health maintenance. In April 2003, the AHA Bill of Rights was updated with a version titled *The Patient Care Partnership*. This document outlines what patients may expect during a hospital stay and encourages patients to ask questions if they have concerns. *The Patient Care Partnership* can be reviewed at *http://www.aha.org/aha/issues/Communicating-With-Patients/pt-care-partnership.html.*

Social and Cultural Factors

Changes in the attitudes of society as a whole profoundly influence each of its segments. For example, the changing roles of women, the shifting attitudes toward marriage and the family, and the increasing emphasis on culturally competent care and evidence-based practice have all required nurses to reexamine their personal feelings and alter their approach to providing nursing care.

Ethical concerns are the by-products of many factors at work in our society today, including the role of the individual and the family. In the healthcare field, this is most pointedly illustrated by the use of the terminology "healthcare" as opposed to "medical care." Healthcare suggests much greater involvement of others in care delivery, whereas medical care places the physician in the key role. We see similar language being applied to "telehealth" as opposed to "telemedicine." The meaning of "consumer unit" is shifting from an individual to a whole family or even a whole community. The focus of care also has shifted from disease to prevention and wellness, even when encountering chronicity.

The size of the group being affected by ethical decisions has a bearing on the decision-making process. The smaller the group, organization, or society involved in or affected by the decision making, the easier the process of arriving at an acceptable alternative. When a larger group is affected by a decision, it becomes more complex because more divergent views are encountered. Many of our ethical considerations now involve our society as a whole or, in some cases, the world; therefore, solutions are difficult. An excellent example is the difficulty the United States has encountered in trying to develop and implement a national health plan. The value a society places on the individual or the family directly influences the standard of care (Fig. 8.2). In Western society, we believe in each person's right to exercise choice based on individual beliefs and conscience. We also place high value on preserving individual life; therefore, we often use tremendous resources to try to achieve additional years, months, or even days of life, for example, in the case of heart transplantation. A society that placed greater emphasis on the community good than on the individual may not choose to use resources in that way. The standard of care might aim for comfort without the use of expensive treatment modalities.

A culture's religious values and belief in an afterlife directly affect ethical issues. The Hindu belief in rebirth after death and the immutability of fate affects decisions about using healthcare resources. Those who believe that an outcome is predetermined by fate will not choose to commit major resources and efforts toward altering that outcome.

The population, or, more accurately, the overpopulation, of a country relative to its resources also may have a direct bearing on the value placed on life. The material resources to provide many health services may not be available. Decisions may be made to eliminate certain costly healthcare procedures even though they are known to be effective and desired by individuals.

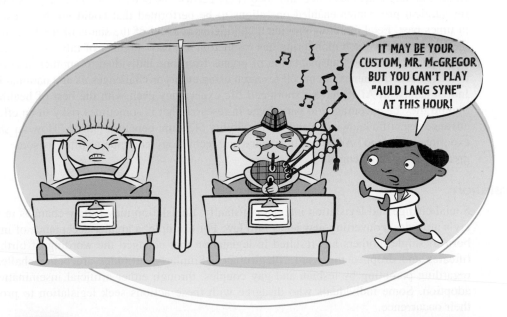

FIGURE 8.2 In providing care, the nurse respects the beliefs, values, and customs of the individual.

Critical Thinking Activity

Identify two sociocultural factors with which you have had personal experience that could affect ethical decision making. How is your view of this different than it might have been 5 years ago? In what ways have your views remained the same? Why do you think your views have changed or remained the same? What implications does this have for the way you will view things in the future? If you are comfortable doing so, discuss these with a classmate.

Science and Technology

Scientific advancement and technology have left us wrestling with concerns that would have been considered science fiction 50 years ago. Before the development of kidney dialysis, we accepted the fact that people with nonfunctioning kidneys would soon die. After machines that could filter body wastes were invented, a genuine dilemma arose over who would have dialysis and who would not; the number of people needing treatment far exceeded the personnel, time, and equipment available to treat them. As the technology increased the availability of equipment to treat those needing it, the ethical questions refocused on decisions to end treatment rather than on issues related to initiating treatment.

Other technology has had similar effects. The advent of machines that could artificially breathe for someone challenged the medical and legal professions to examine their definitions of life, and brought into focus problems of whether and when to turn off a ventilator. Heart and lung machines that could adequately perfuse the body while the heart was stopped for surgical procedures enabled operations to be performed that could not be considered in times past. Fetal monitors provide a continuous readout of the status of the fetus during the labor process. Such monitoring has resulted in a greater number of infants delivered by cesarean section. The transplantation of organs from one individual to another has created untold ethical dilemmas. Stem cell research using embryos challenges us at a national level. Individuals with AIDS have a shortened life expectancy even with the best of healthcare. Should they be encouraged to participate in research that is sometimes risky in an effort to advance scientific knowledge and the possibility of future benefit to others? How far should experimentation go? Advances in science and technology continue to offer us some of the greatest ethical challenges.

Legislation

Social change and legislation interact constantly. Legislation may follow changes in society's attitudes, converting new ideas into law. For example, a greater acceptance of infants born to single mothers has resulted in legislation that changed the wording of birth certificates and dropped the word "illegitimate." Similarly, attitudes are being challenged regarding parenting by lesbian and gay couples, through either artificial insemination or adoption. Some individuals who disagree with these actions seek legislation to prohibit their occurrence.

When social change is desired, legislation may be actively sought to require people to talk and behave in new ways. This was true for civil rights legislation. A change in society was desired, and supporters of civil rights sought legislation as one step toward change. Recent legislative action that addresses the needs and opportunities available to the disabled has brought about changes in public policies, procedures, and even architecture.

Judicial Decisions

The judicial system provides a major avenue for debating and trying to solve ethical problems. More issues are being taken to court, and judicial decisions are used more often as the basis for determining appropriate action. As you continue to study this topic, note that we have cited landmark decisions regarding ethical issues. The process does not stop there, however. Some people may disagree with a judicial decision and continue to oppose it, appealing the decision to a higher court. Higher courts may overturn judicial decisions. Meanwhile, the questions regarding the individual's role in carrying out a judicial decision remain. For example, although the law in the past forbade abortions, some physicians believed strongly in the right of the individual to have the procedure done. These physicians were upset by the results of abortions performed by individuals who lacked the necessary education and skill to do it safely, and therefore were willing to perform abortions despite the law prohibiting the procedure. These physicians were, of course, liable to prosecution if it were discovered they were performing illegal abortions, and some were prosecuted. The issues of abortion and government funding of the procedure are still controversial, and it is unlikely that these issues will be resolved in a way that is satisfactory to everyone.

Funding

The financing of healthcare represents a major area of conflict that has ethical dimensions. The government has become increasingly involved in providing funds for healthcare. Some people are asking how much time, money, and energy we should allocate to healthcare, and how those resources should be divided. How obligated are we as a society to make some form of healthcare available to all? Should that care be provided to illegal immigrants who live in this country as well as to legal residents? What is it that healthcare can and cannot provide? Which is more important, prevention or cure? Healthcare includes controversial procedures as well as high-cost options, such as abortion, sterilization, transplantation, and gene therapy. This challenges the basic values of some taxpayers who do not ethically sanction these procedures and do not want their tax dollars used to fund them.

Personal Religious and Philosophic Viewpoints

Religious beliefs form the basis for ethical decision making for most people; however, a person who is a member of a particular religious group may not ascribe to all of the beliefs of that group. Some individuals make their own decisions regarding each situation, which, in some cases, may not parallel the doctrines of their religious group. For example, some Muslims maintain that women should be completely separated from men and wear veils when in the presence of men. They would find any healthcare setting that did not respect this belief to be in conflict with their basic values. Other Muslims do not adhere to this strict interpretation of Islamic law and believe women should wear modest clothing but need not wear veils. They would be more comfortable in most Western healthcare settings because they would not feel a conflict with their personal values.

Your personal viewpoint certainly will be a major factor influencing your ethical decision making. As stated earlier, values are the product of our life experiences and are influenced by family, friends, religion, culture, environment, education, and many other factors.

PERSONAL VALUES AND THE WORK ENVIRONMENT

Nursing offers a variety of job opportunities to the new graduate, and you will want to consider your personal values when choosing a position after graduation. You certainly cannot expect to avoid all conflict or problem situations, but you will want to avoid working in an area in which conflict is constant.

Seeking Employment

Before you accept a position, consider whether it has the potential to conflict with your basic beliefs. For example, if you believe that no individual should be denied lifesaving techniques, you might be unhappy working in a research institution where the effects of treatment or no treatment are studied. In this situation, making your views known and refusing certain assignments after you begin employment might result in termination, because the employer may justifiably assert that you agreed to fulfill all the responsibilities of the position when you accepted employment.

Similarly, you might choose to work in an area that supports your personal value system or strong ethical commitment. For example, religious groups that saw value in the life of the dying person began the hospices for the dying in England. Their religious beliefs were and have continued to be part of their approach to care. If you strongly value your own ethnic or cultural approach to healthcare, you might choose to work in a healthcare setting where that approach is part of the philosophy.

Workplace Influences

By virtue of the positions they hold in the healthcare system, nurses experience special pressures as they try to make decisions. An awareness of these factors may help you as you grapple with personal problems in decision making and will be significant in your choice of jobs.

Status as an Employee

Most nurses are not in independent practice but are employed by hospitals, nursing homes, community agencies, or outpatient facilities. Codes do not speak of responsibilities to the employer, yet, from an ethical standpoint, you have certain loyalties and obligations to the employer who pays your salary and makes decisions regarding your work. You may feel pressures of loyalties divided among your patient, your employer, and yourself.

When discussing ethical decisions in the abstract, most people say that, of course, the patient's best interest should be the only priority. In real situations, however, the issues often are not so clearly defined. If a nurse's decision affects the employer adversely, the result may be job loss, poor references, and a severely curtailed economic and career future.

▶ *EXAMPLE*

Blank Surgical Permits

Carrie Lipton worked on a surgical unit in a community hospital. At the request of one of the chief surgeons, it was the practice on that unit for the nurses to sign blank surgical permits on admission to the unit. Carrie did not believe that it was ethical to require patients to sign blank documents because they were not informed of alternative methods of treatment. She discussed her concerns with the surgeon. He became angry and complained to the hospital administration stating if something wasn't done he'd take his surgeries elsewhere. Carrie was called to the office of the Chief Nurse Executive to discuss the issue.

Had the surgeon gone elsewhere, this might have created a considerable economic loss for the hospital, and, depending on the action of the hospital administrator, the nurse might have been labeled a troublemaker and discharged to placate the physician.

Critical Thinking Activity

If you were in Carrie's position, what would have been your next step? What are your alternatives? Who might serve as your advocate in this situation? Is there any other way the situation might have been handled for a more positive outcome? What would that have been?

When nurses are consistently faced with situations such as the one described above, it is referred to as the human condition of **moral distress**. Moral distress has been defined as occurring when one knows the ethically correct action to take but feels powerless to take that action (Epstein & Delgado, 2010). The sources of moral distress are many and varied, but Saver (2009) has listed three common areas: end-of-life situations (particularly where there is disagreement about treatment), fair distribution of resources, and protecting patients' rights. Situations in which the patient or family make decisions that the nurse does not agree with and yet require the nurse's participation fall into this category. We discuss this in greater depth in Chapter 9.

Collective Bargaining Contracts

Collective bargaining contracts can protect nurses in making ethical decisions. By formalizing reasons and procedures for termination of employment, and outlining grievance measures to provide a mechanism by which the individual nurse can be protected, a contract may provide greater freedom. Others believe that contracts hamper individual freedom because of the lengthy processes that are required. See Chapter 5 for more discussion of collective bargaining and grievance measures.

Collegial Relationships

An excellent climate for ethical decision making can be provided when nurses who work together support one another, share in decision making, and present a unified approach to others. All too often, such relationships are lacking in healthcare institutions, especially as we move into a time when several generations of nurses are working in the same unit. Nurses feel alone and are not experienced in seeking and providing support to one another. Greater collaboration and support on the part of all nurses in this area might be rewarding and is certainly long overdue. This is discussed in greater detail in Chapter 13.

Authoritarian and Paternalistic Backgrounds

The historically authoritarian and paternalistic attitudes of physicians and hospitals often have relegated nurses, most of whom are women, to dependent and subservient roles. These role differentiations have discouraged nurses from taking independent stands on issues and continue to affect relationships in the healthcare field. In some settings, ethical decisions are made without the participation of nurses, yet nurses are expected to implement the decisions.

More nurses are speaking out against an approach that leaves them out of the decision-making process. Nurses today might expect a physician to discuss the possibly futile treatment of a critically ill patient with the patient, family, and nursing staff. The patient would be encouraged to express personal needs, the family's views would be included, and the nurses' input would be part of the decision-making process regarding the medical plan of care. The advent of ethics committees, in which nurses have a voice, has created a positive environment for discussions in many institutions.

Institutional Supports for Ethical Behavior

An institution or organization that recognizes the individuality of all employees and treats them with respect in regard to decisions may provide a working climate that supports ethical behavior. When nurses are respected and there is no fear of reprisal or adverse response, ethical concerns can be voiced and issues raised.

For years, many hospitals have had ethics committees composed of physicians. With a major goal of monitoring physician behavior, they acted when a physician's inappropriate behavior, such as arriving at the hospital intoxicated, was reported to them. Today, the structure and mission of ethics committees have enlarged considerably. Composition of the committee often includes physicians, nurses, social workers, hospital administrators, a community representative, an ethicist, a chaplain or minister, and perhaps an attorney.

Three major roles of the ethics committee include education, policy review and development, and case review. Through case review, the group provides guidance to the hospital community, patients, and their families on matters that may involve ethical concerns such as end-of-life care, consent for medical interventions when the patient is unable to participate in the discussion or decisions regarding the termination of treatment. Using their expertise and experience, the members of ethics committees help individuals who must make ethical decisions to identify whether they have all the relevant information, to determine other options they have not considered, and to compare the situation with basic ethical principles and theories. Often, the committee acts in an advisory capacity to medical staff members and families struggling with difficult decisions.

Consumer Involvement in Healthcare

With consumer involvement in healthcare, nurses again may face situations in which they are expected to take action based on the conclusions of others. Many nurses may find this problematic. For example, an elderly diabetic who has gangrene of the foot may refuse amputation, saying, "If I'm going to die, I'm going to die whole." The nurse, recognizing the lifesaving benefit of the amputation, may have difficulty maintaining effective communication and rapport with the patient and family because of his or her own conviction that an amputation is the best treatment. Mental health is another area in healthcare in which nurses may struggle. Patients may refuse to comply with the recommended treatment and, as a result, live in a homeless, psychiatrically unhealthy situation. This also is very difficult for family members.

A FRAMEWORK FOR ETHICAL DECISION MAKING

When faced with ethical decisions, most of us hope to find the right answers. Unfortunately, a right answer may not exist for everyone or every situation; such is the nature of dilemmas. However, you can proceed from a basic framework that encourages you to look beyond your first thoughts or feelings to basic issues. A great deal has been written about the decision-making process in the past two decades—more in recent years than before. Along with this, several models have been developed to assist us when ethics are involved (Curtin, 1978; Jameton, 1984; Milner, 1993; Thompson & Thompson, 1981; Velasquez, Moberg, Meyer, et al., 2009). Over time, the steps have remained somewhat alike, and you will see a similarity to the steps of the nursing process with which you are already familiar. When patients and families must make ethical decisions, you may assist them in working through this process within the framework of their own values.

Identify and Clarify the Ethical Problem

To define the ethical concern, the situation needs to be reviewed so as to gain as clear a perception of the problem as possible. What is the decision to be made? Does the decision involve a choice between good and bad? Two "goods"? Two "bads"? Could this be damaging to someone or some group? Who are the relevant parties to this decision? What are their values? Are there legal or institutional concerns? Consider what ethical principles might be involved. Are those principles in conflict? Who should assume responsibility for this decision? Is this an individual's decision or is it one in which a collaborative decision must be made? What is your role and relationship to the problem? Are there time constraints on making this decision? What other factors influence the decision? Once a clear picture of the problem has been achieved, more information can be gathered about the situation.

Gather Factual Data

It is important to have as much information about the unique situation as possible. The facts of the situation make a difference in what options are possible. Remember that there is no magic pattern or formula to facts in most situations; they are screened through each person's background and experience. What clearly appears to be a true fact to one person may seem to be opinion to another or perhaps even a falsehood. Therefore, seeking other viewpoints may help everyone involved to see the situation more clearly. Who are the relevant people in the situation and what are their concerns and perspectives? Have they all been consulted? Consider whether legal cases might affect decision making in this case.

Identify and Evaluate Options

Most ethical problems have more than one possible solution. If only one solution existed, there would be no ethical dilemma because there would be no choice. In some cases, more than one solution may be satisfactory; in others, none of the options will seem satisfactory. The more options identified, the more likely those involved will find one they can support. What is the range of actions that could be taken? What would be the anticipated outcome of those actions?

For each option, consider its impact on each person involved. Also think about the impact on society as a whole if this option were chosen. Consider the ethical theories presented and explore how each option compares with the basic principles of each theory. In this way, it might be determined that one option is basically a utilitarian approach (seeking the greatest good for the greatest number), whereas another clearly supports a deontological position of doing one's duty. Which option does the greatest good while at the same time doing the least harm? Which option respects the rights and dignity of all persons involved? Is one approach more appropriate than another in this situation? Is this approach in keeping with your own moral and ethical position? Helping others to explore these questions (without necessarily using the terminology of formal ethical theories) requires personal involvement and interpersonal skill.

Make a Decision

At some point, a decision must be made. Patients and families, as well as care providers, may find this difficult and, in some instances, painful. However, to not make a decision is, in fact, making a decision. There will never be enough time, data, or alternatives in some situations. No matter how thorough the analysis or how carefully people weigh all competing claims, there may still be uncomfortable feelings. When dealing with these feelings, it is helpful to plan ahead to the action that will be taken. What would a respected and admired individual say? This strategy may be helpful to you as well as to patients and families.

Act and Assess

Once a course of action is chosen, it must be carried out. This may involve working with others or personally carrying out plans. Patients and families need ongoing support as they carry out their decisions. Assess the outcomes as the processes go forward. Unforeseen outcomes are common in ethical situations. Share your thoughts and concerns with others as you proceed, and continue to seek new insights into the situation.

As you assess the outcome in any particular situation, consider its relevance for a wider range of situations and concerns. Use this situation as a foundation from which to grow and develop. Ask yourself, "What have I learned from this experience that will be useful in the future?" "What would I do in another situation?" "What would I change?"

SPECIFIC ETHICAL ISSUES RELATED TO THE PROFESSION OF NURSING

Some ethical issues of concern to nurses relate specifically to the nursing profession; others relate to bioethical issues confronting all of society. In this section, we discuss the issues facing nurses through commitment to the patient, commitment to personal excellence, and commitment to the nursing profession as a whole. Bioethical issues that relate to the whole society are discussed in Chapter 9. We present a definite viewpoint regarding ethics in the nursing profession. We feel strongly about the individual nurse's responsibility for nursing practice and place high value on personal integrity in professional relationships.

Commitment to the Patient

Nursing has a strong history of being committed to the well-being of patients who need care. Both codes of ethics—from the ANA and ICN—clearly point out the nurse's obligation to fulfill this commitment. In the past, this obligation has been used to try to persuade nurses that they must not be concerned for themselves, their working conditions, their salaries, or other aspects of their employment. However, rejection of the handmaiden philosophy and the adoption of more nurse autonomy do not require rejection of a basic philosophy that nursing is focused on providing patients and their families with support for growth toward maximum health and well-being. Patients can never become the objects of nursing care but must be approached as unique individuals who deserve concern, respect, and culturally competent care that evolves from evidence-based practice.

Commitment to Your Employer

Once you have accepted a position in a healthcare organization, you also have accepted the responsibilities that the position encompasses. Some of these responsibilities may be spelled out in the contract, if a formal contract exists between the employer and the employee. Others are more or less taken for granted. It is these latter responsibilities that can present problems.

Responsible Work Ethic

First, it is understood that you will arrive at work on time. When you arrive late, you obligate others to remain overtime to ensure continuous patient care. If you find yourself in an emergency situation that is going to cause you to be delayed, it is important that you notify your supervisor that you are going to be late.

Second, it is also expected that you will not abuse breaks or sick leave. When one extends a break beyond the usual time allowed, it jeopardizes the opportunity for others to have a full break. Your patients also receive less than optimum care if you are unavailable. Likewise, the fact that you have a given number of paid sick days each year does not mean that you are entitled to that many more days off. They are intended for use if you are ill. Often, it is difficult to find replacements when staff members do not report for work. This means that others must pick up additional work assignments and that the quality of care provided that day may be less than desired.

Many healthcare facilities operate 24 hours a day, 7 days a week. This means that there are at least two or three shifts to be covered, as well as weekends and holidays. Be prepared to take your share of weekend and holiday shifts, as well as evening and night rotations, without grumbling if this is part of the staffing pattern. Most employers have developed some system of rotation, with employees able to make requests for the time that works best for them. Some employees for whom the holiday carries less significance may prefer to work, especially if there is additional pay for those days.

If you work in an area where you have a fair amount of privacy, remember that you should not conduct personal business during your work shift. Scheduling appointments, telephoning friends or business associates, writing notes, and similar activities should occur during your break or after you have finished your shift.

When you decide to terminate your employment, it is expected that you will give appropriate notice. Please refer to Chapter 4 for further discussion regarding resignation.

Responsible Use of Supplies

Pilfering includes stealing in small amounts or stealing objects of little value. Many people who are scrupulously honest in other aspects of their lives do not recognize that taking small items from a place of employment is indeed theft. Employees often take home adhesive bandage strips, pens, and other such objects so routinely that they do not even consider whether this is right or wrong. This constant petty theft may total thousands of dollars, the cost of which must be passed on to those who pay the bills—the patients. As a leader in the care setting, the registered nurse (RN) is often in a position to communicate clearly to all employees that pilfering is unacceptable. The nurse can set an example of careful stewardship of the hospital supplies.

Sometimes removing supplies is an oversight rather than a planned action (Fig. 8.3). To make efficient use of time, nurses commonly place many small items such as alcohol wipes, extra Band-Aids, and pens in their pockets. One hospital unit found that its yearly supply budget for black pens was almost exhausted in the first 6 months of the year. The simple action of placing a basket in the lounge into which nurses dropped everything from their pockets before leaving cut the pen costs dramatically. Perhaps you can be equally creative in helping to solve such problems in your work setting.

As the costs of healthcare soar, it is important that everyone associated with healthcare be mindful of the use of resources. You can help reduce costs by being judicious in your use of resources. For example, supplies that will not be used should not be taken into patient rooms, only to be discarded later. Using extra linens such as bath towels to clean up spills adds to costs. Determining that a clean glove is acceptable rather than reaching for sterile gloves reduces costs. Ensuring that all charges are processed for supplies that are used is also important. Operating equipment in a knowledgeable manner to reduce breakage or repairs is the responsibility of all workers. When all persons do their part, the cumulative effect can be significant.

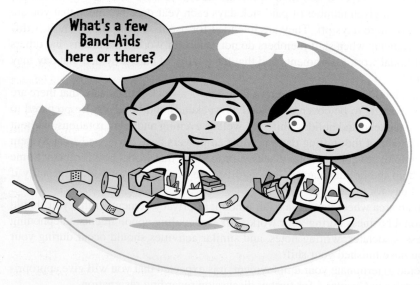

FIGURE 8.3 Many people who are otherwise scrupulously honest do not recognize that taking small items from a place of employment is theft.

Commitment to Your Colleagues

It has been suggested that a strategy to improve the nurse shortage is to improve the quality of the work environment. Many factors influence the climate of the work environment. One of the most noteworthy is our relationship with colleagues. As a new graduate, how do you affect this area?

One approach is to model those behaviors that you wish to see in others. Develop a collaborative approach. Maintain a positive attitude; respond to others in a pleasant, courteous manner; be sensitive to others; and be a positive ambassador for nursing. Be supportive of others and avoid opportunities to gossip about your colleagues and their activities. Compliment others on things they do well and provide assistance with things they are still learning. This is especially important as you become a more seasoned employee and have responsibility for helping to orient others. Give new employees time to learn skills that are new to them and to become efficient in their execution. Show care and compassion to fellow workers as well as to your clients.

Today, the workforce in nursing consists of individuals from four different generations, resulting in differences in attitudes, beliefs, work habits, and expectations (see Chapter 13). This can result in greater conflict in the workplace, especially in the area of work ethics and the use of technology. It is critical to the work environment that all nurses exhibit respect and tolerance for one another that will promote an atmosphere in which all viewpoints are considered legitimate (Sherman, 2006). All nurses must assume shared accountability for establishing and maintaining intergenerational relationships that foster a positive work environment. Nurses must seek to understand each generational cohort, communicating in a manner that will accommodate and capitalize on generational differences.

Commitment to Personal Excellence

Nurses must be committed to personal excellence and assume responsibility for maintaining competence. You are the one who is best able to identify your weaknesses and practice deficits as well as your strengths. Your careful and genuine self-evaluation is the patient's best protection against poor or inadequate care.

When we are truly honest with ourselves in the self-evaluation process, we often uncover areas we wish were not there. These weaknesses, once identified, provide the greatest opportunity for growth and improvement. Fortunately, when it is done informally, these weaknesses do not have to be shared with anyone. On the other hand, do not hesitate to ask for assistance if you think you need it.

Many institutions now include self-evaluation and the establishment of personal goals in the formal evaluation of employees. In this process, you might be asked to prepare a written self-evaluation that will be shared with your immediate supervisor and may be incorporated into your records.

So how do you proceed? One approach to self-evaluation is the use of the nursing process format. Begin with a thorough personal assessment, objectively gathering data about your own performance and keeping notes on yourself. For example, if you want to increase your efficiency in carrying out treatments, you may want to time yourself on several occasions to determine how long you are taking and whether you improved with performance.

After data have been collected, give yourself time to analyze it thoroughly. The self-assessment outline includes questions you should ask yourself (Display 8.3); however, the

DISPLAY 8.3 Self-Evaluation Plan

Assessment of Patients
- Do I gather enough data about patients and families, including both strengths and deficits?
- Is there sufficient depth and breadth in the data I gather?
- Do I listen closely to the patient and attend to what is being said?
- Do I regularly use all available sources for information about my patients (eg, patient, family, other staff, chart, Kardex)?
- Have I recognized problems quickly so that they did not become worse through inattention?
- Do I recognize physiologic, social, and psychological problems?
- Is my assessment free of personal biases and viewpoints?
- Do I separate relevant from irrelevant data?

Planning for Patient Care
- Do I routinely seek more information on which to base decisions about patient care?
- Are my assumptions correct?
- Do I include the patient in decision making whenever possible?
- Do I consult with others on the healthcare team when planning?
- Are my written plans clear, concise, and reasonable to carry out?
- Do I take into account the realities of the situation when planning care?
- Are my plans for care sound and appropriate to the individual patient?
- Do I employ principles from the biologic and social sciences in planning?
- Have I considered all alternatives?

Intervention
- Is my work organized and finished on time?
- Do I maintain optimum safe working habits?
- Do I perform technical skills in an efficient and safe manner?
- Do I communicate clearly and effectively with patients, family, and staff?
- Do I use therapeutic communication techniques appropriately and effectively?
- Do I use teaching approaches appropriate to the individual patient and family?
- Do I keep accurate and complete written records?
- Do I understand and perform any administrative tasks that are my responsibility (eg, ordering supplies, planning for laboratory tests)?
- Do I make the effort to learn about new techniques and procedures?
- Do I function as a team player?
- Do I incorporate critical thinking into all of my activities?

Evaluation
- Do I routinely evaluate the effectiveness of the nursing care I give?
- Do I effectively assist in evaluation of the patient's response to medical care and to ordered therapies?
- Do I encourage the patient to participate in evaluating both the process and the outcome of care?
- Have I evaluated all aspects of care fair-mindedly?

Personal Growth and Relationships
- Have I established a sound trust and working relationship with coworkers?
- Do I support and assist my coworkers when possible?
- Do I communicate effectively with others on the healthcare team?

DISPLAY 8.3 **Self-Evaluation Plan** (continued)

- Do I seek answers to questions for which I have no answer?
- Have I sought opportunities for learning and personal growth?
- Is my attitude helpful and productive?
- Do I have sound working habits (eg, appearing on time, limiting coffee and lunch breaks to the correct time)?
- Is my appearance appropriate to the working environment?
- Do I use appropriate channels of communication within the institution?
- Do I handle criticism constructively?
- Do personal biases interfere with the care that I provide or my relationship with colleagues?
- Am I doing my share in overall professional activities (eg, serving on committees, assisting with development projects)?
- Am I honest with myself, being neither too harsh nor too easy on myself?
- Do I have personal values and beliefs that interfere with providing quality nursing care?

criteria that you use to determine whether your answers reflect the quality of performance you want to attain are not included. Those specific criteria must be individualized to the setting in which you work and the nature of your role in that setting. For example, the breadth of data that represent excellent practice for the nurse in the emergency department differs from what would represent excellence for the nurse working in a rehabilitation setting. Thus, criteria specific to your work situation are needed.

Your analysis can reveal strengths, weaknesses, and areas for growth or improvement. Congratulate yourself on the strengths identified and then clearly delineate those areas in which you want to change or to improve. Identifying and stating the problems or growth needed helps you to plan more effectively, just as it has in nursing care planning.

Next, establish a plan of action. The plan will be more helpful to you if it contains clearly defined goals. Once the goals are set, you will be better able to plan the appropriate action and timeline to meet them. You might consider such things as requesting in-service education, taking continuing education courses, consulting with colleagues, and doing independent reading and study. Some plans need to include specific things related to your daily nursing care. To do this, you may want to request assignments that provide opportunities for practice of the desired skills. Perhaps you are interested in transferring to a specialty area of care. This will involve communication with your immediate supervisor and may involve enrolling in special classes.

Implementing this plan will require you to remain focused on what you are trying to accomplish. Keeping records on your progress is often helpful and provides positive reinforcement when you realize that some of your goals have been met.

Periodic evaluation of your progress is necessary so that you do not become discouraged. Sometimes it is hard to identify gradual change. Any records you have kept are valuable for this purpose. Plan rewards for yourself for improvement that occurs. Try not to become discouraged if you do not see the improvement you desire. Remember that just as a reassessment and a new plan are often necessary in patient care planning, a revised plan also may be needed in the self-evaluation process. Keep in mind that your overall goal is personal excellence in nursing practice.

Commitment to the Nursing Profession

Commitment to the nursing profession requires that each individual nurse be concerned not only about personal performance but also about how nursing is practiced. This involves participation in formal and informal evaluation of nursing care, dealing with poor care, and identifying the impaired nurse. Nurses always have evaluated one another in both formal and informal ways. The main purpose of peer evaluation is to maintain consistent high-quality nursing care and not simply noting error or deficiency. This is an ethical, professional obligation.

Formal Evaluation

Formal evaluation of nursing care occurs in most settings under the title of quality assurance and quality improvement. Quality assurance is a planned program of evaluation that includes ongoing monitoring of the care given and outcomes of care. It includes a mechanism for instituting change when problems or opportunities for improvement are identified. Quality assurance programs are required by The Joint Commission (see Chapter 6). Special nursing projects such as the work done on nursing outcomes (see Chapter 1) have a focus on the quality of care provided.

All types of evaluation first call for establishing specific criteria to be used in the evaluation. These criteria may refer to process, outcome, or both. The creation of the criteria is a professional nursing responsibility.

The process begins by determining whether the nursing actions taken are complete and appropriate. Criteria developed to evaluate this aspect are called process criteria. One basis for developing process criteria is *Nursing Professional Development Practice: Scope and Standards of Practice*, published by the ANA (2010), which is a revised version of *Standards of Clinical Nursing Practice*, published in 1991 and again in 1998 and 2004. General standards refer to all settings; more specific ones exist for more than 20 specialty areas of nursing. Some specialty organizations, such as the Intravenous Nurses Society, also have published standards that refer to their specialty.

Another basis for formal evaluation is the use of outcome criteria for patient care. Outcome criteria are specific, observable patient behaviors or clinical manifestations that are the desired results of care. *Nursing Professional Development Practice: Scope and Standards of Practice* identifies six standards of nursing practice, one of which is outcomes identification (ANA, 2010).

Typically, nurses working in groups develop the criteria. They consult nursing literature so that they establish the appropriate criteria. Several methods have been used to evaluate both the process and the outcomes of nursing care. These may include conferences designed to discuss the matter to be evaluated, interviews with patients or staff, direct observation of patients, and review of the record. This record review, which is gaining wider acceptance in nursing, involves comparing the patient record with the criteria and is often completed by medical records personnel. The accuracy of the review depends on the adequacy (that is, the completeness) of the documentation. If information does not appear in the record (other than situations in which "charting by exception" are employed), then, for the purposes of the audit, the appropriate observations were not made or the actions were not taken.

This is just one of the reasons why you must recognize the importance of your documentation and make sure that you maintain a high standard in records. The record review has raised serious concerns, which have resulted in greater attention to documentation and even revision of record systems. Nurses then have taken the initiative to determine the meaning of the data in relationship to enhanced patient well-being. Changes in policies and procedures and in-service education classes often occur. Once remedial action has been taken, reevaluation is done to determine its effectiveness.

Informal Evaluation

An important day-to-day evaluation of patient care occurs informally as peers observe the performance of others. Watching other nurses also helps you to grow in your own practice. When you observe coworkers, strive for objectivity. A common mistake is to let personal feelings influence what we see, such as viewing a close friend in a positive light or seeing only the negative aspects of a nurse with whom we have a poor relationship. Remember to examine the results or outcomes of care. Two nurses may use different approaches or techniques in similar situations, but both may achieve positive results. In most instances, you will see good care. Do not hesitate to commend others and share your positive feelings. Everyone benefits from positive reinforcement of skill; it helps nurses to create a good climate for personal growth and sharing.

Addressing Substandard Care

Concern for the welfare of patients requires that nurses acknowledge the existence of substandard care and work toward improving that situation. It is not a matter of whether the nurse should become involved, but rather how to most effectively accomplish the goals of better care.

If faced with a situation where patient care is less than desired, consider whose care you are criticizing. If it is the care of another nurse, or a care provider with less educational preparation than you possess, the situation is more straightforward. If you have questions about medical care delivered or the action of a physician, it becomes more difficult, because medical actions are outside the scope of practice of nursing. Be careful about how you proceed, referring to hospital policy manuals, trusted colleagues, your supervisor, or possibly the chief of the medical staff for advice before taking action.

When you observe a colleague practicing what you think is poor patient care, such as poor sterile technique, it is not as difficult. The action you choose to take will depend on the seriousness of the situation you have observed. Usually, the simplest and most effective solution is to go directly to the person involved and discuss what you have observed. As mentioned in other sections of this textbook, this should occur in a private setting, away from others, and as soon after the occurrence as possible. This approach allows the nurse to give a rationale for the action taken. When you understand the situation more fully, you may have a different point of view. If you disagree with your colleague and the situation is not critical, you might want to state simply that you disagree. If the situation is critical, the two of you will want to seek resources that will outline the best approach. If you observe poor care a second time, and it has been determined that your colleague's care is substandard, you should again approach the person. State what you have seen and note that it is the second time. If the person still disagrees that a problem exists, state that you feel obligated to discuss this with your immediate superior because it is not in the best interest of the patient. You should then follow through on this.

If you have a reputation on the unit for maintaining a focus that enhances the welfare of patients, and you have been quick to praise the good care provided by others, your action in response to poor care will be more readily accepted. Remember that your attitude when approaching another nurse is crucial. Facial expressions and tone of voice, as well as words, need to be considered. If you are perceived as friendly and caring, your comments probably will be accepted in a far different manner than if you are seen as being negative and critical.

However, you cannot always count on this reaction. Many nurses feel threatened by the idea of evaluation or have had bad experiences in which evaluation only involved pointing out deficiencies. These nurses may be angry and upset with any colleague who considers evaluation part of the colleague role. Therefore, it is wise to have thought out how you will proceed.

A Basic Pattern for Action. The first step to be taken in any situation in which you believe substandard care exists is to collect adequate, valid information on behavior that you have personally observed. Do not make decisions based on gossip, hearsay, or an isolated instance, unless the single incident was very serious. If this is the case, be certain of your facts before taking action.

Also be certain you understand both the formal and the informal systems of authority and responsibility within your facility and the laws of the state in which you practice. In some states, laws exist requiring that poor practice be reported directly to the relevant licensing board. In others, reporting to your supervisor is considered adequate reporting. You need to know which people have the authority to make decisions and changes, what the official prescribed route of change is, and what the hidden priorities of the institution might be. It is most commonly recommended that once you are certain of your data and know how the system works in your organization, you should take concerns to your immediate supervisor, who would forward the concern until it reached the individual or body with the authority and duty to act. Many people believe that reporting to a supervisor fulfills your ethical responsibility as well as your legal responsibility.

When you approach a supervisor, give specific information that includes the dates, the situations, and the action you took. Do not indulge in generalities or sweeping statements; stick to specific observed instances by simply describing what you saw. Let the supervisor know that you have talked with the person under discussion and have informed the person that you would speak with the supervisor. It is important to specify the action you would like to see occur. You might ask the supervisor to discuss the matter with both of you, or you might ask the supervisor to discuss the matter with the other nurse or observe the nurse. It is also important to remember that once you have initiated this action, you may or may not be involved in some follow-up. You may never learn what was done, even when positive action was taken, because of the constraints of confidentiality for the affected employee. If the manager decides to observe and take corrective action, that will be confidential for the employee involved. Occasionally, results emerge only much later, when a change in procedure and policy occurs.

If you observe an incident that has the potential to cause a patient danger (eg, an unreported medication error) or one that has legal ramifications (eg, the falsifying of narcotic records), you have a legal as well as an ethical responsibility to go immediately to a supervisor with your information. In a situation that has the potential for legal involvement, keep an exact personal record of your observations and actions. Include in the record the times and dates of incidents and of your reporting efforts (see Chapter 7).

Alternative Approaches for Action. At times, the system does not always work as expected. Your concern regarding what you perceive as poor practice may be dropped or ignored at any one of many points.

Often, there are good reasons for this. Perhaps, the persons in authority want to collect more specific data about a situation, with as little general discussion as possible. Sometimes, there are aspects of a legal contract or a collective bargaining contract of which you are unaware that must be considered in the actions that are taken. Other times, professional confidentiality may make it seem that nothing is being done, when, in fact, steps have been taken to correct a situation. It is easy as a newcomer to the healthcare scene to see only part of a picture. Simply checking back with a manager, acknowledging that information may be confidential, and asking for reassurance that the matter is being addressed may be an appropriate action.

If your initial approach is not effective, a formal route for seeking further change would lead you through the official lines of authority within your facility. After discussing your concern with your immediate supervisor and receiving no satisfactory response, tell the supervisor formally that you intend to carry your concern to the next higher authority. Informing your supervisor of your plans should help to avoid problems, but be prepared to listen to some words of warning from the supervisor or efforts to discourage you from taking action. There are reasons this individual has chosen not to pursue the issue; some of these may be valid.

However, there are times when an alternative approach is more appropriate than formal action. Another route for seeking further change is through designated committees or procedures within your facility. As hospitals move into models of shared governance, this may be your best alternative. Discussing or sharing a problem (without naming names) with a particular committee might require a carefully written and documented report explaining your concern. You then might be called to answer questions that the committee believes are important.

You may volunteer to serve on committees that deal with peer review. If there are no such committees, you may work to have them established, perhaps through a bargaining unit. This route of action will require a considerable investment of your own time and effort, a factor you need to consider.

Another alternative approach is to use the informal system within the facility. You may discuss your concern with a trusted person (or mentor) who has influence within the system. You may learn that you are not alone in your concerns, that efforts toward change are being made, and that your input of data is welcomed. Another approach would be to seek the assistance of another individual with power within the organization. However, we must caution you about using informal systems, as they can backfire. Therefore, we suggest that you use these alternative approaches only when the ones suggested earlier have failed to bring about the desired results.

A final alternative to a problem in your work setting is to offer your resignation if a change is not made. Continuing to work in an environment in which poor practice exists may place you in conflict with your ethical standards and values. If you find it necessary to do this, be careful that you do not jeopardize your own future with angry letters or intemperate remarks. Render your resignation in a polite and professional manner, even when expressing dissatisfaction with the system.

Reporting directly to a state licensing board or professional organization's disciplinary committee is an avenue of action outside of the employment setting. The licensing board exists to assure the public of safe practice; therefore, these organizations and agencies usually deal with serious problems that represent a breach of the public trust or serious harm. They may not have the capacity or desire to pursue minor (though still important) problems. The same constraints apply when reporting to these organizations. Remember that their investigation and decisions may be done in a judicial or legal manner. This may involve the requirement that you provide legal testimony regarding your complaints.

Personal Risks in Reporting. If you decide to pursue any of these routes, be fully aware of the possible consequences. You may be labeled a troublemaker, or worse. You may lose the opportunity to be promoted because you are seen as being antagonistic to the system. Although officially it should not happen, it is possible that you could lose your job for raising too many issues. We do not mean to be unduly discouraging, but we want to warn you that the role of change agent is not easy, and you should be aware of the consequences and weigh them before you decide to act. Above all, be certain that your perceptions are correct and that your concerns are well grounded.

Whistleblowing. The ultimate step one might take in a situation in which negligence or maltreatment is allowed to persist would be whistleblowing. **Whistleblowing** is an effort made by a member or past member of an organization to warn the public about a serious wrongdoing or danger created or masked by the organization (Lachman, 2008). In healthcare, Ray (2006) has identified whistleblowing as the revelation of an ethical failure in which the organization has lost its moral compass. Lachman (2008) emphasizes the importance of establishing an ethical organizational culture. In the business world, whistleblowing that resulted in high-profile cases involving manipulation of gas prices, breast implants, accounting fraud, and insider trading alerted the public to ethical wrongdoing. If you encounter a situation that you consider so serious that whistleblowing actions need to be taken, do so only after thoughtful consideration, because exposing unethical and incompetent healthcare providers is not without risk. The worst-case scenario might be legal retaliation; an individual identified as giving substandard care might sue you for slander, which could be expensive to defend. There may be unpleasant reactions from coworkers or you may place your job in jeopardy. Some states have enacted legislation that protects nurses and other healthcare staff members from retaliation when they report a case, but others have not. There is no federal legislation that specifically protects nurses.

Because there can be serious ramifications to whistleblowing, do not go public until all the avenues to address concerns through the system have been exhausted, with no response. The following should guide your activities:

* Consider contacting an attorney before taking any steps.
* Learn as much as you can about your state's policies by contacting your state nurses association, the ANA, or your state board of nursing.
* Be certain of your facts and have them well documented. Be confident that a wrongdoing has occurred.
* As you pursue your concern within the system, follow the healthcare organization's chain of command.
* Be professional when dealing with others.

Recommending a Care Provider

Patients and acquaintances may ask you to recommend a physician or other care provider because they believe that, as a nurse, you have special knowledge and insight in such matters. If you have no personal knowledge about the requested information, then honestly tell the individual requesting information that you have no personal or professional knowledge regarding a particular care provider. However, if you do have knowledge, you could recommend several competent persons, pointing out characteristics of each that might be factors in personal choice.

▶ *EXAMPLE*

Recommending an Obstetrician

Your next door neighbor exuberantly greets you when you return from work one after-noon with the news that she believes she is pregnant. Because you work in the Birthing Rooms at the local hospital she asks you if you can recommend an obstetrician. After letting her know you, too, are excited about the news, you state, "There are three who are very popular at our facility. One is an older physician who has a fairly traditional approach to childbirth, another is a young and innovative physician who strongly advo-cates partner participation and natural childbirth, and the third is new in the community but appears to allow patients a great deal of choice in their approach to childbirth." After this, you explore with her some of her expectations regarding care and allow her to make a personal choice.

If you are asked specifically about a physician whose care you believe to be less than satisfac-tory, you are faced with a different dilemma. Making severely critical statements might leave you open to a legal charge of slander by the physician (see Chapter 7). However, saying noth-ing is ethically a problem because you are not acting to protect the patient. A safe approach is to state, "I personally would prefer to see Dr. N or Dr. O rather than Dr. X." If pressed to give reasons, you are legally more secure if you say that you would prefer not to discuss specifics or to focus the conversation on the strengths of the doctors you have recommended.

Be careful that any recommendations are not based on hearsay or gossip. If you do not have solid information on which to base a referral, do not be drawn into making one. Being a nurse does not obligate you to be an expert on all healthcare questions.

THE CHEMICALLY IMPAIRED PROFESSIONAL

Chemically impaired professional is a term used to describe that person whose practice has deteriorated because of chemical abuse, specifically, the use of alcohol and drugs. The terms addiction, drug addiction, alcoholism, chemical dependency, and chemical impairment are all names that we associate with the dependence on alcohol, drugs, or other substances. Addiction has been defined as compulsive need for and use of a habit-forming substance (such as heroin, nicotine, or alcohol) characterized by tolerance and by well-defined physiological symptoms upon withdrawal (Merriam-Webster Online Dictionary, 2010).

Dependency refers to the strong desire and impaired control over the use of a substance despite the consequences associated with continued use (Wood, 2006). There is a strong pos-sibility that if you remain active in the profession, at some time you will find yourself working with a chemically impaired colleague; perhaps you already have.

Chemical Impairment in Healthcare Professionals

One would like to believe that nurses, who have studied the physiologic effects of alcohol and drugs on the system, would avoid such abuse. However, this is not the case. As a result of increasing concern about the problem, in the 1980s, nurses began to collect data on the topic (Bissell & Haberman, 1984; Bissell & Skorina, 1987; Sullivan, Bissell, & Williams, 1988). Later studies explored the probable use of alcohol among nursing students (Campbell & Polk,

1992; Marion, Fuller, Johnson, et al., 1996; Sullivan, Bissell, & Leffler, 1990). Some studies would suggest that the prevalence of substance abuse is no higher in healthcare professionals than in the general population, but given the responsibility to the public and the risk of error, it is a serious concern (Kenna & Lewis, 2008).

Later studies examined what substances were abused and in which areas of healthcare the abusers most frequently were employed (Trinkoff, Eaton, & Anthony, 1991; Trinkoff & Storr, 1998). The prevalence of use of all substances was 32%, with emergency nurses 3.5 times as likely to use marijuana or cocaine, oncology and administration nurses twice as likely to engage in binge drinking, and psychiatric nurses most likely to smoke.

Why are nurses affected by this problem? Factors that lead to chemical dependency include the stress of the nursing profession, particularly in intensive care units and emergency departments. Frequent shift changes and staffing shortages resulting in excessive overtime add to the situation. Musculoskeletal injuries and pain and knowledge of medications also contribute to the abuse as do unrealistic personal expectations, frustration, powerlessness, anxiety, and depression. Once the problem exists, denial is a big part of the disease.

All areas of the profession are affected by the problem of chemical dependency in nursing. A significant financial impact, in the forms of sickness, absenteeism, tardiness, accidents, errors, decreased productivity, and staff turnover, is realized by institutions that employ nurses with dependency problems. Problems related to drug abuse are complicated by the fact that the nurse often obtains drugs from the supply available on the hospital unit and is therefore in violation of the Controlled Substances Act. As with other healthcare conditions, early recognition and treatment have been recommended to help offset this problem.

Since 1981, the ANA has worked with the problems of chemical abuse, first establishing a task force to review the concern and then, in 1990, developing suggested state legislation focusing on voluntary treatment rather than disciplinary action (ANA, 1990). Since that time, over 40 states have alternatives to disciplinary action, including peer assistance and recovery monitoring programs (Maher-Brisen, 2007).

Recognizing the Chemically Impaired Nurse

The concerns about the chemically impaired nurse are twofold. The first is a personal concern for the nurse who is afflicted: The illness may go undetected and untreated for years. The second concern is for the patient, whose care is jeopardized by the nurse whose judgment and skills are weakened, thus increasing the possibility of errors.

The major avenue for identifying impaired nurses is through nonimpaired coworkers. However, nurses, by virtue of their education, are socialized into caring roles and have not always dealt with the problem in a straightforward fashion. The impaired nurse was often protected, transferred, ignored, and, in some instances, promoted. None of these actions helped solve the problem. As you enter the nursing field, be aware of the following characteristics, which are commonly seen in impaired healthcare practitioners:

- Mood swings
- Inappropriate behavior
- Frequent days off for implausible reasons
- Noncompliance with acceptable policies and procedures
- Deteriorating appearance

- Inconsistent job performance
- Inadequate documentation
- Unusual prescribing practices
- Alcohol on breath
- Poor judgment, concentration
- Dishonesty
- Missed appointments
- Boundary violations

(Washington Health Professional Services, 2006)

Reporting the Chemically Impaired Colleague

As an RN, what should you do if you suspect that a colleague has a chemical dependency problem? First of all, you need to know what the law in your state requires of you. In many states, every professional is legally obligated to report a chemically dependent healthcare professional. This reporting most commonly is done through channels at the place of employment but also may be done directly to the state board of nursing. If you do not know the requirements, you should immediately learn what they are. In some states, failure to report can result in disciplinary action toward you.

When planning to report, you do not have to be sure beyond any doubt that a problem exists. You need to have enough data to present a reasonable concern. The investigation to clearly establish the problem is the responsibility of the employing agency or the state board.

To establish reasonable concern, collect and document data, including objective facts, dates, and times when the situation occurred. For several good reasons, you should not confront the person whom you suspect at this time.

First, the person may become more secretive about the behavior because of the danger of being caught. This will make collection of data difficult, if not impossible. Personal defenses and denial may become stronger. The suspected person may ask for a transfer to another shift or to a different part of the facility, or, if truly feeling threatened, may seek employment in another facility.

Second, the person may feel attacked and rejected. To ensure that it will not end in a disaster, a confrontation needs the support of an appropriate and knowledgeable healthcare professional to ensure that the individual is guided to appropriate choices for treatment and rehabilitation. If the person is someone you know well, who confides in you regarding personal problems and is likely to follow your suggestions, you might use those occasions to refer the individual to appropriate resources for personal assistance and counseling.

Another reason why you should not confront the suspected person at this time is that you are still collecting data and documenting them. You cannot be sure from a single observation that a problem exists. There are often reasons why things are not what we initially perceived them to be.

Once you feel you have data to support a realistic concern, report them to a supervisor to validate your observations. Usually, once you have notified your supervisor, he or she will assume responsibility for the problem, but may ask for your continued assistance with data collection or with confrontation (see earlier discussion on reporting to your supervisor).

Once adequate information has been gathered, agency administrative personnel will notify the state board of nursing. In addition, they usually must notify the state board of pharmacy if drugs are involved. More investigation will be carried out; records will be examined. If a problem exists, actions appropriate to the situation will be taken. These usually include a carefully planned confrontation by an intervention team, a requirement that treatment be sought, and a presentation of the consequences of not seeking treatment.

The worst thing you can do if you suspect a problem is to ignore it or help a colleague cover for inadequacies. The colleague will not get better if the problem is not recognized and treated. The longer the delay, the greater the chance that an innocent patient will be placed in jeopardy.

Fortunately, help and rehabilitation are being made available to those who need it through state nurses associations and state licensing authorities. These programs usually provide a specific contractual agreement regarding professional practice during the treatment and monitoring period. This is often done without formal disciplinary proceedings. The goal of this process is restoration of the individual to effective functioning.

In some states, the licensing boards may institute formal disciplinary proceedings to suspend a license or issue a license with limitations on practice, and to provide monitoring and supervision while the individual seeks treatment. When treatment is completed, the board may reinstate the license with temporary limitations and continued monitoring and support. The goal is the eventual full rehabilitation of the healthcare professional to the service of the community. Reporting a chemically dependent colleague may be the most caring action you can take.

If, as a nursing student, you suspect that a fellow classmate (or worse yet, an instructor) has a problem with chemical abuse, you would be wise to discuss your concerns with your instructor (or with the director of the program if you suspect an instructor). Because such problems typically worsen with time, the earlier they are addressed and corrected, the better it is for everyone. Again, it is important that you have accurate information to report, along with times, dates, and examples of the behavior that caused your concern.

Critical Thinking Activity

Assume that you have serious concerns that a colleague is delivering poor patient care because of problems with chemical dependency. Where would you begin? What is your personal responsibility? What is your responsibility to your colleague? What is your responsibility to the patients? What steps should you take? Do you have a personal liability in the situation?

BOUNDARY VIOLATIONS

The term **boundary violations** is used to refer to situations in which nurses move beyond a professional relationship and become personally involved with a patient and the patient's life. It is of particular concern because it represents a violation of the trust relationship that exists between the patient and the nurse. In nurse–patient relationships, the nurse necessarily holds power, creating a vulnerable situation for the patient. The nurse also has access to confidential and privileged information about patients and their families. It is the nurse's responsibility to define the boundaries of the relationships and ensure that they are maintained. The nurse must be warm and empathetic but should not try to be friends with the patient (Fig. 8.4).

Perhaps the most extreme boundary violation is professional sexual misconduct. Professional sexual misconduct has been defined as "a specific type of professional misconduct which involves the use of power, influence and/or special knowledge that is inherent in one's profession in order to obtain sexual gratification from the people that a particular profession is intended to serve" (National Council of State Boards of Nursing, 2009).

Although sexual misconduct is the major focus of this concern, boundary violations expand into other areas of conduct, such as overidentifying with a particular family member or moving into pseudofamily relationships with the patient's family. If this happens, the family may question the nurse's motives, wondering whether the nurse is looking for a bequest in a will or other tangible benefit. Such overinvolvement will interfere with the nurse's personal life and even could result in legal actions on the part of the family.

Some early indications that boundaries are beginning to break down include situations in which the nurse spends extended time with a patient beyond assigned duties or visits the patient when not on duty. Showing favoritism or possessiveness of a patient, meeting patients in isolated areas in a manner that has nothing to do with direct patient care, or personal disclosure by the care provider are other indicators that boundaries are being violated (Ellis & Hartley, 2009).

It is important that you are able to recognize situations in which a colleague may cross sexual boundaries. If you believe sexual misconduct is occurring on the unit where you are employed, the steps you would follow are similar to those you learned to use in dealing with chemical abuse. It is extremely important that you document the behavior carefully, noting dates, times, and the names of the individuals involved. Keep your documentation focused on factual information and objective data. You would then share this information with your immediate supervisor.

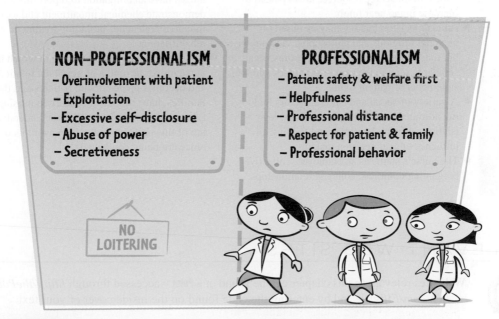

FIGURE 8.4 Everyone benefits when boundaries are clearly established and maintained.

KEY CONCEPTS

- Ethics is a branch of philosophy referred to as moral philosophy. It seeks to provide answers to some of the questions of human conduct that arise in our life, and attempts to determine what is right or good.
- Inherent in the study of ethics is an appreciation of individual values that are derived from societal norms, religion, and family orientation. We can better understand our own value system through the process of values clarification.
- The basic ethical concepts of beneficence, non-maleficence, autonomy, justice, fidelity, veracity, and the standard of best interest underlie ethical decision making and may be in conflict in an individual situation.
- The ethical theories of utilitarianism, deontology, natural law, and social equity and justice may be used to examine the implications of ethical decisions.
- The concept of justice has been expanded to include distributive justice that is applied in situations requiring the allocation of scarce resources. The problems associated with the allocation of scarce resources are expected to increase in the near future.
- Ethical decision making may be based on personal religious and philosophic viewpoints, but must always be grounded in professional standards seen in the Codes for Nurses and the statements of patient rights.
- A variety of social and cultural factors including attitudes, science and technology, legislation, judicial decisions, and funding all influence ethical decision making.
- The nurse's status as an employee, collective bargaining contracts, collegial relationships,

the authoritarian and paternalistic backgrounds of healthcare, deliberations of ethics committees, and consumer involvement create pressures regarding ethical decision making.
- A basic framework for ethical decision making emphasizes identifying and clarifying the problem, gathering data, identifying options, making a decision, acting, and assessing.
- Nurses have ethical obligations to the patient and to the employer and must maintain an objective stance regarding other healthcare providers, and when confronting substandard care. Commitment to personal excellence and to the profession of nursing are also desired characteristics of the professional nurse.
- In serious situations, when using the chain of command doesn't invoke response to voiced concerns, one might use whistleblowing to bring attention to the circumstances. This should be used as a last resort because of the possible ramifications to the individual blowing the whistle.
- The chemically impaired nurse is a concern to the profession and a danger to patients. All nurses have an obligation to report those who demonstrate chemical impairment and to assist impaired colleagues in finding treatment and rehabilitation.
- Boundary violations, a situation in which the nurse moves beyond a professional relationship and becomes involved with patients and their families, have become a concern in nursing. Educational programs to increase understanding of this problem and to help avoid its occurrence are being conducted.

RELEVANT WEB SITES

Web sites relevant to this chapter can be found at **thePoint** accessed through *http://thePoint. lww.com/Ellis10e* and by entering the code found on the inside cover of your text.

REFERENCES

American Hospital Association. (1992). *A patient's bill of rights*. Chicago, IL: Author.

American Nurses Association. (1990). Suggested state legislation: Nursing Practice Act, Nursing Disciplinary Diversion Act, Prescriptive Authority Act (Pub. No. NP-78). Washington, DC: Author.

American Nurses Association. (2001). *Code for nurses with interpretive statements*. Silver Spring, MD: Nursesbooks.org.

American Nurses Association. (2010). *Nursing: Scope and standards of nursing practice*. Silver Spring, MD: Author.

Bennis, W. (2009). *The essential Bennis*. San Francisco, CA: Jossey Bass—A Wiley Imprint.

Bissell, L., & Haberman, P. W. (1984). *Alcoholism in the professions*. New York, NY: Oxford University Press.

Bissell, L., & Skorina, J. (1987). 100 alcoholic women in medicine. *Journal of the American Medical Association, 257*(2), 939–944.

Boyd, A. D. (2006). *Physician-assisted suicide: For and against*. Retrieved August 10, 2010, from willamette.edu/cla/.../Physician-Assisted Suicide.htm

Campbell, A. R., & Polk, F. (1992). *Legal and ethical issues of alcohol and other substance abuse in nursing education*. Atlanta, GA: Southern Council on Collegiate Education for Nursing.

Chaffee, M. W. (2006). Making the decision to report to work in a disaster. *American Journal of Nursing, 106*(9), 54–57.

Curtin, L. (1978). A proposed model for critical ethical analysis. *Nursing Forum, 17*(1), 12–17.

Distributive Justice. (2010). Retrieved January 10, 2010, from http:legal-dictionary.thefreedictionary.com/Distributive+justice

Ellis, J. R., & Hartley, C. L. (2009). *Managing and coordinating nursing care* (5th ed.). Philadelphia, PA: Wolters Kluwer· Lippincott Williams & Wilkins.

Epstein, E. G., & Delgado, S. (2010, September 30). Understanding and addressing moral distress. *Online Journal of Issues in Nursing, 15*(3), Manuscript 1. Retrieved October 8, 2010, from http://www.nursingworld.org/search.aspx?SearchMode=1&SearchPhrase=Moral+distress&SearchWithin=2

International Code for Nurses. (2006). *The code of ethics for nurses*. Geneva, Switzerland: Author.

Jameton, A. (1984). *Nursing practice: The ethical issues*. Englewood Cliffs, NJ: Prentice-Hall.

Kenna, G. A., & Lewis, D. C. (2008). Risk factors for alcohol and other drug use by healthcare professionals. *Substance Abuse Treatment, prevention, and Policy 3*(e-article 3), 2008 Abstract. Retrieved August 10, 2010, from http://www.projectcork.org select bibliographies, from list selectImpariedProfessionals

Lachman, V. D. (2008). Whistleblowing: Role of organizational culture in prevention and management. *Demotological Nursing, 20*(5), 394–398. Retrieved August 10, 2010, from http://www.medscape.com/viewarticle/582796_5

Maher-Brisen, P. (2007). Addition: An occupational hazard in nursing. *American Journal of Nursing, 107*(8), 78–79.

Marion, L. N., Fuller, S. G., Johnson, N. P., Michels, P. J., & Diniz, C. (1996). Drinking problems of nursing students. *Journal of Nursing Education, 35*(5), 196–203.

Milner, S. (1993). An ethical nursing practice model. *Journal of Nursing Administration, 23*(3), 22–25.

Merriam-Webster Online dictionary. (2011) addiction. Retrieved April 9, 2011 from http:www.merriam-webster.com/dictionary/addition

Merriam-Webster Online Dictionary.(2011) beneficent. Retrieved April 9, 2011 from http:www.merriam-webster.com/dictionary/beneficent

Merriam-Webster Online dictionary. (2011) futility. Retrieved April 9, 2011 from http:www.merriam-webster.com/dictionary/futility

National Association of Practical Nurse Education and Service. (2007). *NAPNES standards of practice for licensed practical/vocational nurses*. Falls Church, VA: Author.

National Council of State Boards of Nursing. (2009). *Practical Guidelines for Boards of Nursing on sexual misconduct cases*. Retrieved August 10, 2010, from www.ncsbn.org type Sexual_Misconduct into search box

Rawls, J. A. (1971). *Theory of justice*. Cambridge, MA: Harvard University Press.

Ray, S. L. (2006). Whistleblowing and organizational ethics. *Nursing Ethics, 13*(4), 438–445.

Saver, C. (2009). Life-and-death scenarios lead to moral distress in nurses. Retrieved August 18, 2009, from http://news.nurse.com/apps/pbcs.dll/article?AID=/20090601/NATIONAL01/90529002/-1/

Sherman, R. O. (2006). Leading a multigenerational nursing workforce: Issues, challenges and strategies. *Online Journal of Issues in Nursing, 11*(2), Manuscript 2. Retrieved August 10, 2010, from www.nursingworld.org click on OJIN - type Multignerational Nursing Workforce in the search box.

Sullivan, E., Bissell, L., & Leffler, D. (1990). Drug use and disciplinary actions among 300 nurses. *International Journal of the Addictions, 25*(4), 375–391.

Sullivan, E., Bissell, L., & Williams, E. (1988). *Chemical dependency in nursing: The deadly diversion*. Menlo Park, CA: Addison-Wesley.

Thompson, J., & Thompson, H. (1981). *Ethics in nursing*. New York, NY: Macmillan.

Trinkoff, A. M., Eaton, W. W., & Antony, J. C. (1991). The prevalence of substance abuse among registered nurse. *Nursing Research, 40*(3), 172–175.

Trinkoff, A. M., & Storr, C. L. (1998). Substance use among nurses: Differences between specialties. *American Journal of Public Health, 88*, 581–585.

Values. (2010). Retrieved January 10, 2010, from www.businessdictionary.com/definition/values.html

Velasquez, M., Moberg, D., Meyer, M. J., Shanks, T., McLean, M. R., DeCosse, D., et al. (2009). *A framework for thinking ethically*. Retrieved January 14, 2010, from http://www.scu.edu/ethics/practicing/decision/framework.html

Videbeck, S. L. (2010). *Psychiatric mental health nursing* (4th ed.). Philadelphia, PA: Wolters Kluwer: Lippincott Williams & Wilkins.

Washington Health Professional Services. (2006). *Symptoms*. Retrieved January 18, 2010, from http://www.doh.wa.gov/hsqa/Professions/WHPS/default.htm

Wood, D. A. (2006). Nurses poised to assess patients' alcohol use. *Nurse Week: Mountain West Edition, 7*(17), 22.

9

Bioethical Issues in Healthcare

LEARNING OUTCOMES

After completing this chapter, you should be able to:

1. Explain how nurses and their clients benefit from an understanding of bioethical issues.
2. Discuss the reasons that family planning in the United States has been an issue and discuss how various value systems and beliefs have affected it.
3. List some of the ethical and legal problems associated with assisted reproductive technology (ART).
4. Discuss the problems associated with determining when death has occurred and how decisions regarding healthcare are affected by it.
5. Analyze the multiple factors in right-to-die issues, including physician-assisted suicide and the difference between active and passive euthanasia.
6. Analyze the various points of view related to withholding and withdrawing treatment.
7. Discuss the ethics that establish the foundation for providing clients with informed consent and involving them in decisions regarding treatment.
8. Identify the major issues associated with organ transplantation.
9. Identify possible bioethical issues that could evolve from the Human Genome Project.
10. Discuss the limitations of gene therapy.
11. Analyze the reasons that controversy surrounds stem cell research and outline the positive and negative outcomes that could result from that research.
12. Discuss the multiple concerns that affect decisions regarding the treatment of the mentally ill.
13. Outline concerns related to the rationing of healthcare.

KEY TERMS

Abortion
Advance directive
Age of consent
Amniocentesis
Artificial insemination
Assisted reproductive technology (ART)
Assisted suicide
Behavior control
Bioethics
Chorionic villus sampling (CVS)

Durable power of attorney for healthcare
Emancipated minor
Eugenics
Euthanasia—negative and positive
Futile treatment
Gene therapy
Genetic screening
Genome
Human Genome Project (HGP)
Living will

(key terms continues on page 332)

Bioethics is defined in the Merriam-Webster Online Dictionary (2010) as a "discipline dealing with the ethical implications of biological research and applications, especially in medicine." This area of study is also called biomedical ethics because of its association with medical practice. It is a subdiscipline within the larger discipline of ethics, which (as discussed in Chapter 8) is the philosophic study of morality, or what is right and what is wrong. The word "bioethics" was coined by the biochemist Van Rensselaer Potter (1911–2001), a researcher at the University of Wisconsin in Madison, in 1970.

Today more than ever, nurses and their patients need to keep pace with the technologic changes occurring in healthcare. This chapter discusses some of the choices with which nurses and their clients must grapple. It should be read, studied, and discussed within the framework of the information concerning ethical decision making that was provided earlier. The content of the chapter should provide a basis with which you can look at judicial rulings, legal mandates, and social standards and understand how they can be used to assist in resolving concerns that face us in healthcare delivery. You have had some experience in looking at what is right or wrong regarding your personal professional practice. This chapter examines more specifically the issues that apply to the bioethics of patient care.

THE HISTORY OF THE EVOLUTION OF BIOETHICS

A number of factors contributed to the interest in and the development of bioethics. Evolving in the last decades of the 20th century, awareness of bioethical issues was heightened by abuse of human subjects who were unknowingly coerced into participating in research and by the rights movement for self-determination that occurred in the 1950s and 1960s. Media addressing the topic drew attention to practices that many believed were wrong.

Some would suggest that the birth of bioethics occurred with the publication of a magazine article in *Life* titled "They Decide Who Lives, Who Dies" (Alexander, November 9, 1962). This article told the story of a group of individuals in Seattle whose duty it was to select patients for the first hemodialysis program to treat chronic renal failure. Many more patients needed treatment than could be accommodated; those not selected would likely die. This event was followed several years later by an article about the ethics of medical research that provided the impetus for examining these issues.

Soon after, centers for research in bioethics emerged, most notably the Institute of Society, Ethics, and the Life Sciences, located in Hastings-on-Hudson, New York (often called The

Hastings Center), which was founded in 1969, and the Kennedy Institute of Ethics, located at Georgetown University in Washington, DC. The Kennedy Institute of Ethics, founded in 1971 by Joseph and Rose Kennedy, is a teaching and research center that provides ethical perspectives on major policy issues. It boasts the largest university-based faculty in the world devoted to research and teaching biomedical ethics. Journals such as the *Hastings Center Report* and the *Journal of Medicine and Philosophy* have come into being, and an encyclopedia, *The Encyclopedia of Bioethics*, has been published. Web sites devoted to the topic of bioethics are so numerous that they cannot be listed in the confines of this textbook. Today, bioethicists are included in many important task forces and special committees.

Entire textbooks have been devoted to bioethical considerations. Initially, most of these were written for medical students, but now just as many are written for nursing students. Some nursing programs include a course in ethics and bioethics in the curriculum. This chapter can only introduce the topic and, we hope, broaden your perspective and deepen your interest. You are encouraged to read about and study these issues further as they affect your nursing practice.

Most of the bioethical issues have evolved as a product of the technologic advances occurring in medical practice and research and were not a concern 50 years ago. Table 9.1 lists some

Table 9.1 Some Medical Milestones of the 1900s

WHEN	WHO	WHAT
1928	Alexander Fleming	This British bacteriologist noticed that one of his culture plates had grown a fungus and the colonies of staphylococci around the edge of the mold had been destroyed. Because this fungus was a member of the *Penicillium* group, he named it penicillin.
1938	Howard Florey and Ernst Chain	These two pathologists took up the work of Fleming and demonstrated the efficacy of penicillin in treating infection. In 1945, the three were jointly awarded the Nobel Prize for Physiology of Medicine.
1951	Forrest Bird	The first Bird breathing device was developed (Bird Mark 7), and breathing treatment machines were introduced. Inhalation (respiratory) therapy rapidly developed as a health profession (Pilbeam, 1998).
1953	James Watson and Francis Crick	These two geneticists deciphered DNA's double-helix structure. Researchers began to focus on the internal functioning of the cell, and molecular biology developed as a specialty.
1954	Physicians in Boston	Transplanted the kidney from one twin to the other, thus moving kidney transplantation from the experimental stage it had occupied since 1902. Kidney transplantations have been the most successful of transplantations (Kidney Transplantation: Past, Present & Future, n.d)
1955	Jonas Salk	Public health officials began immunizing children against polio with Dr. Salk's vaccine, which contained dead virus.
1957	Albert Sabin	A polio vaccine was developed, which was based on weakened live virus that could be administered orally.
1967	Christiaan Barnard	This South African surgeon performed the first human heart transplant.
1972	British engineers	The computed tomography (CT) scanner, which assembles thousands of x-ray images into a highly detailed picture of the brain, was developed in England. It was later expanded to provide scans of the entire body.
1978	English physicians	The process of IVF was developed. Louise Brown became the first person to be conceived in a test tube, and then implanted into her mother's uterus.
1979	World Health Organization	This group declared that smallpox had been eradicated 2 years after the last known case was identified. This occurred because of worldwide immunization against the disease.

(table continues on page 334)

Table 9.1 **Some Medical Milestones of the 1900s** (continued)

WHEN	WHO	WHAT
1981	Physicians in San Francisco and New York	Doctors from these two cities reported the first cases of what would later become known as acquired immunodeficiency syndrome (AIDS). To date, no cure exists.
1982	The US Food and Drug Administration	The first drug developed with recombinant DNA was approved by this group. It was a form of human insulin; its availability saves thousands of lives.
1995	Duke University surgeons	Hearts from genetically altered pigs were transplanted into baboons, proving that cross-species transplantations can be done. Transmission of animal viruses to humans emerges as a serious concern.
1998	James Thomas and scientists from University of Wisconsin—Madison	Culture embryonic stem cells (cells that are the parent cells of all body tissues) from donated human blastocysts, opening the door to potential repair or replacement of diseased tissues or organs (All About Popular Issues, 2002–2010).

Material for this table was gathered from an article by Sherwin B. Nuland, *Time Special Issue,* Fall 1996 except as otherwise noted.

of the significant medical milestones that have occurred since 1920, some of which we have come to take for granted (eg, antibiotics and DNA). You readily can see that in 1960 there was no quest for human organs or critical decisions regarding the life status of a possible donor. We were not able to fertilize ova outside the human body and transfer the fertilized eggs in a woman's uterus until 1978. Certain lifesaving machines (eg, ventilators) and miracle drugs (eg, some of the chemotherapeutic agents used today) were not available to offer extension of life. Technologies such as magnetic resonance imaging, which gives us information about the structure of tissues and allows for early diagnosis and treatment, were not available. Positron emission tomography was to follow. As advances occur in medical practice and technology, we must challenge ourselves to think through our own beliefs and feelings about these practices, especially as they relate to quality of life and patients' choices.

MAJOR AREAS WHERE BIOETHICS IS APPLIED

The bioethical issues surrounding the delivery of healthcare grow in number each year, constantly changing and taking on new scope and proportions. For years, we have debated issues related to birth and death; today, those topics represent just the tip of the iceberg. Of equal or greater concern are such matters as universal access to healthcare and insurance for all, rationing of healthcare, cost containment and quality of care, where and how federal dollars should be spent with regard to the nation's health, and the obligation of others to assist the homeless. Our media thrive on issues created by recent biomedical research, such as concerns regarding stem cell research. Biotechnology opens many doors, and as more and more possibilities become a reality, new issues must be addressed. How far should a society go in memory boosting or its suppression? Is it appropriate to carry out sex selection? What about cloning? Should assisted reproduction be regulated? To what extent should drugs be used on children to control their behavior? Should we extend life through age retardation? These are but a few of the questions for which our society must find answers.

Each year, the percentage of America's gross domestic product (GDP) spent on healthcare increases. It has been estimated that the national health spending grew 5.7% to reach $2.5

trillion in 2009, raising the health share of GDP to 17.3%. This represents the largest 1-year increase since the National Health Expenditure Account (NHEA) began recording health spending in 1960 (Truffer, Keehan, Smith, et al., 2010).

Because of lifestyle changes and medical breakthroughs, more people today live to reach old age, thus placing a greater burden on an already stressed system. Life expectancy has increased 1 to 2 years in each recent decade. In the United States, the life expectancy for females born in 2009 is 80.69 years and for males it is 75.65, compared with 47 years at the beginning of the 20th century (Central Intelligence Agency [CIA], 2010). Diseases such as Alzheimer and multiple sclerosis, for which cures are still being sought, have increased in prevalence. With globalization have come new threats to our well-being, such as that created by the H1N1 flu pandemic.

New technologies have led to treatments that were not available even 5 years ago. But rather than decreasing healthcare needs, the new technologies have resulted in increased needs because these specialized services are in high demand. Many treatments require use of technologies so expensive that they are priced beyond what an individual or family can afford without help from third-party payers. Finding new and better ways to treat life-threatening conditions challenges medical researchers, and the treatments that become available often invite debate among bioethicists. For example, stem cell research is forcing our society to make distinctions about life's beginnings that have enormous scientific and religious implications.

BIOETHICAL ISSUES RELATED TO THE BEGINNING OF LIFE

Many bioethical issues with which we wrestle today are focused on the process by which conception occurs, the products of conception, and the beginning of life, including whether it should occur. Family planning methods and issues related to conception have been a subject of debate for many years.

Family Planning

Family planning refers to the various methods used to control the size of one's family or to space births. Although we often think of it as synonymous with contraception, in reality it is much broader; for example, for some it might involve adoption. It can employ natural methods, pharmaceutical preparations, or barriers. The religious beliefs and personal values of individuals usually influence the methods and approaches used.

In 1798, in an essay titled, "On Population," Thomas Malthus, a minister in the Church of England, expressed deep concern about a population that was growing faster than were the resources to support it. To offset this problem, he advocated late marriage, no marriage, or sexual abstinence in marriage. No forms of contraception as we know them today were available, although women sometimes developed homemade devices in an effort to prevent pregnancy, such as pessaries inserted vaginally.

In 1873, the US Congress passed the Comstock Act, prohibiting the selling, mailing, or importing of "obscene literature and articles for immoral acts." All contraceptives and any material teaching about sexuality or birth control were included in this prohibition. Those who continued to import and distribute birth control literature or contraceptives were breaking the law. You may have read about Margaret Sanger (1883–1966), a nurse who championed for contraceptive practices in the early 1900s. Although charged and sentenced for disseminating information about birth control, she went on to establish the National Committee on Federal Legislation for Birth Control, the forerunner of the Planned Parenthood Federation. In 1938, in Sanger's landmark case, a federal judge dismissed this federal law as unconstitutional, thus ending the federal ban on contraceptives.

Although some states were more liberal than others, and some changed sooner than others, the state that had prohibitions against contraceptives for the longest time was Connecticut. It was not until 1965, in the case of *Griswold and Buxton vs. the State of Connecticut*, that the Supreme Court of the United States overrode the state law forbidding sale or teaching about contraception and established the right of the individual to obtain medical contraceptive advice and counseling (*http://womenshistory.about.com/library/ency/blwh_comstock.htm*).

Much of the controversy over birth control is related to the theological teachings of some religious groups, who believe interference with procreative powers is wrong. The Roman Catholic Church has strongly advocated that the natural purpose of sexual activity is to create new life and nothing should try to interfere with that potential. The members of the Church of Jesus Christ of Latter Day Saints (Mormons), although less adamant in their teachings, also discourage the use of artificial birth control under normal circumstances. Some conservative Protestant Christians and conservative Muslims also advocate allowing God to plan families and do not use birth control methods. Orthodox Judaism has specific rules about when sexual intercourse may or may not occur; these rules have the effect of supporting sexual activity when a woman is fertile. The Orthodox Jewish population is so small in proportion to other groups that the impact is not significant.

The opposite end of the spectrum is found in those who are strong advocates of zero population growth and encourage individuals to limit families to one or two children in all instances. Others are so concerned about population growth and the state of the world that they decide to not have children.

During your career as a nurse, you will care for patients who represent many differing viewpoints. When caring for individuals whose personal beliefs prohibit the use of artificial birth control, you must be knowledgeable about natural methods of family spacing, such as fertility awareness methods, that will meet the patient's needs. If your personal views regarding contraception differ, your values must be set aside as you focus on assisting the patient in selecting a method that is compatible with the patient's personal values and beliefs. If you are unable to do this, find a colleague who can provide answers to the questions and supply the needed information.

Among the methods of birth control available to those who have no religious sanction against their use, not all methods are acceptable to all people. Central to all discussions of contraception is the issue of freedom of a woman to control her own body. This immediately raises a second question: Who has that right? Is it the woman's right because it is her body? What if the partners disagree about family planning practices? Does one have more say than the other? What if one partner wants to have a family and the other does not?

Problems of Consent and Family Planning

The ability to have children precedes what is generally considered legal age; therefore, we find ourselves grappling with problems related to age of consent, its definition, and the role of the parents and the family. In legal terms, the **age of consent** is the age at which one is capable of giving deliberate and voluntary agreement. This implies physical and mental ability and the freedom to act and make decisions. The age of consent is established state by state and varies from age 14 to age 18 and may be different for males and females. Many states have age-gap provisions that make teen sexuality legal as long as the participants are within a certain age range, for example, the male is 18 and the female is 16. Most states have established age 16 as the age of consent (Age of Consent Chart for the US, 2009).

Until children reach the age of consent, parents are required to give consent for the care of their children. Implicit in this is the assumption that the parents have the best interests of the child at heart and that they are better qualified than the child to make decisions in the child's best interest. Generally speaking, the parents are responsible for the care (including medical costs) and education of the minor. However, today's trends cloud the issue, as we struggle with individual rights.

With regard to research, federal guidelines required that children with a mental age of 7 years or older be informed about proposed treatment or research and agree or concur with the decision made by the parent or guardian. This is referred to as *assent*.

Another example is the concept of the **emancipated minor**. As previously discussed, emancipated minors (an individual legally under the age of majority), who are financially independent, married, or in the military, may give consent for medical treatment, including all treatment for sexually transmitted diseases (STDs), contraception, and pregnancy-related concerns, regardless of their parent's or legal guardian's knowledge or agreement. Most states recognize some form of emancipation of minors.

The term **mature minors** is generally applied to individuals in their mid- to late teens who are considered mature enough to understand the treatment being recommended and provide informed consent. Under this definition, most states allow mature minors to seek treatment for STDs, drug or alcohol abuse, contraception, and pregnancy care without the consent of a parent or guardian. The most liberal legislation applies to the treatment of STDs and is endorsed by most states. Minors of any age can consent to diagnosis and care for STDs. However, the definition of the word "mature" varies from state to state, so some ambiguity continues to affect this area of care. For more discussion of age of consent and informed consent, see Chapter 7.

In some instances, this autonomy of the mature minor may bring health providers into a conflict between two laws. Although the mature minor may be able to consent to treatment for an STD, if the health provider believes it to have been contracted through sexual abuse of the minor, the provider is required to report that abuse. Most authorities direct that child abuse laws take precedence over privacy laws.

Certainly, there are times when a healthcare provider's ethical and moral convictions prevent him or her from complying with adolescents' requests for care. This occurs most commonly in response to requests for contraceptive pills and abortions. In such cases, the care provider often discusses his or her beliefs with the adolescent and refers the patient to another provider for assistance.

A major controversy exists around the role of the school in the sex education of high school students and the dispensing of contraceptives through high school health clinics. Those who are concerned about the high incidence of teenage pregnancies and STDs argue that the information must be disseminated, regardless of who does it. Others believe that this promotes erosion of the role of the family and worry that dispensing contraceptives encourages promiscuity and secrecy among teenagers. Concern about the spread of AIDS has done much to alter thinking, particularly regarding the dispensing of condoms.

The advent of emergency contraception in the form of birth control pills taken in high dose for a limited time after intercourse has added another dimension to these ethical issues about birth control. In some states, emergency contraception is available directly from a pharmacy without a physician's prescription. The pharmacist, therefore, is drawn into the decision-making web. Some pharmacists have refused to fill birth control prescriptions for college students, and others have refused to fill prescriptions for emergency contraception. Although many believe that people should not be compelled to engage in work they regard as unethical, others view this position as one of dispensing morality. Nurses working in emergency departments, student health services, family planning clinics, and similar environments find themselves in a comparable dilemma when it comes to administering these medications or counseling about their availability. If the nurse is the only care provider available, this would leave the patient without care and could constitute patient abandonment. With this in mind, some nurses choose not to apply for or accept positions where such care is required. In other instances, as long as there is another care provider present who can administer or dispense the medication, the concern is resolved.

Abortion

In medical terms, **abortion** is the termination of pregnancy before the viability of the fetus—that is, any time before the end of the sixth month of gestation. An abortion may occur spontaneously as a result of natural causes (spontaneous abortion). A pregnancy may be interrupted deliberately for medical reasons (therapeutic abortion) or for personal reasons (elective abortion). It is the latter two classifications (especially the last) that induce bioethical debate. Ethically, the entire debate revolves around the definition of human life and when the fetus should be considered a human being. There are two major schools of thought about the nature of the fetus: One supports the belief that new life occurs at the moment of conception; the other contends that human life does not exist until the fetus is sufficiently developed biologically to sustain itself outside the uterus. However, even the definition of the moment of conception differs between individuals with some stating that if the sperm has entered the ovum, conception is present, while most reproductive scientists state that conception has not occurred until implantation of the ovum because many fertilized ova never implant. One's position on this affects one's beliefs about whether emergency contraception should be considered potential abortion because there might have been a fertilized ovum that was prevented from implanting due to shedding of the uterine lining.

The legal aspects of abortion were set forth on January 22, 1973, when the US Supreme Court ruled in the case of *Roe vs. Wade* that any state laws that prohibited or restricted a woman's right to obtain an abortion during the first 3 months of pregnancy were unconstitutional. In this case, the Supreme Court identified that, during the first trimester of pregnancy, a privacy right exists that allows an individual woman to make the final decision with regard to what happens to her own body (*Roe vs. Wade*, 1973). Certain time limitations as to when an abortion can be performed were determined to be necessary because of the state's interest in protecting potential life. At the period of viability, the state's interest took precedence over the mother's desire for an abortion. Supreme Court Justice Blackmun, in writing an opinion that met with agreement from six other justices in *Roe vs. Wade*, decided that a woman's decision to terminate a pregnancy was encompassed by the right to privacy, up to a certain point in the development of the fetus (Blackmun, 1981). It was established that this lasted until the end of the first trimester. Thus, the courts ruled that the state could not prevent abortions during the first trimester, but could regulate abortions during the second and third trimesters of pregnancy, at which point the interests of the fetus took precedence over those of the mother. In 1992, the Court reaffirmed the basic principles of the 1973 decision.

Despite these rulings, the issue of abortion continues to surface, with new legislation and rulings being considered each year and the issue being debated before each presidential election. In 1977, Congress barred the use of Medicaid funds for abortion, with the exception of those done for therapeutic reasons and in other specific circumstances. Abortion was a major issue in discussions regarding national health insurance in 2009 and 2010.

However, the legal positions do little to help us deal with bioethical concerns. Many people view termination of life at any point after conception as murder. The Roman Catholic Church firmly upholds its traditional position of opposition to abortion. Many conservative Protestant Christian groups also are active in opposing abortion.

Some believe that although abortion is not desirable, under certain circumstances it would be justifiable—for example, in cases of rape or incest, or in instances where amniocentesis indicates that a fetus would be born retarded or genetically defective. Others think that early termination of a pregnancy might be acceptable but that termination after the fourth month would not be appropriate.

Those who support abortion without restriction usually do so because they believe that women should have control over their own bodies, which is tied to issues of privacy. They further argue that the quality of life of an unwanted child, or a child born with a deformity or genetic defect, may be minimal. Interesting and challenging cases have emerged with respect to this concept. These are generally known as **wrongful birth** cases, and they are based on the principle that it is wrong to give birth to children (such as those with birth defects or limitations that can be diagnosed or anticipated before birth) who will not have the same quality of life as other children.

As a nurse, these issues present difficult questions you will need to answer. To what extent do you believe you can personally participate in the abortion procedure? Would the stage of pregnancy and type of procedure make a difference? As a nurse, you have the right to refuse, based on your own ethical beliefs, to be involved in abortion procedures or the care of patients seeking abortion. Employment in certain areas (eg, labor and delivery rooms), however, may rest on the nurse's willingness and ability to assist with abortions and to give conscientious care to the patient who has had an abortion. Some religiously affiliated hospitals have elected to close their labor and delivery services rather than perform abortions.

Although textbooks traditionally have defined the age of viability (the earliest age at which fetuses could survive outside the uterus if they were born at that time) as 20 to 24 weeks' gestation, technology has increased the ability to enable very–low-birth-weight and premature babies to survive. The age of viability is less clear than it once seemed. Attention has been focused on incidents in which an abortion was attempted toward the end of the fifth or sixth month of gestation, and the fetus was born showing signs of life. Is the doctor or nurse obligated to try to keep the infant alive? Is the doctor or nurse guilty of malpractice, or even murder, if he or she does anything to hasten the infant's death? Should this infant be considered a human being? Does the infant have rights? Does the mother have legal possession of and responsibility for the child if, in fact, she attempted to abort the fetus? This issue, like so many others, probably will be settled in a court of law while we continue to debate it ethically.

The abortion issue also is complicated by consent problems. Many states have recognized the special problems related to parental consent for teenagers and to healthcare involving pregnancy and have legislated special exceptions. Nurses practicing in areas that provide abortions to minors must be concerned about parental consent and counseling issues because of the wide variations in state statutes governing abortions.

In the past few years, the abortion issue has been made more complex by research that would use the fetal tissue resulting from an abortion for stem cell research and therapeutic purposes. We will discuss stem cell research later in this chapter.

As a society, it seems likely that we will continue to debate the issue of abortion. Ultimately, the decision rests with the individual who must make the choice. Certainly the legal entanglements become more complex with each court ruling and will be limited only by our willingness to challenge other aspects of the question.

Critical Thinking Activity

Select one of the positions taken regarding abortion. Defend your position, providing a strong rationale for your thinking. Examine your thinking for biases. Why did you develop those biases? Has your position on abortion changed any over the past few years? If so, why? Discuss the topic of abortion with a classmate who holds a different position, remembering that all persons are entitled to their own viewpoints.

Prenatal Testing

A major breakthrough in our ability to detect genetic abnormalities in the fetus occurred in the 1970s with the development of techniques to carry out amniocentesis and has created a different dimension in the abortion debates. **Amniocentesis** involves aspirating and analyzing amniotic fluid and is performed between 14 and 20 weeks after the woman's last menstrual period. From these cells, many genetic problems of the fetus can be diagnosed prenatally, including such conditions as Down syndrome (which accounts for about one third of the cases of mental retardation in Western countries), hemophilia, Duchenne muscular dystrophy, Tay–Sachs disease, and problems related to the brain and spinal column (eg, anencephaly and spina bifida).

The potential for Down syndrome, a condition occurring with higher frequency in mothers in their early 40s and older, is the most common reason for performing an amniocentesis. When amniocentesis reveals a genetic condition, a woman may choose to have an abortion. Some of the diseases that have resulted in the parents choosing the alternative of an abortion include muscular dystrophy, cystic fibrosis, alpha and beta thalassemia, hemophilia, and sickle cell anemia, as well as congenital and genetic defects. Some couples request amniocentesis if they are in an at-risk group, but state that they would not abort the fetus under any circumstances; instead, they believe that an additional 5 months will give them time to adjust to the presence of a serious condition before the baby is born. **Chorionic villus sampling (CVS)** involves securing a sample of chorionic villi from the developing placenta. A sample of the placenta is obtained either vaginally or percutaneously and then analyzed genetically. Like amniocentesis, these tests can predict birth defects and certain diseases. CVS can be performed earlier than an amniocentesis, usually in the 10th or 11th week of pregnancy, but carries with it a risk to the developing fetus that increases the miscarriage rate.

Today, almost all pregnant women who are receiving prenatal care have a sonogram (ultrasound). It is used for fetal assessment at least once in a normal pregnancy, more often in those who have a risk factor. The sonogram can detect abnormal conditions that are manifested in abnormal anatomy in addition to ensuring that the pregnancy is progressing normally.

The advent of amniocentesis, CVS, and ultrasound heralded the development of yet another medical specialty: prenatal surgery. Although the specialty is still new, some corrective surgery is being performed on infants while they are in their intrauterine environment.

Some people are concerned about prenatal testing because of where it might lead. Is mass genetic screening a possibility? **Genetic screening** makes it possible to determine whether persons are predisposed to certain diseases and whether a couple might have the possibility of giving birth to a genetically impaired child. Ethicists have expressed concern about the possibility that the government may make diagnostic amniocentesis and abortion of all defective fetuses mandatory. Others argue against genetic screening, counseling, and amniocentesis because of the stress it places on a couple and because of the guilt placed on the partner carrying the defective gene (when that can be determined). They argue that there are some things we are better off not knowing. Genetic screening also may result in at least one of the partners (often the carrier) seeking voluntary sterilization to prevent pregnancies with less-than-favorable outcomes. As genetic screening of a fetus becomes more available, the tests may also be used to identify gender. China, India, and some other Asian countries have traditional societies in which sons are highly prized and daughters are an economic liability. As gender identification has become more widespread, the ratio of boys to girls born in those countries is changing as couples choose to abort female fetuses (Practical Ethics, 2009). In a study published by Wei Xing Zhu, Li Lu, and T. Hesketh (2009) in 2005, the births of boys in China exceeded births of girls by more than 1.1 million. The long-term effects of the imbalance in sexes are viewed as socially disruptive, as is the low value placed on female children. In the United States and Europe, most providers do not include this as a valid reason for termination of pregnancy.

As a nurse, you may care for clients with varying viewpoints regarding prenatal screening and abortion, and you will also have your own values to consider. Will your values conflict with those of your clients? Are you obligated to advocate for a client when the client's request is squarely in opposition to what you believe to be right? Should you try to sway a woman who is indecisive toward either decision?

COMMUNICATION IN ACTION

When Others Seek Advice

Your cousin Edwina, age 37, has just learned that she is pregnant. Because of her age, it was recommended that she have an amniocentesis. Because you are in nursing, she asked what you think she should do. You sit with her and listen. After you have determined that she understands what is involved in an amniocentesis and the information it provides, you say, "It is not uncommon for women who become pregnant after age 35 to have an amniocentesis. Perhaps, to help you to decide if this is something you want to have done, you should make two lists—one listing the advantages to you of having this done and the other listing the disadvantages. This might also help you develop a list of questions you would want to discuss with your obstetrician."

Sterilization

For years, surgical operations resulting in permanent **sterilization**, such as the removal of reproductive organs to halt the spread of cancer, have been performed for therapeutic purposes. Although problems may arise for the patient and family as a result of such surgeries, usually they are resolved without serious ethical debate, depending on the family's religious values, the patient's body concept, family plans, and personal values.

With increasing frequency, voluntary sterilization has been requested by individuals to terminate reproductive ability with more women seeking the surgery than men. Although sometimes reversible, patients are counseled that these surgical procedures, whether performed on men or women, should be considered permanent and irreversible. Many people see it as the prerogative of an individual; others find any type of sterilization in conflict with their religious and moral beliefs. Sterilization may pose few problems for those who are satisfied with the number of children they have had or who are adults who have determined that they do not want to have children. People may decide not to have children for a variety of reasons, including personal health status, familial genetic disorders, or simply not wishing to parent. Full and informed consent is required of the person being sterilized; however, healthcare providers often prefer also to obtain assent from the spouse if the person is married to avoid subsequent emotional and family problems. Some people question whether a man or woman should be free to make such a decision without consulting the partner, but doing so is completely legal. A few states still have laws forbidding voluntary sterilization for contraceptive purposes, but these laws may not be enforced. Chemical sterilization, sometimes called chemical castration, refers to providing drugs, often a form of progesterone, to decrease sexual drive by lowering the testosterone level. The effects are reversible when the medication is discontinued. Initiated by California and soon followed by Florida, chemical castration is slowly gaining ground throughout the country as a means of sentencing and treating sex offenders. Passage of such legislation was made easier by the Child Protection Act of 1999 that mandates "two strikes and you're out" and by Megan's Law that requires that sex offenders be registered with local authorities. Offenders may prefer the treatment to other alternatives. This approach has been used in individuals with a history of repeated rape, who are often incarcerated during the time they are receiving chemical sterilization. In some instances, this has been recommended or even requested by those individuals who were convicted of repeated sexual offenses, particularly those against children. Despite the criminal history, some challenge the ethics of this action.

Because sex crimes are related to power and aggression, and not just to sex drive, this remains a controversial issue.

Eugenics

Eugenics is a term that has had different meanings in different eras but is generally thought of as the study of methods to improve inherited human characteristics. The idea of improving the quality of the human race is at least as old as Plato, who wrote on the topic in his *Republic*. The philosophic beliefs of certain 18th-century thinkers about the notion of human perfectibility were central to the eugenics movement, which is thought to have started in the 19th century. Charles Darwin's cousin, Francis Galton, who created the term "eugenics," based his work on Darwin's theory of evolution. When Mendel's law provided a framework for explaining the transmission and distribution of traits from one generation to another, the eugenics movement took hold. Organizations focusing on eugenics were created around the world.

The center of the eugenics movement in the United States, which grew until the early 1930s, was the Eugenics Record Office in Cold Spring Harbor, New York, and its leader was geneticist Charles Davenport. Eugenicists presented a two-part policy. Positive eugenics encouraged increasing the desirable traits in the population by urging "worthy" or "superior" couples to have more children. Negative eugenics advocated the elimination of unwanted characteristics from the nation by discouraging "unworthy" couples from procreating.

Negative eugenics included a variety of approaches, such as marriage restriction, sterilization, and permanent custody of "defectives." Many eugenicists were actively involved in other issues of the day, including prohibition, birth control, and legislation that would outlaw miscegenation (ie, marriage between two persons of different races, especially between white and black people in the United States). Indiana enacted the first law permitting sterilization on eugenic grounds in 1907; Connecticut followed soon after. In 1914, Harry Laughlin, who worked at the Eugenics Record Office, published a Model Eugenical Sterilization Law that proposed sterilization of the "socially inadequate," a group that included "feebleminded, insane, criminalistic, epileptic, inebriate, diseased, blind, deaf, deformed and dependent," including "orphans, ne'er-do-wells, tramps, the homeless and paupers." By the time the law was published in 1914, 12 states had enacted sterilization laws; by 1937, 31 of the 48 states had compulsory laws. By 1924, approximately 3,000 people in America had been involuntarily sterilized (Lombardo, n.d.). By 1979, this number increased to more than 60,000. The Immigration Restriction Act of 1924 also was passed at this time, dramatically limiting the immigration of people from southern and eastern Europe on the grounds that they were "biologically inferior." The trend in recent times has been for states to modify, repeal, or ignore sterilization laws.

The eugenics movement also grew in Germany. In 1933, Hitler sanctioned the Hereditary Health Law, or the Eugenic Sterilization Law, thus ensuring that the "less worthy" members of the Third Reich did not pass on their genes. This action provided the legal basis for the sterilization of more than 350,000 people (Lombardo, n.d.). By the late 1930s, eugenics in the United States began a tremendous decline. Americans became concerned about the concept of a "master race."

The eugenic movement was rekindled in the 1960s with a different focus—one related to genetic counseling and genetic research. Today, a couple giving birth to a child with a congenital anomaly (or who realize that one of them is carrying a genetic trait that could cause a child to have a congenital anomaly) might voluntarily seek genetic counseling, and possibly opt for the sterilization of one of the partners. Again, this approach offends the religious and moral values of some, but generally, it is viewed as the couple's prerogative.

In states that permit sterilization of a person who is not competent to give consent, questions can be raised about who may request sterilization, who may sign the consent, and who must fund the procedure as in the case of a parent requesting surgical sterilization of a mentally retarded adolescent. Some states allow a guardian to make such a decision, but other states specifically prohibit guardians from consenting to sterilization. As the result of a court decision, federal dollars may not be used for sterilization of a person who cannot give personal consent. However, the taxpayer contributes to the cost of institutionalizing people who are not capable of living independently in today's society, and caring for those with severe illnesses and disabilities. The question must be raised regarding the ability of two individuals who are mentally retarded to care for children they may parent. Therefore, it is not only a personal concern, but also society's concern.

The use of prenatal testing to determine characteristics of a child and to abort fetuses without desired characteristics is a matter of concern to those who are skeptical of the use of this high technology. Where should lines be drawn between what is an acceptable variation and what is not? What happens to a society that suggests that those who do not conform to a "norm" should not live?

Artificial Insemination

Artificial insemination involves the planting of sperm in the woman's body to facilitate conception. Although we tend to think of this as a fairly new procedure, the first time artificial insemination is said to have been used was in Philadelphia in 1884. There are two kinds of artificial insemination: homologous (Artificial Insemination Homologous), in which the husband's sperm is used, and heterologous (Artificial Insemination Donor), in which a donor's sperm is used. Using the husband's sperm is by far the most common and creates the fewest problems legally, ethically, and morally. In some instances, the sperm from the husband and the sperm from a donor with similar physical characteristics are mixed together. As a result, if conception occurs, the couple could easily believe it was the husband's sperm that fertilized the ovum; however, with DNA testing available to determine parentage, this may not have the desired outcome.

Although some religious groups may have objections, few concerns arise when the husband's sperm is used. That is not true with donor sperm. If the woman is artificially inseminated with donor sperm without the knowledge and consent of her partner, the problems are multiplied. If conception occurs and the child is not biologically that of the husband, can one say that adultery has occurred? Others suggest that the husband should legally adopt the child. To some extent, this helps to clarify issues of inheritance, child support (if the couple should later divorce), and the legal status of the child.

A growing concern relates to the problem of the donor remaining anonymous and depriving children of knowledge of their parental and family background. Anonymous donors are usually guaranteed that their anonymity will be permanent, but courts sometimes overturn this when there is a need for genetic information for the child. Should this anonymity be guaranteed or do children have a right to know who the biological father is and what familial disease tendencies or their ethnic heritage might be? When an anonymous donor has been used for insemination many times in one community, the potential exists for children with the same donor father to meet and marry.

Assisted Reproductive Technology

Assisted reproductive technology (ART) includes fertility treatments in which both the egg and the sperm are handled in the laboratory. In vitro fertilization (IVF) is an example. Ova for IVF may be gathered from the mother or from a donor who sometimes is a member of the family. IVF and similar procedures help many infertile couples, with new techniques and approaches being developed every year.

Many herald this as one of medical science's great advances. For others, it raises many concerns. Several fertilized ova are usually returned to the uterus to ensure that at least one will survive. If more than one implants successfully, it is possible for the mother to have multiple births. Multiple births seldom go full term, resulting in financial and emotional costs. When the number of implanted embryos is too great, consideration is given to aborting several of them to improve the chances of full development for the remaining ones; this creates additional ethical dilemmas for the family.

▶ *EXAMPLE*

Multiple Births

In 2009, world attention was focused on a 33-year-old unmarried, unemployed woman with six small children, who was living with her parents. This mother had begun IVF treatments in 1997 when she was still married (the couple separated in 2000), and all her pregnancies resulted from the IVF treatments. Knowing there was a risk of multiple births if she had all six remaining embryos transferred at one time, she requested that all her embryos be inserted. All six embryos did implant and two apparently split, resulting in the birth of eight premature babies, all of whom required intensive care before joining their siblings at home.

Fertility treatment guidelines call for women under 35, who have favorable chances for a successful pregnancy, to have no more than two fresh embryos transferred. Although this mother's embryos had been frozen, there was still no justification for transferring more than two or at most three. Some experts further state they "would not agree to treat a single mother on disability with six small children at home" (Boyles, 2009). In addition to all the other concerns this situation creates, one must ask, "Should there be sanctions on physicians who will carry out such procedures?"

What should be done with fertilized ova that are not returned to the uterus? (There are an estimated 500,000 such embryos in the United States.) Should they be thrown away? Given to a donor? Used for research? Should tax dollars be used to fund this type of research? If frozen, how long should they remain frozen? What should be done with them at the end of that time? Is discarding the embryos the moral equivalent to having an abortion?

Some couples with embryos to spare have chosen to give the embryos to another infertile couple. The fertilized ovum is implanted into the uterus of the infertile female and often results in a full-term pregnancy. Although opponents of abortion rights may view this as a better alternative than stem cell research, in which embryos are destroyed, the moral and legal implications comprise a gray area. Are these embryos people, property, or their own entities worthy of respect? Like other adoptions, should a home study and background check be completed on the family receiving the fertilized ova? Some believe embryo donation is different, because most state laws presume that a woman who carries and gives birth to a child has earned the right to be a parent.

Other offshoots of IVF allow people who are carrying a severe genetic disease to be assured that their children will not be affected by the condition or carry the defective gene. Fertilized ova are examined for possible disease before being implanted in the uterus; those that are diseased are not implanted (see later discussion). As wonderful as this may seem, concerns exist regarding what some would call the misuse of IVF. This technique has allowed women in their 60s and 70s to become pregnant.

▶ *EXAMPLE*

A 72-year-Old Mother

In 2008, a 72-year-old woman in India who had two children and five grandchildren gave birth to twins—a boy and a girl—by cesarean section, making her the world's oldest mother. Lacking a son in a society in which sons are greatly valued, the septua-genarian couple spent their life savings and took out a loan from the bank to enable the mother to undergo in vitro treatments. For the couple, the desire to have a son was most important because they wanted to carry on the family name (Russo, 2008).

In some countries, legislation has been passed to prevent such situations. One can readily identify some of the difficulties in starting the mothering process at a later age, not the least of which would be living long enough to see the child reach adulthood. Quality-of-life issues also may be involved.

In 1988, another technological advance, **preimplantation genetic diagnosis (PGD)** was developed. PGD enables families to have a child free from a specific inherited genetic disease or, less often, to have a child with specific genetic characteristics. PGD allows physicians to pluck a single cell from an eight-celled embryo and determine whether that embryo has specific genetic alleles or the proper number of chromosomes. Using this technique, only healthy embryos can be selected for implantation. By testing embryos before a pregnancy has begun, the need to terminate a pregnancy in which a fetus is found to have a genetic mutation can be avoided. PGD has been used to test for dozens of inherited diseases, to select embryos that will be a matched tissue donor for an ailing sibling, and to select embryos based on sex (Baruch, Javitt, Scott, et al., 2010). Some of the conditions PGD can identify are Duchenne muscular dystrophy, hemophilia, Tay–Sachs disease, Down syndrome, and cystic fibrosis.

Concerns focus on the fear that PGD will be used to make perfect babies (sometimes referred to as "designer babies" or "custom babies"), to create babies that are an immuno-logical match for a seriously ill sibling, or to select embryos of one gender in preference to the other—a practice that is referred to as "family balancing," even when there is not a medical reason (such as hemophilia, Tay–Sachs, or sickle cell anemia) for such action. An additional concern is one mentioned in the discussion of IVF—the analysis of fertilized ovum and the implantation of only those that are most likely of producing a child free of a genetic condition.

The Genetics and Public Policy Center has studied these concerns and points out that PGD raises a number of scientific, ethical, and policy issues. First, there are questions about the safety of the IVF and embryo manipulation required for PGD and about the accuracy of the genetic tests that are used. The second relates to the fact that some find PGD, or its uses, morally unacceptable because it involves the creation, selection, and destruction of human embryos. Third, there are questions of equity: many cannot afford PGD, and it is not clear whether and to what extent health insurers will cover it. The last issue relates to broad ethical questions about the impact of PGD on family relationships, people living with disabilities, and society as a whole. The goal of their work is to ensure that policy decisions, even decisions to maintain the status quo, have been undertaken with a clear-eyed understanding of their potential impact (Baruch, Javitt, Scott, et al., 2010).

Choosing Children Outside of Marriage

As social mores regarding unmarried mothers have relaxed and as younger women have placed career ahead of marriage and motherhood, the number of women aged 35 and older who desire to have a family has increased. Some of these women are in relationships with partners who father their children, or they are partnered with another woman and use donor insemination. A large number of these women choose to have and raise children independently and see artificial insemination as a logical solution to their desire to become pregnant.

While some argue against the artificial insemination of any unmarried woman on the basis that the traditional two-parent family composed of a man and woman is in the best interests of all children, others focus on the importance of having wanted children with parents who are thoughtful and committed to their well-being. This is an area in which people are choosing for themselves with little interference by society as a whole.

Recent years also have witnessed the adoption of children by those who are single or unmarried partners of both opposite sexes and the same sex. Such instances do not involve artificial insemination but, rather, a formal adoption process through the courts. Again, some of the same arguments are set forth against this process as against single women bearing children.

Surrogate Mothers

A **surrogate mother** is one who agrees to bear a child conceived through artificial insemination or IVF and implantation and to relinquish the baby at birth to others for rearing. Surrogacy first became commercial in the United States in the late 1970s. Between 1976 and 1988, 600 babies were born to surrogate mothers. The number of surrogate births soared to 5,000 in the next 4 years, as infertile couples found it to be a way to have children. While initially the individual who agreed to be the surrogate was a friend or family member, now it is more often a contractual arrangement with a stranger to the family.

The number of surrogate births has continued to rise, and the structure of the parentage has taken unique avenues, creating interesting challenges. It is possible that there may be a biological mother (the individual who provided the ovum for implantation), a biological father (who provides the sperm), a gestational mother (the individual who carries and gives birth to the child), and the individuals (who may or may not be married) who plan to parent the child (one or both of whom may have been one of the biological parents as well). Some writers also refer to an egg donor as a surrogate. On at least one occasion, a woman agreed to serve as surrogate for her daughter, thus making her the gestational mother as well as the genetic grandmother to the triplets she carried (Christ, 2008).

One of the most important aspects of the process is finding a good match between the surrogate and the contracting family. Surrogate mothering within a family has caused fewer problems than have been seen when a stranger serves as the surrogate mother. Ethically, carrying a child for a family member out of love and concern and planning to remain in that child's life as part of the family reflect a commitment to the child and respect for the personhood of the child. The majority of serious conflicts have occurred in situations in which a woman has been paid to serve as a surrogate mother. A formal, contractual relationship is usually established. The couple who wishes to have the child agrees to pay all expenses associated with the pregnancy and to pay the surrogate mother an agreed sum for her time and involvement—usually between $25,000 and $75,000. The contract must be carefully drawn up because it is illegal in

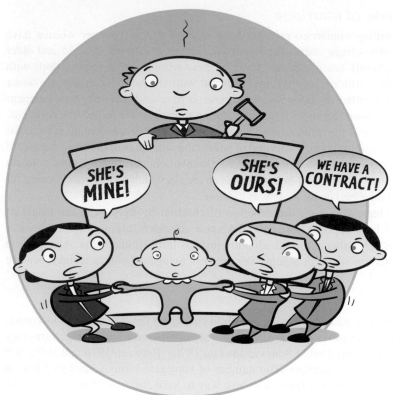

FIGURE 9.1 Complexities arise when surrogate mothers are unwilling to relinquish the infant after birth.

all states to sell a child. Paid-surrogate arrangements are illegal in some states and countries, including Arizona, Minnesota, New York, Utah, Washington State, and Washington, D.C. Many ethicists view parenting for pay as a gray ethical area that may fail to value the person-hood of the child. This becomes apparent when things do not go as planned. What happens if the child is born with an anomaly and the family refuses to take the child? What if the surrogate becomes attached to the child and refuses to give up custody? What if the parents divorce before the child is born and wish to nullify the contract? How are these dilemmas to be solved? What is to happen to the child? Who bears the responsibility? Recently, problems associated with surrogate mothering have centered on the surrogate mother's unwillingness to give up the child after birth (Fig. 9.1).

 Critical Thinking Activity

What safeguards would you recommend regarding IVF, artificial insemination, and surrogate mothers to ensure respect for the human condition? Be specific about how you believe these safeguards would be effective. Reflect on your proposals. Are there any you would change? Discuss your proposals with a classmate.

Sperm Banks

Sperm banks or cryobanks have been springing up across the nation since the late 1970s, with about 25 major ones currently operating in the United States (Herscher, 2009). They have been established for various reasons. Men who want to have a vasectomy may contribute to a sperm bank if there's a chance they may change their minds in the future. Men who will be exposed to high levels of radiation in their work, or during treatment of disease, may wish to have sperm stored because radiation may cause mutation of the genes or result in sterility. This allows them to father children at a later date without concern about the effect on the sperm.

In most cases, the medical community establishes sperm banks so that sperm is available for artificial inseminations. Sperm banks collect sperm from willing donors, who are reimbursed for their sperm. The sperm is frozen and then sold to individuals or families who, for various reasons, desire to become pregnant but cannot without the help of the sperm bank. Concerns have been raised regarding the possible number of offspring in a single community who might be genetically related without knowing it. In California, a sperm bank was developed that contained only sperm of outstanding and brilliant men. The idea was to create children with this sperm who would be genetically endowed with greater intelligence and creativity. Many find this unacceptable because it brings up the issue of creating a superior race.

Are there ethical implications for the man who becomes a sperm donor and is the biologic father of a child, but assumes no ethical responsibility for who receives that sperm or for the resulting child and, in fact, has no knowledge regarding the use of his sperm? Some ask how a man can ethically father offspring and have no responsibility for their well-being.

Although there are strict safeguards for privacy of a sperm donor, the donor is known to the woman by a code number. In California in 2000, an organization called the Donor Sibling Registry was formed for individuals seeking half-siblings who share their donor father. Through identifying the sperm bank and the code number of the father, others with that same father can be identified. This organization (*DonorSiblingRegistry.com*) successfully links individuals who strongly believe that ties of family are strong and want to know these half-siblings. These donor-conceived children seek the same rights to know the identity of their biologic fathers as adoptive children have. This movement may create major changes in the area of donor insemination.

The Right to Genetic Information

All the issues of artificial insemination using donor sperm, IVF using donor sperm, surrogate mothering, single parenting, and sperm banks are further complicated by a recent trend toward providing individuals with information regarding their familial background, makeup, and history. You can readily anticipate the problems that would be created if donor sperm were used for insemination. In some instances, no record has been maintained regarding who donated the sperm.

As society emphasizes the importance of the role of fathers and the rights of children to know their family heritage, will anonymous sperm donation remain an option? How many individuals would be willing to donate sperm if it were to necessitate detailed background information? What might be the ultimate legal involvement? On the other hand, what are the rights of the child to know what genetic factors he or she carries? Whose rights should take precedence? Several states have passed legislation opening birth records for adults adopted as infants to learn of their backgrounds, even though anonymity of the birth mother was guaranteed at the time of the adoption. Will tracking of sperm donors also become a concern in the future?

BIOETHICAL ISSUES CONCERNING DEATH

One of the most important areas of ethical debate revolves around the topic of death and dying. As mentioned earlier, the advent of lifesaving procedures and mechanical devices has required redefinition of the term "death," caused us to examine the meaning of "quality of life," and created debates about "death with dignity."

Also associated with the issue of death are several companion concerns that did not exist before the technologic advances that occurred over the past 30 years. Some of these concerns relate to euthanasia, the right to refuse treatment, and the right to die. Other concerns relate to organs retrieved from the dying, because of the scarcity of these medical resources. Generally, the demand for donated organs far exceeds the number of organs available to meet the needs. Superimposed on all these issues is that of informed consent.

Death Defined

Until recently, the most widely accepted definition of death was from *Black's Law Dictionary*, which defines death as the irreversible cessation of the vital functions of respiration, circulation, and pulsation. This traditional view of death served us well until the development of ventilators and other advances in medical science that made it possible to sustain life functions. We also have learned that various parts of the body die at different times. The central nervous system is one of the most vulnerable areas, and brain cells can be irreversibly damaged if deprived of oxygen, while other parts of the body will continue to function.

Newer definitions of death have been built around the concept of human potential—meaning the potential of the human body to interact with the environment and with other people, to respond to stimuli, and to communicate. When these abilities are lacking, there is said to be no potential. Because this potential is directly related to brain function, the method most often used to assess capability is electroencephalography. Brain activity, with few exceptions, is said to be nonexistent when flat electroencephalographic tracings are obtained over a given period, often 48 hours. After this point, the person may be considered dead, although machines may be supporting the vital functions of respiration and circulation. Many institutions now accept this definition of cerebral death and use it as a basis for turning off respirators and stopping other treatments. It is also used as a basis for determining death when there is a desire to recover organs from the patient.

Planning for End-of-Life Issues

Increasing emphasis is being placed on prior planning for end-of-life issues. Identifying futile treatments is one aspect of this process. Another important consideration relates to patient self-determination regarding these issues. Many hope that the use of such planning will decrease the ethical dilemmas in end-of-life situations.

Futile Treatments

Futile treatments (medications, devices, or therapy) are those that are evaluated by the healthcare team, the family, or both as being nonbeneficial or harmful to the patient in as much as they cannot cure or reverse the underlying disease (Grossman, 2009). For example, when an individual is dying of terminal cancer, treatment for a respiratory infection may be deemed futile because it will not alter the fact that the person is dying and will not restore a satisfactory quality of life. Identifying whether further treatment is futile may be extremely difficult. It is related to many assumptions about quality and quantity of life and, based on the best interests principle, places high demands on the individual responsible for decision making. However, Schneiderman, Jecker, and Jonsen (1996) suggest that if, in the past 100 cases of the same nature, there was no change in the outcome based on the treatment, it can be considered futile. Others take a position that treatment never can be declared futile. In their thinking, the future cannot be predicted accurately, and if there cannot be absolute certainty about the outcome, then futility cannot be clearly identified.

Other problems may arise when futility is declared. To what extent should the patient be involved in the decision making? Does a patient have a right to treatment even if it has been identified as futile? What about cost considerations? Should insurance companies be required to pay for treatment that has been classified as futile? What about Medicare or Medicaid? Should there be differences in decisions based on age or quality of life?

Critical Thinking Activity

Do you think that factors such as ability to pay, treatment of children or younger adults versus the elderly, the cost of the treatment, and the percentage of time the treatment is effective should be issues considered when deciding whether treatment is futile? Provide a rationale for each answer. What are your biases?

Ethical Issues Surrounding Advance Directives and Living Wills

In December 1991, the federal **Patient Self-Determination Act (PSDA)** went into effect. Passed by Congress in 1990, this legislation requires that all Medicare and Medicaid providers inform patients on admission of their right to refuse treatment. The intent of this legislation was to enhance an individual's control over medical treatment decisions by promoting the use of advance directives (see Chapter 7). The entire process has not been without its problems. The time of admission to a healthcare facility is often filled with anxiety, making it almost impossible to consider such matters.

The American Nurses Association emphasized that nurses should facilitate informed decision making and should occupy a critical role in education, research, patient care, and advocacy. The organization's 1991 position statement of nursing and patient self-determination remains in effect today (American Nurses Association [ANA], 1991).

In an attempt to gain greater control over the area of dying, several documents have been developed to assist with this process. **Advance directives** are legal documents that indicate the wishes of an individual with regard to end-of-life issues and were described and discussed in Chapter 7. A **living will**, a form of advance directive, allows individuals to identify what measures to include in care if they become terminally ill. The living will is often used to request that no extraordinary measures be implemented, although it can be used to indicate a preference that all possible actions should be taken.

Some have voiced concern that advance directives have failed to achieve their goals. Often, this is because they are not available or are misunderstood, are not clear, or are not as specific as needed. There is also a tendency for family members, when faced with the real situation, to say, "Well, he didn't really mean that." Providing competent assistance in filling out the forms and creating documents that are easier to use can help with this concern (Brooks, 2010).

Another approach being used with increasing frequency is the signing of a **durable power of attorney for healthcare**. In this type of an agreement, an individual (referred to as the principal) may designate another person to have the power and authority to make healthcare decisions for the principal should the principal be unable to make those decisions. Durable power of attorney documents were discussed in detail in Chapter 7.

Euthanasia

Euthanasia, meaning "good death," may be classified as either negative or positive. The word, as it is generally applied, refers to the act or method of causing death painlessly so as to end suffering.

Negative Euthanasia

Negative, or passive, euthanasia refers to a situation in which no extraordinary or heroic measures are undertaken to sustain life. The concept of negative euthanasia has resulted in what are called "no codes" (also designated as DNR—do not resuscitate) in hospital environments. In these situations, hospital personnel do not attempt to revive or bring back to life persons whose vital processes have ceased to function on their own.

It is difficult to describe what constitutes extraordinary measures, and to determine on whom they should or should not be used. Is it one thing to defibrillate a 39-year-old man who is admitted to an emergency department suffering from an acute heart attack, and quite another to defibrillate a 95-year-old man whose body is riddled with terminal cancer and whose heart has stopped? Often, people who are involved in giving medical and emergency care develop an almost automatic response to lifesaving procedures and have difficulty accepting dying as an inevitable part of the life process. This is particularly true when emergency personnel receive a 911 call and rush to the home of an individual who has requested that no extraordinary measures be taken to sustain life. Often, cardiopulmonary resuscitation or other such efforts are started before the rescuers know of the request.

It is difficult to know when it is permissible to omit certain life-supporting efforts, or which efforts should be skipped. If the 95-year-old man who is dying of terminal cancer were also to develop pneumonia, should his physician prescribe antibiotics? This brings us to the distinction between stopping a particular life-supporting treatment or machine, and withdrawing treatment or not starting a procedure in the first place—that is, withholding treatment.

Some ethicists do not differentiate between withholding treatment in the first place and withdrawing treatment once it has been determined to be inappropriate or futile. They would see both as having the same position in terms of right and wrong. Those who support negative euthanasia support both withholding and stopping treatment. The general public often sees these as separate issues and may support withholding treatment, while not supporting the termination of treatment once it has begun. Increasingly, the legal system has supported withdrawing treatment that is determined to be futile. A landmark case in 2005 was that of Terri Schiavo, who was in a persistent vegetative state (PVS) following a heart stoppage due to a chemical imbalance that occurred 5 years earlier. Her husband wanted her feeding tube removed, which would ultimately result in her death; her parents wanted the treatment continued. Finally, the courts decided that the husband was the legal decision maker. He then had the feeding tube removed.

Positive Euthanasia

Positive, or active, euthanasia occurs in a situation in which the physician prescribes, supplies, or administers an agent that results in death. On some occasions, a physician prescribes strong narcotics for a terminally ill patient and requests that the medication be given frequently enough to keep the patient comfortable. Although this is not legally considered positive euthanasia, nurses may be reluctant to administer a medication that they realize has a potentially fatal effect when given in that dosage. Medications given for the comfort of the dying patient may be ethically justifiable even if they hasten death to some extent. This is based on the ethical concept of double effect, in which the acceptable effect (such as pain relief) is the purpose of the medication and the secondary effect (such as depressing respiration) is not the intended effect. When nurses have difficulty with this issue, a patient conference with an oncology specialist or with a nurse skilled in the area of death and dying can help the staff to clarify values and deal with individual feelings.

Rights Issues Surrounding Death

Rights issues surrounding death are gaining much more attention than in previous years. These include the right to refuse treatment, a right to death with dignity, and the right to choose the time and manner of one's death, and even a right to assisted suicide. These may be grouped together under the terminology "**right to die.**"

A great deal of controversy surrounds the issue of maintaining the lives of persons considered to be in a PVS. Some of the issues that arise are the patient's rights stated above (if their wishes are known), the family's wishes, and the cost to society. In most cases, the problems emerge when the life of a person is being maintained through support measures that might be considered extraordinary. Healthcare providers and families may fail to communicate effectively when physicians continue to emphasize that the patient may be helped to *survive* while not clearly explaining that this does not indicate that there will be *recovery* to any prior level of function.

Withdrawing and Withholding Treatment

Withdrawing treatment is defined as stopping treatment that is considered medically futile, that is, will not provide a cure or control the disease. **Withholding treatment** occurs when this type of treatment is not provided at all. Although withholding and withdrawal of therapies have been described mainly in situations related to technical interventions (ventilator, hemodialysis), they can also be applied by extension to chemotherapy, artificial hydration, and nutrition as long as the aim of these therapies is to prolong life beyond expectation, to delay death. Landmark cases are numerous with some of the most notable ones being the case of Karen Quinlan, a young comatose woman on a ventilator whose parents sought to have the treatment stopped, and the Terri Schiavo case mentioned earlier.

Of particular concern to nurses are their own feelings when a decision is reached to remove life-supporting measures, whether the measures are tube feedings or ventilators. Strong emotional attachments often form between the nurse and patient, even when the patient is in a vegetative state. Nurses who have worked to preserve the patient's dignity have great difficulty letting go. In some instances, patients are transferred to other facilities to die in an environment where the nurses are not so emotionally involved with the patient.

Positions on Withholding and Withdrawing Treatment

Several organizations and groups have issued guidelines for their members and others who would find them useful, with regard to the issue of withholding or withdrawing treatment. Key to all of these guidelines is whether the patient is legally competent (able to make decisions for himself or herself) or incompetent (in need of someone else to make those decisions). Table 9.2 outlines the date, organization, and major tenets of some of those positions.

Table 9.2   Positions on Withholding and Withdrawing Treatment

	ORGANIZATION	POSITION
1983	President's Commission Report—*Deciding to Forego Life-sustaining Treatment*	Focused on the ethical, medical, and legal issues in treatment decisions. Distinguished between withholding (not starting) and withdrawing (stopping after it started) treatment without making a moral distinction between the two. Suggested that withholding may require more justification because the positive effects would not be known.
1986	American Medical Association—*Statement on Withholding or Withdrawing Life-prolonging Medical Treatment*	Stated that life-prolonging medical treatment and artificially or technologically maintained respiration, nutrition, and hydration could be withheld from a patient in an irreversible coma even if death was not imminent (Fry, 1990).
1986	Office of Technology Assessment of the US Congress—*Life-sustaining Technologies and the Elderly*	Issued the results of its study on the use of life-sustaining technologies on the elderly. Report noted that the most controversial of the technologies was that of nutritional support. Identified that the most troublesome aspect of nutritional support is whether it is intravenous feeding and hydration or a tube feeding (Fry, 1990).
1987	Hasting's Center—*Guidelines on the Termination of Life-sustaining Treatment*	Provided clear definitions of key terms and a general guideline for making decisions regarding treatment. Viewed nutrition and hydration as medical interventions, much as other life-sustaining measures. Placed emphasis on the patient's ability to make decisions and required case-by-case assessment (Fry, 1990).
1988	American Nurses Association—*Guidelines on Withdrawing or Withholding Food and Fluid*	Indicated that there were few instances under which it would be permissible for nurses to withdraw food or fluid from their patients. No- distinction was made between withdrawing and withholding (ANA, 1988).
1992	American Nurses Association—*Position Statement on Foregoing Medically Provided Nutrition and Hydration*	Stated that the decision to withhold medically provided nutrition and hydration should be made by the patient or surrogate with the healthcare team. The nurse continues to provide expert and compassionate care to patients who are no longer receiving medically provided nutrition and hydration. Distinguished between medically provided nutrition and hydration and the provision of food and water (ANA, 1992).
1994	Alzheimer Association	Stated that if such a patient is unable to receive food and water by mouth, it is ethically permissible to choose to withhold nutrition and hydration artificially administered by vein or gastric tube. Spoon-feeding should be continued if needed for comfort (Alzheimer's Association, n.d.).

	ORGANIZATION	POSITION
2005	National Hospice and Palliative Care Organization (NHPCO)	Indicated that is always acceptable to withhold or withdraw artificial nutrition and hydration when a competent patient refuses or when adequate evidence exists that an incompetent patient would have found the balance of risks and potential benefits to be unacceptable or when it is in the patient's best interest (NHPCO, 2005).
2009	American Pediatric Association	Supported the position that withdrawal or withholding medical interventions is morally permissible when requested by competent patients, or, in the case of patients without decision making capacity, when the interventions no longer confer a benefit to the patient or when the burdens associated with the interventions outweigh the benefits received. (Diekema & Botkin, 2009).

Assisted Suicide

Assisted suicide involves helping another end his or her life. In June 1997, the US Supreme Court rendered a decision on physician-assisted suicide (PAS). This decision took the position that there was no constitutionally protected right to PAS on behalf of terminally ill patients.

The activities of a retired Michigan pathologist, Jack Kevorkian, who is alleged to have assisted patients in their suicide, received much media attention in the 1990s. Although eluding criminal charges for a number of years, in March 1999, Dr. Kevorkian was convicted of second-degree murder and the delivery of a controlled substance after CBS televised a video showing him administering lethal drugs. Dr. Kevorkian's release from prison in 2007 brought renewed attention to the issue of assisted suicide.

In April 2001, The Netherlands became the first nation to fully legalize euthanasia, a process that was 3 years in the making.

Currently two states, Washington and Oregon, have set aside the Supreme Court ruling to the extent that residents have supported Death with Dignity Acts allowing PAS, and California has proposed such legislation at least once. On December 31, 2009, the Montana Supreme Court determined that nothing in state law prevents patients from seeking PAS, making Montana the third state that will allow the procedure. The Montana law falls far short of the reform standard established by Oregon and Washington where the legislature has immunized doctors from having to stand trial if challenged so long as they comply in good faith with a set of rigorous procedures (Bowden, 2010). Oregon first passed such legislation in 1997 and reconfirmed it in 1994; Washington's legislation became effective on March 5, 2009. Both Oregon and Washington released their 2009 reports on the use of the Death with Dignity law in each state. In Oregon in 2009, 59 terminally ill patients used the law to hasten their deaths, and 36 terminally ill patients used the law in Washington (Death with Dignity National Center, 2011). Further details of the reports may be obtained by going to *http://www.deathwithdignity.org* and clicking on the state's report. Montana has not had time to accrue any statistics.

The ANA has developed a position statement in which it states that the nurse should not participate in assisted suicide. Such an act is viewed as a violation of the Code for Nurses (see Chapter 8). It is the position of the ANA that the challenge for nurses should not be in legalizing assisted suicide. Rather, the role of the nurse should be directed toward reversing the despair and pain experienced in the last stages of life, and in fulfilling the obligation to provide competent, comprehensive, and compassionate end-of-life care (ANA, 1994).

The Right to Refuse Treatment

The **right to refuse treatment** is an issue closely aligned with the right to die. However, it carries special implications that require separate consideration. Although we discussed some of the parameters of this issue in the previous section on the right to die, other aspects can create even bigger problems for the nurse. Support of the right to refuse treatment is based on a basic belief in and respect for the autonomy of the patient. Cases such as one in which a patient refuses to have a leg amputated, even though not having the surgery undoubtedly will result in death, often will make the news. When the patient refuses treatment but does not withdraw from the role of being the patient, the matter becomes more complex. By refusing one type of treatment, the patient is essentially demanding alternative medical management. An example would be the patient who refuses to have a gangrenous toe surgically removed and demands to have it treated otherwise. One form of treatment may be more accepted than another, but both may be successful. When children are involved, it is even more newsworthy, and again points out that there is as yet no consensus about when minors should be allowed to refuse treatment. Often, cases involving children are related to cases in which the parents refuse to have the treatment started, many times because of religious beliefs. The courts usually become involved in reaching a decision. When time is not a factor, the court may recommend that treatment be delayed until the child is 15 or 16 years old and can make a decision as an older minor. Other judges will rule just the opposite, deciding that it is cruel to place the burden of the decision on this older minor.

Because nurses have the most contact with patients, they must examine their own feelings and attitudes when patients refuse treatment. Nurses must recognize that patients also have the right to attitudes and beliefs. If a nurse decides that his or her feelings are so strong that they might interfere with the ability to give compassionate care, it would be wise to ask to be assigned to other patients (Fig. 9.2).

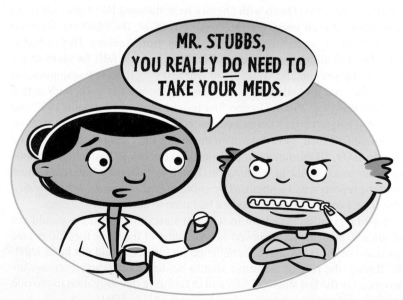

FIGURE 9.2 People working in the healthcare field are frequently confronted with the dilemma of patients who may wish to refuse treatment.

BIOETHICAL CONCERNS RELATED TO SUSTAINING QUALITY OF LIFE

With the increase in technology, bioethical concerns have expanded significantly to include issues related to maintaining or sustaining the quality of life through such procedures as organ transplantation, xenotransplantation, and stem cell research. We cannot discuss all of these in detail, but will provide an overview of the topics. We encourage those interested in this area to explore the topic further on the related Web sites listed on thePoint.

Organ and Tissue Transplantation

Developments in the area of organ transplantation have created several issues deserving consideration. **Organ transplantation** is the process by which an entire organ is removed and replaced by a corresponding part. Tissue transplantation involves the use of tissues such as skin, bone, cartilage, and corneas. Developments in the area of organ and tissue transplantation have created several issues deserving consideration. Transplants can be done using tissue from one's own body; this is called an autograft. Transplantation using organs or tissue from a donor's body is known as homograft or allograft; it might involve organs such as the kidney, liver, pancreas, and heart, and tissues such as cornea, bone, or skin of another individual. Some organs (eg, the heart) must be transplanted immediately, or the tissue will die. Others, such as the kidney, can be stored for short periods. Many tissues, such as bone and skin, may be preserved for long periods of time. Organs require matching between the donor and the recipient, while most tissues do not require a match. According to the United Network for Organ Sharing (UNOS), there are more than 106,397 individuals waiting for an organ transplant (UNOS, 2010).

Initially, the replacement for a diseased organ was obtained from a donor who had died. More recently, organs have been received from living donors. In 2009, UNOS listed 6,609 living donors, compared with 21,853 deceased donors. Transplants performed during this period numbered 28,462 (UNOS, 2010). In a landmark study conducted by Johns Hopkins researchers and published in the March 2010 issue of the Journal of the American Medical Association of more than 80,000 live kidney donors from across the United States, it was found that the procedure carries very little medical risk and that, in the long term, people who donate one of their kidneys are likely to live just as long as those who have two healthy ones (Segev, Abimereki, Muzaale, et al., 2010).

The supply of organs that can be used for transplantation has not been able to keep up with the demand. Individuals who wish to donate organs should check what is required in the state in which they reside. Many states allow people to indicate their wishes on their driver's licenses, or they can sign up online at that state's organ and tissue donor registry. A model donor card, which includes provisions for designating whether all organs and tissues may be donated, as well as lines for signatures by two witnesses has been developed (Fig. 9.3). This card may be downloaded from the Internet site *http://www.organdonor.gov/donor/index.htm*.

Concerns About Organ Procurement

Organ procurement refers to all the activities involved in obtaining donated organs. The idea of consent becomes important when we talk about organ transplantation and procurement. It is preferable to have the consent obtained from the donor. This has been facilitated in many states by the Uniform Anatomical Gift Act, which was drafted by a committee of the National Conference of the Commissions of Uniform State Laws in July 1968.

Organ/Tissue Donor Card

I wish to donate my organs and tissues. I wish to give:

☐ **any needed organs and tissues** ☐ **only the following organs and tissues:**

____

Donor Signature ______________________ **Date** __________

Witness ______________________________

Witness ______________________________

FIGURE 9.3 Organ/tissue donor card.

In most instances, the next of kin also must grant permission for the removal of organs and tissues after death. However, the time factor is crucial; the deaths are often accidental, and the relatives are often so emotionally distressed that the process of obtaining permission may be uncomfortable. Hospitals that receive Medicare funds are mandated to have required request policies in place. Typically, they have developed a procurement team that has received special preparation related to requesting organ donations. These are persons skilled in recognizing the stress being felt by the family and experienced in providing information that will be important to them. A growing number of hospitals are designating a nurse as transplantation coordinator to facilitate this process.

In an effort to increase the number of donated organs, some federal grants have been awarded to obtain organs from emergency room patients—an action that has been considered off-limits in the United States. In this project, surgeons would take organs from individuals who had agreed to become donors by checking off a box on their driver's license or by signing up on a state registry and would not seek a family member's consent if one is not present. This process, known as "donation after cardiac death" or DCD, would be done within minutes from the time a patient being treated in the emergency department (ED) is declared brain-dead. Doctors must wait two minutes after death has been pronounced before taking steps to retrieve organs. Although this practice may have occurred in intensive care units or other parts of the hospital when death was anticipated and family members could be consulted, it has not been common in emergency departments. Experts worry that the practice of DCD in EDs could influence how hard nurses and doctors might work to save patients (Stein, 2010).

Children and young people experience the most critical need for human organs. This has caused us to challenge previous decisions. A good example is that raised when considering organs removed from an anencephalic infant. An anencephalic infant is one born with only enough brain to support such vital functions as heartbeat and respiration. It has been estimated that about 60% of these infants are stillborn, and of those born alive, only about 5% will live longer than 3 days. Because anencephaly affects only the brain, other organs can be used for transplantation if the infant is kept alive on a respirator until an organ recipient is located. This challenges our definitions of death. How can current definitions of "brain" death be applied to a condition in which there is no brain as we normally recognize it?

Artificial Organs

The skill of modern technology has resulted in the development and implantation of artificial organs such as the heart. Such technologic advances once were viewed as science fiction. As a result, historic cases such as the implantation of an artificial heart in Barney Clark in 1982 received a great deal of publicity. Over the years, the use of artificial organs has not proven effective for long-term use, but artificial organs have made it possible for individuals to live with the hope that a transplantable organ will become available. Over the past few years, a heart assist has been developed and used to provide the patient's heart a rest and an opportunity to heal, in some instances reducing the need for heart transplantation. Work and research to develop better organs continues, and recipients are living longer, although the promise is far less than that with donated organs. The use of artificial joints, heart valves, and other prostheses continues to grow and to be successful.

Minority Groups and Organ Donation

Another issue that has emerged is that of minority differences regarding organ donation. Of the persons awaiting an organ for transplantation, minorities form more than half the kidney transplant waiting list with blacks accounting for 34.2% of the list (Organ Procurement and Transplantation Network [OPTN], 2011). More minority donors are needed to increase the chances that a well-matched organ will be available to minorities awaiting transplants.

Several factors may affect reticence of minorities to donate organs. Some groups have identified religious beliefs and cultural customs as forbidding organ donation, although no major Western religion prohibits organ donation. Religious objection often stems from the high value attached to keeping the body intact. African Americans listed distrust of the medical community, fear of premature death, and racism as major barriers. Hispanics experienced language barriers and identified the importance of having the entire extended family involved in all decision making regarding donations. Puerto Ricans verbalized denial of death and fear of mutilation of the body as critical factors. Barriers to organ donation in Asian American cultures included the belief that the body should remain intact to the grave and lack of respect during the handling of the body after death. Although Native Americans are theoretically supportive of organ donations, their rate of donation is low, probably due to lack of knowledge. Although no single approach to organ donation fits all groups, efforts to decrease barriers to donation are being instituted.

The Minority Organ and Tissue Transplant Education Program (MOTTEP) has a number of sites across the country focused on educating the minority community in an effort to increase the number of minority donors and transplant recipients. MOTTEP represents African

American, Hispanic/Latino, Native American, Asian, Pacific Island, and Alaskan Native populations. It includes a health promotion and disease prevention component designed to reduce the incidence of conditions that can lead to organ failure. It can be reached at the Web site *www.mottep.org*.

Critical Thinking Activity

Have you signed an organ donation card? If not, discuss the reasons why you have chosen not to do so. If you have, discuss the reasons why you have. Is there a possibility you will change your mind? Why or why not? What solutions can you suggest to help the nation deal with the shortage of organs needed for transplantation?

Concerns About Allocation of Organs

How will we determine who receives donated organs? Does elitism exist in their distribution—that is, does a wealthy individual have a better chance to receive an organ than someone who is poor? Medicaid and most insurance policies refuse to pay for the cost of many organ transplants, although Medicare usually covers the costs of corneal transplants and kidney transplants. Transplants are expensive procedures, often running into several hundreds of thousands of dollars, and success is not guaranteed. If money is required up-front, as it sometimes is, where can the needy person procure such funds?

Other questions involve both donor and recipient. Should the donor or the donor's family have the right to say who will receive the organ? How does one get onto the list for an organ, and how can that need be made known? What about selling a healthy organ, such as a kidney? Current law makes it a crime to sell body parts.

Much has been written about the problem of selecting recipients for organ transplantation when the number of applicants exceeds the number of available organs. Many criteria have been suggested, and as one might anticipate, these criteria have arguments both pro and con; the criterion requiring medical acceptability is probably the only exception. Many transplants require that compatibility exist in the tissue and blood type of donor and recipient. In response to this problem, some centers transplant organs that are less well matched. This results in a higher rejection rate, but as immunosuppression improves, this is less marked than it was formerly. Other centers do not believe it appropriate to give a much-needed organ to a person whose body would have a high potential for rejection.

The criterion of the recipient's social worth is probably one of the hardest to defend, although it was used in the Pacific Northwest in the early 1960s to decide who should be allowed to live by kidney dialysis. Social worth, including past and future potential, was considered, and even such factors as church membership and participation in community endeavors were considered.

Some suggest a form of random selection, once the criterion of medical acceptability has been met. This could be either a natural random selection of the first-come, first-served variety, or an artificial selection process such as a lottery. A criticism of this method is that it removes rational decision making from the process.

We offer no suggestions to solve this problem but merely demonstrate the difficulty it presents. Even the issue of who should serve on the decision-making committee can be problematic. The potential for personal biases is a big concern.

In an effort to gather donations and disseminate information about individuals who need various organs, an Organ Procurement Program was started in Pittsburgh, Pennsylvania. This program was established to facilitate the matching of donor with recipient and to provide a central listing agency for those in need of transplants. Today, organ procurement agencies are located in all regions of the country. These groups carry out many activities related to organ procurement, including establishing groups for individuals who have received donated organs and their families, publishing newsletters, developing educational materials, increasing public awareness of the need for organs, and serving as a clearinghouse for organ procurement and matching. They are connected through the federally funded UNOS.

Xenotransplantation

Xenotransplantation refers to the practice of using animal organs, cells, and tissues for transplantation into human beings. Some scientists believe that having a reliable supply of organs from pigs or other animals could solve the great shortage from human donors. It is in the stage of experimentation around the world.

Xenotransplantation usually involves organs or tissues from pigs and nonhuman primates. The transplants done to date have, for the most part, been unsuccessful. In addition to the obvious problems associated with immune system rejection, of particular concern to some is the possibility of transmitting serious animal viruses and other microbes, so-called zoonotic diseases, to people, particularly from primates. This has prompted pigs to become the donor of choice and has led to attempts to alter pigs genetically so that tissues would be more adaptable to transplantation.

Concerns in England over the communicability of bovine spongiform encephalopathy through the ingestion of meat from ill animals has prompted the discussion of the potential for all animal organs to transmit diseases that would appear only years later. Even raising animals in a sterile environment has its limitations, because it is now being discovered that some diseases are transmitted from mother to fetus in utero. Some groups in England are urging that the xenotransplantation project be abandoned and that research into xenotransplantation be stopped because of the social cost and because of ongoing suffering of animals inherent in such an approach.

In September 1996, the federal government proposed strict safeguards to provide protection. Representatives from the Food and Drug Administration (FDA), the Centers for Disease Control and Prevention, and the National Institutes of Health (NIH) developed the guidelines. The guidelines urged that patients and their families be fully informed of potential risks and further required that any planned procedure be thoroughly screened and approved by a series of local institutional review boards and by the FDA. The recommendations also require that transplants take place at a clinical center associated with an accredited biology and microbiology laboratory.

The Human Genome Project

A **genome** may be defined as an organism's complete set of deoxyribonucleic acid (DNA), a chemical compound that contains the genetic instructions needed to develop and direct the activities of every organism, including the genes that carry information for making the proteins required by all organisms. These proteins determine such things as how the organism looks, how well its body metabolizes food and fights infection, and sometimes even how it behaves. DNA molecules are made of two twisting, paired strands. Each strand is made of four chemical units, called nucleotide bases, abbreviated A, T, C, and G, and are repeated millions or billions of times throughout a genome. The human genome contains approximately 3 billion of these base pairs, which reside in the 23 pairs of chromosomes within the nucleus of all our cells. Each chromosome contains hundreds to thousands of genes, which carry the instructions for making proteins (National Human Genome Research Institute, 2009). The order of As, Ts, Cs, and Gs is important because it underlies all of life's diversity, including whether an organism is human or of another species.

The **Human Genome Project (HGP)**, first proposed by Nobel prize–winning virologist Renato Dulbecco in 1986, started in October 1990. The goal of the project was to map the entire human genome and involved at least 18 countries in the international effort. It was coordinated by the Department of Energy and the NIH. The project was completed in April 2003.

Genomes have been studied for many reasons, including disease prevention, determination of the effects of radiation and chemicals on living species, and more recently, genetic therapy. Genome-based research will eventually enable medical science to develop highly effective diagnostic tools, to better understand the health needs of people based on their individual genetic makeups and to design new and highly effective treatments for disease. Individualized analysis based on each person's genome will lead to a very powerful form of preventive medicine.

The ethical and bioethical concerns that can evolve from this research are many and varied. Among them are the issues of access to and use of new genetic information and technology to improve health, research that would involve human participants, and the implications of the discovery of genetic contributions related to diseases, nondisease attributes, and various behavioral traits such as cognition, mental illness, diurnal rhythms, and aging for how we understand health and illness. In preparation for these challenges, the National Human Genome Research Institute's (NHGRI) Ethical, Legal, and Social Implications (ELSI) Research Program was established in 1990 as an integral part of the HGP. Its purpose was to foster basic and applied research on the ELSI of genetic and genomic research for individuals, families, and communities. The ELSI Research Program funds and manages studies and supports workshops, research consortia, and policy conferences related to these topics.

More information regarding the HGP and related issues can be obtained from the Web site, *www.genome.gov/HGP/*.

Gene Therapy

An estimated 4,000 disease genes have been identified that reside with the genome. Identification and isolation of defective genes, and their replacement with functional genes (gene therapy), could result in the elimination of diseases that have plagued society for generations. Several significant conditions currently under study are cystic fibrosis, Huntington disease, myotonic dystrophy, gout, and adult polycystic kidney disease.

Gene therapy is an experimental technique that uses genes to treat or prevent disease. It is anticipated that this technique may allow doctors to treat a disorder by inserting a gene into a patient's cells instead of using drugs or surgery. Researchers are testing several approaches to gene therapy, including

- Replacing a mutated gene that causes disease with a healthy copy of the gene
- Inactivating, or "knocking out," a mutated gene that is functioning improperly
- Introducing a new gene into the body to help fight a disease

Although gene therapy is a promising treatment option for a number of diseases (including inherited disorders, some types of cancer, and certain viral infections), the technique remains risky and is still under study to ensure its safety and effectiveness. Gene therapy is currently only being tested for the treatment of diseases that have no other cures.

To date, gene therapy is primarily experimental and has produced far more failures than successes. Positive results in mice do not necessarily promise positive outcomes for humans. Many of the basic problems with gene therapies have not been worked out. A mechanism to insert the new gene into the body needs to be found. Scientists need a better understanding of how genes function. The problems associated with multigene disorders must be solved. As research has progressed, it has become apparent that even genetically based diseases have multiple causative factors that may affect whether the disease is actually expressed in a given individual. Questions regarding the repair of genes versus the replacement of genes are yet to be answered. The high costs associated with this new technology present another concern. However, gene therapy offers a wide array of possibilities and undoubtedly will gain momentum in the near future.

Stem Cell Research

A **stem cell** is a special kind of cell that is able to renew itself and give rise to specialized cell types. These cells, unlike most other cells in the body, such as those of the heart or skin, are not committed to conduct a specific function. The cell remains uncommitted until it receives a signal to develop into a specialized cell. Scientists are looking at a type of stem cell that is called "pluripotent," because pluripotent cells have the ability to differentiate into any type of cell found in the body. Until recently, stem cells have come from three main sources: embryonic cells, umbilical cord cells, and adult cells. Out of these three cells, the form with the least amount of controversy is the adult type—doctors extract cells from the bone marrow of the patient's body, which causes some pain and some destruction to bone marrow. The advantage is that the DNA is an exact match to the patient's, and is used to replace other dead or damaged cells in the body. Adult cells are also plentiful.

The second type of stem cells is extracted from the umbilical cord, which is then stored using a process similar to storing donated blood. The infant and immediate family are the best ones to receive these stem cells because of the close genetic match, but other people with similar blood types can also benefit.

The most controversy comes from embryonic cell use. These cells are extracted from the embryo before these cells start to differentiate. The embryo at this state is known as a "blastocyst." Most of the 100 cells in the "blastocyst" are stem cells. These can be grown and kept alive in cultures indefinitely, and will replicate and double about every 3 days in number. In order to get these cells, the embryo must be destroyed—a process that is unacceptable to those who believe life begins at fertilization. Researchers and scientists believe that embryonic stem cells hold the future cures for a variety of medical illnesses and diseases such as cancer, Alzheimer disease, Parkinson disease, and diabetes. The list of possible cures that can be found through this research is very lengthy (NIH, 2010).

Recently scientists have discovered that stem cells can be extracted from amniotic fluid. These amnion stem cells can form three-dimensional aggregates of cells known as embryoid bodies (EBs). It is believed that cells at this stage of development can be directed to become virtually any cell in the human body. They also can be grown in large quantities and are readily available during gestation and at the time of birth (Biology News Net, 2009).

Because research of this nature needs federal funding and approval to move forward, stem cell debate is a national issue. On March 9, 2009, President Obama issued Executive Order 13505 which removed the barrier to embryonic stem cell research established in August 2001 by former President George W. Bush (NIH, 2009). In October 2010, researchers in California announced the injection of stem cells derived from human embryonic tissue in a clinical trial involving patients with thoracic spinal cord injuries (First Human Trials with Stem Cells Begin, 2010). This was followed by the government approval, in November 2010, of the testing of the use of embryonic stem cells in the treatment of individuals suffering from Stargardt disease, which affects about 30,000 Americans and attacks central vision. The hope is that it can be expanded to treat age-related macular degeneration that affects millions (Stem-Cell Study to Treat Blindness OK'd, 2010).

Critical Thinking Activity

Given the arguments for and against stem cell research, what position would you take? Why do you hold this position? What are your biases? Discuss your position with someone who holds the opposite point of view. What are that person's strongest arguments?

OTHER BIOETHICAL ISSUES

Although our discussion cannot be exhaustive of the topic, certain events occur frequently enough in the healthcare delivery system that we would be remiss in not mentioning them.

Truth Telling and Healthcare Providers

The issue of whether to share specific information with a patient may not carry the emotional and bioethical impact that one experiences with concerns such as euthanasia, but it is often encountered in the healthcare environment. Although informed consent has forced a more straightforward approach between physician and client, the problem of having the patient fully understand the outcome of care still exists (see Chapter 8). Sometimes, the question about telling the client the expected outcome of care results from a request made by a close relative, but most of the time it results from the persistence of past medical practices.

In such instances, the physician operates in a paternalistic role in relation to the client. Under this model of care, the locus of decision making is moved away from the client and resides with the physician. "Benefit and do no harm to the patient" is the dictum often cited as the ethical basis for this approach. It rationalizes that complete knowledge of his or her condition would place greater stress on the client. More recent discussions of medical ethics explore the rights of clients, particularly their right to make their own medical decisions. These discussions emphasize that in our pluralistic society, which also has fostered medical specialization to keep up with advances in knowledge and technology, physicians may be unable to perceive the best interests of their clients and to act accordingly.

Physicians do not agree on how much information should be provided to patients regarding their conditions. We usually experience a major controversy relating to this issue when a client has a terminal diagnosis such as cancer. Physicians may feel concerned that sharing bad news will result in unhappiness, anxiety, depression, and fear, and that the client suffering from a terminal illness will give up. In some cultures, such as Japan, this approach is widely considered appropriate, and both physicians and families strongly believe that those who are ill should be protected from bad news.

Physicians who argue the other side of the issue state that there exists a common moral obligation to tell the truth. They believe that the anxiety of not knowing the accurate diagnosis is at least as great as knowing the truth, especially if the truth is shared in a humane manner. These physicians also argue that one needs to have control over one's life and, if the news is bad, to have time to get personal affairs in order.

Regulations regarding informed consent and more aggressive treatment for all life-threatening conditions have minimized situations in which patients are not provided full knowledge of their condition. However, these situations still arise. Sometimes, care providers are challenged as to the best ethical and legal approach when a family is from a different cultural background and strongly disagrees with giving full information to a patient.

Thus far, we have discussed situations in which information regarding a terminal illness may be shared with the client and family. At least one other circumstance that involves telling the truth is worth mentioning, although many examples could be included. One that we often see in the obstetric area of the hospital deals with sharing information with the parents of a newborn who is critically ill or who has a malformation. Sometimes, physicians want to spare the mother unpleasant news until she is stronger. This occurs frequently enough for obstetric nurses to have labeled it "spare-the-mother syndrome." In some instances, the physician may want to delay giving information until suspicions can be validated. If the doctor is waiting for the return of laboratory tests to confirm suspicions of genetic abnormalities, several days may be required. If good communication exists between nurse and physician, so that the nurse is well informed, the nurse can provide emotional support and meet the client's need for information.

Another situation in which sharing the truth may be a concern occurs when a parent is diagnosed with a degenerative disease (such as Huntington disease) for which there is no cure and that is an autosomal dominant trait (ie, there is a 50% chance that an offspring also will develop the disease). Should this information be shared with the offspring? Because there is also a 50% chance they will not develop the condition, is it wrong to compromise the individual's good life with bad news? What if the parent does not want the information shared and the physician believes it should be? Is ignorance bliss? What about the right to make informed choices and decisions?

Although to tell or not to tell (or to delay telling) is a problem that exists between client and physician, nurses often become involved. Because the nurse is in contact with the client for a more extended time, he or she may be put on the spot by the client's questions. The nurse may feel that hedging on a response compromises the ethics of nursing practice. In such instances, a conference, whether formal or impromptu, that would involve the physician, nurses, and other appropriate members of the health team, may help everyone deal with the situation. The nurse who is a novice in the healthcare system should realize that anyone may initiate a client care conference, although appropriate channels of communication should be followed in organizing it.

The question of whether to tell has been applied to another issue in the healthcare delivery system in recent years. That controversy pits the rights to privacy of the individual who is HIV positive against society's right to be protected.

Many express concerns about privacy and confidentiality. If universal testing for AIDS were to be mandated, what would be next? Others argue that if healthcare providers exercise proper precautions, little danger exists. Still others would find the cost of universal testing too great to make it realistic. There is no agreement among healthcare providers, activists, civil libertarians, and all concerned citizens regarding this issue, and the controversy is certain to continue.

Ethical Concerns and Behavior Control

Many people experience extreme discomfort when contemplating research into human behavior and **behavior control**. Although it may be one thing to work with atoms, molecules, and genes, it seems quite another to look at the science of human behavior.

Some of the problem seems to center around the fact that people define "acceptable behavior" in different and sometimes conflicting ways. When is behavior deviant? When is the client mentally ill? An excellent example is that of homosexuality, which the American Psychiatric Association at one time listed as a mental illness. Although many people may not approve of homosexuality, they would not classify all homosexuals as being mentally ill. Increasingly, society looks on sexual orientation as a personal matter.

The world has benefited from the work of many people whose behavior might not be looked upon as normal. Van Gogh cut off his ear; Tchaikovsky had terrible periods of depression; Beethoven was known for his uncontrollable rages. Some have suggested that Florence Nightingale's flights into fantasy could better be described as neurosis. Should this behavior have been changed? If so, by what methods?

We now can change behavior by several methods. Certainly one of the most common methods in which nurses will be involved is the administration of pharmacologic agents. Psychotropics are now one of the largest classifications of drugs in the United States. Many of these such as antianxiety agents and antidepressants are prescribed for people who wish to modify their feelings and behaviors. Other chemicals, such as alcohol, marijuana, cocaine, and methamphetamine also change mood and/or behavior. Some of these are considered socially acceptable, whereas others are not. Some are socially acceptable to some people or to some cultures yet unacceptable to others.

Electroconvulsive therapy (ECT), known earlier as electric shock therapy (EST), has been used for years to treat severe depression. Although antidepressant drugs are more commonly used today, ECT is still used in many areas of the country for depression that does not respond to drugs. Opponents of this form of therapy, who see it as inhumane, are becoming an organized political force. Proponents point out that with the current safeguards, it can be an effective therapy.

Psychosurgery—for example, frontal lobotomy (portrayed in *One Flew Over the Cuckoo's Nest*)—was used in the 1930s. This is undoubtedly one of the most criticized treatment modalities because of its effect on the person. It is rarely used today, although another type of brain surgery is now being suggested for obsessive–compulsive disorder (OCD) that will not respond to other forms of treatment. The surgery involves the use of radio-frequency waves to destroy a small amount of brain tissue, which disrupts a specific circuit in the brain that has been implicated in OCD.

Psychotherapy can change other behaviors. Techniques include verbal and nonverbal communication between the client and the therapist. Although psychotherapy requires considerable time, it is widely used.

When are any of these methods justified? Who makes the decision? What behavior is beyond the realm of acceptability? Who determines this? How does behavior control mesh with our beliefs about the autonomy of the individual or with concepts of self-respect and dignity? The issues of power and coercion pose a concern at this point. Problems related to involuntary commitment have moved this from the arena of ethics to that of legal determinants.

Many of the issues related to controlling the behavior of human subjects have been eased with the passage of legislation such as the Self-Determination Act and emphasis on informed consent and patients' rights. It is important to remember, if working on a mental health team, that clients receiving care retain all civil rights afforded to all people with the exception of the right to leave if involuntarily committed. Each state has laws specific to how such cases are managed and how long an individual can be detained.

Critical Thinking Activity

What do you see as the major issues related to controlling the behavior of others? Under what circumstances do you feel it is justified to take action? Why do you believe these circumstances warrant action? If action is taken, which of the ethical theories (ie, autonomy, beneficence, veracity, fidelity, and utilitarianism—[see Chapter 8]) are at risk?

Rationing of Healthcare

Perhaps no issue in healthcare causes more distress than the **rationing of healthcare**. Rationing is restricting the availability of some desired commodity (healthcare) to limited amounts for each individual. Most consider rationing to be a planned, thoughtful approach to a limited supply. Some would argue that we currently ration healthcare by restricting its availability to those with the financial means to pay, although none would argue that this is a carefully planned approach. Insurance companies ration by limiting what they will pay for and how much they will pay. Medicare and Medicaid have strict payment rules that might be considered rationing.

Closely related to rationing is the concern for scarce medical resources, especially as seen with regard to the need of organs for implantation. Technology has allowed people to live longer. New treatment modalities have become more expensive. Dollars do not exist within our current social system to make all forms of healthcare available to all who wish to receive it. What should be treated and what should not? Who should receive the treatment and who should not? Should age be a factor? Mental status? Ability to contribute to society?

Some states have begun to address these issues. In 1989, the Oregon legislature passed several statutes that, among other things, created a process to establish healthcare priorities so that Medicaid and state-encouraged private coverage could provide the most cost-effective and beneficial forms of care for the largest number of persons. Explicit in this legislation was the involvement of the public in the process of building consensus on the values to be used to guide health resource allocation decisions. Oregon has continued to lead the nation in healthcare reform, especially at the consumer involvement level.

In Vermont, a statewide public education and discussion project was initiated to explore public attitudes and values that underlie healthcare and the public's priorities in the allocation of health resources. The project focused on the need for individuals to make known their preferences with regard to personal treatment.

In New Jersey, a Citizens' Committee on Biomedical Ethics has taken the position that citizens have the right and responsibility to insist that their preferences and values influence the development of healthcare policies and the allocation of medical resources. They have launched a community health program to clarify the ethical and social issues surrounding the provision of healthcare in that state.

Other states are following these examples. Citizens are being asked to make informed decisions regarding healthcare. As a nurse, you have a vital role to play in the sharing of information regarding the delivery of health services. It is critical for you to anticipate some of the questions you may be asked and to analyze your own values (Fig. 9.4).

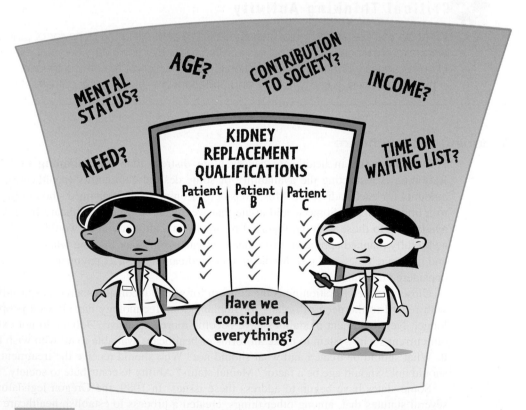

FIGURE 9.4 It is critical that you analyze your own values.

Critical Thinking Activity

What do you see as the major issues regarding the rationing of healthcare? Develop a list of the major health conditions for which you believe care should be funded. Identify those that should receive partial funding. List those that you believe should not be funded. Give a rationale for placing the various conditions on one of the three lists.

KEY CONCEPTS

- Bioethics is the study of ethical issues that result from technologic and scientific advances, especially in biology and medicine. The number of bioethical issues surrounding the delivery of healthcare is growing.
- Many bioethical issues are associated with conditions related to the beginning of life and/ or with those related to the end of life.
- Family planning (and the associated concern regarding age of consent) is one issue related to the beginning of life. Personal preferences and religious beliefs are critical determinants, and nurses should be prepared to meet the needs of all clients without imposing their personal values on clients.
- Abortion, amniocentesis, chorionic villus sampling, prenatal diagnosis, genetic screening, sterilization, the concept of eugenics, artificial insemination, assisted reproductive technology, and the right to genetic information are additional topics presenting concerns.
- Fundamental bioethical issues concerning death are affected by the changing definition of death and the decision about when it occurs.
- Although many courts, based on individual circumstances, have accepted negative euthanasia, positive euthanasia remains controversial.
- Surrounding the discussion of right to die are many issues, including those related to patient self-determination, futile treatment,

withholding or withdrawing treatment, assisted death, and the right to refuse treatment.
- Bioethical concerns associated with the process of organ transplantation include procurement of organs, availability of organs for minorities, allocation of organs, individual property rights, and the appropriateness of xenotransplantations.
- The area of human genetic research has raised many ethical questions, including how this knowledge should be used, rights to privacy, and who in the healthcare delivery system carries the responsibility for making testing, diagnosis, and cost-effective care available to patients.
- Stem cell research, which holds great promise for diseases and conditions for which there is no cure, is also laden with bioethical concerns, particularly those related to whether a blastocyst should be considered a human life.
- Debate and controversy have long surrounded determining what degree of information should be shared with clients and their families.
- The area of behavior control is subject to bioethical review. Recent legislation focused on patient self-determination and rights have provided guidance in this area.
- Rationing of healthcare commands major attention now. Many states have begun to establish citizen committees to respond to this concern.

RELEVANT WEB SITES

Web sites relevant to this chapter can be found at **the Point**✷ accessed through *http://thePoint. lww.com/Ellis10e* and by entering the code found on the inside cover of your text.

REFERENCES

Age of Consent Chart for the US. (2009). Retrieved March 10, 2010, from http://www.ageofconsent.us/

Alexander, S. (1962). They decide who lives, who dies. *Life. 53,* 102–125.

All About Popular Issues. (2002–2010). *History of stem cell research.* Retrieved March 19, 2010, from http://www.allaboutpopularissues.org/history-of-stem-cell-research-faq.htm

Alzheimer's Association. (n.d.). *Ethical Issues in Alzheimer's disease: Assisted oral feeding and tube feeding.* Retrieved August 12, 2010, from http://www.alzdsw.org/pdf_documents/factsheets/oralfeeding.pdf

American Nurses Association. (1988). *Guidelines on withdrawing or withholding food and fluid.* Washington, DC: Author.

American Nurses Association. (1991). *Position statement on nursing and the Patient Self-Determination Act.* Washington, DC: Author.

American Nurses Association. (1992). *Position statement on foregoing medically provided nutrition and hydration.* Washington, DC: Author.

American Nurses Association. (1994). *Position statement on assisted suicide.* Washington, DC: Author.

Baruch, S., Javitt, G., Scott, J., Hudson, K. (2010). Genetics and public policy center - Center reports. *Preimplantation genetic diagnosis: A discussion of challenges, concerns, and preliminary policy options related to the genetic testing of human embryos.* Retrieved March 12, 2010, from http://www.dnapolicy.org/pub.reports.php?action=detail&report_id=7

Biology News Net. (2009). *New research shows versatility of amniotic fluid stem cells.* Retrieved August 11, 2010, from http://www.biologynews.net/. Click on archives and type "amniotic fluid stem cells" into search box.

Blackmun, H. (1981). Majority opinion in Roe vs. Wade. In T. A. Mappes & J. S. Zembaty (Eds.), *Biomedical ethics* (2nd ed.) (pp. 478–482). New York, NY: McGraw-Hill.

Bowden, T. (2010). *Montana addresses physician-assisted suicide.* Retrieved August 11, 2010, from http://blog.aynrandcenter.org/montana-addresses-physician-assisted-suicide/

Boyles, S. (2009). *Octuplets birth sparks fertility debate.* Retrieved August 11, 2010, from http://www.webmd.com/infertility-and-reproduction/news/20090210/octuplets-birth-sparks-fertility-debate

Brooks, M. (2010). Advance directives—What's worked and what's failed: An expert interview with Bernard Hammes, PhD. *Medscape Medical News.* Retrieved March 12, 2010 from http://www.medscape.com/viewarticle/717944?src=mp&spon=24&uac=101399FV

Central Intelligence Agency. (2010). *The world factbook.* Retrieved August 11, 2010 from http://www.cia.gov/. Click on World Factbook, then type "Life expectancy" into the search box.

Christ, G. (October 28, 2008). Mother gives birth to triplets for her daughter. *The Daily Record.com.* Retrieved March 13, 2010 from http:www.the-daily-record.com/news/article/4453907

Death with Dignity National Center. (2011). *Living with dying: Just what are death with dignity laws anyway.* Retrieved April 10, 2011 from http://www.deathwithdignity.org

Diekema, D. S. & Botkin, J. R. (2009). *forgoing medically provided nutrition and hydration in children.* American Pediatric Association. Retrieved August 12, 2010 from aappolicy.aappublications.org/cgi/reprint/.../2/813.pdf

First Human Trials with Stem Cells Begin. (2010, October 12). *The Herald,* p. A3.

Fry, S. T. (1990). New ANA guidelines on withdrawing or withholding food and fluid from patients. In C. A. Lindeman & M. McAthie (Eds.), *Readings: Nursing trends and issues* (pp. 499–507). Springhouse, PA: Springhouse.

Grossman, A. (2009). An offering of comfort—A contemplative response to futile treatment. *New York Zen Center for Contemplative Care: June 2009 Newsletter.* Retrieved March 13, 2010 from http://www.zencare.org/newsletter/0905a.html

Herscher, E. (2009). Sperm Banks. *A Healthy Me.* Retrieved March 13, 2009 from http://www.ahealthyme.com/topic/spermbanks

Kidney Transplantation: Past, Present & Future. (n.d.). *History.* Retrieved August 11, 2010, from http://www.stanford.edu/dept/HPS/transplant/index.html

Lombardo, P. (n.d.). *Eugenics sterilization laws.* Retrieved March 11, 2010 from www.eugenicsarchive.org/html/eugenics/essay_8.html

Merriam-Wabster Online Dictionary, bioethics. Retrieved April 10, 2010 from http://www.merriam-webster.com/dictionary/bioethics

National Hospice and Palliative Care Organization. (2005). *Commentary and position statement on artificial nutrition and hydration.* Retrieved August 12, 2010, from http://www.nhpco.org/files/public/ANH_Statement_Commentary.pdf

National Human Genome Research Institute. (2009). *The human genome project completion: Frequently asked questions.* Retrieved March 18 from http://genome.gov/1106943

National Institute of Health. (2009) *Stem Cell Information: US Policy on Stem Cell Research*. Retrieved March 19, 2009 from http://stemcells.nih.gov.

National Institute of Health. (2010). *Stem cell basics*. Retrieved August 11, 2010 from http://stemcells.nih.gov/info/basics

Nuland, S. B. (1996). An epidemic of discovery. *Time Magazine Special Issue*, Fall, pp. 8–13.

Organ Procurement and Transplantation Network. (2011). *National data* Retrieved April 11, 2011 from http://optn.transplant.hrsa.gov/latestData/rptData.asp

Pilbeam, S. P. (1998). *Mechanical ventilation: Physiological and clinical applications* (3rd ed.). St. Louis, MO: Mosby.

Practical Ethics. (2009) *Prenatal sex selection—When prenatal testing can threaten social harmony*. Retrieved August 11, 2010 from http:/www.practicalethicsnews.com. Type "prenatal sex selection" into the search box

Roe v. Wade, 410 U.S. 113 (1973).

Russo, K. (2008) *World's oldest mom*. Retrieved March 12, 2010 from http://abcnews.go.com/Health/ActiveAging/story?id=5309018&page=1

Schneiderman, L. F., Jecker, N., & Jonsen, A. (1996, October 15). Medical futility: Response to critiques. *Annals of Internal Medicine, 125*(8), 669–674. Retrieved March 21, 2010 from www.annals.org/cgi/content/full/125/8/669

Segev, D. L., Abimereki, D., Muzaale, B. S., Caffo, S. H., Mchta, A. L., Singer, S. E., et al. (2010). Perioperative mortality and long-term survival following live kidney donation. *Journal of the American Medical Association, 303*(10), 959–966.

Stein, R. (March 15, 2010).Project to get transplant organs from ER patients raises ethics questions. *The Washington Post*. Retrieved August 11, 2010 from http://www.washingtonpost.com. Type "transplant organs from ER patients" into the archive search box.

Stem-Cell Study to Treat Blindness OK'd. (2010, November 22). *The Herald*, p. A6.

Truffer, C. J., Keehan, S., Smith, S., Cylus, J., Sisko, A., Poisal, J. A., et al. (2010). Health spending projections through 2019: The recession's impact continues. *Health Affairs, 29*(3). Retrieved March 10, 2010 from http://www.politico.com/static/PPM136_100203_health_projections.html

United Network for Organ Sharing. (2010). Data. Retrieved March 14, 2010 from www.unos.org

Zhu, W. X., Lu, L., & Hesketh, T. (2009). *China's excess males, sex selection abortion & one child policy: Analysis of data from 2005 National Intercensus Survey*. Retrieved January 2, 2011 from http://www/bmj.com/cgi/content/abstract/338/apr09_2/b1211

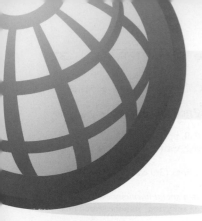

10

Safety Concerns in Healthcare

LEARNING OUTCOMES

After completing this chapter, you should be able to:

1. Identify at least three national organizations that have studied the issue of adverse events and medical errors in healthcare and describe the findings of each study.
2. Discuss the safe practices as outlined by the National Quality Forum and indicate how each would play a part in decreasing errors.
3. Describe actions taken by the Joint Commission to encourage healthcare organizations to reduce the incidence of errors.
4. Explain what is meant by the term "sentinel event."
5. List at least five occurrences that could be labeled adverse events.
6. Describe what a "time-out" involves.
7. Analyze the relationship between "failure to rescue" and nurse staffing.
8. Describe the sources and types of medication errors and explain how medication errors can be interdisciplinary.
9. Discuss the role of the nurse in preventing errors and providing a safe healthcare environment.

KEY TERMS

Culture of safety
Failure to rescue
Handoff
National patient safety goals (NPSG)
Root cause analysis (RCA)

Safe practices
Sentinel events
Serious reportable events (SRE)
Time-out
Universal Protocol

No one—patient, family, or healthcare provider—enters a healthcare setting anticipating that an error will alter that experience and have potentially life-threatening effects. Despite the best intentions, however, a high rate of largely preventable adverse events and medical errors occur that cause harm to patients. There is no immunity from these mistakes: adverse events and medical errors may occur in any healthcare setting and in any community in this country. In this chapter, we discuss some of the more common errors and the nurse's role in prevention of those errors. Nurses as managers of patient care must be actively involved in preventing medical errors.

Table 10.1 **Major Organizations Studying Healthcare Errors**

ORGANIZATION	DESCRIPTION	GOAL
Institute of Medicine	Independent, nonprofit organization, established in 1970 that works outside the government to provide authoritative advice to decision makers and the public to improve health.	To help government and the private sector make informed health decision by providing reliable evidence.
National Quality Forum	Private, nonprofit, open membership public benefit corporation established in 1999 that brings together leaders from every sector of the industry in national dialogue.	To set national priorities, endorse national consensus standards for measuring and publicly reporting on performance, and promoting attainment of national goals through education and outreach.
Joint Commission	Independent, nonprofit organization that accredits and certifies more than 17,000 healthcare organizations in the United States.	To improve healthcare.
Center for Medicare and Medicaid Services	Established in 2001 and previously known as the Healthcare Financing Administration, a federal agency within the U.S. Department of Health and Human Services.	To administer the Medicare program and work in partnership with state governments to administer Medicaid, the State Children's Health Insurance Program, and health insurance portability standards.

NATIONAL ORGANIZATIONS AND ACTIONS

As providers, as well as the general public, became more and more concerned about the errors occurring in the healthcare environment, organizations whose focus was data collection and advising initiated studies to gain information about the problem. Some of the major organizations involved in this process are described in Table 10.1

The Institute of Medicine Study

In response to the growing concern about medical errors, in November 1999, the Institute of Medicine (IOM) released a groundbreaking report estimating that between 44,000 and 98,000 patients die as the result of preventable medical errors in hospitals each year (IOM, 2000). The data presented in the 1999 IOM study caught the attention of the general public as well as that of healthcare providers. Neither patients, providers, nor payers (insurance companies, Medicare, Medicaid, and health maintenance organizations) were totally aware of the safety concerns or, if aware, had not recognized their responsibility to create change. The study also reported that hospital-acquired infections, many of which can be prevented, take another 100,000 lives, while mistakes involving medication injure 1.3 million patients annually in the United States (Landro, 2010). In addition to the human suffering and/or deaths that result, errors are tremendously costly. The total annual cost of preventable medical errors (including expense of additional care, disability, lost income, and productivity) in the United States is estimated between $17 and 29 billion (John Hopkins Medicine, n.d.). The report did not stop with identifying the problem: it also provided an analysis of the multiple causes underlying the safety problem. The report noted that the healthcare system is not a coordinated system at all but is fragmented. Areas of care have been traditionally isolated from one another with ineffective communication between various specialties and agencies as the patient moves from provider to provider.

In March 2001, the IOM released another report titled *Crossing the Quality Chasm*, which focused more broadly on how the healthcare system could be reinvented to foster innovation and improve the delivery of care. It defined six aims—care should be safe, effective, patient centered, timely, efficient, and equitable—and 10 rules for care delivery redesign. Toward this goal, the committee presented a comprehensive strategy and action plan for the coming decade (IOM, 2009).

Subsequently, two campaigns were initiated to increase attention to safety in healthcare. The campaigns focused on precise data collection and numerical improvement with the slogan "Some Is Not A Number. Soon Is Not A Time." The first "Saving 100,000 Lives" campaign was designed to save that many lives in the 2005–2006 time period through eliminating medical errors (Institute for Healthcare Improvement, 2005). After the success of that campaign, the "Protecting 5 Million Lives From Harm" was initiated for the 2006–2008 time period (Institute for Healthcare Improvement, 2006). These two campaigns helped to focus attention and resources on identification of actions that would make a positive difference in patient outcomes and create a safer healthcare environment.

The National Quality Forum

In 2002, The National Quality Forum (NQF) created and endorsed a list of **serious reportable events (SRE)**—also referred to as adverse or "never events"—to increase public accountability and consumer access to critical information about healthcare performance. Initially, 27 events were identified; in 2006, one additional occurrence was added. The 28 were each classified under one of six categories of events: surgical, product of device, patient protection, care management, environment, or criminal. The SRE list reflects a consensus among representatives of all parts of the healthcare system. A listing of the SREs can be found at *http://www.qualityforum.org/Publications/2008/10/Serious_Reportable_Events.aspx*.

In 2003, the National Quality Forum, with support from the Agency for Healthcare Research and Quality (AHRQ), identified 30 safe practices that evidence shows can work to reduce or prevent adverse events and medical errors. It was published as *Safe Practices for Better Healthcare: A Consensus Report*. **Safe practices** were defined as practices that reduce the risk of harm from the processes, systems, or environments of healthcare (AHRQ, 2003). These practices, which were not prioritized because all were viewed as important, were organized under five major categories (AHRQ, 2005). The original safe practices were updated in 2006 and 2009. The latest manual, published in 2010, listed 34 practices that are organized into seven functional categories for improving patient safety and are listed in Display 10.1.

 DISPLAY 10.1   Categories for Improving Patient Safety

• Creating and sustaining a culture of safety
• Informed consent, life-sustaining treatment, disclosure, and care of the caregiver
• Matching healthcare needs with service delivery capability
• Facilitating information transfer and clear communication
• Medication management
• Prevention of healthcare-associated infections
• Condition- and site-specific practices

An executive summary detailing the 34 safe practices can be found at *www.qualityforum.org/ Publications/2010/04/Safe_Practices_for_Better_Healthcare_%e2%80%93_2010_Update. aspx* and by clicking to download the abridged report (Simmons, 2010).

The Joint Commission

To address concerns about errors in healthcare, the Joint Commission established patient safety goals for each year beginning in 2002 through the present time (Joint Commission, 2010a). Agencies that were accredited by The Joint Commission were required to begin targeting high-incidence preventable safety problems, such as falls, misread physician orders, and communication errors. An example is the Joint Commission requirement that each hospital or surgical center adopts procedures designed to eliminate instances of wrong patient, wrong site surgeries (Joint Commission, 2010b).

The Joint Commission requires that accredited institutions investigate all **sentinel events**. A sentinel event is an unexpected occurrence involving death or serious physical or psychological injury, or the risk thereof. Serious injury specifically includes loss of limb or function. The phrase "or the risk thereof" includes any process variation for which a recurrence would carry a significant chance of a serious adverse outcome. Serious adverse outcome is defined as instances of error that have the potential for serious harm or death to the client (The Joint Commission, 2010). Some examples of sentinel events, both errors and near misses, are presented in Display 10.2. As you can see, not all sentinel events are errors; rather, some can be considered a near miss. More information can be obtained on sentinel events by visiting *www.jointcommission.org* and clicking on Sentinel Events. At this site, the number of specific events can be found along with recommendations for prevention.

As a critical method by which to promote and enforce major changes in patient safety in thousands of participating healthcare organizations, the Joint Commission has established **National Patient Safety Goals (NPSG)**. There is a separate set of safety goals for each type of agency providing care; the goals are structured in the same way for each type of agency and have used a consistent numbering system. Each year, the Joint Commission reexamines the sentinel event data and the safety goals and revises them by deleting those that have been largely achieved and adding new safety goals. When a goal appears to be no longer an area of concern

DISPLAY 10.2   Some Occurrences Considered Sentinel Events

- Surgery on the wrong body part
- Tubing and catheter misconnections
- Overdosing with commonly used anticoagulants
- Death resulting from a treatment-related or medication error
- Patient suicide occurring in a setting in which around-the-clock care is provided
- Assault, rape, or homicide of patients or visitors perpetrated by staff, other patients, visitors, or intruders
- A maternal death
- Discharge of an infant to the wrong family
- Unprofessional provider behavior

or is not appropriate to that type of agency, the goal and the number are omitted and moved to standards. These patient safety goals are available online at *www.jointcommission.org*.

In efforts to reduce sentinel events and adverse outcomes, in 2002, accredited hospitals began collecting data on standardized—or "core"—performance measures. In 2004, the Joint Commission and the Centers for Medicare & Medicaid Services (CMS) began working together to align measures common to both organizations. These standardized common measures, called "Hospital Quality Measures," are integral to improving the quality of care provided to hospital patients and bringing value to stakeholders by focusing on the actual results of care. With these oversight organizations working together, institutions benefit because the same data set can be used to satisfy both CMS and Joint Commission requirements, thus decreasing the cost of collecting and reporting.

Centers for Medicare and Medicaid Services

In October 2008, CMS demonstrated their commitment to safety by announcing that they would not reimburse hospitals for the costs associated with six serious hospital-acquired complications. The initial six conditions include pressure ulcers, two hospital-acquired infections (HAIs) (catheter-associated urinary tract infections [CAUTIs] and *Staphylococcus aureus* septicemia—methicillin-resistant *Staphylococcus aureus* [MRSA]) and three "never events" (air embolism, blood incompatibility, and foreign object left behind in a surgical patient).

The underlying rationale was a belief that these are preventable complications and denying reimbursement provides a strong incentive for quality improvement actions to avert them. Some have argued that conditions such as pressure ulcers may have begun before admission and that for some debilitated patients it may not be avoidable. However, the plan went into effect, and health insurance plans in several states are considering adopting a similar policy.

Federal Safety Legislation

Almost immediately after the 1999 IOM report was released, federal legislation was introduced in relation to patient safety. Although bills were submitted in the House of Representatives and Senate each year, it was not until 2005 that the Patient Safety and Quality Improvement Act was finally passed by both legislative bodies and signed into law by President Bush (Patient Safety and Quality Improvement Act, 2005). The goal of the Act was to improve patient safety by encouraging voluntary and confidential reporting of events that adversely affect patients. This law provided protection for individually identifiable healthcare data that might be used in assessing safety concerns and created and provided for the certification of Patient Safety Organizations to collect, aggregate, and analyze confidential information reported by healthcare providers. It also set up a plan for a network of patient safety databases that could be used for research and development without fear of disclosure of data about individual organizations and established mechanisms to provide technical assistance to facilitate work on patient safety data.

ADDRESSING SAFETY CONCERNS

Although it is not possible within the scope of this chapter to discuss each of the categories and guidelines that have been set forth for safe practice, we want to expand on those that most seriously affect nursing practice.

Organizational Culture

One of the areas identified among the 34 safe practices listed by the NQF that affects health-care organizations is the need to create a "**culture of safety**." The culture of an organization is a product of its history, its mission and values, its beliefs and customs, the structure of the organization, and the manner in which providers of healthcare carry out their roles (see Chapter 1). A culture of safety is one in which trust and mutual respect encourage healthcare providers to report errors, near misses, and other adverse events without fear of retribution.

Sammer, Lykens, Singh, et al. (2010) identified seven properties within an organization considered important to the development and maintenance of a culture of safety. These include leadership, teamwork, evidence-based practices, communication, a hospital that learns from its mistakes, a system that recognizes errors as system failures rather than individual failures (referred to as a "just culture"), and patient-centered care. We discuss these throughout this chapter but two of the attributes are critical at this point: (1) the organization must actively encourage and support people who report situations that threaten or could threaten the safety of patients or care givers, and providers, and (2) the organization must view errors as opportunities to improve the delivery of care. Organizations embracing these characteristics focus on how and why a problem occurred rather than on the person who may be viewed as responsible for the occurrence. Mistakes that threaten a patient's safety are often related to faulty systems. However, in organizations that have a strongly bureaucratic approach to management, a tendency exists to view errors as singular events, place responsibility on a particular individual, and spend little time determining why the event occurred. Therefore, the root cause of the error may never be identified and corrected.

In response to the recommendation regarding a just culture, the Joint Commission requires a **root cause analysis**, a comprehensive, in-depth process that seeks to identify all the underlying factors that contribute to an error and to identify their role in causing the error. For example, if a nurse were to give the wrong medication to a patient, what were all the aspects surrounding the error? Did the nurse fail to follow the six rights? Was he or she interrupted while preparing the medication? How was the medication stored? How was it labeled? How was it obtained from the pharmacy? How was the order received and transcribed? These are a few of the factors that might affect the outcome. Root causes frequently are interrelated and objective analysis may uncover a deeper root cause (Habel, 2009). In order for error reporting and follow-up to be truly effective, it is critical that nonpunitive actions be taken. Individuals who are worried about job security, embarrassment, and legal ramifications are less likely to report an error.

Most facilities are encouraging individuals to report "near misses" where error could have occurred. An example could be two medications stored side by side in a crash cart that have similar looking labels but very different actions. A nurse may mistakenly pick up the wrong one and prepare to give it but on the third check note the discrepancy and give the correct medication. Noting this as a near miss might result in changes to the crash cart to decrease the likelihood that this error could occur in a stressful situation.

As a new graduate, you may feel that there is little you can do as a newcomer to the scene to influence a culture of safety. That is not the case. You will soon have the responsibility for directing, overseeing, and evaluating the care provided by those with lesser preparation than you have. There will be occasions when you will want and need to advise or correct members of your team. How you go about that is critical. You want to create a pattern of safety, at least with those with whom you work. When you make suggestions and corrections, keep them system oriented rather than person focused. As mentioned above, use this as an opportunity to improve the quality of care the patient receives rather than a time to let a team member know what he or she is doing wrong. Working with team members is discussed in detail in Chapter 13.

Matching Needs With Delivery Capability

Another practice identified by the NQF was to match healthcare needs with service delivery capability. Research has consistently demonstrated that patients undergoing certain high-risk procedures have lower-than-expected mortality rates in hospitals that perform large numbers of those procedures and, conversely, higher-than-expected mortality in institutions that perform low volumes of those procedures. Some examples of high-risk procedures include coronary artery bypass graft, coronary artery angioplasty, abdominal aortic aneurysm repair, pancreatectomy, and esophageal cancer surgery. Safe practice guidelines require that patients be fully informed of the reduced risk at high-volume institutions and encourage their referral to such facilities.

Communications

The area of communication is discussed in many areas of this text and in detail in Chapter 12. This said, it so significantly affects patient safety that we will discuss some specific areas where communicating effectively is critical to safe practice. Breakdowns in communication have been cited as a root cause in the majority of cases reported to and studied by the Joint Commission's Sentinel Event Database since 1996. Within the healthcare environment, communication failures can result from a variety of issues including hierarchy differences, conflicting roles, ambiguity in responsibilities, and power struggles (Nadzam, 2009). It has been estimated that communication errors are factors in more than 70% of sentinel events. This has resulted in the inclusion of the need to improve the effectiveness of communication among caregivers in the Joint Commission's NPSG every year since their inception in 2005 (Federwisch, 2007). Links to the safety goals can be found at *http://www.jointcommission.org/PatientSafety/NationalPatientSafetyGoals/*.

Patient Safety During Handoffs

In our fast-paced and technologically-enhanced healthcare systems, patients are frequently transferred from one area of the hospital to another. An individual admitted through the Emergency Department could easily have received care in at least five different areas of a hospital. Each time that patient is moved, clear and detailed information sharing is required. This is referred to as a **handoff**—a process in which information about the patient, client, or resident is communicated from one healthcare provider to another. Handoffs typically occur at change of shifts, which occur two or three times a day, 7 days a week. If team communication skills have been developed, practiced, and maintained, it can mean the difference between an optimal outcome and an adverse event.

In 2006, the Joint Commission included a new patient safety goal requiring facilities to implement a standardized, interactive approach to "handoff" communications, which includes the opportunity to ask and respond to questions. They defined handoff as "a process in which information about patient/client/resident care is communicated in a consistent manner" from one healthcare provider to another (Joint Commission, 2006). In response, healthcare institutions are attempting to develop shift-to-shift reports that efficiently and effectively communicate the patient's condition, needs, and plan of care. Many of these are models that use evidence-based strategies to ensure that information vital to the care of the patient is communicated to those who need to know it.

In an effort to attain better communications, the healthcare industry has taken a lesson from the aviation industry that more than 20 years ago improved teamwork and communication among those who staffed aircraft by using crew resource management (Hohenhaus, Powell, & Hohenhaus, 2006). One strategy that has emerged is referred to as situation-background-assessment-recommendation (SBAR). The first two components address objective facts and relate succinct briefings regarding the patient situation. The last two are subjective information that can include opinion and a specific intervention. This system builds in a pattern to the relaying of information that allows the receiver to quickly notice the omission and ask for correction.

▶ *EXAMPLE*

Briefing Using SBAR Technique

(**S**ituation) Mr. Tom James is in Room 25 and has just returned from the postanesthesia room.

(**B**ackground) He was admitted through ED with a comminuted fracture of the right tibia and fibula, which was set and casted in OR. Thirty minutes ago, he received 2 mg of morphine I.V. for pain.

(**A**ssessment) He is now resting comfortably with a pain scale of 2. He has a saline IV lock in place. Circulation, motion, and sensation of right foot are within normal limits. No visible swelling of foot distal to cast. Leg elevated to reduce swelling.

(**R**ecommendation) For the next hour, he will need to have his vital signs checked, be reassessed for pain, and have CMS checks every 15 minutes. He can begin oral pain meds when he does not have any nausea and is taking fluids well.

Using a structured and repetitive system such as this, the person receiving the information can respond indicating acknowledgment of the data. For example, the nurse receiving the information in the above example might say, "I understand that there have been no indications of swelling or other problems with the cast, is that correct?" to indicate she understood the assessment. These forms of sharing information during handoff can be practiced or rehearsed so that all members of the nursing team become familiar with the process.

Systems such as SBAR are effective because they are easy to understand and follow. The redundancy helps to mitigate failures, makes it difficult for people to work around the system (to be discussed later), and minimizes reliance on human memory (Nadzam, 2009).

Another is a mnemonic device called I PASS the BATON, which provides a structure for exchanging important information and acknowledging who is responsible for what. The structure includes an introduction, patient, assessment, situation, safety concerns, background, actions, timing, ownership, and next. Implementation of any of these programs involves team training programs that include opportunity to practice the interactive process (Guimond, Sole, & Salas, 2009).

Tools to Improve Communication

Nurses and physicians work closely to foster positive outcomes with those for whom they care. Yet they sometimes have difficulty communicating. Nurses have been educated to be narrative and descriptive in their messages. Physicians, on the other hand, may be action oriented and want the main subject matter of the problem so prompt action can be taken. In facilities that lack a structure or procedure for verbal reports, individuals differ in what they see as critical to report. Communications frequently are interrupted or pressured by time. In 2008, a study by Nelson, King, and Brodine (2008) found that ineffective communication between physicians and nurses resulted in job dissatisfaction and safety breaches on the part of nurses. In efforts to better this situation, many healthcare institutions have initiated specific programs to improve communication.

A whole-system approach to communication that is adapted to the unique characteristics of an organization provides the best results because the culture of the organization is a critical component of safe care. Team training must be provided, elements contributing to organizational hierarchy eliminated, roles and responsibilities delineated, and a zero-tolerance policy enforced with regard to disruptive behavior. All healthcare team members are educated about professional behavior and are held accountable to modeling desirable behaviors.

One such program that helps an organization make changes resulting in efficient and respectful exchanges of information that improve patient safety and nurses' job satisfaction is the TeamSTEPPS (Team Strategies and Tools to Enhance Performance and Patient Safety). It was developed in 2006 by the U.S. Department of Defense Patient Safety Programs and AHRQ. It is based on the concept of a "just culture" (mentioned above) in which all persons—including the patient—regardless of their place in the hierarchy are expected to monitor and speak out about the care provided. TeamSTEPPS targets four competencies: team leadership focusing on a positive environment, situation monitoring in which the entire team must be aware of the environment and team performance at all times, mutual support, and communication.

Another useful tool is the "Call-Out," which simultaneously informs team members of important information and assigns responsibility for tasks at times such as cardiac codes or labor and delivery emergencies. For example, at a code, one nurse might call out "I have started the recording: arrest began at 0900."

A communication tool called the "Check-Back" employs repetition of verbal directives to verify that the information received is correct such as when care is delegated to another provider. For example, "O.K. I will begin the discharge process for Samuel Wilson in Room 202," provides a check that the charge nurse's instructions were clearly understood. A simple "Yes" does not give the charge nurse the feedback that instructions were heard accurately.

When using a communication tool such as any of those mentioned above, the focus of the exchange of information should be positive, conflict-free, and concise. Consistent use will help keep messages precise and complete.

Adopting Safe Practices in Specific Clinical Care Settings

Certain areas of healthcare facilities experience unique problems by virtue of the service provided in that area. Surgery departments are prime examples. To reduce the incidence of wrong site, wrong procedure, or wrong person surgeries, a **Universal Protocol** (which is part of the NPSG) has been developed by the Joint Commission that must be followed by accredited hospitals and surgery centers. The protocol involves three steps to be taken prior to the surgery and includes conducting a preprocedure verification process, marking the procedure site, and performing a "**time-out**" as detailed below. When possible, the patient is involved in the process. Each facility must develop an individualized plan for the steps as they will be used for their facility.

A standardized list is used for the preprocedure verification process, which includes checking for coexisting health problems that might be of consequence and assuring that medications, supplies, blood, and fluids needed before, during, and after the surgery have been obtained. All tests results should be on the record and available.

Sites on which the surgery is to be performed are marked (unless it is on bilateral structures), ideally by the licensed independent practitioner who is ultimately accountable for the procedure and will be present when the procedure is performed although the responsibility for doing the marking may be delegated to a medical resident, physician assistant, or advanced practice nurse.

The standardized "time-out" is conducted immediately before starting any invasive procedure or making the incision. The time out involves the immediate members of the procedure team: the individual performing the procedure, anesthesia providers, circulating nurse, operating room technician, and other active participants who will be involved in the procedure. All relevant members of the team actively communicate during the time-out and agree, at a minimum, that the patient identity is correct as is the site and the procedure to be done. The surgical procedure is not started until all questions or concerns are resolved. If more than one procedure is to be done or the person performing the procedure changes, another time-out needs to be done. Completion of the time-out must be documented.

Infection Control

It has been estimated that about 5% to 10% of patients admitted to acute care hospitals and long-term care facilities in the United States develop a hospital-acquired, or nosocomial, infection with an annual total of more than 1 million people making it the most common serious hospital complication. One of the reasons these infections are such a concern is that they frequently occur in people whose health is already compromised by disease, age, or injury. Nosocomial infections are usually related to a procedure or treatment used to diagnose or treat the patient's initial illness or injury. The Centers for Disease Control of the U.S. Department of Health and Human Services has shown that about 36% of these infections are preventable through the adherence to strict guidelines when caring for patients. The importance of good hand hygiene has gained new momentum including the use of hand sanitizers.

The increasing frequency with which hospitals are reporting cases of MRSA has helped to highlight the need to control infections in healthcare institutions. However, the three most frequently reported HAIs are urinary tract infection, wound infection, and pneumonia. There is evidence to suggest that infection rates increase in hospitals or nursing units where the nurse–patient ratios are the highest. A study sponsored by the US AHRQ found that components of working conditions including a hospital's organizational climate, staffing, and overtime influenced outcomes in elderly patients hospital intensive care units. Conditions studied included central line–associated bloodstream infection (CLBSI), ventilator-acquired pneumonia, CAUTI, pressure ulcer, and 30-day mortality (Stone, Mooney-Kane, Larson, et al., 2007).

Many hospitals have adopted a series of practices called a "bundle" to address each type of HAI. The use of all the practices in the "bundle" has been shown to decrease the incidence of the target infection even though the evidence for each part of the bundle may be limited. For example, many hospitals are adopting a "bundle" approach to preventing CLBSI. This bundle includes the entire procedure for insertion, the daily cleaning protocols, and the protocols for use of the central line catheter. Failure to use all the measures prescribed in the "bundle" may adversely affect patient outcomes. Although the cost of implementing a bundle is significant, its effectiveness in improving quality of care may offset the cost.

Although issues such as staffing are problems to which the hospital administration must respond, as a new graduate, there are steps you can take to reduce the incidence of infection. First, you will want to practice all the precautions you have been taught during your years as a nursing student. You likely will find the pace of the unit on which you begin your work as a registered nurse to be accelerated from that of your student days. You may be tempted to take short cuts in order to keep up. (Short cuts will be discussed in more detail later.) That is where the breaks in the chains of infection can begin. Wash and sanitize your hands before and after contact with each patient for whom you care. When a protocol or "bundle" has been adopted by the institution, learn all the steps and practice them consistently. Remember, all of the steps are important to the outcome.

New graduates have the advantage of having the most recent exposure to nursing literature. Perhaps, there are nurses working on your unit who are unfamiliar with evidence-based practice or are uncomfortable seeking information even if the tools for doing so are on the unit. It is no longer acceptable for nurses to carry out a procedure using techniques that reflect a "that's the way we have always done it" philosophy (Fig. 10.1). Once you are settled in your new position, you can share the information you have with others, some of whom have not had the education from which you have benefited. This sharing can be incidental, as you work together on the unit, or it might be more formal as you present a topic at the time of change of shift report or a team conference. You may choose to share an article with your manager or team as a method of introducing a possible change in practice. You also will have the opportunity once you are settled in your position to serve on hospital committees. Committees provide an excellent opportunity for staff nurses to have input into policy making within the organization. Issues such as nurse–patient ratios may first be introduced at the committee level. Take advantage of this chance to influence change and improvement in your facility.

Failure to Rescue and Nurses' Time at the Bedside

Failure to Rescue has been defined as "deaths per 1,000 patients having developed specified complications of care during hospitalization" (AHRQ, 2007). It is considered a patient safety indicator by the AHRQ and is 1 of 15 nursing-sensitive performance measure identified by the National Quality Forum in 2004. Beginning in 2010, CMS has indicated that it will require reporting of failure to rescue defined as "death among surgical patients with treatable serious complications" as a quality indicator (CMS, 2009).

Failure to rescue has been tied to the amount of time that the nurse spends at the bedside with incidence of failure to rescue decreasing when nurses spend more time at the bedside and less on other activities. An IOM report in 2004 estimated that RNs working a 12-hour shift are

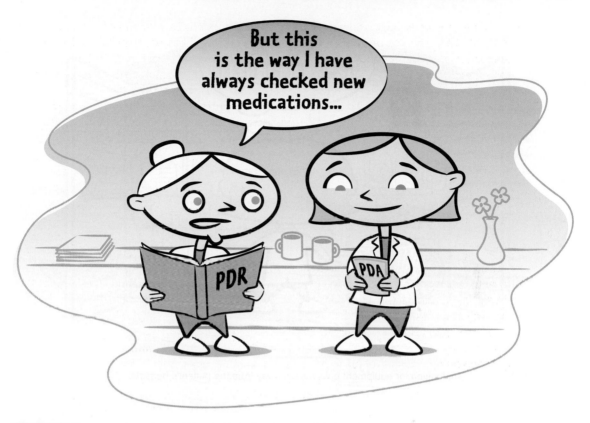

FIGURE 10.1 Some nurses are uncomfortable using new methods or equipment.

only in patient rooms for 1.5 hours (Hendren, 2010). If life-threatening conditions are to be prevented or immediately treated before irreversible damage is done, they need to be recognized. If early recognition is to happen, the nurse must be with the patient. Studies show a direct correlation between increasing the number of nursing hours spent with patients and the reduction of complications such as urinary tract infections and pneumonia experienced by the patient.

VHA, Inc., a national healthcare alliance of more than 1,400 not-for-profit hospitals, identified activities that pulled nurses away from the bedside. Included were actions such as hunting, gathering, and waiting for information. They found that nurses spend a lot of time looking for equipment, going to the pharmacy to get drugs, and waiting for doctors or another department (such as the laboratory or x-ray) to call back results (Fig. 10.2). In some instances, nurses may pick up any tasks that other departments cannot complete such as going to the other department to get supplies instead of having them delivered if the other department is short staffed. This can imply a devaluation of the work of nurses by expecting that their work with patients is less valuable than the work of others. After identifying how nurses spend their time, they initiated measures to return the nurse to the bedside. Table 10.2 identifies successful strategies discussed by Hendren (2010) and outlines how they can be helpful.

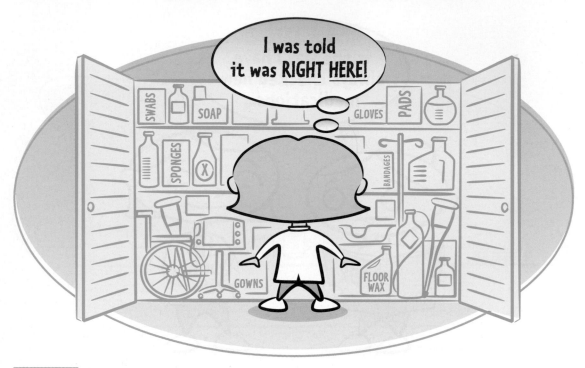

FIGURE 10.2 Time spent looking for equipment pulls nurses away from the patient's bedside.

Table 10.2   Strategies to Increase Nurses' Time at the Bedside and Benefits

STRATEGY	BENEFIT
Rounding hourly	Patients understand their nurse will be around regularly and therefore do not use the call bell as often.
Conducting bedside change-of-shift report	Saves time over taping report and allows the nurse coming on duty to ask questions. Improves patient safety by involving the patient and ensures the patient and nurse are working together.
Streamlining documentation	With the help of technology, improves patient safety and saves time.
Addressing medication administration inefficiencies	Electronic medication administration records and bedside medication administration improves safety and removes inefficiencies if developed with input from users.
Using standardized tools for patient handoffs	Tools, such as SBAR, provide communication checklists and ensure complete information transferred efficiently.
Keeping supplies in close reach	Reduces the time nurses spend hunting and gathering supplies. Locating supply closets in central locations decreases the miles nurses walk each day.
Outsourcing discharge follow-up calls	Assigning to others the task of follow-up calls to discharged patients frees the nurses on the unit.
Seeking physician input	Having physician involvement at the development of system improvements helps assure success of the project.
Asking nurses	The easiest way to learn what will help nurses save time is to ask them. It also decreases frustration.

Adapted from Hendren (2010)

Nurse Staffing

The quality of care provided to patients is dependent on the healthcare workforce. Registered nurses comprise the largest single component of hospital staff and are the primary providers of hospital patient care—nearly 57% of RNs in the United States work in general medical and surgical hospitals (AACN, 2010). Because of the key role nurses play in patient safety and quality of care, the U.S. DHHS and the AHRQ conducted several studies to examine the association between nurse staffing and patient outcomes. The result of the investigation indicated that higher registered nurse staffing was associated with less hospital-related mortality, failure to rescue, cardiac arrest, hospital-acquired pneumonia, and other adverse events. The risk increases quickly as the patients per RN per shift ratio rises above four to five. Increased registered nurse staffing improved patients' safety especially in intensive care units and with surgical patients. When the registered nurse hours spent on direct patient care were greater, there was a decreased risk of hospital-related death and shorter lengths of stay. More overtime hours were associated with an increase in hospital-related mortality, nosocomial infections, shock, and bloodstream infections (Kane, Shamliyan, Mueller, et al., 2007).

Closely related to staffing patterns and nursing workloads is the relationship between overtime and patient safety. Researchers have found that the incidence of errors increases with fatigue. In the example of a tragic maternal death discussed later in this chapter, the nurse who committed the error had worked two 8-hour shifts the day before. She had ended her shift the previous day at midnight and began her shift the following day at 7 AM (Collins Sharp & Clancy, 2008).

Also tied to nurse–patient ratios, staffing, and safety is the matter of patient satisfaction. A study conducted by Aiken, Clarke, Sloane, et al. (2002) found that the nurse–patient ratio was significantly associated with patients' ratings and recommendation of the hospital to others, and with their satisfaction with the receipt of discharge information. They suggested that improving nurses' work environments, including nurse staffing, may improve the patient experience and quality of care (Aiken, Clarke, Sloane, et al., 2002).

The American Nurses Association (American Nurses Association [ANA], 2010) has campaigned strongly for safer staffing patterns supporting nurses who rank staffing as their biggest problem. Linking insufficient nurse staffing with poorer patient outcomes, lengthened hospital stays, and increased chance of patient death, the ANA advocates solving the problem by requiring hospitals to set nurse staffing plans for each hospital unit based on changing conditions:

- Patient acuity (severity of illness)
- Patient numbers
- Nurse skills and experience
- Support staff
- Technology

Using this as a foundation, the organization is working with legislators to pass legislation that empowers direct care nurses to contribute to staffing plan development through hospital staffing committees. As of June, 2010, seven states had passed nurse safe staffing laws that mirror ANA's approach. Some nurses desire a more prescriptive approach in the law. California is an example of a state that has legislated specific nurse–patient ratios for different settings that must be used by all institutions.

Preventing Falls

Falls occur in all types of healthcare institutions and to all patient populations making them a common cause of morbidity and the leading cause of nonfatal injuries and trauma-related hospitalizations in the United States. Patient falls are among the most common occurrences reported in hospitals and are a leading cause of death in people aged 65 or older. Nearly half of all residents in nursing homes fall each year, with many sustaining fractures. Fall-related injuries recently accounted for 6% of all medical expenditures for people aged 65 and older in the United States (Premier, 2010).

Patients fall for several reasons. First, they may fall accidentally. They may trip, slip, or fall because of a failure of equipment or by environmental factors such as spilled water or urine on the floor. Falls may also occur due to physiologic conditions, such as fainting, a seizure, or a pathological fracture of the hip. These types of falls usually cannot be anticipated. Patients can also fall from causes that can be anticipated such as a weak or impaired gait, use of a walking aid, intravenous lines, impaired mental status, or a history of previous falls.

Facilities often have a very specific fall assessment tool. This includes a thorough and sound assessment of patients, their abilities, and their limitations. Knowledge of the effect of the medications they are taking is vital to safe care. Based on the data obtained through this tool, a graduated series of fall prevention measures are instituted. These are termed the "Fall Prevention Protocol." This might include environmental changes such as bed or chair alarms, placing the bed in a low position and putting foam pads on the floor, or locating the patient next to the nurses' station. Nursing care modifications might be instituted such as toileting every 2 hours, visual checks at least hourly, or the provision of assistance any time the patient gets out of bed.

Because of the nature of patients' falls, no single prevention plan is effective for all patients. Although some prevention strategies are obvious and may be used with most patients, other patients present a greater challenge and demand more creative and innovative solutions to ensure patient safety, particularly in long-term care settings. Fall prevention remains a nursing challenge and a nursing responsibility.

Increasing Safe Medication Administration

In 2006, the IOM of the National Academies reported that medication errors were among the most common medical errors, harming at least 1.5 million people every year. The extra medical costs of treating drug-related injuries occurring in hospitals alone were conservatively estimated to amount to $3.5 billion a year, and this estimate did not take into account lost wages and productivity or additional healthcare costs (Stencel, 2006).

In 1995, United States Pharmacopeia (USP) spearheaded the formation of the National Coordinating Council for Medication Error Reporting and Prevention (NCCMERP). The NCCMERP defined a medication error as any preventable event that may cause or leads to inappropriate medication use or patient harm while the medication is in the control of the healthcare professionals, patients, or consumers. The U.S. Food and Drug Administration (FDA) monitors medication error reports that are forwarded to FDA from the USP and the Institute for Safe Medication Practices (ISMP).

In seeking solutions for medication errors, experts in the healthcare field have recommended key areas on which healthcare professionals focus their efforts. These include elimination of ambiguous abbreviations, computerized physician order entry (CPOE), computerized decision support systems (CDSS), computerized adverse drug event monitoring (CADM), barcode point-of-care (BPOC) medication safety systems, and IV administration "smart pumps."

Eliminating Ambiguous Abbreviations

The FDA and the ISMP have launched a national education campaign to eliminate the use of ambiguous medical abbreviations that are frequently misinterpreted and lead to mistakes that result in harm to the patient. The goal of the campaign is to promote safe practices among those who communicate medical information (USFDA, 2009).

The Joint Commission has established a NPSG that specifies that certain abbreviations must appear on an accredited organization's "do-not-use" list; ISMP has highlighted those items on their list with a double asterisk (**). You may be aware of some of the abbreviations that are easily confused such as IV and IU. Other issues in writing out dosage abbreviations are included in this list such as errors in dosage from a misreading of decimal points. Thus, there is the requirement that leading zeros before the decimal point always be included and trailing zeros after a decimal point never be used. A listing of the abbreviations identified as problematic by ISMP can be found at *http://www.ismp.org/tools/errorproneabbreviations.pdf*.

Computerized Physician/Provider Order Entry

Computerized physician/provider order entry is defined as the computer system that allows direct entry of medical orders by the person with the licensure and privileges to do so. The computer system accepts the prescriber's order electronically rather than in writing and checks that order against standards for dosing, interactions and allergies with other medications the patient may be taking, and warns the prescriber about potential problems. Directly entering orders into a computer has the benefit of reducing errors by minimizing the ambiguity of handwritten orders (CPOE, 2010). Use of CPOE is being increasingly encouraged as an important solution to the challenge of reducing medical errors and improving healthcare quality and efficiency. Some of the additional benefits of CPOE include current information that helps physicians keep up with new drugs as they are introduced into the market, drug-specific information that eliminates confusion among drug names that sound alike, improved communication between physicians and pharmacists, and reduced healthcare costs due to improved efficiencies. Despite the considerable benefits, fewer than 5% of U.S. hospitals have fully implemented CPOE systems. The upfront cost of implementing CPOE is one major obstacle with estimated costs as high as $1.9 million and maintenance costs estimated at $500,000. Cultural obstacles also exist with some physicians resisting the use of computerized decision support tools, relying instead on practice experience (The Leap Frog Group, 2010).

Computerized Decision Support Systems

CDSS provides a review of orders as they are written and compares new and existing orders while it scans for possible drug interactions, appropriate dose schedules, and alerts the provider to pertinent lab results. This information will impact the physician's decisions and the plan of care for the patient. CDSS can enhance clinical performance related to prescribing practices and provide important reminders and alerts. This system can also recommend less expensive alternative medications to decrease patient care costs and has the means to identify and prevent duplications related to medications, testing, and imaging.

Computerized Adverse Drug Monitoring

Adverse drug events continue to be the single most frequent source of healthcare errors that place patients at risk of injury. This can be anticipated because drug treatment is the most common medical intervention, and medication use is a highly complex process. It is also multidisciplinary involving the skills of the provider, the pharmacist, and the nurse and is largely a manual process. Historically, the process for assessing the actual safety of drug use has been difficult, mainly because traditional methods such as chart audits and voluntary reporting of data have been shown to be expensive, insensitive, and largely ineffective for detecting mistakes in drug administration and drug-related adverse clinical events (ADEs). The process has been simplified by using computerized methods for detecting ADEs when computerized patient records are in use. The computerized systems employ sentinel words or "triggers" in a patient's medical record. Although these CADMs are effective, they are expensive and require customized software linkage to pharmacy databases. CADM has been a feature in most hospital pharmacy information systems for years although in a limited form. It is now moving beyond pharmacy as a standard offering in CPOE and electronic health record systems.

Barcode Point-of-Care

BPOC systems use a bedside computer, a server with interfaces to the admission-discharge-transfer and pharmacy systems, and medication administration software to cross-check bar codes printed on patient wristbands, nurse identification badges, and medication labels. The system matches the provider's orders with the patient identification and verifies the "six rights" of medication safety by comparing the bar code on medications with the prescribed medications. BPOC software systems have varying levels of sophistication; some systems offer additional clinical alerts regarding sound-alike/look-alike medications or other clinical advisories particular to a specific medication. Following proper dosage administration, some BPOC systems produce an electronic medication administration record, providing legal documentation of the facts of the administration. BPOC is expensive and carries the additional cost of educating employees in its proper use and monitoring that use.

A study reported in the New England Journal of Medicine in 2010 reported that using a bar code on patient's wristbands cut drug errors by more than half. The study was initiated 6 weeks after the new system was phased in. Concerns that hospital workers might try to bypass the system were mitigated when workers once saw they were catching mistakes (Emery, 2010).

"Smart Pumps"

Smart pumps are becoming more prevalent as older IV pump systems are replaced. For several years, infusion pumps have been manufactured with software that can alert users to potential errors. The pumps with this additional software are often referred to as "Smart Pumps" or "Intelligent Infusion Devices." The software associated with the pumps allows an organization to create a library of medications that provides medication dosing guidelines, by establishing concentrations, dose limits, and clinical advisories. Because it can be programmed, it can be tailored for the specific needs of an organization and for different patient groups within the facility, based on patient location, acuity, or weight. The smart pumps provide clinical advisories, soft alerts, and hard stops. Clinical advisories contain relevant information about a specific medication that is displayed on the smart pump screen when the drug is selected from the library. Soft stops notify the user that the dose selected is out of the anticipated range for this medication. However, soft stops can be overridden by the user, and the medication can still be infused without changing the smart pump settings. Hard stops notify the user that the dose is out of the institution-determined safe range and will not allow the infusion to be administered unless the pump is reprogrammed within the acceptable range. These alerts are especially critical when medications classified as *high-alert medications* are being given because the smart pump can reduce administration errors associated with miscalculated doses.

Smart pump technology is not without limitations. If the smart pump drug library is bypassed, and the infusion rate and volume are manually entered, the dose error reduction software will not be in place to prevent a potential error. There is also a risk of choosing the wrong medication from stock or selecting the wrong medication from the smart pump's drug library. Alerts can be overridden. Hard stops that aren't set appropriately can create a barrier to care delivery and may result in nurses using work-arounds (to be discussed later) such as programming the infusion device using the rate/volume mode rather than using the drug library. Failure of users to understand or critically evaluate the information provided by the alert can also result in an error. Organizational resources must also be considered when selecting smart pumps due to the time that must be set aside to develop, maintain, and update drug libraries and reviewing other data (ISMP, 2010).

Nurses' Role in Medication Safety

Safe medication administration is not a new topic to you. From your first practice laboratory sessions to where you are today, your instructors have emphasized the importance of the six rights (right patient, right drug, right dose, right route, right time, and right documentation) and other techniques that will prevent medication errors from occurring. And it is appropriate that they do so—on an international basis, the administration of medications is primarily the responsibility of nurses with up to 40% of their time spent in this activity. With that, the frequency of administration error can range from 2.4% to 47.5% depending on the drug distribution system in place (Shane, 2009). However, there are many factors that play a part in that error other than mistakes made by the nurse. Table 10.3 identifies some of the other areas that contribute to medication error.

Because the administering of medications is one of the major responsibilities of the nurse, many of the medication errors are made by nurses. As the healthcare environment has become more complex and demanding, the error rate has increased. In response, various steps have been taken to reduce the opportunity for errors to occur. There are many places in the process of providing a medication to a patient for mistakes to take place. For example, the provider can err in the drug or dosage ordered, the handwritten order may be difficult to read, it may be inaccurately transcribed, or it could be improperly dispensed or labeled by the pharmacist. However, the final step in most healthcare settings is the administration of the medication by the nurse.

The incidence of medication error can be reduced. When administering medications, always be certain you are giving the right medication to the right patient. Rely on at least two pieces of information, such as name and date of birth, which can be verified both on a medication administration document and on the patient's wristband or from the patient's verbal statement to ascertain accurate patient identification.

If you offer a patient a medication and that person questions it or says, "I've never taken a pill that looks like this before," stop and listen to what is being said. When a patient objects to

Table 10.3 **Common Areas that Contribute to Medication Errors**

AREA OF CONCERN	REASON FOR CONCERN
Calculation errors	Studies have indicated that one in six medication errors involve a calculation error.
Look-alike–sound-alike medications—similar packaging	Many medications sound alike when spoken and/or look alike when dispensed.
Catheter and tubing misconnections	Improper connections and control of intravenous medications result in serious problems.
Interruptions and distractions during time of administration	Medication errors decrease significantly when nurses can administer medications with minimum interruption.
Illegible written medication orders	Handwritten orders are often difficult to read and decipher.
Unclear verbal orders	The pressure of busy units in which verbal orders are frequently given results in increased errors.
Failure to check the patient's name with MAR	Studies have identified this as a frequent cause of medication error despite the five rights.
Overly tired nurses	Errors increase when the individual giving the medications is overly tired.
Inadequate staffing and high nurse–patient ratios	When nurses are rushed or have responsibility for too many patients, errors increase.
Dispensing of medication	In the United States, medications are generally dispensed on patient-specific basis. Internationally, only 18% of the countries require unit dose dispensing.
Verifying absence of drug allergy	National Patient Safety Agency reported that 5.4% of errors leading to harm or death were associated with allergy.
Absence of pharmacists in patient care area	Administration error rates decrease when pharmacists make daily visits to the units.
Confusing or misleading drug labeling	Drugs must be properly labeled to ensure safe administration.

or questions whether a particular drug should be administered, the nurse should listen. Answer any questions the patient may have and (if appropriate) double check the medication order and product dispensed before administering it to ensure that no preventable error is made. If a patient refuses to take a prescribed medication, that decision must be documented in the appropriate patient records. All medications must be labeled, including those in syringes, cups, and basins. The following example chronicles a tragedy that occurred in 2006 that might have been avoided at multiple points by changing the system itself. At several points in the system as it existed, the nurse had an opportunity to recognize the error.

▶ *EXAMPLE*

Mistaken Medication

A bag of bupivacaine (a medication meant to be given as an epidural) was mistaken for normal saline and hooked up to an IV line that pumped the medication into the blood stream of a 16-year-old who was about to deliver a baby. The teen suffered seizures and cardiac arrest and could not be resuscitated. The baby was delivered successfully by emergency Caesarean section. Both medications, which looked alike and were stored in the same drawer, were brought into the patient's room in anticipation of orders for their use. It was found that the nurse had failed to put an identification bracelet on her patient or use the hospital's bar coding system. Problems existed with the bar coding system and nurses had not been adequately trained in its use so they often bypassed it.

The nurse who administered the medication in the example above was fired and eventually lost her license. Felony charges were brought against her but were later reduced to two misdemeanor counts. The hospital paid $1.9 million to settle a malpractice suit brought by the patient's family (Landro, 2010).

Assuming that you conscientiously and consistently follow all the information you have acquired while a nursing student regarding safe medication administration, what other factors in the healthcare environment may make you subject to error? One of the occurrences most frequently reported by nurses is that of interruptions while administering medications. One study found that for each interruption, there was a 12.1% increase in procedural failures and a 12.7% increase in clinical errors (Barclay & Lie, 2010). Interruptions require an individual to switch attention from one task to another. The basis of the interruption must be dealt with and then the context of the original task must be recovered. Redding and Robinson (2009) found that there were six major themes associated with interruptions: (1) employees asking questions, (2) distracting peripheral conversations, (3) supplies not on hand requiring the nurse to go elsewhere to acquire them, (4) phone calls, (5) family questions, and (6) patient call lights. Because of the seriousness of medication error, much attention has been directed toward reducing its occurrence. One group of researchers noted that nurses who prepare medications for all of their patients and then deliver the medications from room to room experienced fewer interruptions than did those who prepared and delivered the medication individually (Potter, Wolf, Boxerman, et al., 2005).

In some facilities, nurses are addressing this concern by alerting others that they are not to be interrupted during the time they are administering medications. Some hospitals have set aside areas for medication preparation that are not to be entered by those not preparing a medication. Posting "Please do not disturb" signs on the automated medication dispensing machines and medication carts has proved helpful (Fig. 10.3). In still other settings, the nurse wears a vest, a hat, an apron, or some other visual indicator that they are in the midst of medication administration and are not to be disturbed.

Additional Responsibilities of the Nurse for Safety

As an individual working in healthcare, you are greatly affected by the attitudes toward patient safety that exist in the workplace. Part of your role as an RN includes your recognition of responsibility for the safety of all patients. It is not enough to make sure that you are personally careful. You need to look at systems and processes to identify areas that need to be studied and changed to be safer. An example is the storage locations for look-alike or sound-alike drugs, especially in emergency areas. Look-alike drugs may be mistakenly confused and administered. While as an individual nurse you might focus on more careful reading of the label, addressing the system concern toward moving the storage areas would protect all patients.

In light of these concerns, another pitfall for the nurse is the attempt to become faster and more efficient by omitting some of the safeguards that the institution has put in place because they are time-consuming. These short-cuts are sometimes referred to as *work-arounds* because the person is working around rather than within the system. Work-arounds

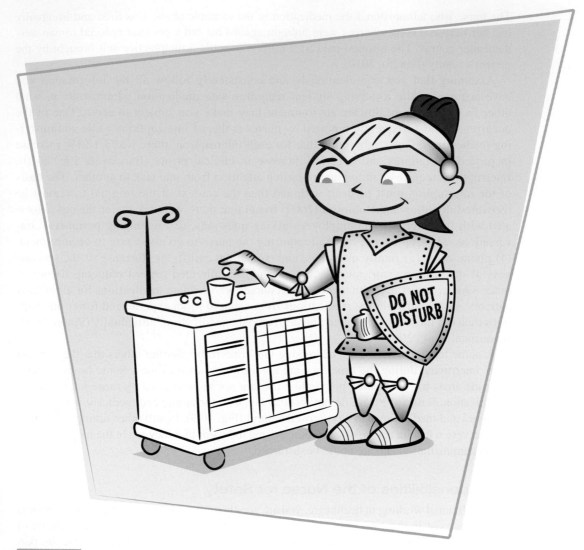

FIGURE 10.3 Nurses in the process of administering medication may wear apparel that indicates they are not to be interrupted.

also are used when something else in the system is not functioning well, such as pharmacy deliveries being routinely slow so that needed therapy is delayed. If safety precautions are too burdensome, the issue needs to be addressed through processes established by the agency to determine quality of care. Omitting safety features or bypassing system safeguards puts the patient in jeopardy.

COMMUNICATION IN ACTION

Refusing to Adopt a Work-Around

Joyce Means had recently begun working as a new RN on 7-Center. Her regular preceptor was out sick, and she was working with Melody, another nurse on the unit. As she was beginning to prepare her 9:00 am medications from the automated machine, Melody said, "Oh, you know you will never get everything done if you go in and out of that machine every time you turn around. When the drawer opens for 9:00 am, I just take out stuff for other times during the day, put them in a little container and put them in the cupboard right here with the patient's name. It saves tons of time." Joyce replied, "I guess I'll just have to learn to be faster at the machine, because I wouldn't be comfortable doing that. The safeguards in the machine help me to not make mistakes, and I really appreciate that. I think it is safer for my patients, too."

▶ EXAMPLE

An Inappropriate Work-Around

In Mercy Hospital, all medications are dispensed from the pharmacy for the individual patient. The computer system used by the pharmacy has information on appropriate dosages, allergies, and incompatibilities and provides a warning to the pharmacist if the order does not conform to safe practice. A patient was admitted with an acute problem. The physician ordered a medication. The nurse noted that this was a medication that another patient was also taking and that there was a dose available in that patient's drawer. She decided that treatment could be initiated more quickly if she gave the available medication and replaced it when the medication for the new patient arrived from the pharmacy. Her intent was to improve the speed of responding to the patient's problem. Her actions circumvented the safeguards that included a pharmacist's double check of dosages, drug interactions, allergies, and other factors that could affect safety that had been built into the system. This really endangered the patient rather than increasing therapeutic effectiveness. While this might not cause a problem in an individual situation, it sets in place a practice that increases the risks to patients overall.

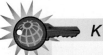

KEY CONCEPTS

- A 1999 study conducted by the IOM found that between 44,000 and 98,000 Americans die each year from preventable errors in hospitals alone. This spurred the AHRQ and the Joint Commission that grants accreditation status to hospitals to take action.
- In 2003, with the help of AHRQ, the National Quality Forum identified 30 safe practices that

were defined as practices that reduce the risk of harm from the processes, systems, or environments of healthcare.
- The Joint Commission has taken steps to encourage hospitals to reduce the incidence of errors and has established NPSG as well as a list of sentinel events that must be reported by hospitals wanting to maintain accreditation.

- A sentinel event is an unexpected occurrence involving death or serious physical or psychological injury, or the risk thereof. Serious injury specifically includes loss of limb or function. The phrase "or the risk thereof" includes any process variation for which a recurrence would carry a significant chance of a serious adverse outcome.
- Serious adverse events or outcomes are defined as instances of error that have the potential for serious harm or death to the client. This could include occurrences such as things such as surgery on the wrong body part, a maternal death, tubing and catheter misconnection, overdose with commonly used anticoagulants, or discharge of an infant to the wrong family. They are what the Joint Commission refers to as sentinel events.
- The Universal Protocol includes preprocedure verification process, marking the surgical site and performing a "time-out" before each surgery when all members of the team review a check list developed to prevent surgical errors from happening.
- Nursing practice must support safe practices. This could include modifying the organizational culture, participating in effective communications, carrying out infection control, preventing failure to rescue, identifying staffing issues, and assuring safe medication administration.

- Failure to rescue is decreased when there is more nursing time spent at the patient's bedside.
- Nurse–patient ratios play a significant role in patient safety with lower nurse–patient ratios contributing to positive outcomes. ANA strongly campaigns for safer ratios and nurse input into staffing patterns.
- Many healthcare workers are involved in the process of providing medications to patients including those who order the medications, those who dispense the medication, and those who administer the medication. Nurses are largely responsible for the administering of medications in healthcare facilities.
- The types and sources of medication errors are many and varied. Technological approaches have been used to decrease the number of errors that occur. These include eliminating ambiguous abbreviations, CPOE, CDSS, CADM, BPOE, and use of smart pumps.
- Additionally, nurses have devised methods to reduce errors.
- Work-arounds jeopardize patient safety by eliminating steps in a process or creating ways to manage outside of the system.
- Because nurses constitute the largest proportion of healthcare workers, their role in the prevention of errors is critical. In one way or another, they touch all aspects of patient care from fall prevention to infection control, or safe medication administration.

ACKNOWLEDGMENT

The authors wish to thank Linda Goodwin, RNC, M.Ed. Manager, Patient Safety and Regulatory Compliance at Evergreen Hospital Medical Center, Kirkland, WA, for her review of this chapter.

RELEVANT WEB SITES

Web sites relevant to this chapter can be found at thePoint·x accessed through *http://thePoint. lww.comEllis10ed* and by entering the code found on the inside cover of your text.

REFERENCES

Agency for Health Care Research and Quality (2003). *Safe practices for better healthcare: Summary.* Retrieved April 13, 2011 from http:www.ahrq.gov/qual/nqfpract.htm

Agency for Healthcare Research and Quality. (2005). *30 safe practices for better care.* Retrieved May 28, 2010, from http://www.ahrq.gov/qual/30safe.htm

Agency for Healthcare Research and Quality. (2007). *Guide to patient safety indicators.* Retrieved July 14, 2010, from http://www.qualityindicators.ahrq.gov/downloads/psi/psi_guide_v31.pdf

Aiken, L. H., Clarke, S. P., Sloane, D. M., Sochalski, J., & Silber, J. H. (2002). Hospital nurse staffing and patient mortality, nurse burnout, and job dissatisfaction. *Journal of the American Medical Association, 288,* 1987–1993.

American Association of Colleges of Nursing. (2010). *Nursing fact sheet.* Retrieved June 27, 2010, from http://www.aacn.nche.edu/Media/FactSheets/nursfact.htm

American Nurses Association. (2010). *Safe Staffing Saves Lives - ANA's National Campaign to Solve the Nurse Staffing Crisis.* Retrieved July 7, 2010 from *http://www.safestaffingsaveslives.org/.*

Barclay, L, & Lie, D. (2010). *Interruptions linked to medication errors by nurses.* Retrieved June 18, 2010, from http://cme.medscape.com/viewarticle/721136?src=cme_mp_top&uac=101399FV

Center for Medicare and Medicaid Services. (2009). *Inpatient and SNF 2010 IPPS. Proposed rule.* Retrieved July 14, 2010, from http://www.scha.org/images/stories/finance/FFY%202010%20Proposed%20%20IPPS%20SNF%20Bullets.pdf

Collins Sharp, B. A. & Clancy, C. M. (2008). *AHRQ commentary: Limiting nurse overtime, and promoting other good working condition influences patient safety.* Retrieved June 15, 2010, from http://www.nursingcenter.com/library/journalarticleprint.asp?Article_ID=778613

CPOE.org. (2010). *Welcome to CPOE.* Oregon Health & Science & University. Retrieved July 1, 2010, from http://www.cpoe.org/

Emery, G. (2010). *Bar-code system lowers medication errors: study.* Reuters. Retrieved June 18, 2010, from http://www.reuters.com/assets/print?aid=USTRE6445NV20100505

Federwisch, A. (2007). Passing the baton: bedside shift report ensures quality handoff. *NurseWeek Northwest Edition,* 8(19), 8–9.

Guimond, M. E., Sole, M. L., & Salas, E. (2009). TeamSTEPPS. *American Journal of Nursing,* 109(11), 66–68.

Habel, M. (2009, February). Promoting a culture of safety to prevent medical errors. *NurseWeek West,* 22, 20–24.

Hendren, R. (2010). Ten ways to increase nurses' time at the bedside. *Health Leaders Media.* Retrieved July 5, 2010, from http://www.healthleadersmedia.com/content/NRS-248033/Ten-Ways-to-Increase-Nurses-Time-at-the-Bedside

Hohenhaus, S., Powell, S., & Hohenhaus, J. T. (2006). Enhancing patient safety during hand-offs. *American Journal of Nursing,* 106(8), 72A–72B.

Institute for Healthcare Improvement. (2005). *Saving 100,000 lives.* Retrieved July 14, 2010, from http://www.ihi.org/IHI/Programs/Campaign/100kCampaignOverviewArchive.htm

Institute for Healthcare Improvement. (2006). *Protecting 5 million lives from harm.* Retrieved July 14, 2010, from http://www.ihi.org/IHI/Programs/Campaign/

Institute of Medicine. (2000). *To err is human: Building a safer health system.* Washington, DC: National Academies Press.

Institute of Medicine. (2009). *Crossing the quality chasm: A new health system for the 21st century.* Retrieved May 28, 2010, from http://www.iom.edu/Reports/2001/Crossing-the-Quality-Chasm-A-New-Health-System-for-the-21st-Century.aspx

Institute of Safe Medication Practices. (2010). *Proceedings from the ISMP Summit on the Use of Smart Infusion.* Retrieved July 1, 2010, from http://www.ismp.org/tools/guidelines/smartpumps/comments/

John Hopkins Medicine. (n.d.). *Innovation in quality of patient care: Fact sheet.* Retrieved September 28, 2010, from http://www.hopkinsmedicine.org in Search box type innovation in quality patient safety—Fact sheet

Joint Commission. (2006). *National patient safety goals: 2006 critical access hospital and hospital national patient safety goals.* Oak Brook Terrace, Illinois, author.

Joint Commission. (2010a). *2010 National patient safety goals.* Retrieved June 15, 2010, from http://www.joint-commission.org/PatientSafety/NationalPatientSafetyGoals/

Joint Commission. (2010b). *The Universal Protocol for prevention of wrong site, wrong procedure and wrong person surgery.* Retrieved June 16, 2010 from *http://www.jointcommission.org/NR/rdonlyres/F8046F2C-A8A2-412F-88D4-E1762BCC5C26/0/UP_Poster.pdf.*

Kane, R. L., Shamliyan, T., Mueller, C., Duval, S., & Wilt, T. (2007). *Nursing staffing and quality of patient care* (Evidence Rep/Technology Assessment No. 151) (Prepared by the Minnesota Evidence based Practice Center under Contract No. 290-02-0009.) AHRQ Publication No. 07-E005. Rockville, MD: Agency for Healthcare Research and Quality. March 2007. Retrieved July 6, 2010, from http://www.ahrq.gov/downloads/pub/evidence/pdf/nursestaff/nursestaff.pdf

Landro, L. (2010, March 15). New focus on averting errors: Hospital culture. *The Wall Street Journal.* Retrieved September 30, 2010, from http://online.wsj.com/search/term.html?KEYWORDS=New%20Focus%20on%20 Averting%20Errors%3A%20Hospital%20Culture.- type in date of the article

Nadzam, D. M. (2009). Nurses' role in communication and patient safety. *Journal of Nursing Care Quality, 23(3),* 184–188.

Nelson, G. A., King, M. L., & Brodine, S. (2008). Nurse-physician collaboration on medical-surgical units. *MEDSURG Nursing, 17(1),* 35–40.

Potter, P., Wolf, L., Boxerman, S., Grayson, D., Sledge, J., Dunagan, C., et al. (2005). Understanding the cognitive work of nursing in the acute care environment. *Journal of Nursing Administration,* 35(7/8), 327–335.

Premier. (2010). *Fall prevention.* Retrieved July 19, 2010, from http://www.premierinc.com/safety/topics/ falls/#Extent

Sammer, C. E., Lykens, K., Singh, K. P., Mains, D. A., & Lackan, N. A. (2010). What is patient safety culture? A review of the literature. *Journal of Nursing Scholarship, 42(2),* 156–165.

Shane, R. (2009). Current status of administration of medicines. *American Society of Health-Systems Pharmacy, 66(5* Suppl. 3), 42–48.

Simmons, J. (April 13, 2010). NQF endorses 34 safety practices in latest manual. *Health Leaders Media.* Retrieved June 13, 2010 from *www.healthleadersmedia.com/content/QUA-249470/NQF-Endorses-Safety-Practices-in-Latest-Manual.*

Stencel, C. (2006, July 20) *Medication errors injure 1.5 million people and cost billions of dollars annually.* News from the National Academies. Retrieved July 1, 2010, from http://www8.nationalacademies.org/onpinews/news-item.aspx?RecordID=11623

Stone P. W., Mooney-Kane C., Larson E. L., Horan T., Glance L. G., Zwanziger J., et al. (2007). Nurse working conditions and patient safety outcomes. *Medical Care, 45(6),* 571–578.

The Joint Commission. (2010). *Sentinel events.* Retrieved May 28, 2010, from http://www.jointcommission.org/. Type sentinel events in search box

The Leap Frog Group. (2010). *Fact sheet: Computerized physician order entry.* Retrieved January 3, 2011, from http://www.leapfroggroup.org/for_hospitals/leapfrog_safety_practices/cpoe

The Patient Safety and Improvement Act of 2005. (2005) Retrieved April 13, 2011, from www.ahrq.gov/qual/pso-act.htm

U.S. Food and Drug Administration. (2009). *Drugs: medication errors.* Retrieved July 1, 2010, from http://www. fda.gov Type medication errors in search box

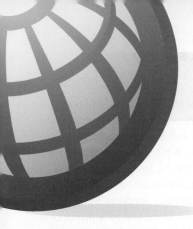

11

The Nursing Profession and the Community

LEARNING OUTCOMES

After completing this chapter, you should be able to:

1. Outline how moving care into the community will affect nursing practice.
2. Analyze the philosophy behind community-based care to determine how that relates to your own philosophy of nursing.
3. Explain approaches to patient/client empowerment.
4. Differentiate primary, secondary, and tertiary prevention and how these concepts can be applied in different nursing settings.
5. Outline the various components of disease management and how those provide for health promotion.
6. Discuss how Healthy People 2020 priority areas and leading health indicators relate to the goals of Healthy People 2020.
7. Explain the nurse's role in disaster response in the community.
8. Differentiate the major categories of complementary/alternative healthcare medicine.
9. Discuss major issues that surround the use of complementary/alternative medicine.
10. Describe ways in which you could use your knowledge of complementary/alternative therapies when working with clients.

KEY TERMS

Alternative healthcare
Biologically based practices
Community-based nursing
Complementary healthcare
Continuity of care
Disaster management
Disease management
Energy medicine
Health disparities
Healthy People 2020
Herbal medicine

Homeopathy
Integrative medicine
Manipulative and body-based practices
Medication reconciliation
Mind–body medicine
Naturopathy
Primary prevention
Secondary prevention
Tertiary prevention
Transition planning
Triage

The emphasis in healthcare has increasingly moved out of the institutional setting and into the community. Individuals are treated in ambulatory centers or even in workplaces and return to their homes or perhaps to work. This has both financial and health advantages. Care in a hospital in-patient setting is the most expensive type of care. While the high-technology care and constant surveillance are essential for the seriously ill, for the less seriously ill, that environment poses a myriad of hazards such as infection, medication errors, and lack of rest. In the home, family members must become caregivers, and healthcare workers have a new relationship with patients and families. In all settings, healthcare has moved to a promotion and prevention model and goals are broader than simply curing illness. This whole movement has impacted nursing in many ways.

UNDERSTANDING COMMUNITY-BASED NURSING

The nursing profession has unique privileges that include a trusted relationship with patients and families, access to individuals when they are most vulnerable, and legal status as a profession. In response, as the community's needs change, the nursing profession has an obligation to expand its knowledge base for practice, enlarge its repertoire of skills and abilities, and commit to meeting newly identified needs in innovative and creative ways.

Community-based nursing refers to the wide variety of settings other than in-patient institutions in which nursing is practiced. Public health, home health, ambulatory care, occupational health, and school nursing all reflect community-based practice. From the inception of modern nursing, community-based care has been part of the nursing profession. Graduate nurses of the first hospital training schools worked in homes nursing the sick. In the early part of the 20th century, the public health nurses working in settlement houses in the immigrant neighborhoods of New York and other large cities brought health education, direct care, and advocacy skills to bear on the many health problems confronting the community. As more aspects of healthcare moved into hospitals and other institutional settings, more nursing took place in those environments. However, public health and home care continued the long tradition of nursing in the community.

Care in the community is cost-effective and often more acceptable to the client because it causes less disruption in life. New opportunities arise as the understanding of care in the community enlarges. The principles of community-based care include an emphasis on advocating for patients, promoting patient education and self-care, focusing on health promotion and disease prevention, and recognizing the importance of family, culture, and the community.

Community-based care requires effective communication and collaboration. The key in all of these community settings is that the patient/client is in charge. The client decides to work with the nurse, to accept or reject advice and suggestions, and to enter and leave care. The nurse serves as an educator, a guide, a resource person, and an advocate, but health action is taken by the client and family. In addition to those who see themselves as working in a community-based setting, all nurses need to be aware of the community in which the client resides and be able to provide care that fits within the scope of the person's life rather than simply an "episode" of illness. Care must be family-centered and culturally competent. Nurses working in all environments must be aware of community health organizations, knowledgeable about availability and accessibility of services and supplies, and familiar with the location and specialty of healthcare providers. An interdisciplinary team approach in which the nurse may serve as a collaborator and coordinator takes on new meaning. As all nurses become more community-focused, the boundaries between the institutional nurse and the community-based nurse blur. All need an understanding of how the client functions in each setting, and each setting must adapt to facilitate transitions from one care environment to another.

CLIENT EMPOWERMENT

A community-based philosophy rests on a fundamental belief in the right of the client to control his or her life, including situations related to healthcare. Giving over control to clients removes healthcare professionals from a position of power over others and requires instead that they participate by empowering clients and families. It requires a partnership or alliance between the nurse and the individual and family that is much different from the traditional hierarchical nurse/patient relationship.

Empowering others requires possessing knowledge of the alternatives available, the ability to teach based on that knowledge, and the skills to help others make decisions and take appropriate action based on their decisions. Nurses can empower others when they assure that those people have the information necessary to make choices within their lives and when they enable patients and families to make their own choices and manage their own health.

Clients are often fearful of making healthcare decisions because so much is unknown. In addition, not everyone has the same interest in decision making. While some patients want to make decisions and need the information to do that, others do not want the burden of decision making. Nurses must navigate these difficult situations and recognize that the patient's decision to NOT have information or to not be burdened with certain types of decisions also represents the patient's autonomy. In such situations, determining what type of information and the depth of information a client wishes to receive is an important aspect of providing care. The nurse then has the additional responsibility of determining to whom the patient has delegated decision making.

Empowerment supports patients/clients in remaining who they are, not in remaking them into some ideal of a person. The elderly woman who asks that her son make decisions for her is empowered when caregivers respect her enough to allow her to live her life as she chooses. Trying to persuade this woman to change who she is and become the model of an independent person does a disservice to her and increases the distance between her and her caregivers when she most needs to be able to trust in them (Fig. 11.1).

HEALTH PROMOTION AND DISEASE PREVENTION SERVICES

Health promotion and disease prevention have long been the major focus of public health nurses, who concentrate on entire populations. This same focus on health promotion and disease prevention is now expanding to nursing in every setting. By recognizing that the determinants of health lie outside of the institution and are found in the community, nurses in the acute care setting enlarge their practice to make it more community-based in philosophy. The various levels of prevention can be addressed wherever the nurse practices.

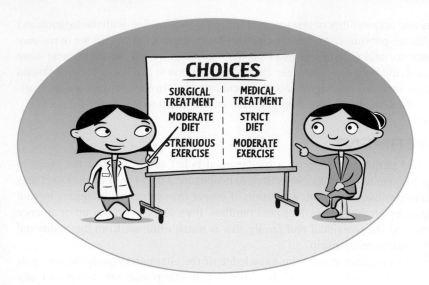

FIGURE 11.1 Teaching people to manage their own health, giving them the information to make choices within their lives, and helping them to carry out those choices empower them.

Primary Prevention

Primary prevention involves the efforts to prevent disease from ever occurring. Primary prevention can be aimed at stopping the cause of disease. On a community-wide level, water treatment and sanitation prevent the spread of communicable diseases by eliminating their sources for the entire population. Helping individuals to be more successful in resisting disease and maintaining health represents another aim of primary prevention. Generalized efforts to educate people regarding healthy diets are aimed at this type of primary prevention. Some efforts involve the individual client and family as the primary focus, although they may benefit the entire community. Immunizations prevent disease not only in the people immunized but also in others by lowering the overall existence of communicable disease throughout the community. Smoking cessation campaigns are aimed at primary prevention and help the individual who quits smoking, but also benefit those who might otherwise be subject to second-hand smoke.

Primary prevention can be a focus of nurses in acute and long-term care settings as well as those who work in the community. Nurses need to think in terms of life span development and identify the common preventable diseases and disorders that occur at any point in life. For example, when the patient must stop smoking to have surgery and remain in the hospital, the impetus may exist to stop smoking for good. Nurses may help patients to examine their options, consult with physicians for medications to manage withdrawal, point out available smoking cessation programs, and in other ways help the patient to quit smoking. Some facilities focus on each contact with a patient as an opportunity to review immunization history and encourage updating of immunizations before leaving the hospital. This is particularly important in ensuring that the elderly have pneumococcal pneumonia immunization or flu vaccine. When planning for discharge, nurses can build in teaching regarding better dietary practices and help patients understand how those will help in long-term health as well as recovery from the current episode of illness.

Long-term care environments have steadily increased their emphasis on health promotion for even the most disabled individuals. Immunizations, fall prevention through strengthening and balance exercises, and activity programs to prevent social isolation and the accompanying depression serve as primary prevention interventions. Nurses are typically the professionals championing these programs, teaching clients and their families, and increasing public awareness of the concerns.

Secondary Prevention

Secondary prevention involves early identification of health problems through screening and the prevention of complications and adverse consequences of illness. Nurses in ambulatory settings help clients to identify screening tests that are important for them and facilitate scheduling those tests. When admission histories are obtained, the nurse in the acute care setting can attend to information about screenings that are needed and encourage the patient to value that activity. To do this effectively, the nurse must understand the current recommendation for screening in specific groups within the population. Asking about screening emphasizes its importance to clients and reinforces other information they may have. It may also create an opportunity for clients to gather additional information. Similarly, in the long-term setting, it is important that nurses continue their focus on prevention activities among the residents. Screening of the elderly population includes different priorities based on the incidence of problems in that age group and the potential years left.

Complications of illness greatly increase morbidity and mortality. Nurses in both acute and long-term care focus on preventing complications as a consistent part of their practice. Careful assessment and timely nursing intervention can prevent the formation of pressure ulcers, falls, and hypostatic pneumonia. These are only a sample of the many secondary prevention actions taken in the institutional care environment.

Tertiary Prevention

Tertiary prevention focuses on preventing long-term disability and restoring functional capacity. Rehabilitation efforts often have been singled out as the major place where tertiary prevention occurs. However, long-term care has a regulatory mandate to prevent deterioration of elderly individuals. Although some argue that decreased functional status is a realistic process that happens at the end of life, the increased emphasis on maintenance of function has revealed that even the extremely debilitated elderly may be helped to avoid the complications of dependency and to maintain functional independence in the face of disability longer than was previously thought.

Disease Management

One approach to increasingly sophisticated and targeted prevention services is found in disease management programs. **Disease management** focuses on providing the best evidence-based care for an individual with a specific chronic illness, such as diabetes. These programs are often instituted by health plans or clinics that recognize that failure to manage chronic illnesses knowledgeably results in increased rates of hospitalization, increased demand on the system for high-cost care, and increased incidence of potentially life-altering complications.

By targeting high-impact diseases such as diabetes for special attention, the aim is for both secondary and tertiary prevention. The person with diabetes who is enrolled in such a program receives comprehensive nutrition education, teaching regarding the management of blood glucose through medication and activity, and regular diagnostic evaluations that include hemoglobin A1c and blood glucose measurements to monitor blood sugar control over time, urine analysis to identify renal function, regular eye examinations to identify and treat retinal complications, and regular foot exams to prevent and treat lesions that might progress to gangrene and amputation. While the intensive involvement in prevention services is costly, the process saves overall through the lowered incidence of hospitalization, blindness, renal failure, and amputations, not to mention the cost of human suffering all of which have monetary costs as well.

Computerized documentation systems facilitate the activities of nurses who are charged with tracking individuals enrolled in a disease management program. They alert the nurse to contact the person through telephone calls, e-mails, or letters when screening services are needed. This same nurse meets with the person to discuss test results. By providing a consistent contact person, the patient feels more comfortable asking questions and is more motivated to maintain needed health practices and lifestyle changes.

HEALTHY PEOPLE 2020

The nation has been addressing health objectives for the whole population through a series of efforts that began with its first set of goals published in 1980 as Healthy People 1990. These have been updated at 10-year intervals and **Healthy People 2020** was released in January of 2010 (US-DHHS, 2010). While the goals of each campaign have not been reached, attention has been focused on them and strategies to work toward them are being refined.

Vision, Mission, and Goals of Healthy People 2020

Display 11.1 presents the statements of vision, mission, and goals for the Healthy People 2020 campaign. The vision provides a single comprehensive statement that defines the entire Healthy People effort. The mission points to actions that will be needed to achieve the goals. The overarching goals provide a framework in which outcomes can be developed.

Achieving these goals will require a policy focus at all levels of government. Healthcare providers, both individual and institutional, will need to examine their processes and policies. In addition to the roles they have in patient teaching, health professionals must recognize the importance of motivation in taking action to improve health. Exploring motivation and the structures that support positive health behaviors will facilitate the engagement of individuals in health promotion activities. To achieve the goals of Healthy People 2020 individuals must become aware of their own responsibility for their health. They need to be knowledgeable about what promotes health and what interferes with health. They must make informed choices that lead toward greater health.

Priority Areas of Healthy People 2020

The priority areas for action under the Healthy People 2020 plan include promotion of healthy behaviors, promotion of a healthy and safe community, improvement in the systems for

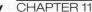

 DISPLAY 11.1 Healthy People 2010–2020 Vision, Mission, and Goals

VISION: A society in which all people live long, healthy lives.

MISSION: To improve health through strengthening policy and practice, Healthy People will
• Identify nationwide health improvement priorities
• Increase public awareness and understanding of the determinants of health, disease, and disability and the opportunities for progress
• Provide measurable objectives and goals that can be used at the national, state, and local levels
• Engage multiple sectors to take actions that are driven by the best available evidence and knowledge
• Identify critical research and data collection needs

GOALS
• Eliminate preventable disease, disability, injury, and premature death
• Achieve health equity, eliminate disparities, and improve the health of all groups
• Create social and physical environments that promote good health for all
• Promote healthy development and healthy behaviors across every stage of life

(USDHHS, Healthy People 2010, *www.healthypeople.gov/hp2020/advisory/PhaseI/summary.htm*)

personal and public health that will provide access and eliminate **health disparities**, and the prevention or reduction of major diseases and disorders that account for a large proportion of the healthcare problems in society. All of these areas for action will help to achieve the four overall goals.

Healthy behaviors are easy to identify and hard to put into practice. These include adding physical activity to life, managing nutrition well, avoiding being overweight and obese, ceasing tobacco use, practicing safe sexual behaviors, being judicious in the use of alcohol, reducing injury and violence, and maintaining a healthy environment. These are primary prevention behaviors that nurses in all settings can address. The challenges of behavioral change on a large scale have led to increased use of media, such as television advertisements, to impart to individuals information regarding healthy behavior. However, behavioral change is a complex phenomenon and whether these broad strategies are effective is not clear.

Promoting healthy and safe communities has long been considered the province of public health departments. As our understanding of safe communities broadens, the role of domestic violence as a health problem has become more prominent. Many agencies promote awareness of what constitutes domestic violence through posters in public rest rooms, through television spots that highlight resources for help for those facing this problem, and by adding routine assessment for abuse to health histories.

Addressing individual behavior is only successful when the systems of the community support it. Access to health services is essential for people to obtain the screenings and preventive care they need. For example, family planning services contribute to the health of both mothers and infants. Medical products must be safe and a public health infrastructure must be in place to support a healthy community. Nurses recognize that many individuals never visit a dentist and that assessment of oral health can be part of physical assessment done in other settings, with referral to dental professionals when obvious problems are identified.

While the number of different diseases and conditions fills volumes of books, there are a limited number of conditions that account for the majority of illness and disability. The successful identification and treatment of these diseases create a substantial move toward greater health and quality of life for millions.

Leading Health Indicators for Healthy People Initiatives

Leading health indicators are classifications for measurement to determine the success of the Healthy People initiatives (Display 11.2). Measures for each category have been devised and are being tracked to determine trends and to evaluate specific strategies for targeted groups. Some are indicators for which a decrease indicates progress—such as tobacco use. For others an increase indicates success—such as access to healthcare. Specific measurements that will reveal prevalence in the population must be devised for each indicator.

Nurses' Roles in Supporting Healthy Communities

While many nurses work professionally in the community, all nurses can support personally the health of their communities. One personal role is as a supporter and advocate for political measures that would improve the health of the community. This might include contacting representatives at local, state, or national levels and advocating for passage of important health-related laws or projects. Strategies for this are discussed in Chapter 15.

Another personal role includes being active as a community service volunteer in a homeless shelter, school, or other community agency. Blood drives, blood pressure screening events, and educational programs may all seek the services of nurses as community volunteers. Within a neighborhood, church, or other setting, nurses are often asked to be a resource person for health-related questions. While nurses need to be careful not to give medical advice or make recommendations without adequate information, they can advise healthy behaviors, suggest health-related screening, help identify that a problem exists, suggest seeing a healthcare provider for a problem presented, help individuals understand the directions given to them by their physician, or teach people about their medications. Some have suggested that nurses can also be role models of healthy lifestyles for those around them. Although many

DISPLAY 11.2 The Leading Health Indicators

- Physical activity
- Overweight and obesity
- Tobacco use
- Substance abuse
- Responsible sexual behavior
- Mental health
- Injury and violence
- Environmental quality
- Immunization
- Access to healthcare

USDHHS, Healthy People 2020

nurses reject the idea that their lives should be lived with this in mind, others recognize that actions often speak to others much louder than words. The nurse who persists in smoking has less credibility when suggesting healthy lifestyle behaviors to others. Some nurses have used this situation to illustrate their understanding of the difficulty of undertaking lifestyle changes and have entered into groups that work together on healthier living.

COMMUNICATION IN ACTION

Talking With a Neighbor About Health Concerns

Joe Reynolds is a nurse who works on the surgical unit of a local community hospital. While he works in his yard, a neighbor approaches him and begins to chat. After a few minutes of talking about yard maintenance, the neighbor says, "Uh—Joe, do you know much about these PSA tests?" Joe replies, "A bit. Do you have a question about them?" "Well, I went in to see my doctor. He did some tests and said my PSA is too high and I should go see a urologist. What the heck is it anyway and why should I see another doctor?" Joe asks, "What explanation did the doctor give you?" The neighbor replies, "Well, he talked about numbers and said something about cancer and then I don't remember what else he said." Knowing that even hearing the word cancer can cause enough stress that a person might not hear the remainder of the doctor's explanation, Joe decides to do some simple teaching. He explains, "Well, the test means that something is going on in your prostate. It is an important test, but the results can be positive even when you don't have cancer; other things can cause the readings to be high. However, it really should be checked out so that you get the proper treatment. A urologist specializes in this kind of problem and will do more tests to find out exactly what is going on and then talk to you about whether you need treatment." The neighbor says, "Thanks, Joe. Guess I should make that appointment." Joe replies, "Yes, I think you should. Let me know if there is anything I can help with."

MAINTAINING CONTINUITY OF CARE

Continuity of care for the individual means that there is an uninterrupted process across settings in which a person seeks care. In an ideal world, there would never be a duplicated test, a failure to account for medications currently prescribed, or a lack of information upon which the care provider could make decisions. However, the current system is far from ideal. When a mother with young children goes to the emergency room and does not have immunization information, this may affect the care provided. When a person leaves the hospital and does not understand the discharge instructions, that person's health is compromised. When an elderly resident moves from the nursing home to the hospital and information on medications for chronic illnesses does not accompany that person, serious complications may result. The Joint Commission requires that the institutions it accredits study this problem and establish effective policies and procedures to ensure continuity of care.

Transition Planning

Transitions are the movement of the patient from one care environment to another, such as from home care to hospital, from hospital to nursing home, or from one unit in a hospital (such as the intensive care unit [ICU]) to another (such as the general medical unit) as needs for care change. **Transition planning** refers to the planning process that takes place to assure that the patient's well-being is maintained throughout the time of transition. The actual actions of healthcare providers during the transition are often termed the "Handoff." Many facilities are establishing policies and protocols on exactly what actions must be taken during a handoff. Medication reconciliation, discussed below, is a critical part of the handoff.

The transition to a new care environment has been identified as a time in which the potential for error rises. Whether moving from home to an outpatient setting or between units in the same facility, transition planning is critical to effective care. While physicians usually have the authority to prescribe the move, the nurses are the ones who usually serve as the coordinators of transitions.

Discharge Planning

Planning for a transition often begins when a decision is made for the patient's care to be moved to another setting. Some transitions can be predicted before the decision about timing is made. For most patients, discharge from a hospital is an expected event; therefore, planning for discharge begins immediately upon admission, if possible. Upon admission to a hospital, a projected timeline for care may contain specific outcomes to be met along a care pathway. A discharge coordinator may be charged with following the patient to assure that planning is accomplished in a timely manner. The discharge coordinator may be a nurse or may be a social worker. This person works with the family to arrange the appropriate setting for post-discharge care.

All nurses assume responsibility for ensuring that medical orders and nursing plans move with the patient to the next location. Written materials that document these orders and plans are essential for accuracy. Teaching is incorporated throughout the process. When discharge is to a nursing home or rehabilitation setting, the goal is that the receiving setting is prepared to provide the care needed. When the person is going home, the nurse is often responsible for ensuring that needed referrals have been arranged and for providing discharge teaching. Patients going home also need written materials to refer to in relationship to self-care. Family members, when available, are integrated into the planning for discharge. The nurse in the institutional setting may follow up with the patient after discharge to ensure that the patient's healthcare needs are being met in the new environment and that communication has been clear. Appropriate documentation of this process is essential.

Transfers

Whether an individual moves from one unit within an institution to another or from the hospital to a nursing home, a careful plan is still needed. While some transfers occur because of sudden changes in a patient's condition or because the demand for beds has accelerated transfers out of a particular unit, most are part of the ongoing therapeutic plan. For a patient admitted for surgery, this might include an admitting unit, the surgical suite, the postanesthesia care unit, the surgical unit, before discharge to home or a rehabilitation setting.

Many facilities now have a separate transfer form that is initiated by the nurse in the unit where the patient's care begins. This form identifies all the key transition information. During the handoff the transferring professional and the receiving professional can quickly review the key information, assess the patient, and enter the receiving assessment and acknowledgment of the information on the form. This same process also might be used for the aid car person-nel handing off to the nurse in the emergency department or the nurse handing off to a nurse in a nursing home (although this latter process might occur over the telephone with written documentation by fax). The advantage of this process is that the receiving nurse does not need to spend a lengthy time trying to find the most important information in a voluminous medi-cal record. Both people are accountable for ensuring that the key information is identified and acted upon.

Medication Reconciliation

One of the major areas of concern for patient safety at the time of any transition is the continuity of medications that the patient has been taking for the successful manage-ment of health problems. The recognition of the importance of this with regard to patient safety has resulted in the process called **medication reconciliation**, which occurs after a person is admitted to a care facility. This process is the result of recommendations by The Joint Commission Patient Safety Goals and the Institute for Safe Medication Practices (The Joint Commission, 2010).

Medication reconciliation at admission involves carefully documenting all the medications and their dosages, including prescribed medications, over-the-counter medications, vitamin/mineral supplements, and herbal products the person was taking before admission to the care setting. These are then compared to what has been ordered for current care. Any differences are brought to the attention of the medical care provider in order for the best care decision to be made.

This same process is used at all times of transition. Medications change when a person leaves an ICU. Nurses on a surgical unit must be aware of the medications a patient received while in the operating room. When a patient is admitted through an emergency room, the medication given there will affect ongoing care. If additional medications are ordered in that setting, the nurses must know whether they were given or must still be given after the patient comes to the care unit.

Facilities develop a standardized form on which medication reconciliation is documented. These records become part of the patient record and are also used to document quality improvement in maintaining safe medication administration by ensuring appropriate continu-ity of medication orders across transitions.

Critical Thinking Activity

A charge nurse in a nursing home is planning for the transfer to the hospital of an 87-year-old resident who fell and fractured her hip. This resident has a history of con-gestive heart failure, osteoarthritis, and osteoporosis, but had been ambulatory using a cane and cognitively intact before the fall. What concerns should be addressed before the transfer occurs? What are the issues that will be of concern during the transfer? What information will the receiving nursing unit need in order to provide effec-tive care?

Continuity of Care Documentation

Historically medical records for any individual may be scattered among the various offices of a primary care physician, a number of specialty physicians, one or more pharmacies, a physical therapist's office, and a hospital. If an individual has geographically moved more than once, these healthcare record sites are multiplied by the number of cities or areas in which the person lived. This may result in discontinuity in care. Clients may not remember exactly what tests were done or their exact results. They may find it difficult to pinpoint whether a particular episode of symptoms occurred 3 or 5 years ago. Although everyone is encouraged to keep a current list of prescription medications and their dosages with them, how many actually carry through with this? When seeking past records is too cumbersome, tests may be redone; there may be no baseline against which to compare results, or significant problems may be overlooked.

The hurricanes of 2005 that saw tens of thousands of individuals displaced from the Gulf Coast region of the United States brought these concerns to the forefront. Cancer patients were evacuated but needed to continue treatment; however, their records remained in flooded hospitals. Individuals with chronic illnesses ran out of prescriptions and were unable to get needed medications. These and many other problems occurred because health records were no longer accessible.

While electronic health records (EHR) that encompass the documentation of a particular health system, including both inpatient and outpatient settings, are becoming more common, many people still receive care where these are not available. Even an excellent EHR will not be available outside of the system. Two computer programs for solving this problem have emerged. They are the Continuity of Care Record (ASTM International, 2005) and the Continuity of Care Document (Corepoint Health, 2009).

The purpose of these computer programs is the creation of an electronic document that "provides a core data set of the most relevant administrative, demographic, and clinical information facts about a patient's healthcare, covering one or more healthcare encounters. (It) includes a summary of the patient's health status (eg, problems, medications, allergies) and basic information about insurance, advance directives, care documentation, and the patient's care plan" (ASTM International, 2005). The Continuity of Care Document is structured to coordinate with additional healthcare documentation standards and to be more compatible with a wide variety of EHR systems. Either would provide the ability to place the patient's information on some type of media or transfer it electronically to another system to facilitate continuity of care. (Fig. 11.2).

While these computer programs are not in widespread use, they have great potential for alleviating the problems involved in patient transitions. As individuals and healthcare agencies become more familiar with these options, the expectation is that there will be increased use of them and nurses will be required to access and use the information contained in this record.

DISASTER RESPONSE IN THE COMMUNITY

Potential disasters have always been a concern in communities, but they have become a greater focus of attention since the 9/11 collapse of the Twin Towers in New York City, Hurricane Katrina in New Orleans, and the 2010 earthquake in Haiti. Display 11.3 lists the 11 major causes of community disasters. Some disasters, such as a fire, may occur in any community; others, such as an earthquake or a hurricane, occur more frequently in one part of the country than in another. **Disaster management** refers to the plans that are in place designating the community's response to a disaster.

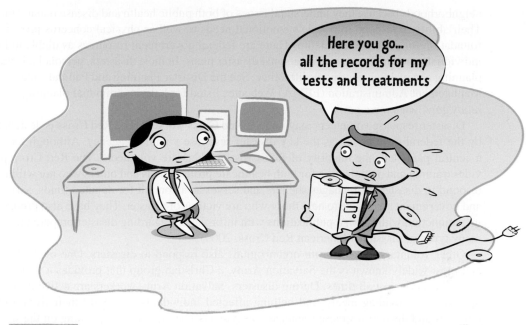

FIGURE 11.2 In an ideal healthcare system, every person would have a "Care Continuity Record."

Volunteers in Disaster Response

Many communities have plans in place to mobilize volunteers for some roles in a disaster. For example, in areas with earthquake potential, community planning focuses at the neighborhood level, with volunteers responding to neighbors. Basic first aid and management of food, water, and shelter cannot wait for professional rescuers to arrive in the event of widespread damage to roads, power, and other infrastructure. Nurses might take a leadership role in their own

DISPLAY 11.3   Types of Community Disasters

- Acts of terror
- Disease—especially epidemic disease
- Drought
- Earthquake
- Fire
- Flood
- Food contamination
- Hazmat (hazardous material spill)
- Hurricane
- Power outages
- Tornado

neighborhoods because they understand issues of both public health and disease management. Their ability to respond to people's emotional needs as well as physical concerns provides a foundation for effective leadership. There are federal government resources available to help individuals and families to make personal disaster plans. In most disasters, personal advanced planning can make an enormous difference. See the Disaster Planning and Federal Emergency Management Administration (FEMA) Web sites listed for help in individual planning (*www. ready.gov/; www.fema.gov/*).

Disaster response volunteers may include Red Cross workers. The Red Cross is designated by the federal government as the key disaster response voluntary agency. Although there is a central paid staff, the majority of Red Cross workers are volunteers. The Red Cross provides training and organization for both healthcare professionals and others who are willing to respond to disasters. It manages shelters and serves as a conduit for donated funds, services, and government assistance to help those who are victims of disaster. They have also produced, in conjunction with FEMA, publications with information regarding disaster preparedness for many types of disasters (American Red Cross, 2009).

Other voluntary and nonprofit organizations also respond to disasters. One of the largest and most widely known is the Salvation Army, a Christian group that provides a wide array of social services at all times. During disasters, Salvation Army workers are active in setting up shelters, providing meals, and helping affected individuals to rebuild their lives. Other religious and disaster response organizations may also be mobilized depending on the size of the disaster.

Institution and Agency Disaster Response

Firefighters, police officers, ambulance drivers, the National Guard, and health professionals are all part of response plans. Most of these individuals are trained for disaster response by their employers.

Firefighters are often the frontline responders to those injured in a disaster. They provide the rescue and emergency medical response skills to save lives. As first responders, firefighters risk the potential for serious injury, smoke or dust inhalation, carbon monoxide poisoning, and heat-related illness from the wearing of protective gear in hot environments. Nurses working in triage must be cognizant of this risk to emergency workers.

Hospitals often serve a pivotal role in managing injuries or illness related to a disaster. Each hospital has plans in place for both internal disasters (such as a fire in one wing of the hospital) and external disasters (such as a tornado in the community). In communities with multiple hospitals, coordination in disaster planning and preparation is essential. Based on their locations and services, each might be designated for a different role.

Learning about their agency's disaster plans should be part of the orientation of all employees. Nurses in hospitals have major roles in responding to disasters. Current patients will be discharged as quickly as possible to open up beds for disaster victims or may have to be moved if the institution is located in an affected area, Units will be reorganized to enable the acceptance and treatment of multiple victims. Nurses may be asked to move to emergency departments to be part of teams that will provide triage. **Triage** involves the initial screening of victims for the purpose of prioritizing treatment and making the most effective and efficient use of both human and material resources. When major triage is no longer needed, nurses may then return to units for patient care.

Part of a disaster plan for any agency is a call-in system. This system is a planned process for notifying staff not on duty that there is a disaster and they should report for work. Building such a call-in list is usually the responsibility of the manager of each unit. There may be a telephone tree with people designated to call others within their neighborhood or geographic area, in order for everyone to be notified more quickly. Healthcare professionals sometimes face an ethical dilemma regarding being called in for a disaster. Their own families and neighborhoods may need them, but the hospital is treating the most seriously injured or ill and needs everyone.

Specific Disaster Concerns

Hurricane Katrina on the Gulf Coast pointed out the tremendous challenges of managing a widespread disaster when the local resources for response are destroyed. Without hospitals, fire departments, and other agencies, all help had to come from outside the community. Transportation and communication were identified as major problems. Moving large numbers of people, arranging for shelters, and communicating among those trying to provide emergency help all became more than the system was prepared to manage. The total resulting effect on people's lives and health is still not known. As a consequence of this situation, communities are looking more closely at their disaster planning and requesting that both the federal and state governments develop better contingency plans. The federal government operates a Web site that is an entry point for learning about the federal government's disaster planning and services (*www.ready.gov/.*)

Communicable diseases that strike large numbers of individuals in a community are considered *epidemics* while those that strike large numbers around the world are termed *pandemics*. Influenza is considered a pandemic when a new strain arises to which most people are susceptible and cases arise in large numbers in multiple countries such as occurred with the H1N1 strain in 2009. Nurses need to become knowledgeable about transmission methods for communicable diseases and the role of immunizations. They must be prepared to give accurate information to those who express concerns. They also need to understand their personal role in any institutional plan for response to an epidemic.

Terrorism, which was most visible in the United States in the 9/11 attacks on the United States, remains a concern. The subway and bus bombings in London in 2005 demonstrated the vulnerability of large cities to the concerted efforts of a few terrorists. A great deal of the federal government's support for disaster planning is focused on terrorism. Part of the disaster planning of every urban community relates to terrorism response. Whole communities may be involved in disaster response drills, and people may be recruited to play the part of victims. A simulated disaster is staged, and all the plans of the various community agencies are activated. A disaster drill provides a mechanism to find out what works and to plan more effectively.

COMPLEMENTARY AND ALTERNATIVE HEALTHCARE

The National Center for Complementary and Alternative Medicine (NCCAM) has defined this field as "a group of diverse medical and healthcare systems, practices, and products that are not generally considered to be part of conventional medicine" (NCCAM, 2010, Defining CAM). Conventional medicine may also be referred to as allopathy, Western, mainstream, orthodox, regular medicine, and biomedicine. This definition of complementary and alternative medicine (CAM) focuses more on what alternative care is *not* than what it *is*, because of the broad range of healthcare practices included in this category. Common among these practices are acupuncture, homeopathy, naturopathy, music therapy, and herbal medicine. NCCAM includes prayer for health reasons as a therapy practice. The list of healthcare practices considered complementary and alternative shifts constantly as some are proven safe and effective, others are proven of little value or even harmful and fade from use, and still others emerge. According to its 2007 survey (NCCAM, 2008), 39.3% of adults in the United States use some form of CAM. Overall, CAM use is greater among women and people with higher education levels. Survey results indicated that CAM is most often used to treat and/or prevent musculoskeletal conditions or other conditions that involve chronic or recurring pain.

These healthcare approaches are considered *alternative* when they are used in place of conventional medical care. The same approaches are considered *complementary* when they are used along with conventional medicine. **Integrative medicine**, as defined by NCCAM, "combines mainstream medical therapies and CAM therapies for which there is some high-quality scientific evidence of safety and effectiveness" (NCCAM, 2010). Thus, integrative medicine supports the higher standard of research evidence for effectiveness.

NCCAM provides training for researchers in the area of CAM, funds grants for research into the effectiveness of all types of alternative care, and disseminates research findings about CAM to both professionals and the public. The National Library of Medicine maintains a database, CAM on PUBMED, which allows for research in relationship to specific diseases, conditions, and therapies (see end of chapter Web sites).

CAM takes place almost entirely within the community, and the client often serves as its primary controlling factor, as opposed to conventional medicine, in which the official healthcare provider controls access to care through ordering diagnostics, prescribing treatments, and determining admission to and discharge from a care facility. As **complementary** and **alternative healthcare** practices remain popular with the public, healthcare providers are challenged to understand these diverse approaches and to work effectively with clients who choose those resources. There is also a need to assist in client education so that choices are made wisely and with sound information.

Major Types of Complementary and Alternative Medicine

NCCAM has categorized CAM into four domains for the purpose of discussion and study. These domains include mind–body medicine, biologically based practices, manipulative and body-based practices, and energy medicine (Tables 11.1 and 11.2). Additionally, CAM studies alternative whole medical systems that cut across many of the domains.

Specific alternative care providers may use more than one type of treatment in their practice. Additionally, there are many areas of overlap between conventional medical practice and CAM. The major types of alternative care available are described briefly in the following sections.

Whole Medical Systems

Whole medical systems represent complete systems of theory and practice that approach healthcare differently than the traditional Western biomedical approach. NCCAM has identified two approaches to entire systems of healthcare that differ from Western medicine: traditional indigenous systems and unconventional Western systems of medicine (NCCAM, 2010). Each system uses a variety of specific therapies.

Table 11.1 **Alternative Whole Medical Systems**

SYSTEM	EXAMPLES
Traditional indigenous systems	Traditional oriental medicine Qi gong Acupuncture Herbal medicine Oriental massage Ayurvedic medicine Native American medicine Other folk medicine systems (Mexican, South American, etc.)
Unconventional Western systems	Homeopathy Naturopathy

Traditional Indigenous Systems. In indigenous medicine, there are complete systems of explanation for health and illness, and therapies are chosen based on these theoretic systems of belief.

Some indigenous systems are quite formal in approach, with individuals studying and serving apprenticeships before practice. These include traditional Asian medicine and ayurvedic medicine from India. Traditional Asian medicine may include the use of qi gong (a form of energy therapy), oriental massage, acupuncture, and herbs. Ayurvedic medicine, a traditional system from India, has existed for more than 5,000 years and has a specific theoretic and therapeutic

Table 11.2 **Types of Complementary and Alternative Practices**

CLASSIFICATIONS	SPECIFIC THERAPIES
Mind–body medicine	Relaxation exercises Hypnosis Meditation Dance Prayer Visualization Biofeedback
Biologically based practices	Herbal medicines Special diets Food supplements Vitamin therapy Biologic substances, such as bovine and shark cartilage
Manipulative and body-based practices	Chiropractic Massage therapy Reflexology
Energy medicine	BEM applications to the body Radiofrequency hyperthermia Radiofrequency diathermy Magnets Nerve stimulators Biofields—manipulations of energy fields originating within the body: Reiki, therapeutic touch

focus on imbalance in the individual's consciousness. Lifestyle interventions are the major form of ayurvedic preventive and therapeutic treatment. As the popularity of Ayurvedic treatment has grown, a number of medical centers, retreats, and spas provide these treatments in the United States.

Informal approaches are often termed *folk medicine*; these traditions usually are handed down by word of mouth and are used by individuals and families to treat common health problems. Indigenous medicine practitioners use a variety of approaches to healthcare, often combining herbs, food, and traditional ceremonies. Little is understood about many of the herbs used, but some have demonstrated therapeutic effects while others may be questionable.

In a given ethnic group, certain people may be designated as healers or as having special knowledge and ability regarding illness. They may have had a period of apprenticeship, but it is informal in nature and not mandated by any outside authority. The advice of the indigenous healer may be sought instead of the advice of a physician. Native American cultures may use a *shaman*, or medicine man/woman. Mexican Americans may use the services of a *curandero*, or healer. A system of understanding hot and cold disorders and foods that help to balance heat and cold in the body is part of many of these folk traditions. NCCAM points out that "other traditional medical systems have been developed by Native American, Australian Aboriginal, African, Middle Eastern, Tibetan, Central and South American cultures" (NCCAM, 2010). To work most effectively with a client who uses folk medicine, you need to learn about the specific beliefs and resources that the client is using.

Unconventional Western Systems of Medicine. Unconventional Western systems of medicine originated in Western society but did not find general support. Some individuals continue to practice in the theoretic precepts of these systems and have reemerged as the public looks for alternatives to conventional medical care.

Perhaps the most common of these unconventional Western systems is homeopathy. **Homeopathy** is based on the belief that exposure to extremely small quantities of either the substance causing an illness or a related substance will stimulate a cure. Of course, this principle is also the basis for immunization and allergy desensitization. The application of this principle to other diseases, however, has not been accepted by the medical community. The dilutions used in many homeopathic remedies are so great that a dosage may contain only a few molecules of a substance. Homeopathy was popular in the early 20th century but fell into disrepute as standard medical research advanced. There is currently a resurgence of interest in this approach to therapy, and new research is being done. Homeopathic practitioners once again are offering an alternative to standard medical care.

Naturopathy gets its name from the natural agents used in treating disease, such as food, exercise, air, water, and sunshine. The naturopathic physician treats people by recommending changes in lifestyle, diet, and exercise, and promoting the use of vitamins and herbs. For many, lifestyle and dietary changes are a successful form of treatment. Naturopathic physicians follow a prescribed course of study that includes clinical experiences with clients and results in the doctor of naturopathy degree. Currently, 15 states, the District of Columbia, and the United States territories of Puerto Rico and the United States Virgin Islands have licensing laws for naturopathic doctors (The National Association of Naturopathic Physicians, 2010). However, questions have been raised about the use of naturopathic physicians in primary care, especially regarding the adequacy of their training in the recognition and treatment of more serious illnesses and the concern that many of the herbal remedies prescribed by naturopathic physicians are untested and unregulated.

Mind–Body Medicine

Mind–body medicine seeks to control physical processes through the mind's capacities. In addition, it treats emotional concerns. Increasingly, mind–body interventions are being incorporated into standard healthcare practice. Traditional psychotherapy, a well-established part of standard healthcare, is a mind–body approach to health. The use of prayer, support groups, yoga, meditation, relaxation, biofeedback, and visualization are all mind–body therapies.

Relaxation exercises, breathing techniques, meditation, and visualization are used to reduce anxiety, reduce blood pressure, and lessen the body's response to stressors. Yoga and other forms of controlled exercise also focus on breathing and mind-calming processes for these same purposes. While yoga originated in Hindu religious practices, most yoga in the United States keeps the techniques but does not include the religious philosophy. These techniques also are designed to prevent stress-related problems from developing; for many people, they are part of a plan to increase health and well-being. These techniques may be suggested for the management of specific health problems such as those causing pain or those related to cardiovascular responses and may be used in conjunction with traditional medical treatment.

Every major religion of the world responds in particular ways to those who are ill. A well-established way for supporting an ill person is through the prayers of others who care. Nurses recognize that spiritual distress has a significant impact on a client's ability to move toward wellness. Supporting the individual's quest for spiritual solace and healing has been a part of the mission of many healthcare agencies that were established by religious bodies. The separation of prayer and spiritual care from other healthcare is a modern phenomenon.

Visualization may be used to help children manage painful medical procedures. Suggestions regarding healing and postoperative recovery are used in the operating room by some anesthesiologists and surgeons. The anesthesiologist may talk to the patient who is still anesthetized, suggesting that pain will be minimal, nausea will not occur, and recovery will be rapid. This is similar to posthypnotic suggestion. Hypnosis has been used in other illnesses for symptom relief (Fig. 11.3).

Biofeedback is a specific mechanism used to assist individuals by altering physiologic responses through mental processes. The machines used for biofeedback provide visual or auditory feedback of physiologic parameters such as blood pressure or galvanic skin response. By observing these parameters, the individual learns to change the underlying physiologic process. Some individuals with migraine headaches use biofeedback control over circulation to abort migraine attacks rather than take medications. Biofeedback is recognized as effective for a variety of processes that are under autonomic nervous system control.

Mind–body interventions in general allow people to participate actively in their own care. People often are changed emotionally and psychologically in the process of treating illness or disease. A big advantage of the mind–body therapies is that they are safe and economical and can be used easily in conjunction with other therapies.

Biologically Based Practices

Biologically based practices include **herbal medicine**, special diets, food supplements, vitamins, and specific biologic substances such as bovine and shark cartilage. Nonvitamin,

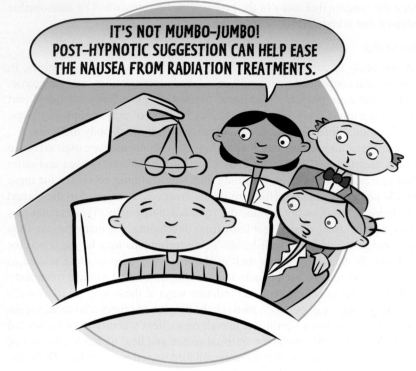

FIGURE 11.3 Alternative healthcare is moving more and more into mainstream practice.

nonmineral natural products such as fish oil and flax seed are the most commonly used alternative medicine (NCCAM, 2008).

Herbal medicines are plant products that are used to treat illnesses. As research into plant products continues, our understanding of the efficacy of herbs increases. Many in the United States who describe themselves as herbalists received their training in herbs during an apprenticeship with an experienced herbalist. There are educational programs for herbalists, but they are not regulated in every state.

Potential problems in the use of herbs and supplements include unreliable dosage and bioavailability, safety and efficacy, and interactions with prescribed medications. The bioavailability of various herbal preparations may vary widely, making it difficult to stabilize dosage. And because plants grow under different circumstances and with different soil and other conditions, the proportion of active ingredient within the plant may vary considerably. This makes accurate and stable dosage of herbs difficult.

While herbal products are available in tablet form with doses listed on the label, at present, there are no laws regulating the potency or purity of herbs sold in the United States. Many herbs are imported from around the world where accurate labeling and content purity may not be monitored. Because herbs are not considered drugs, there are no regulations regarding testing for efficacy or safety, as there are with products that must be approved by the Food and Drug Administration (FDA). This means that some herbs that are sold may contain contaminants. Serious illnesses and even deaths have been traced to contaminants in herbal medicines.

Some countries, such as Germany, have regulated herbal medications for many years. Canada has a system of regulating "natural health products" that includes regulations for herbal and homeopathic remedies. The Canadian system is based on a phased-in process that addresses products with the highest risk potential first (Natural Health Products Directorate, 2006).

Sometimes the active ingredient in an herb may have potent side effects or interact with medications prescribed. The FDA took action to remove the herb ephedra from the market after severe illness, including stroke and cardiac effects, and death were associated with its use (FDA, 2004).

When nurses interview patients regarding their medication history, asking specific questions about vitamins, herbs, supplements, and other therapeutic agents is critical. Patients may not consider these to be "medication" and so may not provide information about these substances being taken. The result may be that the source of an adverse response is missed or a harmful interaction with prescribed medications occurs. With increasing frequency, medical clinics and physicians' offices are asking clients to list on medical histories all over-the-counter medications, vitamins, and herbs as well as those requiring prescriptions.

COMMUNICATION IN ACTION

Assisting With Complete Reporting

Maggie Wilson works in an ambulatory clinic. She is reviewing Mabel Wilson's written new patient information. As she speaks with Mrs. Wilson, she says, "I see that you wrote here that you take supplements. Would you please tell me exactly what supplements you are taking?" Mrs. Wilson says, "Oh, I figured those didn't make any difference; they aren't like real medicine or anything, just like food." Maggie replies, "Supplements need to be considered along with medicines because they all have some effect. Sometimes that is a benefit to you, but sometimes they could interfere with drugs that might be prescribed. Whenever you see a doctor, you need to be sure to let the doctor know all the prescribed medicines, over-the-counter medicines, and supplements that you use. Please tell me what you take so I can add them to your record."

Biologic treatments include a variety of substances not approved as medical treatment by the FDA. These products have been developed by individuals and organizations and are often sold as food supplements rather than as medicines. Cartilage products from sharks, cattle, sheep, and chickens are being used to treat both cancer and arthritis. Peptide fractions derived from human blood and urine, called antineoplastons, are being used to treat cancer. Coley's toxins are killed cultures of bacteria that have been used for treating cancer. Apitherapy is the use of honeybee venom to treat rheumatic diseases, dermatologic conditions, chronic pain, and cancer. Research on the efficacy of these treatments is costly, and sponsors willing to bear that cost are hard to find. Some small studies are being funded with federal grants.

Medical research is beginning to identify some benefits of using food and vitamins in therapeutic ways. We have long known that many individuals who develop type 2 diabetes may be able to manage their blood sugar through dietary control. The role of antioxidants in decreasing cell damage and the effect of certain phytochemicals contained in cruciferous vegetables in preventing bowel cancer are just two examples of the theoretic benefits of nutrients. Some parents have used strict dietary regulation as a management tool for children with attention deficit hyperactivity disorder.

There are hazards in this approach to healthcare, however. Megadoses of vitamins may prove toxic such as liver toxicity from excessive vitamin A. Some nutrients interact with medications, decreasing their effectiveness. Individuals who choose to avoid all traditional medical care and rely on unsubstantiated claims about the therapeutic effects of nutrients may suffer deterioration in health.

All healthcare professionals need to support and encourage healthy dietary practices. Often it is possible to assist clients who rely on the use of nutrients for healthcare by becoming knowledgeable about the research regarding nutrition, accepting what clients believe helps them (as long as it is not detrimental to their well-being), and keeping an open mind. When we are willing to acknowledge the validity of some aspects of their preferred approach to healthcare, these clients may be willing to combine more conventional medical care along with their nutritional approaches.

Manipulative and Body-Based Practices

Manipulative and body-based practices include the physical manipulation of the body to achieve health goals. Some authors refer to these as "manual healing." Manipulative therapy is found in massage therapy and reflexology. Massage therapy uses both fixed and movable pressure and holding by the hands and sometimes the forearms, elbows, or feet. There is evidence that these techniques affect the musculoskeletal, circulatory–lymphatic, and nervous systems. Reflexology is massage of the feet to activate points on the feet that correspond to other body parts or systems.

Perhaps the most commonly known type of manipulative practice is chiropractic. Chiropractic care is based on the theory that disease is caused by interference with nerve function. It uses manipulation of the body joints, especially the spinal vertebrae, in seeking to restore normal function. The chiropractor also may use other treatments commonly associated with physical therapy, such as massage and exercise. There are definite differences among chiropractors. Some state that there are illnesses that cannot be treated through manual healing and do recommend that certain clients seek conventional medical care. Others believe that all illnesses may be treated by chiropractic methods and do not refer clients for conventional medical care. A major concern is that some clients may have more serious illnesses that may be missed altogether or not recognized in time to be given optimal medical attention. Another problem with chiropractic care is the use of chiropractic treatments on infants and young children in place of immunizations and other well-child services. Many people with joint and muscle strain and tension find that chiropractic treatments relieve discomfort and support effective functioning.

Acupuncture, which is a part of traditional Chinese medicine, is growing in popularity as an alternative care practice. While primarily used for managing musculoskeletal pain where evidence of efficacy is accumulating, acupuncture has also been used to control appetite for weight loss. There are few adverse effects; most, including infection from nonsterile needles and penetration of organs, are associated with unskilled practitioners.

Energy Medicine

The use of **energy medicine** (sometimes referred to bioelectromagnetic [BEM] therapies) is based on the understanding that electrical phenomena are found in all living organisms. There are magnetic fields that extend from the body, which can be measured and may be affected by external forces. The mechanisms by which the electromagnetic fields occur in the body, how these can be changed, and the effects of such changes are under study. Many modalities have been used for years without clear studies of their effectiveness. Some believe that BEM may be a unifying theory explaining why such widely diverse therapies as acupuncture and homeopathy produce results.

Some energy medicine is based on applying external energy to the body. There are thermal applications of BEM therapy in the form of radiofrequency hyperthermia and radiofrequency diathermy. Nonthermal applications include magnets and nerve stimulation. One common application is the use of magnets to relieve musculoskeletal problems. Magnetic insoles for shoes and magnets to be worn on the body are widely available.

There are also methods used to manipulate the interior biofields of the individual. These include therapeutic touch and Reiki. Both of these practices are based on a system of changing the energy fields without applying external energy forces to the body. In therapeutic touch, the practitioner moves hands above the body or touches lightly, perceives energy fields, and modifies them through hand movements. While the originator of therapeutic touch (Krieger, 1979) and some practitioners claim that their research supports this practice, others studying therapeutic touch have not been able to discern either the energy fields or methods of change and find the methodology of those studies reporting effectiveness to be flawed (Bullough & Bullough, 1998; Coursey, n.d.). Therapeutic touch has found acceptance by some within the nursing community, and a nursing diagnosis titled "energy field disturbance" has been included in the NANDA-I taxonomy. This is a matter of controversy, and there are strong objections by some to its inclusion without replicable research support. Nurses interested in therapeutic touch should research it further.

Understanding the Use of Complementary and Alternative Healthcare

According to the 2007 survey by NCAM (2008), the use of alternative and complementary therapies is increasing. For many clients with chronic conditions, mainstream medical care offers few options. Long-term treatments with medications often produce their own iatrogenic (treatment-caused) health problems, some of which are as troubling to the individual as the original disease process. A common response of conventional medicine to these problems has been to add more medications and more treatments, each with its own potential adverse effects. Mainstream healthcare providers often give little attention to the problems of daily living that are of greatest concern to the individual. Stress and anxiety also add to the burden of these clients. For clients with acute health conditions, certain treatments or medications may produce unpleasant or harmful side effects. Clients often are looking for alternative treatment methods that do not appear to have the same potential for harm.

Some alternative therapies have been available for many years, and there are people who believe that they have been helped significantly by these approaches. Unfortunately, traditional healthcare providers often have dismissed these therapies without investigating them thoroughly. On the other hand, few alternative therapies have been formally researched, and proponents often rely on undocumented reports of effectiveness.

Research into alternative therapies now is supported by the federal government but only in a small way compared to other research. The federal government has an Office of Alternative Healthcare, the NCCAM, and a Web page of references (see list of Web sites). More attention is being paid to the responses of individuals. Concern about the role of stress in illness has prompted an increased openness to nonmedical methods of managing stress. The possibility of alternative care practices working in a complementary fashion with traditional medical care is gaining wider acceptance. Often these complementary therapies are used to address the whole person and not simply the disease.

Part of the appeal of alternative healthcare is the caring and personalized response that clients often receive. People who have been intimidated by businesslike clinics and made to feel unimportant by impersonal professionals may find that the warm, concerned, accepting atmosphere of the nonconventional setting meets many personal needs. The fact that stress and anxiety play a major role in any health problem may help explain why many people are helped by therapies that may not be based on sound scientific knowledge. Because of the trust placed in nurses, they are in a unique position to relate with people about the issues that surround alternative and complementary therapy. Gallup polls continue to identify nurses as the most trusted professionals when ethics are considered (Gallup Poll, 2010).

To learn more about any specific therapy, or to research alternative and complementary therapies for any condition, use the CAM Citation Index found on the Web site of the NCCAM (see references). You may also search MEDLINE, the database of the National Library of Medicine, through the free PubMed Web site (*www.nlm.nih.gov/nccam/camonpubmed.html*) to research various therapies.

Assisting Clients Who Choose Alternative Healthcare

Many people who support conventional methods of healthcare have long ignored or repudiated the value of unorthodox healthcare traditions. We must recognize that complementary and alternative healthcare practices persist because people find them to be valuable. Acknowledging healthcare alternatives and working cooperatively with them is usually much more productive than trying to oppose them.

NCCAM suggests a five-step process for the consumer considering a particular complementary or alternative therapy. This process has a heavy emphasis on careful information gathering.

Assess Safety and Effectiveness

The first step is for the individual to assess the safety and effectiveness of the therapy in relationship to his or her own condition. One of the difficulties is finding accurate safety and efficacy data. Web sites and other sources of information require close scrutiny to determine the qualifications and bias of the sponsoring individual or group. The NCCAM Web site (*www.nccam.nih.gov*) contains Fact Sheets regarding specific therapies and additional links to research reports and scientific papers. Research reports may also be found through PubMed, the National Library of Medicine's online access (*www.ncbi.nlm.nih.gov/PubMed*). All complementary and alternative therapies are classified there under the Medical Subject Heading of "complementary therapies." The University of Pittsburgh Health Sciences Library System maintains an Alternative Medicine Homepage (*www.pitt.edu/~cbw/altm.html*) that provides links to additional information sites on the Web.

Examine the Expertise of the Therapy Practitioner

The second step is to examine the expertise of any therapy practitioner. Whether this person is a physician or another type of provider, determine whether there is appropriate education and licensing if that is required. Consumers should be encouraged to ask directly about education and credentials for practice. Some consumer organizations will direct individuals to reliable practitioners in the community. Clients who may be reluctant to ask directly about credentials can check whether credentials are available on a Web site or in printed information from the practitioner.

Investigate Service Delivery

Service delivery is the third aspect the client should investigate. How many patients are seen per day? Where is the therapy available and what barriers does that pose? Are standards for safety, privacy, and confidentiality in place? Remember that alternative providers are not included in the federal Health Insurance Portability and Accountability Act of 1996 legislation that mandates confidentiality in conventional healthcare settings unless they are eligible for reimbursement through Medicare or Medicaid. Most alternative providers are responsible for establishing their own standards and policies without outside oversight.

Research the Cost of Therapy

A fourth consideration is the cost of the therapy. Part of this is investigating what coverage may be obtained from an insurance carrier or whether any is available. Are the costs clear? How are payments made? Some unscrupulous practitioners collect large sums of money before any service and then may not provide what was promised. Some types of alternative care (eg, chiropractic care for an acute back injury) may be reimbursable under a traditional health plan.

Discuss the Treatment with Your Regular Healthcare Provider

The fifth step is to discuss this proposed treatment with a regular healthcare provider. The interaction of any traditional treatment and a complementary or alternative treatment may or may not pose a problem. Many healthcare providers support the use of various complementary therapies.

Things that the healthcare provider must also consider are such issues as client choice, informed consent, and the ethical principles of beneficence and nonmaleficence (see Chapter 8). As complementary and alternative therapies move into the mainstream, greater accountability to the public is essential.

Critical Thinking Activity

Identify a specific form of complementary or alternative therapy. Search the health literature regarding this therapy. Review the information available in other sources. Analyze the information to determine whether the data supporting the use of this therapy are weak, moderate, or strong. Provide a rationale for your determination.

KEY CONCEPTS

- Community-based nursing emphasizes advocating for patients, promoting self-care, focusing on health promotion and disease prevention, and recognizing the importance of family, culture, and the community.

- Health promotion and prevention of illness and disease are a part of nursing practice in all settings.

- Client empowerment through teaching, explaining options, and supporting decision making is a foundation for community-based care.

- Primary prevention focuses on preventing disease; secondary prevention focuses on early diagnosis through screening and preventing complications; tertiary prevention focuses on preventing long-term disability and restoring functional capacity.

- Disease management strives to promote health through effective treatment of targeted diseases and health conditions.

- Healthy People 2020 is a federal effort that includes overall goals, priority areas, and leading indicators to measure progress in developing healthier communities.

- Maintaining continuity of care requires transition planning, with special emphasis on reconciling medication records from one setting to another.

- Ensuring that healthcare records are available wherever the client seeks care is becoming a possibility through computerization of medical records and the development of transportable records that contain essential information.

- Alternative healthcare encompasses those types of care outside of conventional Western medicine and includes mind–body medicine, biologically based practices, manipulative and body-based practices, and energy medicine as well as alternative whole medical systems.

- Alternative care therapies are considered complementary therapies when used along with traditional medical care. Integrative medicine involves the deliberative planning for using both traditional medical care and alternative care in a coordinated manner.

- Understanding the different types of alternative healthcare services, why people choose alternative healthcare, and how nurses may assist people who seek this care will form a foundation for more effective relationships with clients.

- Alternative and complementary therapies can be evaluated based on a five-step process that includes safety and effectiveness of the therapy, credentials of the provider, service delivery, cost of services, and consultation with the regular healthcare provider.

RELEVANT WEB SITES

Web sites relevant to this chapter can be found at thePoint, accessed through *http://thePoint. lww.com/Ellis10e* and by entering the code found on the inside cover of your text.

REFERENCES

American Red Cross. (2009). *Preparing and getting trained: preparedness fast facts*. Retrieved January 6, 2011, from http://www.redcross.org/

ASTM International. (2005). ASTM Standard E2369-051. *Continuity of care record (CCR)*. West Conshohocken, PA: Author. Retrieved January 7, 2011, from www.astm.org/Standards/E2369.htm

Bullough, V. L. & Bullough, B. (1998). Should nurses practice therapeutic touch? Should nursing schools teach therapeutic touch? *Journal of Professional Nursing, 14*(4), 254–257.

Corepoint Health. (2009). *The continuity of care document: changing the landscape of healthcare information exchange*. Retrieved January 6, 2011, from http://www.corepointhealth.com/sites/default/files/whitepapers/continuity-of-care-document-ccd.pdf

Coursey, K. (n.d.) Further notes on therapeutic touch. *Quackwatch*. Retrieved January 4, 2011, from http://www.quackwatch.org/01QuackeryRelatedTopics/tt2.html

Food and Drug Administration. (2004). *FDA acts to remove ephedra-containing dietary supplements from market*. Retrieved January 6, 2011, from http://www.fda.gov/NewsEvents/Newsroom/PressAnnouncements/2004/ucm108379.htm

Gallup Poll. (2010). *Nurses top honesty and ethics list for 11th year, 2010*. Retrieved January 5, 2011, from http://www.gallup.com/poll/145043/Nurses-Top-Honesty-Ethics-List-11-Year.aspx

Joint Commission on Accreditation of Healthcare Organizations. (2010). *National patient safety goal on reconciling medication information*. Retrieved January 5, 2011, from http://www.jointcommission.org/npsg_reconciling_medication/

Krieger, D. (1979). *Therapeutic touch*. New York, NY: Prentice-Hall.

National Association of Naturopathic Physicians. (2010). *Licensed states & licensing authorities*. Retrieved January 5, 2011 from http://www.naturopathic.org/content.asp?contentid=57

National Center for Complementary and Alternative Medicine. (2008). *The use of complementary and alternative medicine in the United States*. Retrieved January 4, 2011 from http://nccam.nih.gov/news/camsurvey_fs1.htm

National Center for Complementary and Alternative Medicine. (2010). *What is complementary and alternative medicine?* NCCAM Publication No. D347. Retrieved January 6, 2011 from http://nccam.nih.gov/health/whatiscam/

Natural Health Products Directorate. (2006). *National health products master file*. Retrieved January 5, 2011 from http://www.hc-sc.gc.ca/dhp-mps/prodnatur/legislation/docs/master_file_fichier_principal-eng.php

US Department of Health and Human Services (US-DHHS) (January, 2010) About Healthy People, Washington, DC. Retrieved April 19, 2011 from http://www.healthypeople.gov/2020/about/default.aspx

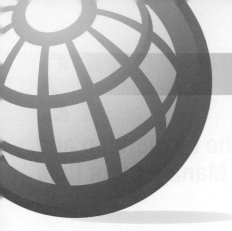

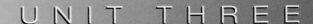

Accepting Greater Responsibility for Nursing Practice

The third and final unit in this textbook is devoted to topics that will assist you to move into the world of employment as a registered nurse (RN). The major goal is to prepare you for the leadership role that you will one day execute as an RN.

Chapter 12 begins with a discussion of leadership, management, accountability, and authority and includes a brief review of theories of leadership. Information is provided about the various leadership and management roles nurses may perform as they fulfill their responsibilities in regard to leading and managing others. You will find helpful information on the distribution and use of power in the healthcare system, a discussion of emotional intelligence, a section on using communication skills effectively, and content related to performance evaluation and time management.

As leaders in the healthcare system, nurses have specific responsibilities regarding delegation within the nursing team and interacting with the interdisciplinary team. Leading requires the ability to build teams and to motivate others. It also requires the ability to bring about change and to manage conflict situations. These topics are explored in Chapter 13.

Chapter 14 helps to prepare you for the challenges you will face in today's workplace. Beginning with a discussion of reality shock and burnout, the chapter goes on to emphasize the importance of workplace safety and its effect on the health of nurses. It concludes with an exploration of the topic of sexual harassment and violence in the workplace.

A discussion of the political process—how it affects nursing and how nurses can affect it—follows in Chapter 15. An understanding of how politics can and does have an effect on the healthcare delivery system can be relevant to your professional experience.

Chapter 16, the final chapter of the unit and the text, emphasizes your role in a healthcare system where nurses are accountable for the development of nursing as a profession. A brief explanation of terms and processes involved in nursing research provides a foundation for fulfilling your responsibilities in this important work. Understanding evidence-based practice and its implementation is essential to providing quality care. The use of technology in healthcare now and for the future is discussed.

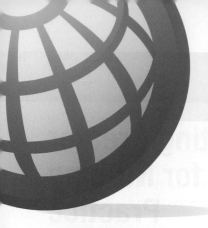

12

Initiating the Leadership and Management Role

LEARNING OUTCOMES

After completing this chapter, you should be able to:

1. Compare and contrast the concepts of leadership and management and make a distinction in the skills involved.
2. Differentiate between the terms "authority" and "accountability."
3. Discuss the major theories regarding leadership.
4. Compare and contrast three prevailing leadership styles.
5. Analyze the factors that have resulted in the development of transformational leadership.
6. Describe the relationship of power and empowerment and identify ways by which one individual can empower another.
7. Explain emotional intelligence and why it is an important quality of a leader.
8. Analyze methods by which the development of leadership style can be enhanced.
9. Describe the basic characteristics of effective communication.
10. Analyze the communication strategies that are essential for effective leadership, identifying the critical role of each.
11. Describe the elements of an effective performance appraisal system, including the conduct of the interview.
12. Analyze the importance of time management and evaluate methods that will help overcome major time wasters and procrastination.

KEY TERMS

Accountability
Authority
Autocratic/authoritarian leadership style
Charisma
Coercive power
Communication
Connection power
Democratic/participative leadership style
Emotional intelligence
Empowerment
Expert power
Informational power
Job descriptions
Laissez-faire/permissive leadership style

Leadership/management style
Legitimate power
Mindfulness
Mentor
Motivational power
Multicratic leadership
Performance appraisal
Procrastination
Professional standards
Referent power
Responsibility
Reward power
Theories of leadership
Time management

The novice in the area of managing a healthcare team can easily be dazzled by the many terms populating the literature that are devoted to the topics of leadership and management. Words such as authority, responsibility, accountability, team building, empowerment, coaching, mentoring, motivating, and collective power are but a few of those incorporated into articles, monographs, and books addressing the topic of successful leadership and management. In this chapter, we define those terms for you and discuss their application to the healthcare environment. This will make them useful to you as you begin your career as a staff nurse and later as you assume a leadership role in patient care.

COMPARING LEADERSHIP AND MANAGEMENT

Although the terms "leadership" and "management" are often used interchangeably, differences exist in how each is practiced in the work situation. At some point in your nursing career, you likely will fill both roles: leader and manager. Understanding the uniqueness of each will help you be effective in either position. Let us explore the differences and how they are applied in the work situation.

Leadership refers to the ability to guide, motivate, and inspire, and to instill vision and purpose. As you read this, you probably can think of individuals you know who possess strong leadership abilities—your class president or the person who arranges and guides your study sessions, for example. To provide leadership, you must be able to influence the beliefs, opinions, or behaviors of others and to persuade others to follow your direction. This can be accomplished in a number of ways, referred to as leadership styles, which we discuss later.

Management refers to activities such as planning, organizing, directing, and controlling with the purpose of accomplishing specific goals and objectives within an organization. Essentially, management involves coordination and integration of resources to accomplish specific tasks. Often, management positions are roles to which one is appointed or hired after a competitive job application and interview. This appointment grants the manager the power to direct others and the responsibility for ensuring that certain tasks within the organization are completed effectively and efficiently. In other words, the authority to act is gained by virtue of the position one holds within the organization.

The very best managers also are leaders, although this may not always happen. Conversely, not all leaders are officially managers in the sense we have defined it. A foremost authority on leadership and organizational management, Warren Bennis (2003), has stated that managers are people who do things right, while leaders are people who do the right thing. Individuals may become leaders because of the way in which they inspire others to follow them. Can you think of a situation in which an individual was a leader but did not have the role of manager? Similarly, can you think of any situations in which the manager lacked the ability to lead a group of people? Can you recall situations in which the manager also was a leader?

DIFFERENTIATING BETWEEN ACCOUNTABILITY AND AUTHORITY

Three terms are frequently associated with leadership and management roles: accountability, responsibility, and authority. Are you clear about the definitions of each of these terms?

Accountability and **responsibility** are terms with similar meanings. They refer to the obligation to answer for one's actions and to accomplish what you have agreed to do. For example, the team leader assigns you the care of four patients and you agree to that assignment; therefore, the patients' care is your responsibility. You have an obligation to provide timely care to that group of patients and to achieve the desired outcome regarding that care.

By virtue of the state Nurse Practice Acts, nurses are held responsible or accountable for their actions. This means they must provide the necessary care competently and in compliance with accepted standards, using sound judgment, thinking critically, and delegating wisely. Failure to perform in a responsible manner could result in legal action being taken against the nurse if harm occurs to the patient (see Chapter 7).

Nurses have always been accountable for the care they give from both a personal and a professional standpoint. However, as we have witnessed the rapid technologic, fiscal, and operational changes occurring within the healthcare system, the term now carries stronger legal implications. Nurses face greater legal vulnerability because of consumer rights, greater access of the public to information regarding health issues, the public availability of records, and increased patient involvement in healthcare decision making. This intensifies the necessity for nurses to be aware of the legal aspects of nursing and of the laws that protect the client. Individuals are accountable for their own actions and also for some of the actions of those they supervise. We understand that tasks can be delegated, but accountability cannot; nurses who delegate tasks to assistive personnel continue to be accountable for that care (see Chapter 13). For example, if you ask the nursing assistant to check the vital signs of four of your patients, you are asking the assistant to act in your place. You are still accountable for that activity (ie, that the vital signs are accurately measured, reported, and documented). This accountability has become a sensitive issue for nurses as, in an effort to contain costs, more unlicensed assistive personnel are hired to replace licensed staff.

Authority can be defined as the power to influence, give directions, command, take action, and make decisions. Traditionally, we have considered it the manager's job to command or make decisions. In this sense, the manager authored all critical decisions. As you read further, you will note that in today's work environment, authority is more often shared. Accompanying this shared authority and decision making is a mutual responsibility for outcomes. We will discuss this concept in greater detail after we have talked about leadership.

In the ideal work situation, workers are given the amount of authority needed to carry out the responsibilities expected of them. However, many nurses experience frustration because they must be accountable for activities without the authority to affect the situation or create change. For example, a nurse has the responsibility of ensuring that all patients receive competent care, but the nurse may have no input into the staffing of the unit or the performance appraisal of nursing assistants working on that shift. Therefore, the nursing assistants may not be as responsive to the nurse's instructions as they should be. Or perhaps a nurse has the responsibility for seeing that there are adequate supplies on a unit but has no opportunity to affect the unit's budget.

► *EXAMPLE*

Accountability Without Authority

John Jones, a RN, works on the night shift with two nursing assistants. All nursing assistants are taught the skills expected in their job description by the staff development department. During his orientation to the hospital, John was informed that all nursing assistants were taught basic care skills and how to measure vital signs and were cross-trained as phlebotomists. The nursing assistants were expected to draw the blood for morning lab work. However, John quickly discovered that one of the nursing assistants on his shift was not able to draw blood successfully. When he spoke with the other RN on his unit about this, she said, "You will find that lots of them really don't have that skill. You will just have to draw the blood yourself. Nobody really says anything to them if they don't do it, and it makes their job easier if they don't draw blood. Some are even afraid to draw blood because they are afraid of the potential for contracting HIV." John replied, "But that really increases my workload at a busy time. Isn't there any way that I can require them to go back and get the skills they need?" The other RN replied, "Nope, you just have to make sure everything gets done on time." John discovered that he was accountable for the care by the nursing assistants but had no authority over their practice.

Critical Thinking Activity

Think for a moment of behaviors you noted in your clinical experiences this past week. What behavior did you observe that was a clear demonstration of authority? What were the characteristics that made it so? Can you recall a situation in which an RN accepted responsibility for an action that had been taken? How was this done?

THEORIES OF LEADERSHIP

Let's talk briefly about the various **theories of leadership** (Table 12.1). Just as knowledge of theories of nursing can help us to understand nursing (see Chapter 1), leadership theories help us to describe and understand the processes of leadership. As a society, we have studied leadership theory since about the mid-20th century, and a number of theories have been set forth, far too many to discuss in detail in this text. The theories of leadership listed in Table 12.1 are those most frequently cited as helpful in understanding specific situations.

As a student preparing for graduation from your nursing program, you may wonder how all the information on leadership theories relates to you. Healthcare represents one of the largest businesses in the United States. Historically, the administrative structure in hospitals has been predominately bureaucratic, with a few decision makers and many followers. That situation is changing as more hospitals adopt different organizational patterns. Having basic knowledge of the various approaches to leadership will help you understand the environments in which you work and will help you determine the leadership approach you wish to develop.

Current emphasis in most management literature is placed on transformational leadership. Today's healthcare work environment relies on teamwork and shared decision making. Many believe that in this environment, the goals of the organization are most likely to be met if transformational leadership is employed. As you study the attributes of transformational leadership in Table 12.1, you will note that the differences in the role of the leader and the followers are de-emphasized. When effectively implemented, transformational leadership can

Table 12.1   Major Theories of Leadership

GENERAL CLASSIFICATION, THEORY, AND THEORIST(S)	ESSENTIAL CHARACTERISTICS AND COMMENTS
Trait	Focuses on certain characteristics of the leader.
Great Man theory	Promotes the concept that certain people were born to be leaders because they inherited a set of special characteristics qualifying them for such responsibilities. Because leaders are "born," this theory suggests that leadership cannot be developed.
Attribution theory	Suggests that leadership relates to personal attributes people tend to characterize leaders as having, such as height, social background, creativity, assertiveness, initiative, integrity, ability, intelligence, etc.
Charismatic theory	Often listed as a quality of other theories, this theory relates to a special charm or allure possessed by the leader that inspires others to follow and give allegiance. Sometimes, this type of leadership is said to emerge in times of crisis and change.
Attitudinal	Theorizes that attitudes of the leader result in the leader's behavior.
Ohio State Leadership Studies	Describes leadership behavior as related to initiating structure and consideration of employees.
Michigan Leadership Studies	Describes leader behavior as employee oriented or production oriented.
Managerial grid (R. R. Blake & J. S. Mouton, 1964)	Identifies five management styles best described on a grid, in which each style combines elements of concern for production and concern for people.
Situational	Suggests basis of leadership is the situation or environment and the behaviors of leaders in response to the situation.
Contingency theory (Fred Fiedler, 1967)	Examines factors in the situation, particularly the skills of the leader and that individual's position of power in the organization, as determinants of leader effectiveness.
Path–Goal theory (Robert J. House, 1971)	Relates effective leadership to leader's ability to minimize obstructions to goals, identify outcomes that workers want to achieve, and reward the followers for high performance and achievement, thereby increasing worker satisfaction and productivity.
Contemporary Theories	Includes theories most commonly in use at the present time.
Transformational leadership (Bass, 1985)	Places emphasis on the collective purpose and mutual growth of both the leader and the follower and de-emphasizes differences in the roles of the leader and followers. Leader activities include creating a vision, building relationships, developing trust, and building self-esteem. Leader makes subordinates aware of how important their jobs are, helps them build skills, and motivates them to work for the good of the organization. Has four major components: idealized influence (attributes and behaviors), individualized consideration, inspirational motivation, and intellectual stimulation.
Transactional leadership (J. M. Burns, 1978; Bass, 1985)	Examines leadership in terms of striking a bargain in which there is a mutual exchange between leaders and followers of benefits for work sometimes referred to as a reward and punishment approach. Maintains stability of organization while offering rewards to employees for performance and met goals.
(Senge, Kleiner, Roberts, et al., 1994)	Identifies the role of the leader as that of a strategic visionary; promotes "learning" organizations in which the leader is the teacher who builds a shared vision.

result in agreements about priorities, shared values, perceived common goals, and meaningful purposes. You can see how this would be desirable in a healthcare environment.

Additionally, because of the demographics of the profession, many positions of leadership in nursing are held by women. A yearlong study conducted by Caliper (2005) found that women leaders were more assertive and persuasive than their male counterparts, had a stronger need to get things done, were more willing to take risks, and demonstrated an inclusive, team-building leadership style of problem solving and decision making. They were also found to be more empathetic and flexible as well as stronger in interpersonal skills, allowing women leaders to bring others around to their point of view because they truly cared about others.

Leadership/Management Styles

Lewin (1951) described three prevailing styles of behavior observed in leaders/managers that we refer to as **leadership** or **management styles** (Display 12.1), which sometimes are

DISPLAY 12.1 Leadership/Management Styles

Autocratic/Authoritative

Majority of decisions determined by the manager

Dictates work to be done and who will do it

Provides little opportunity for input or suggestions from followers

Gives little feedback or recognition for accomplishments

Communication flows downward, with emphasis on completing the task

Works well in emergency situations where time is of the essence

May be preferred style when working with unskilled or uneducated employees

Democratic/Participative

Input to decision making encouraged among workers

Leaders see themselves as coworkers

Communication, consensus, and teamwork stressed

Leader leads by providing information, suggesting direction, supporting coworkers

Communication flows both up and down

Human relationships important

Considered the preferred style in the majority of work situations

Laissez-faire/Permissive

Little or no direction or guidance provided

Coworkers develop their own goals, make their own decisions, and take responsibility

Decision making dispersed throughout the group

Provides maximum freedom for individuals and motivates workers to perform at high levels

If used inappropriately, a leadership vacuum may occur, in which an informal leader may arise

Multicratic

Combines the positive features of authoritative, participative leadership styles

Leader provides a maximum of structure when the situation requires it

Leader provides maximum group participation when needed

Support and encouragement provided to subordinates at all times listed among the behavioral theories of leadership. The focus of these three styles is on the amount of control the manager assumes over the actions of the workers and the beliefs of the leader/manager about the nature of workers (which is why they may be referred to as behavioral theories). The extremes extend from situations in which the manager makes all the decisions to situations in which virtually no direction is given to workers. In addition to the individual characteristics of the leader, several other variables will determine the type of manager a nurse might be. The type of organizational structure will influence leadership styles. How authority is centralized or dispersed throughout the organization also affects leadership styles. The communication patterns, which are directly tied to organizational structure, also will influence leadership styles. Equally important is the situation at hand.

Autocratic or **authoritarian leadership**, in which the leader/manager makes the majority of the decisions, may be essential in emergency situations that call for immediate action. When faced with life-threatening conditions, as we frequently see in emergency departments and critical care units, the leader may be in the best position to make judgments and decisions. Little time exists to contemplate and build consensus regarding the best approach or to allow discussion for alternative actions.

Laissez-faire or **permissive leadership**, in which little or no direction or guidance is provided, is at the other extreme and provides the least structure and control. It is highly effective for situations in which coworkers can develop their own goals, make their own decisions, and take responsibility for their own actions. An example might be seen in an inpatient psychiatric unit where a certain amount of autonomy and self-direction are an important part of the unit's operation.

Democratic or **participative leadership**, in which input to decision making is encouraged among workers, represents the middle ground. The democratic leader focuses on involving subordinates in decision making. There are various methods to accomplish this, such as asking for input, developing a consensus, voting, or delegating decisions to others. It is most effective when the decision or task at hand does not require urgent action and when subordinates have the ability to make meaningful contributions.

A fourth leadership style, not identified by Lewin, is probably the one that is most frequently used in healthcare. **Multicratic leadership** combines the most favorable aspects of all styles as mediated by the circumstances at hand. A multicratic leader provides maximum structure and direction when the situation calls for it and provides for maximum group input into decision making when conditions are conducive to such an approach. Support, encouragement, and recognition of subordinates and their contributions are always present. Learning when to use each of the various approaches is something that a new graduate will need to study and to practice, just as with other nursing skills.

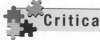

Critical Thinking Activity

In addition to the examples provided in the text, identify a healthcare-related situation in which each of the leadership styles would be appropriately employed. Provide the rationale for choosing that particular leadership style in the situation. What are the advantages of that leadership style? What are its limitations?

Changes in Approaches to Leadership

Nothing operates in isolation or in a vacuum; approaches to leadership are no exception. As you may surmise from the information in Table 12.1 and Display 12.1, the leadership systems have changed as societal values and norms changed.

As a society, we have experienced tremendous growth in information systems and technology. As a result, individuals at all levels within an organization have access to data, which is no longer reserved for a few selected individuals at the top of an organizational chart. Employees at all levels within an organization are knowledgeable about goals, operations, rewards, and critical areas. The information explosion also has brought a more intelligent and informed customer to the healthcare arena, the impact of which can be seen in the changing language by which this person is referred—once patient, then client, now more frequently consumer or customer.

Today, more informed workers are developing into self-directed teams. This has resulted in managers spending time developing the abilities of others rather than directing them. Approaches to leadership have moved from authoritarian styles to a more collaborative leadership style, with the individuals closest to the problem helping to find solutions to it. The strategies used for developing human resources have undergone significant changes. Many organizations, healthcare facilities included, are encouraging employees to be involved in decision making. The leadership required for this type of organization must be much different from that seen in the 1950s, when the manager instructed and directed and the worker acted and followed. Business leaders today would suggest that leadership needs to be visionary, ethical, supportive, facilitative, motivational, and open to new ideas. It also needs to provide for shared decision making and be responsive to the needs of those it serves. The effective leader must be able to communicate clearly and effectively, build consensus and inspire people to do their best, deal well with ambiguity, and maintain diplomatic and productive relationships.

THE CONCEPT OF POWER

Power, as we refer to it in a leadership sense, is the ability to do, act, or produce; the ability to control others. Power connotes having control, influence, or domination; in other words, the ability an individual has to get things done. The concept of power forms a basis for action in transformational leadership.

Types of Power

French and Raven (1959) identified five types of power based on the source of that power (Display 12.2). You can find all of these types of power at work in nursing.

Legitimate power—that which occurs by virtue of the position held in the institution—is based on a specific job description. The most obvious of these forms can be seen in such positions as clinical director of nursing or director of coordinated care management.

Referent power is gained by an individual because others like and admire that person or what the person symbolizes. This can be observed when one selects a mentor or an individual after whom he or she wants to model behavior. The mentor has referent power that translates into the ability to change the behavior of those being mentored. Mentoring has gained much popularity in the past few years, and new graduates are encouraged to find a mentor when they begin their careers. We will discuss mentors in more detail later in this chapter. Referent

DISPLAY 12.2   Types of Power

Legitimate power	Power based on an official position within the organization. Often referred to as authority, in which manager has the right to direct others and workers are obligated to respond. Activities typically include making decisions on behalf of the organization and acquiring or controlling human and material resources.
Referent power	Power an individual has because others identify with the leader or what that leader symbolizes or represents. It also exists because others see the leader as powerful, as in the case of political figures.
Reward power	Power achieved by having the ability to grant favors or give rewards to others. Rewards might be in the form of praise, commendation, respect, or support.
Coercive power	Power that occurs because of the ability to place sanctions on another individual in the form of verbal threats, withholding pay increases, undesired assignments, or warnings. The opposite of reward power, it is based on the fear of punishment.
Expert power	Power gained through the possession of special knowledge, skills, or abilities that are respected by others.
Informational power	Power that is gained by having information or data that are important to others.
Connection power	Power that represents the cumulative effect of more than one person working toward a goal; for example, people working together to bring about a change or influence legislation.
Motivational power	The ability of the leader to stimulate the interest, enthusiasm, or participation of others with regard to a common goal.

power is often associated with **charisma**. Charisma is a combination of characteristics that makes a person appealing and that attracts others. Charisma includes the way the leader acts, talks, walks, and relates to others. It is sometimes listed separately as a theory of leadership and also is included often in the list of traits in the trait theory.

Reward power can be seen anytime one individual rewards another with positive statements, compliments, or other ego-boosting comments. It is also seen in promotions, salary increases, and awards. Even beginning nurses will find reward power available to them if they focus on giving recognition to others' strengths and accomplishments.

COMMUNICATION IN ACTION

Using Reward Power

Jessica Brown was a new RN on the surgical unit. She worked with a charge nurse who had worked at the hospital for many years. After the end of the shift, Jessica stopped to talk with the charge nurse. "I just wanted to take a couple of minutes to thank you for the great job you did as charge this evening. I cannot believe how many details you kept straight and how you were still able to take the time to help me with that difficult IV start. It has really made a difference for me that you are willing to help me learn. Thanks a lot!"

Although Jessica was the newest person on the shift, she found that she could use reward power. Because Jessica was a willing learner and expressed her appreciation for learning opportunities, the charge nurse was very willing to help and felt rewarded for her efforts.

Coercive power involves using threats of punishment to enforce desired behaviors. Coercive power also has its place in nursing. If you fail to practice safe, competent nursing after you are licensed, the board of nursing has the power to compel you to change behavior by the threat of revoking your license to practice (see Chapter 7). For example, if unsafe practice is the result of chemical abuse, an employer can force an employee to enter treatment for chemical dependency, with the threat of job loss for failure to do so.

Expert power involves having specialized skills and abilities that serve to accomplish desired goals or influence others to follow one's leadership. Expert power is observed every day on hospital units. As nursing becomes more specialized, the individual with particular skills, knowledge, and ability will have power in the area where these skills are important.

Two other forms of power other than those originally identified by French and Raven have been described. **Informational power** exists when an individual possesses information that others need or want to accomplish a goal. An individual who has access to information about the unit's budget or one who is more informed about policies that guide behavior of others is an example of someone with informational power.

Connection power is the cumulative effect of more than one individual working toward a goal. Connection power is responsible for the effectiveness seen in networking. Nurses who work collaboratively develop connection power. Connection power also can occur by working with persons who command power, respect, or access to desired positions or places. You will observe nurses using connection power as they work with other professionals in the healthcare system. You will also see nurses who are politically involved exercising connection power.

Motivational power is a new term. It refers to one's ability to arouse in others an excitement and enthusiasm for what they are doing. Because of its inherent or internal nature, motivation must be generated by the individual as opposed to being provided from outside. Motivational power, therefore, refers to the ability of the leader to stimulate the interest, enthusiasm, or participation of others with regard to a common goal. It involves recognizing the elements that drive individuals or creates satisfaction for them. McGregor's (1966) Theory X and Theory Y, Ouchi's (1981) Theory Z, Herzberg's (Herzberg, 1966; Herzberg, Mausner, & Snyderman, 1959) Satisfiers and Dissatisfiers, and Maslow's (1954) Hierarchy of Needs are all examples of approaches to motivation (see Chapter 13). In transformational leadership, motivational power is seen when the leader shares information, involves others in decision making, recognizes accomplishments, and rewards behavior (Fig. 12.1).

▶ *EXAMPLE*

Considering Attributes When Selecting Team Members

The nursing administrative group at Columbia Community Hospital was anticipating a major change in the system of patient care delivery. As they discussed plans for implementing this change, it was decided that a small team to pilot the program would be a sound approach. They then wanted to select individuals to work in the pilot program. Melissa Worth had worked at the hospital for 4 years. A skilled decision maker full of enthusiasm and energy, she was welcomed by all nursing groups. Her positive attitude and ability to relate to others made her a favorite among the staff. When it was suggested that she lead the group to pilot the new program, everyone was in agreement.

Melissa possessed motivational power in that she was able to instill enthusiasm in others as well as herself. In order for a change to take place, those in the administrative group knew that motivation for change would be a key ingredient.

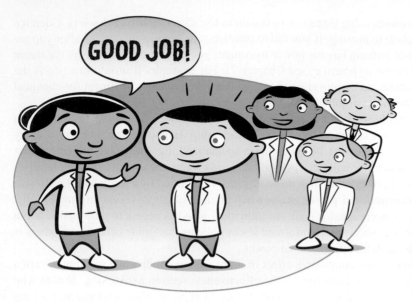

FIGURE 12.1 Motivational power is seen when the leader recognizes the accomplishments of others.

Thus, we see that power is derived from a variety of sources and is used in a number of different situations. It is important for all nurses to realize that they have a power base and to seek positive ways to use it to bring about improvements in the healthcare system that will benefit patients and society as a whole.

Empowerment

The concept of empowerment has received a great deal of discussion over the past 30 years. **Empowerment** refers to the process of increasing the capacity of individuals or groups to make choices and to transform those choices into desired actions and outcomes. It transforms others to partners in the decision-making process by providing them with necessary knowledge and reinforcement.

Kanter (1993) has identified structural conditions as being the key contributors to empowerment. They are: having opportunity for advancement or opportunity to be involved in activities beyond one's job description, access to information about all facets of the organization, access to support for one's job responsibilities and decision making, and access to resources as needed by the employee. Manojlovich (2007) states that three factors must be in place in order for empowerment to occur: A workplace must have the requisite structures that promote empowerment; a psychological belief in one's ability to be empowered; and acknowledgement that there is power in the relationships and caring that nurses provide.

Numerous studies have demonstrated the benefits of an empowered nursing workforce including such factors as increased job satisfaction and intent to remain in the organization (Nedd, 2006). The results of three studies conducted by Laschinger, Almost, and Tuer-Hodes (2003) support the hypothesized relationships between structural empowerment and the magnet hospital characteristics of autonomy, control over practice environment, and positive nurse–physician relationships. The combination of access to empowering work conditions and magnet hospital characteristics was significantly predictive of nurses' satisfaction with their jobs.

We see empowerment at work where transformational leadership is practiced; transformational leaders seek to empower their followers and thus transform the work environment. Transformational leaders openly share information with workers so that everyone is aware of problems and the need for action. The leader provides a vision of what is to be accomplished and helps workers to understand that they are an integral part of the group. Workers are delegated authority for decision making and for helping to find solutions to problems. Transformational leaders work at developing the skills of workers, who then develop a strong sense of self and are motivated toward achievement. Empowered workers have a greater sense of satisfaction derived from goal achievement. None of this could occur if workers were not empowered initially.

Empowerment is not easily achieved. Some organizations do not support empowerment of employees. Supervisors themselves may not be empowered within the organization. Some supervisors lack the self-confidence necessary to empower others and fear loss of control if workers assume greater responsibility in decision making. In other instances, the supervisors may have moved into their roles while working in hierarchical organizations and may find it difficult to shift their approach to management in a new setting. Some employees do not want the accountability and responsibility that are required of the empowered individual.

Organizational Characteristics That Support Empowerment

Senge, Kleiner, Roberts, et al. (1994, p. 51) refer to organizations that support empowerment as "learning organizations" and identify a number of characteristics of the learning organization. They include the following among these characteristics:

- People feel they are doing something that matters and that all individuals are growing and enhancing their capacity to create. Values and visions are shared.
- The belief exists that people are more intelligent as a group than they are individually and that visions of the organization emerge from all levels.
- The knowledge in the hearts and minds of employees is one of the organization's greatest resources.
- Employees are encouraged to learn what is going on at every level within the organization.
- People feel free to inquire about another's values and assumptions, and mutual respect and trust exist among individuals, thus freeing people to take risks and openly assess results.

Tichy and Bennis (2007) strongly support this concept. They contend that winning leaders are teachers who drive their organizations through teaching. Through teaching, leaders invest in the development of leadership judgment in others.

Empowering Others

Nurses are expected to practice according to professional standards. However, nurses function within the constraints of their employment settings, and this affects their ability to engage in true professional practice. As we indicated earlier, if the organization does not support the empowerment of people, it is much more difficult to accomplish. If you want to work in an organization that empowers its employees, you will want to set this as one of your goals when seeking employment following graduation (see Chapter 4). An organization that is involved in transformational leadership styles also will support (and require) the empowerment of employees. The two are intricately interwoven. Manojlovich (2005) found that unit-level leaders who empowered staff nurses enhanced the professional practice behaviors of those nurses. Other employees are also affected by nursing leaders who empower others. When nursing aides in long-term care are empowered by inclusion in decision making, outcomes for residents improve (Barry, Brannon, & Mohr, 2005.)

Empowering others can be accomplished through a variety of strategies that are appropriate for any situation in which the goal is to give others power and control over a situation. For a person to gain more control over a situation, that individual must be knowledgeable. So, a first step in empowering is often the open sharing of information. Everyone must be aware of the underlying situation, the nature of the problems, and why change is needed. Sharing information with others also is an important aspect of gaining the trust of your followers. Without information, others cannot act responsibly. They need to know how the organization works and the factors that impinge upon a situation.

Once individuals are aware of the problems and situations being faced, they can be involved in setting the goal or developing a vision of what is to be accomplished. Through this process, the employee becomes more vested in achieving the desired outcome and buys into the excellence expected and the productivity needed to accomplish it. Along with this, team members need to know the breadth and extent of the areas within which they can act. Another characteristic of empowering others is involving them in finding solutions to the problems once they are aware of the problems being encountered. This is where the collective intelligence of the group is useful. Rather than support the belief that only the leader can propose workable solutions, empowered employees are respected for their contributions and first-hand knowledge of a situation. Ideally, employees will become involved in the development of strategies to accomplish the goal or vision.

Reaching this point in any organization requires that the leader has been able to help workers develop their skills. It involves teaching, team building, and coaching abilities on the part of the leader (see Chapter 13). Workers must gain confidence in their ability to make correct decisions and take appropriate action. Employees need to be able to see themselves as members of influential teams, with the ability to discover new resources. Recognizing the accomplishments of others, sharing credit, valuing honesty and openness, and rewarding behavior are important aspects of this development. As a result of feeling empowered, employees understand the valuable contribution they make.

As you move into positions of responsibility, what are the behaviors and characteristics that you must possess to empower others? How can you motivate others to assume more responsibility and accountability for their actions? Display 12.3 provides a list of personal characteristics that are critical to being able to empower others and identifies some behaviors that help to create those characteristics. How many of those characteristics do you currently possess? Which ones will you need to develop?

Like many other endeavors, empowering others has no straight line to success; do not expect too much success early on. Being successful requires that you maintain an optimistic attitude, persevere in your goals and activities, and remain steadfast in your commitment to them. Continual assessment of yourself and the situation is essential. Be honest with yourself,

DISPLAY 12.3 Personal Attributes That Support Empowering Others

Trustworthiness
- Honest in relationships with others
- Honors commitments, follows through on promises
- Can be relied upon
- Is predictable with regard to responses to others

Integrity
- Accepts responsibility for own actions
- Gives credit to others for things done well
- Is fair and just in relationships with others
- Is sincere
- Possesses sound moral values

Self-Confidence
- Knows one's abilities and limitations
- Models the values and behaviors desired of others
- Maintains a confident body language
- Is able to control one's own feelings and behavior
- Is not arrogant, conceited, or boastful

Sensitivity
- Is kind and thoughtful in interactions with others
- Actively listens to others
- Recognizes things that are important to others
- Is free of cultural and racial biases

Intelligence
- Is reasonable in decision making
- Learns from experience
- Able to respond quickly and successfully to new situations
- Maintains keen approach to problem solving
- Seeks new information regularly

Skill in Communicating
- Communicates clearly and concisely
- Listens to others
- Knows when not to talk
- Maintains positive body language
- Is sensitive to nonverbal cues
- Does not interrupt others when they are speaking

and at the same time avoid being overly critical of your own behavior. Remember that the art of empowering others, like other skills you have mastered, can be learned.

Critical Thinking Activity

Think of a situation you have experienced or observed in which an individual was empowered. What were the factors that resulted in the individual being empowered? How did that individual respond? What additional actions might have made the empowerment even greater? Which of the behaviors that helped empower the person would you want to use? Which ones would you not use? Why did you choose these behaviors?

ENHANCING YOUR EMOTIONAL INTELLIGENCE

With increasing frequency, we hear the term "emotional intelligence," which is sometimes referred to as emotional quotient. **Emotional intelligence (EI)** refers to the essential quality of understanding how emotions function within oneself and others and the ability to use emotions effectively. It is considered by some to be as critical to high performance as is basic intelligence. As a result, a number of large businesses are now assessing an individual's EI before hiring that person into an important position in the organization or before making promotions.

Interest in EI grew when leaders on the topic found that traditional types of intelligence, such as IQ, fail to fully explain cognitive ability. In 1995, Daniel Goleman wrote a best seller titled "Emotional Intelligence: Why it can matter more than I.Q.," and the topic became a part of the approaches to leadership. As you read more about EI, you will find that descriptions will vary among authors. A model developed by Emmerling and Goleman (2003) focuses on personal assessment and development in regard to emotional intelligence. They list five components of EI: self-awareness, self-regulation, motivation, empathy, and social skill. These five components are interdependent, each affects the others, and they create the "whole" that is EI.

Self-Awareness

Self-awareness involves recognizing and understanding your own moods and feelings and includes appreciating how your emotional behaviors affect others. When this skill is well developed, individuals typically see themselves realistically and are able to act confidently. Developing self-awareness requires an ongoing commitment to examining your own feelings and behavior and noting their effects on yourself and on others. It may be likened to holding up a mirror to yourself and inspecting yourself very critically.

▶ *EXAMPLE*

A Targeted Self-Assessment

Jodie Ellington was an RN working in a long-term care facility. She found that she dreaded going to work in the morning. One day, she sat down after work and thought to herself, "What is going on here? I always loved working with the elderly, and now I don't even want to go to work. The nursing assistants have been asking me what is wrong because I am so critical of everything." As Jodie began reviewing what was happening at work, her responses to what was happening, and her dreams for a career in nursing, she became aware that she had always thought in terms of working directly with the elderly, helping them to be more independent, helping them to find joy in the later years. Her job was one of managing documentation, supervising nursing assistants, and organizing the delivery of services. Her unhappiness with a job that had so little resident contact had spilled over into the way she was treating the nursing assistants. She realized that she still loved working with the elderly and that she needed to consider a career change into a different role in gerontologic nursing. Meanwhile, she was going to change how she treated those with whom she worked. They really worked very hard and needed to be appreciated for the care they provided.

Self-Regulation

Self-regulation refers to the ability to control inappropriate impulses and to think before acting (Habel, 2005). Research on mindfulness training indicates it is a positive strategy for managing emotionally charged situations (Kabat-Zinn, 2005). **Mindfulness** is a process of being aware of the present while keeping distressful thoughts away. Persons who have developed skill in this area continue to respond to human emotions such as anxiety, anger, and sadness, but they do not overreact to them and are able to direct them in positive ways. Lack of self-regulation is seen in the person who has emotional outbursts and the one who breaks down and cries and is unable to function if criticized. While tears of sadness can be appropriate, an inability to manage responses in order to function seriously inhibits one's effectiveness.

To increase your ability to self-regulate, try to develop the ability to not take things personally. Managing your own emotions may be the biggest and most difficult to control. You might begin by using stress-management techniques. Deep-breathing exercises, stress relief through physical exercise, and meditation may all help. Using such techniques as deep breathing when faced with an emotional situation may give you time to decide how to react rather than simply reacting from immediate feelings. However, you may still find yourself in a situation where you cannot control your emotions. In such cases, you need to exit the situation. Simply saying, "Please give me a few minutes," may be adequate. Think before you leap. Self-help books and practiced meditation can assist in this process (Habel, 2005). Another important point is that you should not put into writing anything that you would not want to say before a large group of people. This includes writing in e-mail, social networking sites (Twitter, Facebook, MySpace, Linked-In), or on personal blogs. These are not private and may be shared widely, thereby creating many other problems for you in the work environment.

Motivation

Motivation relates to the desire to achieve or get things done. The motivated individual is optimistic and works in self-directed ways toward positive goals (see Chapter 13 for more discussion of motivation). The motivation discussed here is self-motivation, the ability to set goals, standards, and expectations for yourself and meet them. As a new graduate, seeking new learning experiences is an example of self-motivation. Volunteering to serve on committees and accepting a challenging assignment are other activities that demonstrate self-motivation.

Empathy

You are well acquainted with the meaning of empathy from your other nursing courses. Empathy involves the ability to read accurately and respond appropriately to the emotions of others. Expressing empathy for others is important for effective functioning in groups or teams. Individuals who have developed this skill listen carefully to what others say and react in effective ways to this information. You have used this skill in working with patients and their families. You can use it when working with others also. When responsible for directing the activities of others, do not control unpleasant situations by talking. Listen carefully to what is being said. Recognize others' distress with words such as, "I know we are working short-handed this morning, but if we all pull together, we can do it." Maintain eye contact when listening to others; it helps assure them that they have your attention.

Social Skills

Social skills, also referred to as people skills, center on being able to relate to many different types of people and groups. Goleman (1998) calls this "friendliness with a purpose." Greeting people when you meet them, remembering and using preferred names, listening with interest, and using the common courtesies of "please" and "thank-you" are all a part of social skills. Individuals who possess people skills initiate conversations with others, look for opportunities to interact, and respond positively to the communications of others. Being a pleasant and courteous member of the healthcare team demonstrates social skills.

Developing Your Own Emotional Intelligence

Although EI may be learned from life experience, it does not improve greatly without sustained effort and attention. A number of techniques have been suggested to enhance one's EI and can reviewed by browsing the topic "Emotional Intelligence" on your computer and following the links. As we frequently have suggested in this book, EI begins with a thorough self-assessment. Table 12.2 contains statements that will assist you in this exercise.

Critical Thinking Activity

Review the self-assessment you just completed. How did you do on the self-assessment? Did you have many areas where you answered "seldom"? Were most of your responses "usually"? What would you like to improve? Which techniques will help? Improving your ability to identify your own emotions and how they are perceived by others is critical.

▶ ### EXAMPLE

Dealing with a Stressful Day

Dennis Damon is the unit manager on a busy medical unit. Today he met with other unit managers and representatives from hospital administration to discuss budget requests for next year. Each unit manager had prepared an information sheet identifying needs for the coming year with rationale and anticipated cost for each. Dennis was not surprised that it was a stressful meeting and that tempers occasionally flared. Nonetheless, he left the meeting feeling tense and on edge. On his way home, he dropped by the health club and played a fast-paced game of racquetball. When he left the club, he was relaxed and felt more able to think constructively about the concerns of the day.

Table 12.2 **Self-Assessment of Emotional Intelligence**

ITEM	ALWAYS	USUALLY	SELDOM	NEVER
I am able to recognize my emotions and I know what they are.				
I consistently think before I act and do not act rashly.				
I am aware of my own behavior and can describe how it affects others.				
I am able to manage my own feelings in a wide variety of situations.				
I consistently express my negative emotions in an acceptable manner.				
I am able to remain calm and collected when interacting with people who are angry or verbally abusive.				
I am self-motivating and do not require someone else to get me going.				
I find it easy to empathize with others and they frequently share feelings with me.				
I can identify when emotions can be used effectively and when not.				
Others would describe me as an optimistic person.				

DEVELOPING YOUR LEADERSHIP STYLE

In today's healthcare environment, all professional nurses will find themselves involved in working conditions that require some leadership skills. Both acute and long-term care facilities use assistive personnel who have less educational preparation and who require direction from RNs. It is anticipated that this trend will increase. As you move into the world of employment, think about your own leadership style. What approach will you use when directing others? How will you develop those skills? The following suggestions may help to enhance this process:

- *Continue to learn and to grow.* You will be expected to demonstrate competence and knowledge. These attributes can be developed and maintained only when you continue to seek and find answers to problems you encounter, many of which you may not have studied in your nursing program. Subscribe to a nursing journal that focuses on content related to your area of practice so that your clinical knowledge continues to grow. Attend meetings and participate in committees so that you learn more about the organization in which you work. Complete continuing education programs, such as those found in nursing sites on your computer and in nursing magazines, and attend education events and workshops.
- *Seek out a role model or a mentor.* A **mentor** is a more experienced individual who is willing to support and guide an individual who is new to a work environment and who systematically develops a subordinate's abilities through tutoring, coaching, and guidance. It is a fortunate novice who has a good mentor (see additional content on mentors in Chapter 14).
- *Maintain your personal physical resources.* One of the significant criticisms directed at today's healthcare environment by those who are employed in it is the high level of stress encountered daily. This stress can best be managed when a person is physically and mentally fit. Everyone needs time to unwind, to relax and rest, and to find the time and energy to reflect on work activities. It is important to maintain outside interests and relationships that help to balance life and provide diversion from the stresses of work. As you move into the world of employment, be certain that your lifestyle includes a healthful diet, exercise, rest, and relaxation.
- *Retain an open mind and develop flexibility.* Individuals who are open to new ideas and who can cope with unpredictable circumstances have an advantage in the workplace. Remember that there is often more than one way to approach a problem. Locking into only one way of viewing things or one method of dealing with a situation limits one's growth, can create tension in the workplace, and may result in using the wrong approach to solve a problem. Learn as much about the organization in which you are employed as you can. Developing a broad view of how the organization functions will help you to see where you and your unit fit in. Be willing to compromise and to negotiate; these skills are critical to any good team player. Ask questions when you are not sure.
- *Demonstrate respect and consideration for others.* All individuals bring unique perspectives and contributions to the workplace that should be valued. Sometimes encouraging others to do their best requires patience and understanding. Help others to grow just as you want others to assist you. Observe the basic behaviors considered to be social skills. Practice common courtesies and etiquette. Address people by the name by which they wish to be addressed. Be polite and considerate to others, and generally you will find they will

return this behavior. Be sensitive to things that may be distressful to those with whom you work. Trust people and share information—it helps others to know you believe in them.

• *Believe in yourself.* Develop your own self-confidence. Give yourself credit for the things you know you do well. Identify the things that you need to learn more about and do so. Develop a body language that inspires confidence in others; walk tall. Maintain good grooming and dress. Become articulate in your communication patterns and remember the importance of being a good listener. Review the language you use in reference to yourself. Don't discount your own skills and abilities or minimize your accomplishments. In others words, develop a professional demeanor.

COMMUNICATING EFFECTIVELY

After reading the above material, you have an appreciation for how important effective communication is to your ability to provide leadership. The concept of communication is not new to you. In previous studies, you learned that **communication** involves the sending and receiving of a message from one person to another. Let's list some of the other things that you know about the communication process:

• Communication occurs in four settings: intrapersonal, interpersonal, group, and societal. Intrapersonal occurs when you talk to yourself. Interpersonal occurs between two or more individuals. Group communication takes place when a number of persons are involved. Societal communication relates to an entire society or culture.

• Communication takes several forms, notably, verbal, nonverbal, and written. Verbal communication occurs in the use of words. Nonverbal involves one's body language and dress and includes facial expressions, body positions, eye contact, boundaries, and body movements. Written communication is that which is recorded, as in charts, memos, letters, and the like.

• Verbal and nonverbal communication systems interrelate, and may either complement each other or contradict each other. For example, if you say, "It doesn't matter to me" and at the same time shrug your shoulders, the messages complement each other. However, if you say, "Please tell me more" but look away, you have given two different messages. Looking away can suggest you don't really care.

• Certain skills can facilitate the communication process and result in therapeutic communication or communications that are goal directed. Therapeutic communication has a purpose and direction and employs processes to achieve established objectives. It focuses on the needs of the other person and involves active listening and observation.

• The words we use when communicating can mean different things to different individuals. Chief concerns include the use of figures of speech, jargon, slang, and idioms with which not everyone is familiar, such as "She heard it straight from the horse's mouth" (meaning from a reliable source) or "Up a creek without a paddle" (meaning in a difficult situation without a means of exiting). Another example is abstract messages that use vague terms, such as asking a patient in an urgent care center, "What brings you here?" when inquiring about symptoms and receiving the reply, "I came in a car."

• Communication involves feedback that allows us to know which messages were received and understood as intended and which messages need correction. Feedback performs a regulatory function and helps us to evaluate the communication process.

- Communication is influenced by a variety of factors, including a person's perceptions and values. Words represent generalized symbols that may vary from individual to individual. Your perceptions can be altered by crises and anxiety-producing situations.

- Blocks to communication occur when unhelpful responses are made, such as generalizing, labeling feelings, making judgmental statements, or changing the subject. Blocks to communication can involve such things as telling the individual how to do something that he or she has already learned. Belittling others' feelings, disagreeing, disapproving, refusing to admit that a problem exists, or being defensive are other examples of blocking communication.

- Communication is culturally sensitive and culture-bound as a result of impressions formed at an early age about how the world is structured. This applies to both verbal and nonverbal behavior. For example, not all cultures maintain eye contact during communication in the manner of those in the Western culture. In some cultures, such as Native American, Appalachian, Indochinese, Asian American, some Mexican American, and some African American, it is not acceptable to make eye contact when talking because it is a sign of disrespect (Videbeck, 2007). Touch, which is a nonverbal form of communication, may be viewed differently by different cultures. Although it may be comforting to some, others may see it as an invasion of personal space.

In the past few decades, electronic devices have significantly affected our communication systems. The computer, e-mail, faxes, the Internet, cell phones, and smart phones have greatly increased the ease and speed with which we can communicate with one another. At the same time, it has resulted in ethical concerns about the sharing of information, how it is stored, and who has access to it. Increasingly, the care provided to clients is recorded electronically. Be careful with these methods of communication, always thinking about patient privacy and recognizing that brief comments are more easily misinterpreted than are more complete interactions. What may be intended to be matter-of-fact may be misunderstood as being rude.

USING COMMUNICATION SKILLS IN THE LEADERSHIP ROLE

The importance of being able to use communication skills effectively in a leadership role cannot be overemphasized. Ustun (2006) points out that communication skills are an essential element of professionalism and are necessary for being able to affect others. To be an effective leader, one must possess an adequate understanding and application of communication techniques. The following are some basic guidelines for skillful communications:

- *Communications should be clear.* A message being given to others should be free of ambiguities, and the person receiving the message should have no difficulty interpreting what is meant. If messages are not understood, the individual being addressed should ask for clarification. However, in the healthcare environment, we often work with nursing assistants who come from other cultures. They may find it difficult to question a superior, partially because they may not want to offend someone in a position of authority. Sometimes they do not want to acknowledge that they do not understand because they fear it will cost them their job. Instead, they may nod, smile, or give other nonverbal cues that suggest understanding.

COMMUNICATION IN ACTION

Determining Understanding

Alice McAdams worked as the evening charge nurse in a local long-term care facility. Her nursing team was composed mostly of nursing assistants from an Asian culture. Hardworking and eager to please, they struggled with English as a second language. During care planning time, Alice said to two of them, "I would like you to do range of motion exercise on Mrs. Howard and then get her up in a chair for 30 minutes." Both assistants smiled and looked at one another, but Alice was not sure her instructions were clearly understood. She then said, "Now, can either of you tell me how you are going to do that? How will you know it is okay to get Mrs. Howard up?" The assistants rather shyly smiled and one volunteered, "We move her joints and then put Mrs. Howard into chair." "That is correct," said Alice. "And how will you know if it is okay to get her up?" "If she says no, we don't get her up," replied the other. "Well, it is important that she get out of her bed, so if that happens, please come get me so that I can talk with her and explain. But if she says she is dizzy or not feeling well, check with me before getting her up. I will check with you later to see how things are going."

In this situation, Alice clarified that the nursing assistants knew what they were to do and also that they understood the importance of getting the resident out of bed and did so without demeaning them. She also offered her help should it be needed.

- *Communications should be concise.* This applies to both verbal and written messages. We should work at stating the necessary information as briefly as possible while still providing enough data to be clear. The longer messages become, the more extraneous information is included, and the longer it takes for someone to receive the communication. This is particularly important when using e-mail messaging. Learning to communicate in a concise and clear manner is another learned skill that will improve as we become more proficient.
- *Communications should maintain a positive approach or perspective.* When problems arise, individuals respond better to communications that give positive direction, and that focus on finding a solution rather than on fault finding or the problem itself. When people become defensive, their energy is diverted to self-protection rather than to problem resolution, and they become stressed. This detracts from accomplishing the goals.

COMMUNICATION IN ACTION

A Slippery Floor

John Brice worked in a busy urgent care center. After a hectic afternoon of seeing an unusually large number of clients, John noticed a puddle of water on the floor. In the next room, two staff LPNs were relaxing over a cup of coffee. Both would have had to go past the puddle of water to get to the room. John walked into the room and said, "I notice there is a puddle of water in the hall. We can't leave things like that because falls and injuries can result. I need to get to the patient in Room C, but would one of you please see that the water is cleaned up? It is important to maintain a safe environment." Both got up to get a rag to mop up the spill.

In this instance, John did not focus on the fact that the spill had been overlooked in favor of a coffee break, nor did he overlook the hazard because he did not have time to address it personally. He was courteous in his request and explained why it was important.

- *Communication should recognize and accommodate diversity.* Any work environment presents a variety of personalities, cultures, educational experience and capabilities, and gender differences. Maintaining an open mind and being willing to listen to others will help in difficult situations. While being sensitive to cultural values, it is equally important not to stereotype. Recognizing and acknowledging that differences often occur in the communication patterns of men and women is also important. For example, male and female brains are structured and process information differently. Men are more likely to process analytically, while women tend to process things abstractly. Men more often view conversation as a means to exchange information and achieve a particular goal. Women talk to build rapport and make connections (Svecz, 2010). Read more about this topic in an article by Lamb-White (2008) at Suite101: Gender Communication: The Impact Gender has on Effective Communication *http://trainingpd.suite101.com/article.cfm/gender-communication#ixzz0lraKkF00.*
- *Communicating effectively involves active listening.* Active listening tells others that you value both what they have to say and their membership in the team. Active listening involves hearing the facts in the verbal message but also listening for feelings, values, and opinions and observing the nonverbal cues. A busy work situation may not lend itself to this type of communicating. You may need to assess the situation as to its urgency. When time is available, remember to use the communication skills you have learned earlier: accepting, focusing, reflecting, clarifying, questioning, paraphrasing or restating, and summarizing. Listen for vocal cues such as pressured speech or slow, hesitant responses. This will assist you to understand the context of the situation. A major deterrent to active listening is the fact that we often begin to formulate a response to the individual with whom we are communicating before that person has finished talking. This prevents us from listening to all the cues in an individual's message to us.

It is difficult to think of any time in nursing when one would not use communication skills, but certainly some of the situations calling for their effective use include conflict management, negotiations, delegation, assessment, discharge teaching, documentation, and any situation involving interviews. The interview plays a significant role in performance appraisals.

PERFORMANCE APPRAISAL

Performance appraisal represents a formal process by which an individual's performance is reviewed and evaluated against established standards, most commonly a job description. It might also be appropriately referred to as performance evaluation, performance review, or performance assessment. At all times, the focus should be on the performance and not on personality characteristics of the individual being evaluated. At one time it was not uncommon for statements on evaluations to include "cheerful," "smart," "likeable," and "attractive" which, unless critical to the job description, should not be a part of the appraisal. Regular performance appraisal represents one of the standards for approval for many private, federal, and state accrediting agencies.

The primary objectives of performance appraisal are to maintain or improve employee performance and to enhance the development of employees. As a result of the performance appraisal, the employee should know how he or she has been performing and what he or she can expect in the coming months. Performance appraisals also can be a part of identifying individuals for special assignments or for advancement within the organization. Properly

DISPLAY 12.4   **Characteristics of an Effective Performance Appraisal System**

- The appraisal system has administrative support
- Evaluation is based on standards such as job description or other well-defined criteria
- Clear and objective criteria exist for the evaluation used
- Employees know the evaluation standards and who will be evaluating them
- Evaluation procedures are consistently applied
- Evaluations are conducted in a timely fashion at regular intervals
- Evaluators are well trained in the use of the appraisal system
- The appraisal interview is a two-way communication
- All individuals know the related rewards or disciplinary action
- The final disposition of the evaluation is known to the employee

conducted, they can also provide the institution with information regarding the effectiveness of its recruiting and hiring processes.

Guidelines exist for conducting good performance appraisals. Display 12.4 outlines these standards. Please review them carefully.

Often those responsible for conducting the performance appraisal as well as those being evaluated have an aversion to the process. Some of the reasons managers dislike the process relate to the amount of time it consumes, the fact that unpleasant messages may have to be transmitted (many persons are hesitant to criticize others), and fear of legal repercussions. Persons being evaluated may dislike the process because it feels much like receiving a report card or because the process is intimidating. As a new graduate, you should find the process very similar to the end-of-the-term clinical evaluation conference you experienced with your clinical instructors. Hopefully, they helped you to grow and improve your performance, just as performance appraisals in the work situation should help you grow professionally.

Criteria for Evaluation

All performance evaluations, whether formal or informal, should be based on appropriate standards of performance. Standards of performance include job descriptions, policies and procedures, and professional standards of practice.

Job descriptions contain statements that describe the duties for which the employee is responsible. These usually include reporting relationships and accountability. To be useful for evaluation, they should be up-to-date and clearly written to avoid ambiguous interpretation.

Policies and procedures should be taught as part of the employee orientation processes and relate to patient care activities, as well as to timeliness, absenteeism, and participation in agency committees. More institutions are including customer relationship skills in their policies. By this, they usually are referring to what we think of as people skills or soft skills as they are sometimes called. An organization may have an entire program focusing on soft skills. For example, in one facility, the customer relationship procedures include that when meeting a person who looks lost or confused, any employee must stop, ask if there is a concern, offer assistance, and even escort the person to the correct place if that is necessary. This is required of everyone from the custodian to the vice presidents and is being strictly monitored and included in employee evaluations. The goal is that the institution will become known as friendly, helpful, and a place where one would like to receive healthcare.

Professional standards are written statements that describe a minimum level of performance common to the profession and that reflect the values of that profession. In nursing, standards of practice reflect expectations for the behaviors of professionals in relationship to specific areas of practice and may be developed by professional organizations such as the American Nurses Association. Standards of care, which reflect expected processes and outcomes that should occur for individual patients, may be developed by healthcare agencies or by regulatory groups.

Instruments Used in Performance Appraisal

Instruments are the forms and tools used in the performance appraisal process. They should be designed around the predetermined standards described above. A number of different instruments can be used for the performance appraisal. Table 12.3 identifies some of the more commonly used approaches. In nursing, a rating scale is frequently employed. It has the advantage of being easy to use and does not require a great deal of time to complete. The most critical aspect is that the assessment methods and the instruments used should focus on what the person actually does as opposed to personal characteristics of the individual. In many organizations, the appraisal process may also include a self-evaluation. In such instances, the employee and the manager would use the same instrument to guide the evaluative process and would compare ratings during the appraisal interview. Some organizations add peer evaluations to their process for professional employees.

Table 12.3 Commonly Used Performance Appraisal Systems

SYSTEM	DESCRIPTION
Rating scales	Comprises a list of behaviors or characteristics to be evaluated and a rating scale to indicate the degree to which the criterion is met. Rating scales may be numeric (1–5), lettered (A–E), graphic (always, frequently, seldom, never), or descriptive. Rating scales are a widely used type of evaluation instrument in nursing.
Checklist	Describes the standard of performance; the evaluator puts a checkmark in a column (usually yes or no) as to whether the employee demonstrates the behavior. Behaviors can be weighted based on importance.
Essay or narrative	Calls for evaluator to write several paragraphs outlining the employee's strengths, weaknesses, and potential. The evaluator may be provided with a guide for development of the narrative.
Critical incident	Requires that the evaluator observe, collect, and record specific instances of the employee carrying out responsibilities critical to the job. Incidents must be recorded regularly.
Group appraisal methods	May take one of two forms. The first involves using multiple judges. Several people form an appraisal team, typically the immediate supervisor and three or four other supervisors who have knowledge of the work being evaluated. Each person does an independent evaluation and then the results are combined. The second form may be used as a supplement to a supervisor's evaluation. Members of a team evaluate one another and team members' evaluations are included in the final evaluation. All persons use exactly the same job-based criteria for their evaluations.

The Appraisal Interview

As pointed out above, the primary objective of performance appraisal from the organization's perspective is to maintain or improve performance. However, the manner in which it is accomplished can make a significant difference. The interview associated with the performance evaluation should occur in a timely fashion, be held in a setting that provides for privacy, and have a constructive focus. The dialogue may include both positive and negative feedback. Positive feedback is information that communicates to others what they have done correctly. Negative feedback, sometimes referred to as "areas of opportunity," is more difficult because it identifies areas of unsatisfactory performance. Areas for improvement and growth may be included as well.

Negative feedback is best provided at the time the incident occurs and should be objective and accurate. For example, if you see a nursing assistant moving from client to client without washing her hands in between contacts, do not wait until the formal evaluation conference to correct the behavior. Employees usually want frequent and continuous informal appraisal or feedback on their performance, and it should not be left until the formal interview.

As a new graduate, you are more likely to be the one being evaluated as opposed to being the one doing the evaluation, although you may be provided an opportunity to evaluate your superior. There are some steps you can take to assist with the interview aspects of this performance appraisal session.

Preparing for the Performance Interview

Effective performance appraisal is a two-way street. Think about your current role in terms of purpose, skills, and past performance. Assess your past performance evaluating what has gone well and what has not. Think about the goals you set the last time and your career pathways. Before the interview, prepare three or four questions that you can ask during the interview session. These might be as simple as "How do you think I am doing given the time I have been here?" or "Are there ways that you think I might organize my work more efficiently?" "What areas do you recommend I focus on for growth?" These questions would indicate that you are eager to try to improve your performance and meet the demands of the job. Should your manager have a tendency to fill the time with friendly chitchat, the questions will help to focus the interview.

Dealing with Negative Feedback

It is possible that your performance will include some negative feedback or criticism of your behavior. The purpose of criticism should be to help you perform better on the job. Nonetheless, it is often difficult to face. When it occurs, you should strive to listen coolly and without interruption. Remain composed and do not offer excuses. If there is a reasonable explanation to address the shortcoming, offer it in a calm manner. If you believe that some of the statements made by your manager are not accurate or are broad generalizations, it is appropriate to challenge the statements. Of course, you will want to do so in a polite and constructive manner. Ask your manager to talk about the specifics of your behavior and performance. For example, if the manager says, "You seem to have difficulty completing tasks on time," ask for an example of a particular task that should have been done more efficiently. This will bring the conversation back to specifics rather than dealing in generalities. Be prepared for the fact that this could result in more negative feedback than might have otherwise occurred. If

DISPLAY 12.5   Employee Expectations of the Appraisal Interview*

- A feeling that they were dealt with fairly
- An appreciation for their contribution to the organization and its goals
- Recognition of special accomplishments, efforts, or endeavors
- Some indication of how their performance can be improved, with specific recommendations on how it can be achieved
- An honest appraisal of future potential or prospects
- A sense of being fairly rewarded financially relative to others who are in the same position
- A sense that they have been allowed to contribute to the appraisal session and discussion, and that the evaluator actively listened to the comments

*Adapted from McConnell, C. R. (1993).

you receive negative feedback, it should be accompanied with some constructive suggestions for improvement. If the suggestions are not provided, ask for guidance, such as, "Okay, what can I do to work more effectively?" Then set a time frame with your manager for the improvement. If you receive ratings that you believe are inaccurate, negotiate with the manager about the rating. If you can convince the manager that specific aspects were overlooked, he or she may be willing to change the score. It is difficult to predict how the manager will react to this response, but if you truly believe the rating is not accurate, you have nothing to lose. However, you must accept those statements that are a true reflection of your performance, even though they may be negative. These behaviors will be ones you will want to work at improving. Display 12.5 identifies some of the aspects of a performance interview that we all desire. Be certain that you consider these when you are being evaluated or if you are responsible for evaluating others.

COMMUNICATION IN ACTION

Providing Negative Feedback

Patricia Black, unit manager, was not looking forward to the performance interview she had to conduct with Richard Wilson, a new graduate who has just completed his first 3 months of employment. Although obviously trying hard while on the job, Richard was consistently late to work, and his tardiness upset the operation of the entire unit. When Richard arrived at her office, she offered him a beverage and invited him to sit down at the table across from her. Using the standard evaluation form developed by a nursing committee in the hospital, Patricia reviewed Richard's strengths as a new employee. He seemed pleased that his efforts have been recognized. Then she discussed his habitual lateness. She said, "I do have a concern, Richard. You arrive on the unit 20 to 30 minutes late on an average of 2 days a week. For example, this week you were 25 minutes late on Monday and 20 minutes late on Thursday. This disrupts the start of the day for the unit because we count on everyone being here at the start of the shift. Can you explain to me why you believe it occurs?" Richard took a sip of his beverage. "Well," he said, "I know it is a problem. You see, I never was an early riser. Most of my

(display continues on page 452)

jobs in the past have started in the afternoon. As a student, I always tried to get into the afternoon clinicals. Perhaps I am not cut out for a 7:00 am shift."

"That may be true," agreed Patricia. "Nonetheless, the hospital has a policy that all new graduates spend a 6-month orientation on the day shift so that they best can learn the policies and procedures of the hospital. When you have completed that period, we could think about rotating you to the later shift. For now, you need to develop some strategies for correcting your tardiness. Do you have any ideas?"

"Well," replied Richard, "I guess I could begin by setting my alarm clock 30 minutes earlier."

This manager recognized the strengths of the employee but did not neglect discussing areas of concern. While acknowledging Richard's statement of the problem, the nurse manager placed the responsibility for solving it on Richard and did not try to solve the problem for him. The employee, when directly asked to develop a plan, responded with a concrete proposal.

Behaviors to Avoid in the Interview

If you are responsible for evaluating the performance of another, the following lists some of the behaviors that should be avoided.

- Avoid letting the interview deteriorate into an argument. Arguments are counterproductive and destroy communication.
- Steer clear of discussion of personal characteristic or traits other than those that affect or relate to job performance.
- Do not scold or reprimand the employee. Behavior needing a reprimand or correction should have been dealt with when it occurred.
- Do not dispense personally referenced advice. Providing constructive instructions is part of the evaluation and is often considered advice from the supervisor. It should not be confused with advice that has a personal reference rather than advice of a professional nature. Making statements such as "If I were you, I would …" possess a personal reference and should not be a part of the appraisal process (Fig. 12.2).
- Do not wield your authority by making statements designed to coerce, intimidate, or demonstrate your power. The employee already understands your role, and wielding authority in this way will destroy the two-way nature of the process.

Common Problems With Performance Appraisal

In the best of circumstances, performance appraisal probably falls somewhat short of accomplishing the goals for which it is intended. Good evaluation systems require the total support of top management. All persons involved must believe in the process and its value. Often, managers find the process to be unpleasant and time-consuming. Evaluations will be done late, hurriedly, or not at all. Systems work best when someone or some department has the responsibility for ensuring that all the steps in the evaluation process are completed in a timely and appropriate manner. This includes training for those persons who will be doing the evaluations. Training in the use of the evaluation instruments and the process helps to decrease variations in rating from manager to manager and will reduce inconsistencies in

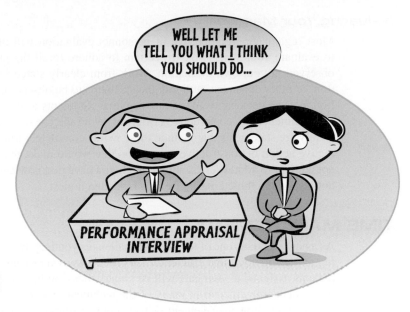

FIGURE 12.2 Personally referenced advice should not be a part of a performance appraisal interview.

application of the process. The discomfort sometimes felt by the evaluators may also present a problem to the appraisal system. Many people dislike giving feedback to others when it is aimed at correcting shortcomings or weaknesses. We shy away from criticizing others, especially when it is discussed face to face. As a result, one of two things may happen. The manager may tend to gloss over the areas that need improvement, or the manager may come down too heavily on the negative concerns. Neither approach is productive. Criticism, when given, needs to be assertive, constructive, and specific and relate to a particular behavior required in the job.

Another problem area relates to fear of legal repercussions. As employee organizations have gained strength and recognition, managers have concerns that actions may be taken against them either in a legal form or in the nature of complaints, grievances, or appeals. Apprehensions of this nature are less common when all aspects of an appraisal can be supported by specific examples. When assessments are completed using specific criteria and definable measures, unsupportable judgments are less likely to occur. Maintaining consistency is as important as avoiding surprises. Evaluations should focus on what an employee does, not who the employee is.

Critical Thinking Activity

Think back to the last time you were evaluated. What were the positive aspects of that evaluation interview? Were there any negative aspects? How did you feel throughout the interview? How could the interview have been made more productive?

Evaluating Your Manager

Most organizations supportive of personnel evaluation will provide an opportunity for you to evaluate your supervisor. Be certain to adhere to all the principles that you would want observed in your own evaluation. Work from clearly stated job expectations, a job description, or other document outlining the standards to be observed. Deal with aspects of the position, not the personality. Word any negative comments as positively as possible. Try to form the comments into constructive criticism. Avoid the use of words like "always" and "never." Rarely are statements that include these words completely true. If you can think of some corrective action or constructive suggestion that would make the situation better, include it. Do not attempt to address areas about which you have no knowledge—just indicate that you cannot respond to those criteria. Be fair, kind, and honest.

TIME MANAGEMENT

As a new graduate, one of the biggest challenges you may face in your first position is organizing and using your time efficiently—a process known as **time management**. The number of patients assigned to your care will be greater than you had as a student, and you have not had time to become efficient in many of the technical procedures required in your job. Because time is finite, time management skills become essential. Time management can be learned.

Principles of Time Management

As you work at learning to manage time more effectively, some general principles will be of assistance to you. The following general guidelines can be applied in every setting and will facilitate your work in any role:

- Plan your activities. This will help you feel more in control as well as help you accomplish more. Keep a schedule. Developing a time schedule or a plan for how you use your time helps you to stay focused and to avoid interruptions.
- Prioritize your list of activities to ensure that you spend your time and energy on things that are important.
- Delegate those tasks that can be passed on to someone else.
- Take time to do things right the first time. Errors result in time spent making corrections.
- Limit distractions. This might involve closing your door, or turning off the phone, pager, or e-mail. Some activities, such as developing a patient's plan of care, require thoughtful attention. Seeking a quiet place where you are least likely to be disturbed will increase your efficiency in completing the plan. Some hospitals now structure units with a room located away from the major area of activity where such tasks can be carried out.
- Take needed breaks. Stress prevents attempts to get organized so take a break from activity and reenergize.

In addition to these strategies we offer these further suggestions. Do an assessment of yourself. This includes a review of your life style: your eating, sleeping, and recreational patterns. Identify things that restore and enhance your level of energy. Analyze your body rhythms and determine when your energy is at its peak. Plan activities requiring the greatest energy output and concentration to coincide with these peaks whenever possible. Take control of your own life. This may mean saying "no" when others ask for assistance. We recognize that it is difficult to say no, especially when a colleague asks for assistance. Offering assistance often means we have to interrupt what we are doing. Interruptions rob us of valuable time. In addition to stopping an action in process, we often have to restart or reorient ourselves to the task at hand before starting again—all lengthening the time it takes for completion. You may need to be assertive with those who have a tendency to interrupt you frequently; explain as kindly as possible that you cannot be interrupted. Sometimes it is easy to refuse assistance. One instance is being asked to do something for which you lack the required skills; for example, being asked by a seasoned nurse to watch a critical patient while she takes a break, and you lack the needed knowledge to safely evaluate that patient. Another example would be assisting another when doing so means you cannot complete your own assignment.

Dealing With Procrastination and Time Wasters

Two final behaviors that help manage time are related to avoiding time wasters and managing the tendency to procrastinate.

We all experience time wasters. Certain occurrences in our day-to-day existence are sure to rob us of valuable time. Perhaps the greatest time waster is social chitchat. Nurses typically are a gregarious group, and while no one intends to waste time, it just happens. Although it is fun and interesting to learn what other team members are doing, it is easy to lose 15 to 30 minutes in such an exchange. If you find yourself frequently involved in such conversation, excuse yourself by saying, "I need to check my patient now, but can we discuss it during break time or over lunch?" If your message is communicated in a kind and genuine manner, feelings will not be hurt and people will not feel put off (Fig. 12.3).

Mackenzie (1997) has identified a list of 20 common time wasters that include telephone interruptions, drop-in visitors, ineffective delegation, personal disorganization, socializing, attempting to do too much, poor communication, and lack of self-discipline. To some extent, time wasters are unique to each individual. One individual spends too much time on the telephone, another makes too many trips to the water fountain, while another only manages by

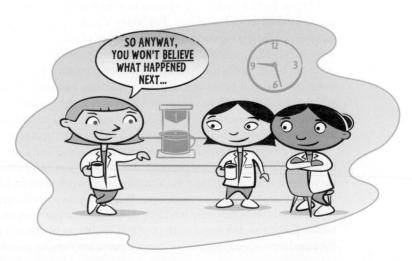

FIGURE 12.3 Perhaps the greatest time waster is social chitchat.

crisis. When you complete your personal analysis suggested earlier, look at ways in which you spend your time and decide which of those activities represent time wasters. Once identified, make plans for eliminating or decreasing the time spent in such activity.

Procrastination is defined as a chronic delay in carrying out actions that are necessary to accomplish important tasks (Ellis & Hartley, 2009). Some individuals are more inclined to procrastinate than others. If procrastination has been a big part of your life, avoiding it may be the most difficult of the tasks we have outlined. Delaying a task can result in it seeming to be much larger, more time-consuming, or more difficult than it actually is. Perhaps you have experienced these feelings in the past when you have put off writing a paper due for class or postponed starting an important assignment. Researchers include fear of failure, lack of interest, and feelings of anger or hostility among the many explanations for procrastination. Regardless of the basis of the behavior, an important step in correcting it lies in making a personal commitment to complete tasks on time. This involves establishing realistic deadlines and adhering to them.

Kanarek (1996) provides five suggestions for dealing with procrastination. First, she suggests that you start working on a project for 10 minutes and quit if tired or bored. Often, at least half an hour will pass and you will have made progress. Second, she suggests that you save the best for the last, a form of reward. Third, make a game out of things: Challenge yourself to handle one task in less than half an hour and make a game of seeing how quickly you can complete tasks you have been putting off. Fourth, break tasks into smaller, more manageable units, and, fifth, tell others of your plans, thus putting pressure on yourself to do what you have indicated you are going to do.

Determine the time of day when you are most productive. When you have determined what works best for you, use this time to initiate projects. This will make the task seem less overwhelming.

Barriers to Effective Time Management

The modern healthcare environment poses many barriers to the individual's ability to manage time effectively. These barriers may be either within the system or within the individual.

One of these barriers is a system in which more is expected of the individual that can be accomplished in the workday. For many nurses, patient care loads have increased both in numbers of patients and in terms of the acuity of patients. In a study by Kalisch (2006), nurses were surveyed in regard to care that was omitted because of time pressures. Routine omissions included basic care measures such as ambulation, turning, feeding, and hygiene, as well as the more professional behaviors of patient teaching and surveillance. For system-wide problems with load and demand, answers must be found in the system. Nurses may influence the system through shared governance or collective bargaining. Examining the work environment before accepting a position may help you guard against this problem.

Another system barrier lies in whether the nurse truly has any control over the personal practice. Those who do not perceive that they have control often give up on planning because they feel it does not change the situation. The work done in Magnet hospitals to give nurses greater control over their practice has been a big step in offsetting this obstacle.

Personal issues that may interfere with time management include both physical and mental health problems. For those with physical health problems, it may not be possible to move at the consistent speed required in many direct care nursing positions. The nurse facing physical health problems may need to consult with the human resources department or with a career counselor to identify positions that mesh with their health status. Mental health problems such as depression cause serious deficits in the individual's ability to initiate and complete tasks (Adler, McLaughlin, Rogers, et al., 2006). When a nurse finds that he or she cannot complete work, a self-appraisal in terms of mental health and possible discussion with a counselor may be needed. Successful treatment of mental health problems will enable the person to function effectively.

Critical Thinking Activity

Identify one activity about which you procrastinated. Using the material discussed above, determine why you delayed completing the task. Does this occur frequently? What steps can you take in the future to avoid such behavior? In what ways will you benefit from avoiding procrastination?

KEY CONCEPTS

- Differences exist in how leadership and management are practiced. Leadership refers to the ability to persuade others to follow your direction, to motivate, to inspire, and to instill vision and purpose, while management refers to activities such as planning, organizing, directing, and controlling resources.
- Accountability and responsibility often are used synonymously and refer to the obligation to answer for one's actions and to do what is promised. Authority can be defined as the power or right to give directions, take action, and make decisions.
- A number of theories exist regarding leadership. The theories can generally be classified as trait theories, attitudinal theories, situational theories, and contemporary theories.
- Three major leadership styles prevail: autocratic or authoritarian leadership, laissez-faire or permissive leadership, and democratic or participative leadership. Each is appropriate in a particular situation or setting.
- A multicratic leadership style that combines the most favorable aspects of all styles is probably most frequently used in healthcare.

- Theories of leadership evolve with social cultures. Currently, a leadership approach referred to as transformational leadership is advocated by many theorists. A transformational leader shares information and decision making with all employees.
- Power refers to the ability an individual has to get things done. Empowerment refers to the process by which one individual who has power is able to share it with another. Both are essential components of effective leadership.
- For individuals to realize their full potential, they must be empowered. Empowerment occurs when information is shared, when individuals are involved in goal setting and finding solutions to problems and decision making, and when efforts are recognized.
- EI refers to the ability to use emotions effectively. This involves recognizing one's emotions and how they affect others. EI is a critical quality in high-performance areas.
- EI has five components: self-awareness, self-regulation, motivation, empathy, and social skill.

- Leadership is a skill that can be developed. You can enhance the development of your leadership skill by continuing to learn and grow, seeking a role model or a mentor, maintaining your personal physical resources, retaining an open mind and developing flexibility, demonstrating respect and consideration for others, and believing in yourself.
- Communication is a critical part of everything we do. It occurs in intrapersonal, interpersonal, and group settings, and is experienced in verbal, nonverbal, and written forms that may complement or contradict one another. Therapeutic communication has purpose and direction, focuses on the needs of others, and involves active listening. Words mean different things to different individuals, and feedback allows us to know which messages are received and how they are understood. Communication is influenced by a variety of factors, and blocks to communication occur when unhelpful responses are made. Communication is culturally sensitive and culture-bound.
- In the leadership role, communications should be clear and concise, should maintain a positive approach or perspective, should recognize and accommodate diversity, and should involve active listening.
- Performance appraisal represents a formal process by which an individual's performance is evaluated. Employees should know who will be conducting the evaluation and where the records will be placed. Good performance evaluation systems are based on appropriate standards of performance, have top management support, are conducted in a timely fashion, involve a two-way communication, and assist the employee to grow in his or her position. Evaluators should have training for this responsibility.
- Effective performance appraisal interviews are a two-way communication system that recognizes an employee's accomplishments and provides direction and motivation for further growth. The interviews are conducted in a setting where privacy can be ensured.
- Time management involves learning to use your time more effectively and efficiently. To accomplish this, you must understand yourself, take control of your own time, develop a time schedule, avoid procrastinating, and avoid time wasters.
- You can avoid time wasters by examining the ways in which you spend your time and then deciding which of those activities were time wasters. Once identified, they can be decreased or eliminated. Making a game of tasks that you want to delay doing can help prevent procrastination. Breaking tasks into smaller, more manageable units can also help.
- When inability to complete required job components is due to system problems, a system change is required. If physical or mental health inhibits individual functioning, that must be addressed in order to manage time effectively.

RELEVANT WEB SITES

Web sites relevant to this chapter can be found at thePoint ✴ accessed through *http://thePoint. lww.com/Ellis10e* and by entering the code found on the inside cover of your text.

REFERENCES

Adler, D. A., McLaughlin, T. J., Rogers, W. H., Chang, H., Lapitsky, L., & Lerner, D. (2006). Job performance deficits due to depression. *The American Journal of Psychiatry, 163*(9), 1569–1575.

Barry, T., Brannon, D., & Mohr, V. (2005, June). Nurse aide empowerment: Strategies and staff stability: Effects on nursing home resident outcomes. *The Gerontologist, 45*(3), 309–317.

Bass, B.M. (1985). *Leadership and performance*. New York: Free Press.

Bennis, W. (2003). *On becoming a leader: The leadership classic—Updated and expanded*. Cambridge, MA: Perseus Books Group.

Blake, R. R., & Mouton, J. S. (1964). *The managerial grid*. Houston, TX: Gulf Publishing.

Burns, J. M. (1978). *Leadership*. New York: Harper & Row.

Caliper. (2005). *The qualities that distinguish women leaders*. Retrieved January 6, 2011, from www.caliperonline.com/womenstudy/WomenLeaderWhitePaper.pdf

Ellis, J. R., & Hartley, C. L. (2009). *Managing and coordinating nursing care* (5th ed.). Philadelphia, PA: Lippincott Williams & Wilkins.

Emmerling, R. J., & Goleman, D. (2003). *Emotional intelligence: Issues and common misunderstandings*. Consortium for Research on Emotional Intelligence in Organizations. Retrieved January 6, 2011, from http://www.eiconsortium.org—Click on Chapters and Articles

Fiedler, F. E. (1967). *A theory of leadership effectiveness*. New York: McGraw-Hill.

French, J., & Raven, B. (1959). The basis of social power. In D. Cartwright & A. Lander (Eds.), *Studies in social power* (pp. 150–167). Ann Arbor, MI: University of Michigan, Institute for Social Research.

Goleman, D. (1995). *Emotional intelligence: Why it can matter more than I.Q.* New York: Bantam Books

Goleman, D. (1998). What makes a leader? *Harvard Business Review* 76(6), 93–102.

Habel, M. (2005). Emotional intelligence helps RNs work smart. *NurseWeek: Mountain Edition*, 6(16), 13–14.

Herzberg, F. (1966). *Works and the nature of man*. New York: World Publishing.

Herzberg, F., Mausner, B., & Snyderman, B. B. (1959). *The motivation to work*. New York: John Wiley.

House, R. J. (1971), A path-goal theory of leadership effectiveness. *Administrative Science Quarterly*, 16(3), 321–338.

Kabat-Zinn, J. (2005). *Wherever you go, There you are: Mindfulness meditation in everyday life*. New York: Hyperion.

Kalisch, B. (2006, October/December). Missed nursing care: A qualitative study. *Journal of Nursing Care Quality*. Retrieved January 6, 2011, from www.nursingcenter.com/library/JournalArticle.asp?Article_ID=668515

Kanarek, L. (1996). *Everything's organized*. Franklin Lakes, NJ: Career Press.

Kanter, R. M. (1993). *Men and women of the corporation*, New York: Basic Books, Inc.

Lamb-White, J. (2008). *Appraisal and Work Performance: Getting the most out of an appraisal interview*. Retrieved January 6, 2011, from http://trainingpd.suite101.com/article.cfm/planning_for_performance

Laschinger, H. K., Almost, J., & Tuer-Hodes, D. (2003, July–August). Workplace empowerment and Magnet Hospital characteristics: Making the link. *JONA: Journal of Nursing Administration*, 33(7/8), 410–422

Lewin, K. (1951). *Field theory in social sciences*. New York: Harper & Row.

Mackenzie, A. (1997). *The time trap*. (3rd ed.). New York: American Management Association.

Manojlovich, M. (2005). The effect of nursing leadership on hospital nurses' professional practice behaviors *Journal of Nursing Administration*, 35(7/8), 366–371.

Manojlovich, M. (2007, January 31). "Power and empowerment in nursing: looking backward to inform the future". *OJIN: The Online Journal of Issues in Nursing*, 12(1), Manuscript 1. Retrieved January 6, 2011, from www.nursingworld.org/MainMenuCategories/ANAMarketplace/ANAPeriodicals/OJIN/TableofContents/Volume122007/No1Jan07/LookingBackwardtoInformtheFuture.aspx

Maslow, A. (1954). *Motivation and personality*. New York: Harper & Row.

McConnell, C. R. (1993). *The health manager's guide to performance appraisal*. Gaithersburg, MD: Aspen Publishers, Inc.

McGregor, D. (1966). *Leadership and motivation*. Cambridge, MA: MIT Press.

Nedd, N. (2006). Perceptions of empowerment and intent to stay. *Nursing Economics*. 24(1), 13–18.

Ouchi, W. G. (1981). *Theory Z: How American business can meet the Japanese challenge*. Reading, MA: Addison-Wesley.

Senge, P. M., Kleiner, A., Roberts, C., Ross, R. B., & Smith, B. J. (1994). *The fifth discipline fieldbook: Strategies and tools for building a learning organization*. New York: Doubleday, a Division of Bantam Doubleday Dell Publishing Group, Inc.

Svecz, A. M. B. (2010). *Gender Communication: The impact gender has on effective communication*. Retrieved January 6, 2011 from http://trainingpd.suite101.com/article.cfm/gender-communication#ixzz0lrc5qAJv

Tichy, N. M., & Bennis, W. G. (2007). *Judgment: How winning leaders make great calls*. New York: The Penguin Group.

Ustun, B. (2006). Communication skills training as part of a problem-based learning curriculum. *Journal of Nursing Education*, 45(10), 421–424.

Videback, S. L. (2007). *Psychiatric mental health nursing*. (4th ed.) Philadelphia, PA: Lippincott William & Wilkins.

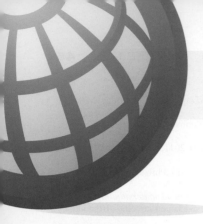

13

Working With Others in a Leadership Role

LEARNING OUTCOMES

After completing this chapter, you should be able to:

1. Discuss why teams are essential in healthcare settings and identify key factors in effective team function.
2. Describe the various roles a nurse may occupy on a healthcare team and discuss why each is important.
3. Describe the team-building process and identify behaviors that will strengthen a team.
4. Discuss the concept of motivation and outline actions that will motivate others.
5. Explain the process of effective delegation explaining why it is necessary in today's healthcare environment.
6. List the five rights of delegation and discuss why each is important.
7. Discuss situations that create a need for change and discuss effective change as it occurs in today's healthcare environment.
8. Discuss how Lewin's theory of change can be applied to situations on a nursing unit.
9. Describe the role of the change agent.
10. Identify strategies that will facilitate change.
11. Outline ways in which a novice nurse can respond positively to change.
12. Identify various sources and types of conflict in a healthcare setting.
13. Discuss the positive outcomes of conflict and strategies of managing conflict.

KEY TERMS

Champion
Change agent
Conflict
Conflict management/resolution
Delegation
Dissatisfiers/hygiene factors
Driving forces
Empirical–rational strategy
Motivation/motives
Movement stage
Normative–reeducative approach

Power–coercive strategy
Reactive change
Refreezing stage
Restraining forces
Role ambiguity
Role conflict
Satisfiers/motivators
Stakeholders
Team building
Unfreezing stage
Unlicensed assistive personnel (UAP)

All healthcare settings require a variety of workers with differing skills in order to meet patient needs. The role of the nurse among these workers is critical and challenging as it is that individual who carries much of the responsibility for organizing and coordinating the activities of the team. This chapter explores and explains some of the challenges of leadership.

TEAMS AND HEALTHCARE

In general, a team is a group of people working together for a common goal. The very nature of healthcare requires the development of healthcare teams and collaboration among all the variously prepared individuals caring for a particular patient or within a given setting. A patient care team could include a nurse, a physician, a pharmacist, a nutritionist, a social worker, clergy, a physical therapist, a speech therapist, a respiratory therapist, and housekeeping staff members, just to name a few. Sometimes their roles overlap. For example, both the social worker and the registered nurse (RN) may see discharge planning as an important part of their work.

What makes a team different from any other group of people who come together for a purpose? A team is a special kind of group. Teams enable us to capture the skills, abilities, and creativity of all persons who work with the group, a factor that can be used to measure the strength of a team. Teams make things happen and create solutions to problems. What one person may not think of, another person very well might. When a team functions as it should, it generates a kind of synergy that makes the work of all members greater than the sum of the contributions of the individuals comprising the group. Teams may be led by facilitators or coaches; have members who share responsibility for decisions, setting goals, and achieving outcomes; use communication patterns that flow both up and down; and have members who share responsibility for decisions and outcomes. Thus, we can expand our definition to say that a team is a group of people working toward a shared goal in ways that maximize the individual skills of each member and for which they all share responsibility.

Nurses are in a pivotal position to affect how the team functions because they contact all the various individuals who are involved in the team. The nurse, with input from other disciplines, develops the patient's plan of care. This role requires finely tuned interpersonal and coordinating skills as well as excellent communication proficiency.

Critical Thinking Activity

Review the number and background of caregivers in the clinical area to which you are currently assigned. How many health careers are represented? What are the primary responsibilities of each area? If responsibilities overlap, what are they? Who is responsible for bringing the individuals together as a team? Who is responsible for coordinating all the various patient care activities, such as x-rays, lab work, treatments, and the like?

Communication Within the Healthcare Team

To be successful in this team environment, the importance and contribution of each person needs to be recognized. Respect should be the hallmark of all relationships within healthcare. Although their education differs significantly, nursing assistants should receive the same respect as a team member as does the physician or the pharmacist. The same characteristics that demonstrate respect toward a patient may demonstrate respect toward coworkers. From using their preferred name when you address individuals, to avoiding intrusion upon privacy, to using language that reflects courtesy and consideration (such as saying "please" when making a request), you have many opportunities to demonstrate respect for others.

Along with respect for all team members, trust in the integrity and purpose of all individuals with whom you work creates the foundation for successful interaction and problem solving, as well as for team building. Others must be able to trust that you will fulfill your obligations and carry through on responsibilities, regardless of the role you play on the team. They need to be able to predict your response to various situations. Conversely, you must be able to trust that they will fulfill their responsibilities. When you find yourself unable to meet commitments, you maintain trust when you are honest with others and address the issue in a straightforward manner. Letting others know that a situation has changed or that you will be unable to complete something promised is the only ethical way to handle the circumstances.

Sharing information is central to building trust and responsibility among team members. When we share information, there is an implied element of trust that the information will be handled appropriately. There is also the indirect message to the person to whom the message is communicated that he or she is valued and is important enough in the scheme of things to have the information.

▶ ◼ *E X A M P L E*

Building Trust Through the Sharing of Information

On 4-North, the schedule of work hours was always posted 2 weeks in advance of the first work day of that schedule. However, the unit manager, Janie Bright, had been unable to complete the schedule because of heavy demands on her time regarding budget issues being addressed by nursing administration. Knowing that this was an important issue with the staff, Janie shared information regarding the delayed posting at the change of each shift, explaining the reason for the delay and giving a date by which the schedule would be available. She also apologized for any problems this might create for her team members.

Relationships Within the Healthcare Team

In healthcare settings, there has been a pervasive tendency for individuals to align relationships into a hierarchical system (see Chapter 1). Thus, some people see themselves as being of higher status or more important than others and develop an expectation of having more power within the system. Those in lesser-paid jobs frequently are assigned lower status and typically have less power. Often, they accept this as the expected way the system will operate. Some are even content with this because they do not want the added responsibility that often accompanies a higher-level position.

The approach to working with teams has changed significantly over the past century, with the quality improvement movement having a major effect. In the early 1950s, interest grew in the area of quality-improvement initiatives. The work of leaders in this movement led to many changes in approaches to management, especially with regard to respect for everyone in the system and trust among various members of the team. Trust and respect, as mentioned earlier, are considered vital factors in creating a work environment that will result in quality products, including quality healthcare.

Nursing Teams

Nursing teams focus on the provision of nursing care. RNs, licensed practical nurses (LPNs) (known as licensed vocational nurses, or LVNs, in Texas and California), nursing assistants (with various titles), as well as nursing students may all be members of a nursing team. In most situations, it is anticipated that the RN will lead the nursing team. However, in some long-term care facilities, LPNs lead nursing teams because there are so few RNs. In that situation, however, an RN must be available for oversight of the nursing care. There are a wide variety of nursing teams in different settings, some small, composed of two or three persons, others quite large.

The Many Roles of the Nurse

Traditionally, the public and even some nurses have thought of the nursing role as being one of providing care. While that certainly remains true in today's healthcare environment, the role of the nurse has expanded to include many other responsibilities and obligations. Nurses often find themselves simultaneously carrying out several responsibilities, each of which might be viewed as "wearing a different hat" (Fig. 13.1).

The Nurse as Educator

An important role filled by the nurse is that of educator. As a patient educator, the nurse is responsible for ensuring that patients and their families have a clear understanding of managing personal healthcare when returning home from the clinic, the hospital, or the long-term care facility. They must be sure the patient and family understand the proper dosage and know when to take medications, what side effects need to be reported, and a host of information related to recuperation and health maintenance. As a leader of the nursing team,

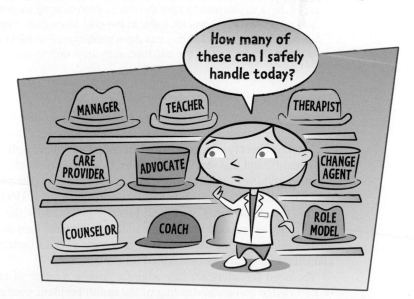

FIGURE 13.1 Many times, the nurse wears more than one "hat" and performs several roles simultaneously.

the RN plays a key role in the ongoing education of team members with lesser educational preparation. RNs improve patient care through coaching and teaching staff on a day-to-day basis. As a member of the community, the nurse is an informal educator who can provide important information related to health issues for friends and others within the community. In an era when health promotion and health maintenance are emphasized, this role takes on new dimensions.

▶ *EXAMPLE*

Assisting a Client to Understand and Comply with Medication Orders

Jane Allard, an 87-year-old female, was being seen as an outpatient in a large health maintenance organization. After a routine physical with blood work, the physician placed Jane on 3 mg of warfarin daily, told her to discontinue taking the 325 mg of aspirin she took each day, and asked her to return for more blood work in 2 weeks. He then hurried on to the next waiting patient. Mary Beth, the nurse in the clinic, talked with Jane following her examination. She learned that Jane had taken aspirin for many years and was convinced that the cause of her blood being "too thick" was related to the fact that she ate too much raw spinach in salads because she liked it so much. Mary Beth realized that Jane planned to adjust the dosage of the warfarin on her own and without the knowledge of the physician. Jane also stated she really did not want to quit taking her aspirin daily. She planned to treat her condition by not eating any more spinach. Mary Beth sat down with Jane and explained why it was very important that she take the medications exactly as ordered. She encouraged Jane to use a soft tooth brush, to watch for any signs of bruising, and to be sure to return to have the blood work in 2 weeks. She further explained that if Jane adjusted the dosage of the medication, then it would influence the results of the blood work and the doctor would not be able to assess whether the dosage prescribed was appropriate for Jane. She was able to get Jane to promise to take the medication exactly as prescribed and discontinue the aspirin for the next 2 weeks. Later in the day, Mary Beth made a special point to seek out Jane's physician and discuss Jane's resistance to taking the medication as ordered so that he might review the situation with Jane during her next appointment.

The Nurse as Patient Advocate

Another role the nurse fills is that of patient advocate. The healthcare system has become so complex (see Chapter 3) that clients may need assistance in moving through it. It is often the nurse who is keenly concerned with ensuring that patient rights are not violated, that care is of high quality, and that service is provided in a timely manner.

When serving in an advocacy role, the nurse can assist the patient to be involved in informed decisions that affect that individual's healthcare. Since 1991, advocacy has been included in the ethical standards of clinical practice prepared by the American Nurses Association (ANA). Because nurses spend more time with patients than do other healthcare workers, they are in a prime position to fill this role, may have a keener understanding of the patient's desires and values, and have an established trust relationship.

The need for advocacy can originate from a number of causes, including patients' lack of knowledge and understanding of the health problem, confusion about the way the healthcare system operates because of the complexity of the system, ethical and legal concerns, frailty or disabling conditions that will not allow patients to speak for themselves, or perhaps inadequate care.

The Nurse as Counselor/Coach

Tied closely to the role of advocate is that of counselor or coach. In their educational programs, nurses are provided with interpersonal knowledge and skills that allow them to assist others to express their concerns, seek alternative approaches and second opinions, and ask questions. Through such activities, the nurse is able to empower the client and family. Assisting those with less experience to move into effective roles within the organization is an important aspect of the responsibility of more senior individuals (see Chapter 14 on mentoring).

The Nurse as Manager and Leader of Teams

Manager and leader of healthcare teams are other important roles nurses occupy. Often, these involve serving as a change agent within the healthcare environment. Leadership and management were discussed in Chapter 12, and we will discuss the change process later in this chapter.

The Nurse in Nursing Informatics and Research

RNs fill a wide variety of other roles in healthcare. Two roles that we are seeing more frequently relate to nursing informatics and nursing research (see Chapter 16). The need for information management in healthcare has never been greater, and nurses are in a unique position to take a key role in data management for decision making. Similarly, as the profession stretches to enlarge to a body of knowledge that is uniquely nursing and as evidence-based practice moves to the forefront, the demand for nurses who will manage and participate in research increases.

Critical Thinking Activity

You have just moved into a new position in the long-term care facility where you have been employed for 6 months. The position requires that you do more teaching and counseling of staff than you have done in the past. What resources will you seek to gain information to increase your skill in these areas? Which persons might you contact? How will you assess your new competencies? How can you be alert to personal biases?

Nurse–Physician Relationships

Nurses work more closely with physicians in the acute care or long-term care setting than any other group. Throughout the 1990's, much was written about the importance of "good" nurse–physician relationships. The relationships of nurses with physicians may be very positive, but they also result in some of the most stressful encounters for nurses. Because this stress plays a key role in patient care, job satisfaction, and retention of nurses, studies were done focusing on nurse–physician relationships (Baggs, Ryan, Phelps, et al., 1992; Larsen, 1999; Nelson, 2008; Rosenstein, 2002). The studies indicated that when these relationships lack respect and trust, the result is a taxing working environment and potential for ineffective patient care. Rosenstein (2002) identified five key circumstances or events that resulted in disruptive physician behavior. These occurred at the following times:

- After placing calls to physicians
- After questioning or seeking to clarify physicians' orders

- When physicians were concerned that their orders were not being carried out correctly or in a timely manner
- After perceived delays in the delivery of care
- After sudden changes in patient status

Disruptive behavior is discussed in detail in Chapter 14. As a manager of nursing care, the nurse can reduce the incidence of disruptive behavior by being certain when placing calls to physicians that you have all necessary information available before placing the call. Be certain that assessments are complete and that you have all needed vital signs and other information. This is doubly important if that call is made in the middle of the night. None of us appreciates being wakened from a sound sleep, especially if we know we have a busy day ahead. A physician might be distressed if the call were made without adequate assessment data to allow a decision to be made. Using a standardized approach to communicating in such situations such as SBAR (Situation, Background, Assessment, Recommendation) will assist you in planning your interaction to facilitate an effective response (see Chapter 10). Some settings require that the nurse consults with a supervisor for verification of the situation and consultation regarding options before making a middle-of-the-night call.

COMMUNICATION IN ACTION

The Patient With a Changing Condition

Patricia White worked the 11 PM to 7 AM shift in a small community hospital. She cared for a patient admitted to the unit during the evening shift who had been involved in a serious motorcycle accident resulting in multiple injuries. Although morphine sulfate 1 mg had been administered intravenously (IV) every hour, the patient continued to complain of pain, particularly in the abdomen. Patricia knew Dr. Whittle, the patient's physician, did not like to be disturbed during the night; however, she was concerned that the medication had not helped relieve the pain. She called Dr. Whittle and said, "This is Patricia White on 3-South at Mercy Hospital. (S) I am calling about your patient Jim Short who was admitted this evening following a motorcycle accident and is experiencing severe pain. Despite the fact that I have given him morphine sulfate 1 mg IV every hour, he continues to complain of pain, particularly in his abdomen, rating it as an 8 on a scale of 1 to 10. (B) As you recall, he has a fractured left leg and multiple contusions and abrasions. His leg was set in surgery after admission and is currently casted and elevated. (A) His vital signs show some change with a slight drop in blood pressure from 130/80 to 122/72 in the past 3 hours. His pulse is slightly increased from 80 to 88 over that same time period. His abdomen is tense and is the site of the majority of his pain. His neuro signs remain normal. He is alert and complaining. (R) I believe that his condition urgently requires a medical assessment of the abdomen." Dr. Whittle replied, "Make him as comfortable as you can, and I will be there in 30 minutes. There may be more injury than we first believed. Please, tell him I am on my way and prefer that he not have more medication until I see him."

In the communication example above, the nurse carried out the responsibility of alerting the physician to the needs of the patient. Recognizing that the phone call would awaken the physician, she reviewed the situation and provided background status about the patient to assist with orientation. She provided the physician with assessment data to help understand the patient's condition. She provided a clear recommendation of the action she was requesting.

Because nurses are held legally accountable if they make medication errors, the nurse must follow through with appropriate communication with the prescriber (most commonly the physician) if there is a lack of clarity about a medication order or if the order does not conform to documented expectations. Communication should be conducted in a collaborative and polite manner. Often it is not what is said, but the manner in which it is said, that will determine the emotional content of the response. Keep in mind that the prescriber also desires that no errors occur and that appropriate care is provided. Provide information such as reference or resource about the medication or assessment data to help substantiate your concern. In some settings, the pharmacist may assist with this process.

When receiving communication from the physician or another leader of the healthcare team, recognize and allow for situations in which the emergency nature of what occurs with the client may affect the nature of communication. Direct orders for action are appropriate in these situations. The tenseness of a crisis may make individuals abrupt, and they may appear somewhat rude. Responding calmly and confidently in your role may relieve tension and help to ensure that care is rendered quickly and efficiently. A difference exists between meeting the demands of the situation and disruptive behavior.

Nurses can positively influence nurse–physician relationships. Sirota (2007) suggests two strategies that will contribute to improving communications with physicians and empowering nurses. Schmalenberg and Kramer (2009) suggest four factors that contribute to positive relationships: a culture in which concern for the patient comes first; constructive conflict resolution (discussed later in this chapter); interactive, interdisciplinary collaborative patient rounds; and competent performance and self-confidence on the part of the nurse.

The importance of interdisciplinary interactions and collaboration can't be overemphasized. This can be fostered by regularly scheduled interdisciplinary rounds in which everyone's participation is encouraged and nurses have the opportunity to share information they have regarding the patient's response to treatment. Nurses must be mindful that they work and communicate within the scope of practice of nursing and remain in the realm of nursing practice when initiating suggestions for care.

Ensuring competence and possessing excellent nursing skills fosters positive nurse–physician relationships. If procedures are not carried out correctly, if medication errors occur, or if the nurse appears inept in a particular situation, patient care is jeopardized, and it can be anticipated that the physician will be critical of the behavior. Nurses are empowered when they feel secure in their knowledge and expertise. Fortunately, the number of physicians who display inappropriate behavior is small.

Critical Thinking Activity

It is 2:00 AM on a busy surgical unit. A new surgery patient, who had a nephrectomy late the previous afternoon, is experiencing a high level of pain. You have administered all the medication for which orders were left without alleviating the pain. You have decided that the patient situation requires that you call the attending surgeon. What should you consider before calling? What information should you have? Are there other persons with whom you should discuss this before making the call?

TEAM BUILDING

In the late 1980s and 1990s, the concept of team building began to receive a great deal of attention in business environments as well as in healthcare. This can be attributed in part to the changes occurring in management strategies, as managers responded to guidelines that had evolved from recommendations designed to improve quality. In implementing a quality-improvement process, managers need to have a concern for the satisfaction of staff and must demonstrate respect for staff and their abilities. Without these attributes, team building will not be successful. Today, we see the concept of team building, especially with interdisciplinary (interprofessional) staff, being added to the curricula of helping professions.

Team building itself sometimes seems rather nebulous. People aren't quite sure what it is. For purposes of our discussion, we will refer to our earlier definition of a team: a group of people working together toward a shared goal in ways that maximize the individual skills of each member and for which they all share responsibility. The goal of team building is to create a type of synergy, in which the effect of everyone working together toward the shared goal results in a greater total effect than could be achieved by the sum of the efforts of everyone working individually.

One of the most obvious forms of team building that exists in today's world can be found in the sports arena, where teams and team functions are integral to the activities that take place. Much of the literature about team building comes from the area of athletics. Team building begins with involving all members of the team in identifying the goal and establishing the steps to be taken to achieve that goal. Through the process of goal setting, members of the team recognize their contribution and its importance in the work of the team. All members of the team have an ownership in the process and the product.

Teams are composed of a diverse membership, with a variety of skills and abilities represented. Each has a special role to play on the team. On the interdisciplinary healthcare team, some have special knowledge of pharmacy, some of medicine, some of respiratory therapy, some of nursing, with each member contributing to the patient's recovery. There are informal roles as well the formal roles. The formal role relates to an individual's contribution to the team goal or purpose and relates to the individual's job preparation (eg, physician, therapist, nurse, or pharmacist). The informal roles are defined by natural skills and talents. For example, some have natural abilities to smooth over potentially volatile situations, some individuals are good at detail, others have a bent for creative ideas, and some are able to energize a team. Team members need to recognize both the formal and informal roles of each of the members.

Many of our life experiences have not encouraged team behaviors. Our early schooling may have emphasized individual achievement, recognizing those who excelled over others. Many of our work experiences may have occurred in environments where decisions were made by a few and passed down to others who were expected to follow though without questioning. Work was accomplished by a group directed by a supervisor. Thus, as we move into a work environment that requires greater teamwork, we need to make mental shifts that place more value on working together and less on personal triumphs.

Central to building effective teams is the belief that those who are closest to problems may best be able to provide the sound solutions to address the concern. All share in the problems that occur; all share in the success that is achieved. In bringing together members of the team, the manager needs to establish a working environment that recognizes and values the contribution of each individual on the team. This serves another purpose as well. It helps each team member to feel necessary and included in the team and that the member's contribution is important. They become engaged, feel valued, and take pride in the activities of the team.

Another part of team building relates to celebrating successes. As we look at building healthcare teams, we need to look for opportunities to celebrate the good things that happen. This will help members appreciate one another and the effort that has been made as a group.

Leaders focus on how problems can be corrected rather than on how they occurred. If one approach to treatment does not provide the outcome desired, a conference is held, and other strategies are discussed and decided upon. The focus centers on how things can be made better rather than on what was not working right.

Team building works to eliminate individual faultfinding. Instead of spending valuable time discussing with a nursing assistant why the dinner trays were not promptly delivered for the evening meal, helping that individual develop an organized approach to tray distribution would have more long-lasting and better results. The role of the manager often becomes more one of coach than that of boss.

Critical Thinking Activity

As a new graduate, you have accepted a position on the medical unit of a community hospital. After working for 1 month, you have determined that the morale among the nurses and nursing assistants on the unit is low, that they do not function as a team, and that they don't have much team spirit. What can you do about this situation? Where would you begin? What are your limitations?

BECOMING A GOOD TEAM MEMBER

Although you eventually may carry major responsibility for leading a nursing team, when you initially move into a staff nurse position, you will likely be a member of a team rather than its leader. How can you best fulfill that role?

Once again, we suggest a self-assessment. How well do you listen to others' opinions and ideas? Sometimes we forget that listening is just as important to effective communication, sometimes more important, than talking. People who are good listeners learn things that others may miss. Good listeners communicate a message to others that they are interested in what is being said and value the individual who is speaking.

Do you communicate your ideas clearly in an open and honest manner? It is important to team effort that you contribute ideas and concerns when appropriate. Contributions should be constructive and should be expressed in positive language that does not imply a lack of respect for previous ideas or approaches.

Can you accept constructive criticism? Part of growing and improving involves having one's actions evaluated. Evaluation should involve feedback and it may not always be glowing. Maintaining a positive approach in such a situation is a mark of emotional maturity. Pouting, clamming up, withdrawing, or having an emotional outburst are not appropriate responses. Feedback and recommendations can be steps toward professional growth. Analyze your performance honestly and make changes where needed.

DISPLAY 13.1 Questions to Assess Your Competence as a Team Member

• Are you a good listener?
• Do you communicate ideas clearly?
• Can you accept criticism?
• Do you support others?
• Do you ask good questions and contribute?
• Are you a team player?
• Can you deal with change and conflict?
• Are you self-motivating?

Do you support others? Just as you want support in the role you play in a group, others need support also. When someone does a task well, let him or her know you noticed. Give credit where credit is due. Statements such as, "I think Warren has a good idea" or "I'd like to try Wendy's approach" are supportive in nature. And when things are going poorly for another, be helpful and encouraging. Offer your assistance if it is appropriate to do so.

Do you ask good questions and contribute? One of the reasons why teams succeed is because they use the collective intelligence of all members. If you fail to share your ideas or ask pertinent questions that will lead to new approaches or prevent poor ones, you are letting down other members of your team.

Are you a team player? Are you willing to give a little to accomplish the goals of the team? This means making team goals your goals and, in some cases, giving up a little of the spotlight. There may be more than one effective path to the goal. Team players are willing to take the path that someone else prefers rather than insisting on their own preference.

Can you deal with conflict? Conflict is a natural part of our lives. When we are unable to deal with conflict, we may become frustrated, jealous, or angry or may withdraw from the situation. Conflict must be dealt with in ways that are constructive and positive rather than negative (discussed later in this chapter). In a study conducted by Osterman, Bertram, and Büssing (2010) focusing on the effects of team building, it was found that the most significant changes following a team-building process occurred in the ability of the team to constructively resolve conflict.

Are you self-motivating? Being able to set your own time lines and commitments and meet them are indications of self-motivation. Demonstrating ability and confidence to manage what you do are important behaviors to nurture. Display 13.1 summarizes these questions you can use to assess your competence as a team member.

THE COACHING ROLE

The activities of the team leader often involve one of coaching less experienced members of the team as we strive to involve all team members in decision making and team effort. Whitworth, Kimsey-House, and Sandahl (1998) describe coaching as a collaborative process that is focused on actions that will move the individual forward through the process of learning and result in helping people achieve goals. The learning may be associated with job skills, understanding the operation of the organization, meeting new challenges, increasing efficiency and productivity, or other issues specific to the organization. The goal is to help the individuals who are being coached to fulfill their potential, thus building a stronger team.

In a coaching role, a more senior nurse supports and nurtures the learner, providing positive reinforcement as well as information. Rather than telling less experienced nurses what to do, the coach might ask how they plan to approach a problem and then help refine the plan so that success will be realized and the team members learn to handle situations on their own. It involves asking reflective questions and providing feedback. Coaching may be consultative, educational, motivational, or a combination of all three.

An individual who accepts the coaching role must possess certain qualities. This individual must be competent and emotionally stable. He or she must be willing to take risks, be honest and credible, communicate clearly, and possess energy and enthusiasm.

In some ways, the coaching role is as much a style of management as a unique approach in and of itself. The unit manager who can coach teams to efficient and effective performance will have a much happier and more motivated group of workers than the manager who tells them what to do. The coaching role is further discussed in Chapter 14.

MOTIVATING OTHERS

Team building and motivating are closely related. What team building is to a group, motivating is to an individual. Motivating others to perform at their best for the benefit of the organization is a huge task. It requires strong people skills, leadership, clear personal goals, and participatory supervision.

Understanding Motivation

Motivation encompasses the sum of all those individual factors that cause or impel an individual to do something. Individual factors, called **motives**, are generally referred to as extrinsic or intrinsic.

Extrinsic motives include things such as salary, the work environment, and recognition by others— in other words, factors outside the individual. As far back as we can remember, society has relied on a combination of threats and rewards (considered external motivators) to get people to do what it wants them to do. Much of our early history saw a predominance of the threat or punishment as a motivator. As time went on, rewards were introduced and those who performed well were rewarded for their action. Today, the use of punishment or threat is considered less effective in motivating individuals than are rewards for work well done. Sometimes, these awards are financial in the form of increased pay, bonuses, or promotions. However, there are times when the organization cannot afford to continue to increase financial rewards. Managers and leaders must then find other types of rewards to motivate workers.

Intrinsic motives are more difficult to work with than extrinsic motives because they arise from within the individual. Some would argue that all motives are intrinsic and that the most we can do is try to foster within the individual the desire to act in a certain way, to perform certain activities, or to strive for certain goals, because the motivation to do so originates from within the person who will be doing the acting. Those who adhere to that approach state that when we talk about motivating others, it is limited to those acts of persuasion that will fire the inner desire within another individual to take the desired action (Fig. 13.2).

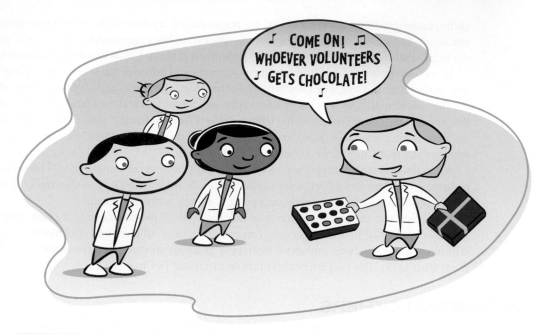

FIGURE 13.2 Rewards provided by the manager are external motivators.

When it comes to grades, why do some individuals strive for A's, while others are satisfied with C's? Why do some seek leadership roles within organizations, while others prefer positions that may capture a lower salary but be less stressful? Why do some people seek doctorate degrees, while others believe a high school diploma will provide them with all the education they need? A lot of study and a number of theories have been set forth to explain why people make the choices they do from among a variety of possible behaviors.

You may already have learned about human needs as motivation and that needs appear in a hierarchy, with unmet needs creating motivation. People engage in actions that help them to meet their needs (Maslow, 1954). Abraham Maslow, an American psychologist whose work has been popular since the 1950s, established the highest level of functioning as self-actualization. The needs for food, shelter, belonging, esteem, and self-esteem (in approximately that order) provide motivation for behavior. Self-actualization, the highest level, occurs when esteem needs are met and the individual is no longer driven by the need to prove himself or herself.

Herzberg, Mausner, and Synderman (1959) and Herzberg (1966) discussed **dissatisfiers** or **hygiene factors** and **satisfiers** or **motivators**, which were essentially independent of one another in his Motivation-Hygiene theory. His theory stated that people focused on the environment in which they were working when dissatisfied with the job. His hygiene factors related to conditions under which the job is performed and include such things as organizational policies, working conditions, salaries, status, and job security. These factors could be considered quite applicable today as nurses leave the profession because they are unhappy with work situations (see Chapter 14). When satisfied with working conditions, they focused on the job. Satisfiers referred to feelings regarding the work itself and included such items as achievement, professional growth, recognition, responsibility, and advancement. When workers are satisfied, work performance increases.

Another approach to motivation suggests that some people are motivated by a desire for affiliation, the desire for power, or the desire for achievement (McClelland, 1953, 1961). Affiliation referred to the desire for friendly, close social relationships—to be liked. Power referred to the need to be in control—to manage things. Achievement related to the desire to excel, advance, succeed, and grow. McGregor (1966) suggested that some managers operate as if people are motivated only by fear of the manager's displeasure or the potential for a concrete reward, such as pay (extrinsic factors). His Theory X supported the concept that most people would rather be directed than assume responsibility for creative problem solving, found work distasteful, were motivated primarily by physical and security needs, and needed to be managed through close supervision. McGregor recommended another approach to managing people that assumes that people want to do well and welcome opportunities to make contributions and can be self-directed and creative. McGregor labeled this Theory Y.

A central concept for you as a beginning nurse is that different factors motivate different people and that one individual might be motivated by one factor at one point in life but by another factor at a different time. Keeping a broad view of what might motivate others will enable you to work more effectively to motivate nursing staff. Table 13.1 summarizes the theories mentioned above and describes how they may be used to motivate people.

Developing Your Ability to Motivate Others

As a team leader, how will you motivate others? What behaviors on your part will encourage others to perform at their best? What people skills can you develop that will assist you in

Table 13.1   Application of Theories of Motivation

THEORIST AND THEORY	DESCRIPTION	APPLICATION
Maslow Hierarchy of Needs	Established a pyramid of human needs ordered from simple to complex. The needs at the base of the pyramid are physiological (food, shelter), then self-preservation, affiliation (love, belonging), esteem (confidence, recognition), and self-actualization (maximum achievement).	Facilitate opportunities for workers to meet as many basic needs as possible in the workplace, thus attracting more workers.
Herzberg Motivation-hygiene	Dissatisfiers/hygiene factors prevent job satisfaction and result in workers focusing on work conditions.	Provide enriching opportunities for workers in the work environment
	Satisfiers/motivators promote work performance and work achievement.	Recognize performance and achievements.
McClelland Affiliation, power, achievement	Major motivators are the need to belong, the need to control, and the need to succeed.	Foster opportunities within the work environment for gratification of needs.
McGregor Theory X Theory Y	Theory X: Workers are dissatisfied and are motivated by fear of the manager's displeasure. Need to be supervised.	Broaden employees' responsibility, involve them in decision making.
	Theory Y: Workers are satisfied, self-directed and creative, enjoy work.	Recognize achievements.

DISPLAY 13.2   Personal Behaviors that Motivate Others

• Inspire trust and confidence from others
• Role model the behaviors you want to see in others
• Treat others with respect
• Give recognition for things done well
• Maintain a positive attitude

working with others? A key aspect of being successful in this area relates to your ability to develop the kind and quality of relationships with others that will positively influence the way they perform. You will want to know your team members well enough to know what things you can do that will bring out the best in them: personal praise may result in outstanding performance in one individual; another may respond best when given new responsibilities or challenging assignments. Some motivating behaviors are discussed below and are summarized in Display 13.2.

Inspire Trust and Confidence

As you examine the personal behaviors that will help you motivate others, give serious consideration to the things that people do to inspire trust and confidence in others. What helps build credibility—the assurance that people can count on you to do what you say you are going to do when you say you will do it? Behaviors that lend credibility to actions include exercising good judgment, and being knowledgeable about procedures, policies, and protocols. Performing in a timely fashion is also critical. You will want to be even-tempered and patient, even in stressful situations. As a result of developing these qualities, others will view you as a person from whom they can seek answers and directions.

Role Model Behaviors

You will want to model the behaviors you want to see in others. In doing so, you set the pace for your team. When you are energized, others also will be energized. When you respond to others in a positive way, it becomes contagious and others respond positively. Avoid any behaviors that would undermine a team member's motivation, such as being arrogant, showing favoritism, telling jokes that put down others, making racist statements, or issuing threats.

Treat Others with Respect

Foster all opportunities to take pride in the accomplishments of the team and share ideas for improvement. Find ways to let your team members know you care about them as individuals. Show a genuine interest in things that are important to them. Be sensitive to problems they may encounter away from the workplace as well as within. Learn what their personal goals and aspirations are and encourage activities that will help them to reach those goals. Avoid gossip or humor that makes someone else the object of the joke. Do not talk about one person with another. When you need to speak to someone about a problem, do so privately.

COMMUNICATION IN ACTION

Avoiding Gossip

One evening at dinner, Sarah, a new graduate, ate with an LPN and a nursing assistant from her unit. The nursing assistant said, "I get so tired of Jennie [another LPN] always showing how smart she is!" The LPN replied, "I know just what you mean—you would think she was the nurse manager or something. Sarah, haven't you noticed how bossy and controlling Jennie is?" Sarah replied, "I feel really uncomfortable discussing Jennie behind her back. It seems unfair. I guess if it is a problem for you, maybe you should try to talk to Jennie about it." She then introduced a new topic of conversation. Sarah has not labeled the others but has indicated she will not participate in gossip and laid the framework for others to expect that she will not gossip about them.

Recognize Achievements

Receiving recognition for things done well helps motivate many people. Even those who answer, shyly, "No problem" appreciate having their efforts acknowledged. Giving praise for accomplishments also means that you will be working closely with individuals, so that you know when they have done something well. Praise and recognition, even in the form of a thank you, serve as great reinforcers and encourage people to keep trying. Most individuals seek to please others by their performance and need to know when that has been achieved. If you can offer this praise in public, it will reap even greater rewards. You have heard before that we praise publicly and correct privately. This is certainly true when trying to motivate others to do their best.

Another aspect of encouraging individuals to perform at their best focuses on having them know that their opinion is wanted and valued. This means involving them in decision making. We talked earlier in this chapter and in Chapter 12 about involving those closest to the action in the decision-making process. People perform better when they believe they are important and contributing to the team effort—that they are valued. You can provide the opportunity for others to have input into decisions and to articulate their thoughts and opinions. When you initially try this, you may run into resistance. When encouraging others to participate in decision making, you may get the response, "That's what they pay *you* for." If this occurs, continue to offer opportunities for input. If this is a new experience for the team member, that individual may doubt your sincerity. Developing a genuine approach when working with others creates the basis of trust and respect as mentioned at the beginning of this chapter.

Maintain a Positive Attitude

When working with others, maintaining a positive attitude will help both you and those with whom you work. If you avoid becoming upset and angry, you can respond to problems or errors more effectively. This may require using your sense of humor when things go awry. The discomfort of many situations can be decreased by being able to laugh at things that fail to meet our expectations. In contrast, becoming upset or angry if something is done incorrectly will only cause your team members to avoid you. They will consider you unapproachable, and communication will decrease. The opportunity to build the strength of the team will be missed.

A final word should be said about redirecting the efforts of others. Especially when working with unlicensed assistive personnel, you may identify techniques that are incorrect or approaches to client care that need improvement. When this occurs, always focus your comments on the observed behavior you believe needs to be changed, not on the individual's personal characteristics. You will find it useful to ask personnel for their own commitment to make the needed change in behavior or performance. This places the responsibility for correct performance on the individual. Then, when you observe the corrected behavior, be certain to positively comment about it. More discussion related to supervising the actions of others follows later in this chapter.

COMMUNICATION IN ACTION

Lost Privacy

John Wilson was making rounds of the patients in a long-term care facility when he noticed a nursing assistant with an elderly resident. The assistant was preparing to move the resident onto a commode, but the curtain was not pulled. John moved to the bedside and simply said, "Here, let me get that curtain for you," and pulled the curtain around to protect the resident's privacy. When the nursing assistant was finished, John approached her privately and said, "I am concerned that you did not pull the curtain when you were assisting the resident to the commode. You must always remember to pull the curtain before providing care to assure that our residents are provided privacy. Will you agree to work on that?" He avoided making general statements such as, "You are inconsiderate and careless of the modesty of our residents," but was specific about the incorrect behavior and the rationale for the correct behavior. Also, John asked the nursing assistant to make a commitment to changing her own behavior.

Learning to Delegate

In today's healthcare environment, the need for all RNs to skillfully delegate, assign, and supervise those who have lesser educational preparation is an essential competency. In response, both the ANA and the National Council of State Boards of Nursing (NCSBN) have developed resources designed to make the delegation process easier to understand and utilize. Two such resources are the "ANA Principles of Delegation" and NCSBN's "Decision Tree on Delegation" that reflects the four phases of the delegation process (NCSBN, 2006).

Delegation may be defined as "the process for a nurse to direct another person to perform nursing tasks and activities" (NCSBN, 2006). An example would be an RN asking that a nursing assistant help a client ambulate in the hall. The nursing assistant assists the client to walk; the RN is still responsible for seeing that the client ambulates and that it is completed safely and documented in the client's record.

In today's healthcare environment, which uses variously prepared caregivers, the importance of being able to effectively delegate responsibilities is critical. Nurses would not be able to complete their duties, tasks, and responsibilities without the ability to delegate some nursing activities. Delegating effectively requires that you have skill in the ability to guide, teach, and direct others. And like other skills you have mastered, it can be learned.

Reasons to Delegate

There are a number of reasons that we delegate certain tasks to others. Primary among these is the current trend in healthcare facilities to allow the RN more time for critical aspects of care by hiring **unlicensed assistive personnel (UAP)** to perform those tasks that they can perform safely. This also results in cost cuts, as a UAP commands a much lower salary than does an RN. At one time in nursing, a primary care model of care delivery was popular in which the RN performed all nursing care activities for a group of patients (see Chapter 5). Although this was a desirable approach from a patient care standpoint, it was very costly. In an effort to contain costs, hospitals restructured and redesigned staffing patterns to change the skill mix—the number of RNs was decreased and those with lesser educational preparation were increased. This change was predicated on the assumption that many tasks occurring on a nursing unit do not require the skills of an RN. Individuals with lesser educational preparation can carry out certain aspects of care such as taking vital signs, ambulating, transporting clients, and performing basic procedures. This allows the RN to focus on activities such as client assessment, care coordination, and teaching. In this way, delegating provides for effective time management.

Another reason to delegate relates to the positive effect it can have on building team spirit. As team members are able to effectively perform the tasks delegated to them, a sense of satisfaction is created and self-esteem is increased. Thus, teams function more effectively.

Critical Aspects of Effective Delegation

For delegation to be effective and to ensure that the quality of patient care remains high, a number of factors must be considered. Review these factors before you begin delegating tasks to others.

It is critical to remember that although you have asked someone else to carry out a nursing task, you are still accountable for the care that is given. You need to be able to ensure that the task will be completed in compliance with accepted standards, in a timely fashion, and that the activity, along with the patient's response, if appropriate, is adequately documented.

Knowing When Not to Delegate

Are there tasks that should not be delegated? When should I not delegate a task? What are the situations in which I should retain responsibility for doing the task? How will I know the difference? These are questions frequently asked by the nurse who is just moving into the role of managing the activities of others.

Certain tasks cannot be delegated. The most obvious of these are activities that are not within the scope of practice of the individual to whom you might delegate the task. Any activity that requires knowledge and judgment that is unique to the function of an RN cannot be delegated to others.

You may not delegate responsibilities that call for professional judgment, skill, or decision-making ability such as asking the UAP to do assessments or evaluations. An RN must complete all assessments of the client and client needs. Information from the assessment that is important to the client's care then needs to be communicated to any person to whom care is delegated. The ability to do a thorough assessment and to not overlook some critical need is part of the nursing judgment acquired through your education. Someone with lesser preparation might overlook that need. For example, if you admit to your unit a patient with head trauma, the assessment of that patient cannot be delegated.

You may not delegate roles that are limited to licensed individuals under the nursing licensure laws. For example, giving medications cannot be delegated in most settings, because medication administration involves assessment, understanding of appropriate procedural

DISPLAY 13.3   Situations in Which Delegation Is Inappropriate

• When the activities to be delegated fall outside the scope of practice of the person to whom they would be delegated. You cannot delegate something the individual is not allowed to do.
• When the activities to be delegated require independent, specialized nursing knowledge and judgment. This protects the safety of the client.
• When the activities to be delegated fall within job description and role of the RN and delegating it would erode that role. This would apply to situations in which the nurse is responsible for evaluating the performance of others.
• When the work situation will not allow time for adequate supervision of those to whom tasks are delegated. Delegated tasks must be supported and supervised at all times.

safeguards, knowledge of pharmacology, and the ability to evaluate the effectiveness of the medication. Because of this, the law limits who may administer medications. In some states, routine medication administration can be delegated to specially trained medication aides in long-term care or to home care aides in community settings. In these instances, the task is delegated, but an RN retains accountability for the assessment and decision-making surrounding medication administration and for assuring that the task is carried out correctly. Display 13.3 summarizes information on what should not be delegated and provides the reason why.

Identifying to Whom to Delegate

You can delegate only to a person who is competent to perform the task delegated. The nurse who is delegating tasks must know and understand the level of care that can be performed by the person to whom the task is being delegated. In other words, you need to understand staff members' competency level or, if they are licensed, their scope of practice—what activities a person with a particular license may legally perform. The scope of practice for RNs and for LPNs is outlined in state practice acts and may vary from state to state (see Chapter 3). You will want to be familiar with the practice acts of the state in which you are employed. When working with someone who is not licensed, you will want to be knowledgeable about that individual's skill level, job descriptions, specific competencies, and agency policies and protocols.

Determining What to Delegate

The tasks delegated to assistive personnel should not require nursing judgment while being carried out. This implies that the tasks should be routine in nature, ones that can be performed according to certain exact standards, and that the client's condition be relatively stable. We have said it before, but it bears repeating—activities that require specialized nursing skill, knowledge, or experience cannot be delegated. It is the use of this specialized nursing judgment that constitutes the heart of professional nursing.

The anticipated outcome of the care that is being delegated should be reasonably predictable. For example, if the responsibility for checking the vital signs of a patient is assigned to an LPN, the result will be the accurate assessment and recording of the patient's vital signs.

Tasks associated with any situation requiring ongoing assessment, complex observations, additional instructions, or critical decisions should not be delegated. Again, these activities require the use of nursing judgment and, therefore, should be completed by the RN. This would apply to any situation in which a client's condition is unstable, changing, or whose acuity level is high.

Matching the Task to the Person to Whom It Is Delegated

When delegating, you have the responsibility for ensuring that a match exists between what care the client needs to have performed and the level of competence and understanding of the person being asked to provide that care. In this way, you are assured that the tasks that are delegated are not beyond the ability of the individual asked to do them. This requires that you know members of your team and their abilities. It also requires that you understand the legal scope of practice of the various members of your team. This can be an important consideration in situations in which an RN is floated into a special care unit to assist during especially busy times. Aspects of care in that unit that are specialized should not be delegated to someone who has not had the additional training and education required to render safe care, even if that person has the RN license. Rather, the floated nurse should be asked to perform only those aspects of care with which he or she is familiar.

Supervising Delegated Tasks

The supervision of delegated activities is essential. The ANA (1997) defines supervision as "the active process of directing, guiding, and influencing the outcome of an individual's performance of an activity." This means that an individual with greater skill and education is available, usually in person, but occasionally through alternate means, such as written or verbal communications, to give directions and ensure that activities are carried out properly. For delegation to be successful, there must be sufficient personnel and adequate time to provide the needed supervision and follow-up. If either of these is missing, problems may result.

The Five Rights of Successful Delegation

If you have followed all these guidelines when delegating responsibilities to others, in all likelihood you will have also followed the five rights of successful delegation. The NCSBN issued these five rights in 1995, when changes in delivery of patient care first included use of UAP and similar care providers (NCSBN, 1995). (Typically, this includes positions with job titles such as nurse aides, certified nurse assistants, nurse technicians, patient care technicians, personal care attendant, or unit assistants.) The five rights as identified by the NCSBN are found in Display 13.4.

DISPLAY 13.4 **The NCSBN'S Five Rights of Delegation**

• Right Task
• Right Circumstances
• Right Person
• Right Direction/Communication
• Right Supervision/Evaluation

Suggestions for Successful Delegation

A number of elements can result in delegation either enhancing or compromising patient care. Following the steps in the nursing process will help ensure the best outcomes.

Assess the Situation

Before you decide which aspects of care you can ask others to do and which you should complete yourself, be certain that a complete assessment of the client has been done. You will want to know what that individual's needs involve, what priorities have been set, the goals of care, the time you have to accomplish the care, and other factors that impinge on the situation.

If you are to make a good match between the skills of the person to whom you delegate responsibilities and the complexity of the task, you must know the abilities of the person to whom you will delegate tasks. This can sometimes be determined through hospital protocols that establish the competencies of various levels of caregivers or via job descriptions that define what an individual in a certain job category is capable of performing. If the individual is licensed, you can be guided by what that category of worker can legally do. The length of time they have worked in that position or on that unit can also give some guidance. The best way to understand what individuals can and cannot do is to have worked with them for a sufficient period of time. If you are unfamiliar with the skills of a particular worker, you will need to provide greater supervision as you begin working with that person.

Initially, you will want to delegate only those tasks that have the highest level of predictive outcome, that is, those that are routine and standard. In so doing, you also are considering the potential for harm to the client and how difficult a particular task is to perform. You will note that your process of assessment has broadened to include the patient, members of your team, and the work situation.

Plan Your Actions

At this point, you will need to compare in your mind the information you have about the skill level of your team and the nursing care activities to be accomplished. Using the information you have gleaned in your assessment, you will then identify the specific persons to whom you may delegate the various tasks. Plan the time to give them their assignments to ensure that you have adequate opportunity to clearly communicate your expectations. Also plan time for them to ask any questions they may have regarding the assignment.

Think about the situations that may require you to provide teaching and guidance to your team members. You will want to create an environment in which those you direct feel comfortable asking for assistance or instruction regarding procedures and skills with which they are less familiar. This could include the actual skill itself, but do not forget areas such as communication, priority setting, and critical thinking.

Implement Your Plan

As you begin to direct the activities of others, your instructions should be complete, easily understood, and able to be followed correctly. What activities need to be completed immediately? Which ones can be done later in the shift? What are the expected outcomes? If you are working with an individual whose primary language is not English, this may take more time (see "Communicating Effectively" in Chapter 12). Be certain that the assistants know what to

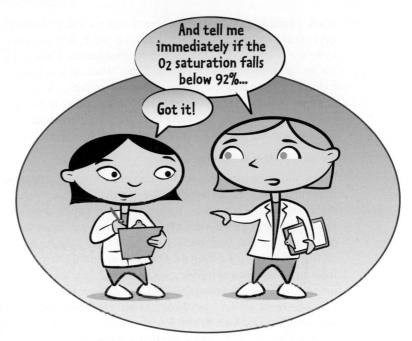

FIGURE 13.3 Good communication skills are critical to delegating tasks, setting down expectations, and providing ongoing evaluation.

report back to you and when you want to receive that information. What information can be left until the end of the shift? What data should be shared immediately (Fig. 13.3)? Listening carefully to their response to your instructions will help you to know that they have understood what you want accomplished. Watch for both verbal and nonverbal cues to their comprehension of your expectations. Ask them to repeat back to you what they plan to do and when. Ask whether they have any questions before beginning their work. Tell them where you will be if they need assistance.

Supervising care constitutes an essential part of delegation; it means that you know what is occurring with the patients and the staff, what has been accomplished, what remains to be done, and what problems may have occurred in the process. This requires that you check with individuals throughout the day to determine how they are progressing, what problems they may be having, or what assistance or instruction they may need. Asking questions such as, "How are you progressing with your task?" or "Are you having any difficulties with care?" or "Is there anything with which you need help?" will provide opportunity for feedback. If you find that a team member is behind in the tasks you have delegated, plan adjustments that will allow completion of the care. You many need to help the individual set new priorities, or you may need to find another person to assist with the completion of care if you are unable to do so yourself.

Sometimes the individual who is a novice in the supervising role finds it difficult to know when to step in and assist and when to step back. Initially, you may be so concerned about doing a good job that you micromanage the situation. When you delegate responsibilities, provide an appropriate amount of autonomy for the person to decide how to accomplish the work. Generally speaking, once you delegate a task you should not take it back. This is a good opportunity for you to use your skills as a coach. Ask questions that will help people to whom tasks are delegated find the answer for themselves. Cueing questions such as, "What did you do the last time you had this to do?" or "What do you think will work best?" stimulate individuals to begin to solve problems for themselves, elevates their self-confidence, and builds stronger teams. If your assistance is required, provide just that—assistance—rather than taking over the situation. You want to develop team members who have confidence in their own abilities and who feel they are valued members of the team.

Evaluate the Results

When you are responsible for the activities of others, evaluating the outcomes of care is more important than ever. Remember, the fact that you have delegated part of it to another person does not absolve you of the responsibility of seeing that it is completed according to established standards and in a timely manner. You will want to evaluate all patients in your care and determine that their needs have been met to the highest degree possible. Be certain that all documentation is complete and done according to standards. Talk with members of your team to obtain needed information about the care they gave and any observations they made in the process of providing that care. Asking questions such as, "Did any problems arise while care was being given?" or "How did Mr. Drummer respond to the range of motion you performed?" or "Did Mrs. Winston seem comfortable when you finished?" or "How much apple juice did Julie drink?" will help elicit responses.

If, in your evaluation, you believe there is some aspect of care that has been done well, comment on it. We all like to know our efforts are appreciated and to receive recognition for a job well done. Positive feedback is a powerful motivator. A pat on the back along with a few positive words lets people know their work is appreciated. On the other hand, if corrections need to be made in the care, be certain that such conversations occur in a private, supportive manner. Display 13.5 summarizes suggestions for delegating successfully.

Blocks to Effective Delegation

Situations exist in today's healthcare environment that result in blocks or barriers to effective delegation. If these blocks can be eliminated or reduced, delegation will be more satisfying to all who are involved.

DISPLAY 13.5   Suggestions for Effective Delegation

- Know what your team members are able to do, including their scope of practice and educational preparation.
- Plan ahead to avoid problems, decide what tasks to delegate.
- Match the task to be accomplished with the abilities of the individual to whom you are assigning the task.
- Communicate clearly the task you are delegating and your expected outcomes.
- Provide the necessary authority and responsibility to accomplish the task to the individual to whom you are delegating.
- Monitor and assess the performance of the task.
- Provide positive feedback as is appropriate; take corrective action when necessary.

▶ *EXAMPLE*

Appropriate Delegation of Tasks

Annett Jordon, RN, is employed in the labor room of a busy metropolitan hospital. The staff members are experiencing a particularly busy morning, with all birthing rooms full and several mothers expected to deliver within the next hour. Nursing administration has sent another RN, Belinda, to the area to assist with care. Annett quickly interviews the floated RN about her experience in the birthing area and determines that it is minimal and occurred 2 years ago when Belinda was a student. She determines that Belinda has had recent experience in recovery room. She decides to assign Belinda to the care of two mothers who have just delivered. She asks that Belinda check their blood pressure every 15 minutes, take their pulse, watch until IVs have been completed and then discontinue them, assess for full bladders, and check lochia. She assures Belinda she will return to check the height and condition of the fundus. In this situation, Annett carefully assessed the situation and the person who had been sent to assist on the unit. By her careful attention to the principles of delegation, she ensured that all the patients had appropriate professional nursing care.

Lack of Job Descriptions

The first serious block to good delegation is the lack of current and complete job descriptions for all employees within the institution. As mentioned earlier, the RN must know the abilities and competency of members of the nursing team. These are most commonly found in the job descriptions of the institution. As new positions are created, management should distribute up-to-date job descriptions. This will help ensure that the individual responsible for delegating tasks has access to the information and can use it for decision making. Similar to this problem is that of job descriptions that are not kept current. Jobs may be changed and tasks redistributed, but job descriptions reflecting these changes may not be completed. Thus, those needing the information find themselves having to make decisions without being fully informed.

Time Required to Delegate and Supervise

A second concern rests with the time required to effectively delegate and supervise. Many nurses believe they do not have enough time to spend with their patients. Time that is taken to plan, implement, supervise, teach, coach, and evaluate activities delegated to others may be viewed as taking even more time away from that spent at the bedside. This is especially true when working with inexperienced UAPs, who may require a lot of teaching and support. The high rate of turnover in UAP positions heightens the frustration. There are no simple answers to this problem. To some extent, these are system problems that need to be addressed at a level higher than the individual nursing unit. The best action you can take in such situations may be to let your supervisor know that the problem exists. Perhaps longer periods of orientation can be planned for the assistants or better screening in the hiring process.

Inadequate Training

A final block to effective delegation rests with inadequate training both for those who will be involved in patient care and for those who are moving into management positions. Formal orientations to the facility and to on-the-job-type skills for the position the employee will fill help ease new employees into their roles. This is also true for those who will be responsible for supervising the new employees or who are new to the management role. It is one thing to know how to provide quality care to a small group of patients and quite another to oversee the activities of a team that is caring for a large group of patients. As with other situations in nursing, you will develop greater skill with experience.

LEADING CHANGE

When referring to **change,** we generally think about something that is altered or made to be different, something transformed or modified. As an individual who will have the responsibility for managing others, you need to know how to deal with change yourself and how to help others deal with the change process.

Origins of Change

Typically, change occurs because of **driving forces** that push individuals and organizations to change and may be internal or external. Internal forces may be twofold; they may come from within the individual organization or the individual. External forces originate outside the entity experiencing the change

Internal changes within healthcare organizations can result from new ideas about the system of nursing care delivery, changes in the way pharmacy will dispense medications, the opening of new units, or the implementation of a new computerized system for charting. All of these might be initiated because of the goal of improving the quality of patient care and/or patient satisfaction. Change might also be required to reduce costs due to economic constraints. Or it could be initiated to improve the work environment, thus creating greater employee satisfaction (eg, the introduction of a shared governance structure).

Internal forces within the individual that create the need for change may include the desire to advance oneself, to retire, to marry, to find a more challenging job, and so forth. Other internal factors, such as a desire for more efficiency, greater competence, and additional education that would give individuals greater knowledge, also create change.

External forces abound in the healthcare environment. Some external factors that create the need for change in the healthcare field include technology, healthcare legislation, medical and nursing research, new standards, and changing population demographics. How many specific examples of each of these can you cite? What would you add to the list? Regardless of the reason for the change, you can anticipate that things will not remain the same. And whether the change is internal or external, whether it is within the individual or the organization, you will want to be able to work with the change and, if in the position of providing leadership, be able to assist others in the process.

Planned and Unplanned Change

Planned change has been defined as "the deliberate design and implementation of a structural innovation, a new policy or goal, or an overt change in operating philosophy, climate, and style" (Thomas & Bennis, 1972, p. 289). Thus, planned change has a definite design and structure established to facilitate the process, including time lines, identification of stakeholders, goals, plans for implementation, and processes for evaluation. Thoughtful planning often results in more effective and efficient change processes and is essential for projects that are complex or large in scope and that require greater time, resources, or skills.

Change also may be unplanned and occur as a reaction to another issue. This is referred to as **reactive change**. Reactive change occurs when some problem or event arises that requires a different way of doing things.

► *E X A M P L E*

A Case of Wrong Medication Setting the Stage for Change

A nurse on a medical unit of a community hospital became concerned when she noticed that the Toprol-XL, a medication to treat hypertension, sent from the pharmacy looked different from the medication she had administered to a patient for the previous dose. She placed a call to the pharmacy, and a pharmacist came to the unit to double-check the medication. The medication order had been filled with Topamax, an antidepressant used in the treatment of seizures. A team was quickly put in place to recommend actions to prevent such incidents from occurring. The final result of this team process was a requirement that prescribers include both the trade and generic names of a drug and that the indication for ordering be written on all medication orders. Additionally, nurses were required to confirm that the drug ordered was appropriate to the patient's condition.

Lewin's Theory of Change

Kurt Lewin's (1951) force field theory of change is one of the most widely accepted theories and remains in current use today, particularly with planned change. In order for change to occur, an imbalance must exist between the forces that call for change—the driving forces, which push the system toward change and the **restraining forces** that pull the system away from change. These may include economic factors that make the change too expensive. It might be the lack of staff who have the knowledge and skills to make the change. In some instances, it may be that the change dramatically affects one group more than others and the group strongly resists the change. Systems may maintain equilibrium through the interaction of the two forces. Equilibrium is reached when the sum of the driving forces equals the sum of the restraining forces. For change to occur, the balance between the driving forces and restraining forces must be altered so that the driving forces outweigh the restraining forces.

Lewin's change theory identified that change has three stages: the unfreezing stage, the moving stage, and the refreezing stage.

The Unfreezing Stage

According to Lewin, the **unfreezing stage** occurs when an individual is motivated by the need to create a change. This person becomes a **change agent**, the person who seeks to create the change and is responsible for facilitating the change process with others. Having gathered data, identified the problem, and decided that change is needed, the change agent sets about making others aware of the need for change. The change agent attempts to "unfreeze" or lessen the resistance to change or selects someone else who can help to unfreeze the current position by notifying those who will be affected of the need for change and garnering their support and cooperation.

The Movement Stage

The second phase of Lewin's theory is called the movement stage. During the **movement stage**, a knowledgeable and respected person responsible for initiating the change identifies strategies that will facilitate the change and then plans and implements them. The process of facilitating change is described below.

The Refreezing Stage

In the final phase, the **refreezing stage**, the changes are integrated and stabilized and become part of the value system of the organization. The change agent helps to stabilize the change that has been made in the organization so that it becomes part of everyday operation. This step is necessary to prevent the system from reverting to old patterns of behavior. Refreezing occurs when the new behaviors have occurred frequently enough that people are comfortable with them and feel rewarded because of them. Most changes need between 3 and 6 months before being totally accepted. During this time, the change agent supports those affected by the change and helps them adapt to it.

Other Theories of Change

A number of other individuals have set forth theories related to change. Each of these theories explores a different aspect of change or addresses change from a different framework. Every theory may have value depending on the situation.

The theory of Lippitt, Watson, and Westley (1958), which built on the work of Lewin, begins by recognizing and diagnosing the problem; determining the ability to change; selecting the change; planning, implementing, and evaluating the change; and then stabilizing afterward. This presents a logical method of approaching change and may sound very much like the problem-solving methods with which you already are familiar.

Rogers and Shoemaker (1971) identified five factors that determined successful planned change: relative advantage, compatibility, complexity, divisibility, and communicability. Relative advantage refers to the change being thought of as better than the status quo. Compatibility refers to the change possessing values that are similar or compatible with the existing values held by the individual or group. Complexity suggests that simple techniques are more readily adopted than more complex ones. Divisibility states that changes attempted on a trial basis will have a greater chance of succeeding. Communicability implies that the easier the change is to describe, the more likely it will grow. The proper balance of all factors would result in achieving the desired change.

Asprec (1975) described four behaviors that help one to recognize resistance to change:

1. Active resistance through frustration and aggression
2. Organized passive resistance or resisting change as a group
3. Indifference by ignoring or attempting to divert attention elsewhere
4. Acceptance on the surface or by not openly opposing change

This writer emphasized the importance of decreasing the resistance in order to reach the goal set forth in the change process.

In 1990, Perlman and Takacs, focusing on the emotions change evokes and using death and dying literature as a base, listed 10 emotional stages or phases that are experienced throughout the change process. These phases include the following:

- Equilibrium—there is a sense of peace or balance before the change occurs
- Denial—the reality of a change is denied, thus draining energy from the process
- Bargaining—effort and energy go into attempting to eliminate the change
- Chaos—energy is diffused with an accompanying loss of identity and direction
- Depression—no energy remains to produce results
- Resignation—energy is used to passively accept the change

- Openness—renewed energy becomes available
- Readiness—energy is used to explore new events
- Reemergence—energy is rechanneled, resulting in feelings of empowerment

This theory focuses on the strong feelings most people have about the change process. As you work with change, explore some of the ideas described by these authors more fully.

Developing Strategies for Implementing Change

Along with the theories that have been developed to explain and facilitate the change process, strategies for implementing change have also been identified. We will discuss some of the most commonly recognized strategies for change.

Empirical–Rational Strategy

The **empirical–rational strategy** suggests that individuals will follow their rational self-interest once it is revealed to them (Benne, Bennis, & Chin, 1976). This means that people will accept change when they see it as desirable and when it fits with their personal interests. This strategy is based on reason and knowledge and is often used to implement technologic changes. This strategy might be useful in helping to shift from paper documentation of care at the nurses' station to one using a computer at the bedside. When individuals understand how much easier and more accurate computer charting will be, they will be more eager to learn how to use it and will learn the process more quickly.

For this strategy to be effective, it is important that every initiative for change have a clear purpose and goal. Those involved in the change process need to know why the change is necessary and what will be gained by completing it. Sometimes this is not easily accomplished, because there may not be adequate information regarding all details involved. Make efforts to collect and share as many facts and figures as is possible.

Power–Coercive Strategy

A **power–coercive strategy** is in use when a leader orders change and those with less power or position comply (Benne, Bennis, & Chin, 1976). The use of this strategy requires that the change agent have official authority to mandate the change. The compliance of those affected rests in their desire to please or with their fear of the sanctions that might accompany noncompliance—things such as loss of employment, rewards, advancement, or other benefits. We may see this strategy used when new laws are enforced, such as occurred when the minimum data set was mandated for use in long-term care.

The power–coercive strategy was more effective when management styles gave great power to individuals at the top of the organizational chart. As newer approaches to management came into place in which more decisions were made at lower levels in the administration, this strategy lost some of its effectiveness.

Normative–Reeducative Strategy

The **normative–reeducative approach** states that change will take place only after changes have occurred in values, attitudes, skills, and significant relationships (Benne, Bennis, & Chin, 1976). To accomplish this, those who will be involved in the change must necessarily be included in working out the plans for the change. Mutual trust and collaboration are hallmarks of the process. If conflict occurs, the process of change must be delayed until the conflict is resolved. Table 13.2 summarizes these three strategies for change.

Table 13.2 **Strategies for Change**

Empirical–rational	Individuals will accept change when they see it as desirable and fitting with their personal interests.
Power–coercive	A leader orders change and those with less power must comply.
Normative–Reeducative	Change will take place only after there have been adjustments in values, attitudes, skills, and significant relationships.

From Benne, K. D., Bennis, W. G., & Chin, R. (1976). Planned change in America. In W. G. Bennis, K. D. Benne, R. Chin, & K. E. Corey (Eds.), *The planning of change.* New York: Holt, Rinehart and Winston.

Selecting the Change Agent

Once the decision has been made to implement a change, some person or group must be responsible for leading that change. A change agent (see discussion above) may initiate change, assist others in understanding why the change is needed and what it involves, recruit support, manage the change process, and/or assist in resolving conflict (Martin, 2009). This may be an individual within the organization who is particularly knowledgeable about theories of change and skilled in assisting people in the process of change, or it may be someone hired from outside the organization who has the skills needed to bring about the process. On occasion, teams are established to bring about a change. To be effective, the change agent must be able to affect the attitudes of others through interpersonal influence, power, or control. In organizations that have adopted continuous quality improvement, the change agent is often referred to as the **champion**. Within that system, anyone could have an idea for improvement of the organization.

Facilitating Change

As with many other management and leadership skills, facilitating change can be learned. One of the first aspects that must be recognized and dealt with relates to overcoming the resistance to the change.

Understanding Resistance to Change

Because making a change will require that we alter the way we have been doing things, most people are initially resistant to change. In 1990, Senge stated resistance to change "arises from threats to traditional norms and ways of doing things" (p. 88). We become comfortable with the way that things have been done and may be apprehensive of new approaches that require us to change established patterns of behavior. The new approaches may take additional time to learn or may be threatening to us if they involve skills with which we are not entirely familiar. Resistance to change may be the basis of sayings such as, "If it's not broken, don't fix it." In some instances, resistance to change occurs because of fear for job security. People may be concerned that the change will eliminate their position or that they will not be able to handle the demands required by the change. Overcoming resistance to change is a major role of the change agent.

Most authorities on change agree that change is most easily implemented when it is the result of a collaborative process (the normative–reeducative approach). This means involving everyone who is going to be affected by the change or those referred to as **stakeholders**. All persons involved need a good understanding of the change, why it is necessary, how it is to be accomplished, and what will be the benefits. Suggestions from those affected by the change need to be built into the change model whenever possible. Mutual trust and respect must exist among all persons working with the change.

DISPLAY 13.6   Communication Skills for Facilitating Change

- Communicate openly, frequently, and honestly
- Provide as much information as possible
- Allow for questions and suggestions
- Accept feedback constructively
- Address rumors quickly
- Supply facts when perceptions are incorrect
- Listen actively to people's concerns, feelings, and objections
- Remain matter-of-fact and avoid being argumentative or defensive

The Importance of Communication

One of the most valuable tools for facilitating change and overcoming resistance to it is communication. Communication should remain open throughout the entire process. The whys and hows of the change need to be communicated frequently, and regular feedback should be provided. When questions arise, answer them in an honest and straightforward manner. Often during the change process, rumors will begin to circulate. Address these rumors as quickly as possible and supply facts where perceptions are incorrect. Listen to and address the concerns of those affected by the change to the best of your ability. People need the opportunity to express their fears and possible losses they believe will occur when the situation is changed. They need time to grieve those losses. Their feelings need to be accepted, not disputed. Provide opportunity for input and suggestions and implement these when possible. Display 13.6 identifies some of the communication skills to be used in facilitating change.

COMMUNICATION IN ACTION

Resistance to Developing New Processes

Janet Chasey, a unit manager on the medical floor, announced, "Hi folks, thanks for taking the time to come to this staff meeting. I'll be very brief because I know you all have things to do and places to go. The only agenda item is to inform you that a committee is being formed by nursing administration to develop and implement a standardized approach to communication between caregivers when patients are moved from one department to another within the hospital." One nurse responded, "It really isn't fair to ask us to take on a committee when we are already overworked." Another said, "It just sounds like more paperwork to me! We don't need that!" A third spoke up, "I think the forms and taped messages we currently use are more than adequate. Why change what isn't broken?" Janet patiently explained, "There is a new standard set by The Joint Commission. It requires that we have a standardized process to ensure that all information about the patient's condition is shared, including allergies, potential problems, medications, and stability of vital signs." She further explained, "The whole purpose of this is to make patient handoff safer, and I know that is your concern too. Maybe one or two of you might like to be involved in developing the process and help shape the direction it takes." Elsa, who had graduated from her nursing program the previous year, spoke up, "I have never been involved in setting up a policy or procedure. It would probably be a good thing to learn. You can put me down for that committee." By respecting their concerns, explaining carefully, and pointing out shared goals, Janet was able to achieve her objective of having a unit member participate.

Assessing the Setting

Before beginning the change process, it is important to have a good understanding of the existing power structure within the setting where the change is to occur. Who within that area gets things done and makes things happen? Where is support typically found? Where—or with whom—can obstacles be anticipated? Are there values one must be sensitive to? Are there factors present that could prevent the change from taking place?

If you are in a position to decide whether to make a change, or when to make that change, consider when the last change occurred in the area. Because change is stressful to individuals, there needs to be downtime between changes. Abrahamson (2004) identifies a condition he calls repetitive-change syndrome, of which change-related chaos is a part. Change-related chaos refers to the continuous state of upheaval that happens when too many changes are trying to be instituted. People lose track of who's doing what and why and may become anxious, cynical, frustrated, and/or burned out. If it is possible, delay making a change if those affected by it have recently experienced other changes.

Thinking and Planning

Successful change is well thought out and planned. A process similar to that which you have used in the application of the nursing process provides good guidance. First of all, once a problem that might benefit from change has been identified, data need to be gathered that will assist with the diagnosis of the problem. Is it a problem? Why is it a problem? Who does it affect? How are they affected? Might there be a better way to approach the situation? What would the costs be in terms of time? What would be the personal cost to those affected? What would be the effects of not addressing the problem? Should we move forward with the change or look for other solutions?

Once a reasonable amount of data have been gathered, begin to plan. Who needs to be involved? Who should be the key players? How might the change best be implemented? When would be the best timing? What resources will be needed? What needs to be done to help those affected to unfreeze? What needs to be built into the plan that will help to ensure that the changes remain in place? What additional training and education will be necessary? Display 13.7 highlights these questions.

Early in this process, those who are going to be affected by the change need to be included. They need to be informed of intentions to make changes and be brought into the collaborative process for planning. Mutual objective setting will help motivate others toward change. Smith (1996) includes, as one of his management principles related to change, ensuring that each person always knows why his or her performance matters to the purpose and results of the whole organization. Providing maximum information about the change is important, as is calming concerns about its personal effects. Those who will be affected need to realize how they can benefit from the change. Positive relationships must be built between the change agent and those experiencing the change.

Implementing the Change

Once plans are well formulated and people who will be affected have full information as well as a role in the process, the change needs to be implemented. Establishing a timetable is often useful.

Generally, it is wise to implement change as quickly as possible. The slower the change process, the greater the opportunity for individuals affected by it to ruminate on how things were,

DISPLAY 13.7 **Questions to Consider When Planning for Successful Change**

Questions About the Situation:
- Is the present situation a problem?
- Why is it a problem?
- Who is affected by the problem?
- How are they affected?
- Is there a better way to approach the situation?
- What would be the costs in terms of time?
- What would be the personal cost to those affected?
- What would be the effects of not addressing the problem?
- Should a change be initiated or should other solutions be sought?

Questions Related to Planning:
- Who needs to be involved?
- Who should be the key players?
- How might the change best be implemented?
- What would be the best timing?
- What resources will be needed?
- What needs to be done to help those affected "unfreeze"?
- What additional training and education will be necessary?
- What needs to be built into the plan that will help to ensure that changes remain in place?

to build up anger, and to develop fears and resentment. Once dates have been announced, it is unwise to change them or to postpone actions, because people will become suspicious and/or critical of the process. If delays are necessary, share the full explanation of the reason(s) for the delay. This is a continuation of the open communication process. Recognize and praise positive efforts toward making a change. Celebrating milestones of accomplishment throughout the entire process can generate team spirit. It helps create feelings of well-being about the change and builds a bond among those who are involved in it.

Evaluating the Change Process

Monitor the change process throughout its implementation and evaluate it after it is completed to determine whether the change is accomplishing the desired outcome. Evaluation provides information about how people are adjusting to the change and how satisfied they are with it—data that are crucial to sustaining the change. When implementing and evaluating change, remember that change does not occur instantly but rather over a period of time. Additionally, the pace of change is not regular. It tends to have periods when it slows down and other periods when there are spurts. The slower periods can be viewed as reflective time, when the individuals involved in the change have the opportunity to assimilate new facts, approaches, values, and other items involved in the change.

Standardizing and Refining the Change

For a change to be sustained, it must be standardized and refined. The change agent, if outside the usual staff, needs to transfer responsibility for the continuance of the project to the participants in the change. If the change requires modifications in policies or protocols, those need to be written and incorporated in organizational manuals. People who have made notable contributions need to be recognized for their efforts.

It is through careful planning, implementation, and follow-up that successful change occurs. Flexibility in addressing and adjusting problems that arise is important. Interpersonal relationships need to be given high priority during this time.

Responding to Change

As a new graduate, you most likely will be one of the individuals affected by change rather than the one trying to implement change. How will you react if a change must occur on the unit to which you are assigned? Will you drag your feet and be one of the last to accept the change, or will you be one of the first to join the change team? How can you be an effective participant?

Learn About the Change

Take all available opportunities to learn about any anticipated changes. Attend scheduled meetings and read all announcements that are circulated. If there are matters that seem unclear to you, ask questions at the appropriate time. Learn what the benefits will be for you and for others. Discuss your thoughts and findings with others and share any suggestions you have. Validate any information about which you may not be certain. Rumors often run rampant during the process of change. Be sure you are dealing with facts rather than rumors.

▶ *EXAMPLE*

Concern for a Job During Restructure

The nurses on 4-South knew that their unit was in serious need of remodeling and updating. Yet, when it was announced that patients would be transferred and the unit would be closed, many became concerned about their positions. Small groups of nurses would gather in corners and ask questions of one another. Nurses discussed it during their coffee breaks. Soon a rumor was circulating that they would all be laid off during the remodel. Several decided to submit their resignations and look for work elsewhere. After receiving three resignations from the same unit within 1 week, the head of the human resources department made an appointment to talk with the surgical supervisor about the resignations. Afterward, the supervisor immediately scheduled a meeting with the unit staff. He explained the plans for the remodel and the time lines and assured the unit staff that during the remodel process, they would all be assigned to other units. He further explained that individual appointments would be made with each employee to determine that person's work preferences.

Express Your Concerns

As you learn about the anticipated changes, you may develop concerns about various aspects. If you have concerns, express them. If you are anxious, there are probably others who share your feelings. Remember that most often those who are closest to a situation are the individuals who understand it best. When setting forth your concerns, think a minute before you speak. Organize your thoughts. Be clear, concise, and unemotional. Speak clearly in a well-modulated voice.

Actively Listen

We often are encouraged to actively listen when working with others. Active listening involves focusing entirely on what the other person is saying and refraining from other mental activities (Fig. 13.4). This works well in many situations, including conflict, which we will discuss later in this chapter.

The following behaviors are usually included in active listening:

- Always be respectful and courteous.
- Use constructive language, both in verbal and nonverbal (eg, body language) communication.
- Remain calm and unemotional.
- Maintain eye contact.
- Do not interrupt.
- Be serious but cheerful.
- Use nondirective techniques to encourage the person to share concerns.
- Ask for clarification as needed to facilitate your understanding.

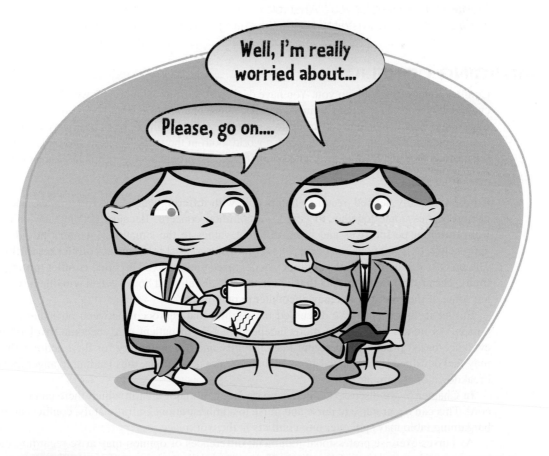

FIGURE 13.4 Active listening means focusing entirely on what the other person is saying and avoiding other mental activities.

Listen very carefully to the responses that are given to your concerns. If you are not clear about what has just been said, ask the other individual to please repeat it. Too often, people are so busy thinking about what they will say next that they do not hear the explanations that are being provided.

You will find that if you actively participate in the change, it will be much easier to move into the new behaviors it may require. Change can be energizing for some individuals. It often opens the door for new opportunities. It can provide empowerment and enjoyment if managed correctly.

Critical Thinking Activity

You have just learned that a new form of charting is being initiated on your unit. As a new employee, you have just become comfortable with the current system, which was quite different from anything you used as a student. You are dismayed that you will now need to learn a new system. What steps can you take to participate effectively in this change? How can you develop a more positive attitude toward this change? What will facilitate the process for you? What role do you see for yourself in the change process? If you become really frustrated during the change process, to whom will you speak?

MANAGING CONFLICT

Conflict is not a new topic to you. You have dealt with it from the time you were a child. Like change, it is a part of everyday living. The very nature of conflict is what keeps attorneys, marriage counselors, mediators, and arbitrators in business. Our ability to work positively with conflict may determine our success in today's world, both in the work situation and outside of it. It is critical that you learn to deal with conflict, because progress stops if it is left unresolved.

Conflict and Nursing

Conflict, broadly defined, results when people with differing values, interests, goals, needs, or approaches come together to address a common concern. Because people view things from different perspectives and bring different values to the situation, incompatible ideas, approaches, or resolutions can occur. The settling of a conflict is known as **conflict resolution**. The process through which the conflict is recognized and resolved is called **conflict management**. The critical element is not that conflicts come about—but how we deal with them. What are some of the conflicts you may encounter in nursing?

Earlier in this chapter, we discussed the conflict that can occur between physicians and nurses. As nurses command a more independent role in patient care, become involved in evidence-based practice, and accept responsibility and accountability for their actions, they may feel devalued if their suggestions for care are not acted upon, thus leading to anger and a breakdown of communications.

In Chapter 5, we discussed collective bargaining, a major area in which there can be discord. This can occur nurse to nurse and nurse to administration. Unfortunately, conflicts at the bargaining table may spill over into conflicts in the workplace.

As nurses exercise professional judgment, differences of opinion may arise regarding the best approach to treatment for a client. There may be disagreements about staffing patterns, particularly during the holidays. Overlapping roles can result in conflict, and not having sufficient resources, either monetary or physical, can cause discord. Often, the utilization of space in the healthcare environment leads to conflict.

These represent just a few of the many situations in nursing in which disagreements can happen. Conflict leads to stress and the disruption of professional relationships. As you will see in Chapter 14, the consequence of all this can be burnout.

The Positive Side of Conflict

Conflict can have positive aspects; not all conflict is serious, ominous, or intimidating. Conflict can result in personal growth and development. We learn by contrasting our values and beliefs with those of others. As we learn about others, we learn about ourselves.

Conflict can provide the impetus for change. It can contribute to innovation and creativity. When conflict is a major part of any operation, reasons for its presence must be sought and alternatives set forth. Thus, new approaches are tried. Conflict also helps employees of an organization to have a better understanding of one another's jobs and responsibilities. As healthcare becomes more specialized, differences become greater and give rise to conflict. Conflict may result in people from different areas sitting down and talking to resolve the problem (Fig. 13.5). As talk continues, a greater appreciation for others can develop, thus creating unification within the organization.

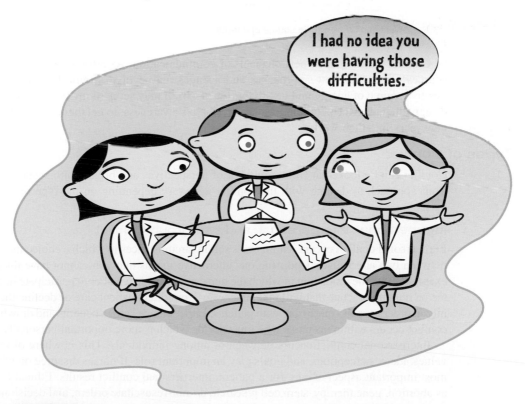

FIGURE 13.5 When people from different areas sit down to talk to resolve a problem, they often gain a greater appreciation for one another.

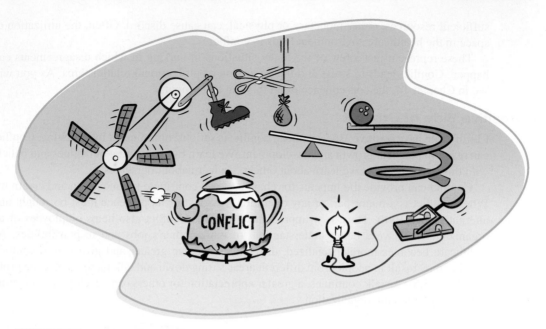

FIGURE 13.6 Conflict can be a positive source of energy.

Conflict can also open new channels of communication. As efforts are made to eliminate sources of conflict, new approaches and avenues may evolve. Similarly, conflict can be a positive source of energy and creativity (Fig. 13.6). It may serve to invigorate people. A good disagreement has the potential to sharpen people's awareness, to get them thinking, and to put new spark into their work.

Types of Conflict

Conflict can be looked at from a number of perspectives and broken into several categories. Your approach to dealing with the conflict may vary depending on the type of conflict that exists.

Intrapersonal, Interpersonal, and Intergroup Conflict

Intrapersonal conflict occurs within one's self in circumstances in which a choice must be made between two alternatives. Choosing one alternative means that you cannot have the other. An example would be a situation in which the nurse must decide whether to participate in a committee on nursing practice that will take time away from direct patient care or decline the opportunity in order to spend more time with patients. Either choice carries benefits and drawbacks. The conflict occurs within the nurse who must decide which is more important personally.

Interpersonal conflict occurs between or among individuals. This is where differences in values, ideas, perceptions, and goals play an important role. If nurses disagree on which is the most important aspect of care for a patient, interpersonal conflict results. Ethical issues such as abortion, gene therapy, stem cell research, do-not-resuscitate orders, and decisions to withdraw or withhold treatment can result in conflict among those responsible for delivery of care. Different leadership styles and organizational climates can also result in interpersonal conflict.

▶ *EXAMPLE*

Too Many Managers

The unit manager on 5-South decided to accept a higher position in the organization. He was replaced by an interim manager. Within a month, a permanent new manager was hired to provide leadership to the staff on the unit. As a result, within a short period of time, nursing staff members on the unit had worked with three different managers, each with a different management style and different expectations. This caused unrest and increased conflict among members of the staff. These confrontations, disagreements, and episodes of anger gave evidence of the stress created by the changes.

Critical Thinking Activity

Think of an interpersonal conflict that you recently observed or in which you were involved. What was the basis of the disagreement? How did the individuals conduct themselves during the heat of the conflict? How were the issues resolved? How might the conflict have been avoided?

Intergroup conflict is seen when two or more groups of people or departments struggle for power, authority, territory, or resources. Each group operates within its own value system, attributing negative stereotypes to the other group. This can be especially true if the group includes racial minorities who feel discriminated against. Today we find conflicts occurring among the four generations of nurses, each with their own orientation to workforce responsibilities, working together on nursing units (Kupperschmidt, 2006). Intergroup conflicts also occur between those who work on different shifts of a nursing unit—the evening shift personnel critical of the day shift and the day shift people believing that their job is harder than that of the evening shift. Intergroup conflicts might also occur between the nursing staff and another department in the hospital, such as housekeeping, over priorities related to work responsibilities. Intergroup conflicts can increase in both number and perception when those in one group spend time recounting to others within their group all the perceived inadequacies of the other group. As they do this, they may gather additional anecdotes to support their own perceptions. Thus, the conflict is maintained and spread.

Organizational Conflict

Some conflicts originate within the structure and function of an organization. Typically, the policies, procedures, channels of communication, and style of management, and similar factors related to organizational operations generate them. These are termed **organizational conflicts**. In organizational conflict, the leader's role and behavior are particularly important to both the origin of the conflict and to the resolution of issues.

Role ambiguity and role conflict are major causes of organizational conflict. **Role ambiguity** refers to a situation in which the role is not clearly defined. **Role conflict** occurs when two or more individuals have role descriptions that overlap. This frequently occurs because of the lack of good job descriptions and clear communications regarding what is expected. An example of role conflict might be seen in the provision of discharge planning. Both the

RN and the social worker clearly may view this as an important aspect of their professional responsibilities, and the job descriptions of both may include this aspect of patient care.

The structure of the organization may also lead to conflict. The term "turf" refers to the territory that one or one's group controls. Turf battles are not uncommon in organizations, with various individuals within the system attempting to protect, expand, or advance the area for which they are responsible. Again, good job descriptions, organizational charts, chains of command, channels of communication, and the like will minimize the advent of this type of problem (see Chapter 5).

Conflict within an organization also can arise when a scarcity of resources exists. Scarcity of resources refers not only to money but also to supplies, equipment, space, personnel, and similar necessities. When the budget for the organization is developed, not all requests are likely to be funded. Competition occurs as various departments vie for the resources that are available. When nursing shortages occur, conflicts related to securing and retaining adequate nurse staffing can be anticipated.

Conflict Outcomes

Filley (1975) identified three positions or outcomes of conflict that have become so well known that they are often included in our everyday language.

One type of outcome addressed by Filley (1975) is the lose–lose outcome, in which there are no winners: the resolution of the conflict is unsatisfactory to both parties. An example can be seen in collective bargaining relationships that stalemate and go to arbitration where a decision is made that neither side finds totally acceptable.

A second type of outcome is referred to as win–lose outcomes, in which one person obtains desired goals in the situation and the other individual fails to receive what is desired. The most obvious example of this would be elections for public office, in which decisions are made by majority rule with only one winner possible. An example in a hospital environment might be one unit receiving all the money available for new equipment, while the other areas receive none. Although this may have been the most prudent approach if the budget for new equipment was very small, it remains an example of a win–lose situation with one department actually getting what it needed (winning) and others receiving none (losing).

The most desirable type of outcome is the win–win outcome. In such situations, both parties walk away from the conflict feeling they have achieved most of the things that were important to them. For example, if we are working on a project and everyone feels good about it when it is done and each individual reaps some rewards, it is a win–win situation for all. If both units received an equal amount for equipment from a constrained budget, both might feel they had won in the situation that existed. In collective bargaining, a collaborative approach may result in both employer and employee feeling that they achieved desired goals, and thus there was a "win–win" outcome.

Strategies for Coping with Conflict

The approach that you use to deal with conflict will depend on a number of factors. The nature of the conflict, the individuals who are involved, your ability to influence the outcome, and the possibility of retribution are all elements that will affect the situation. On occasion, conflicts occur that are not worth the effort of resolving. Thus, a wide variety of approaches to the management of conflict exist. They tend to fall into one of five categories.

Withdrawing From or Avoiding Conflict

You employ the strategy of avoiding or withdrawing from the conflict when you choose not to address the issue at hand. Some would also refer to this as denying the existence of the conflict, sometimes with the hope that if it is ignored it will go away. There are many times when this approach is appropriate. This includes situations in which the conflict clearly is not your problem, when there is little or nothing that you can do about it, when there is more to lose than to be gained by becoming involved, when you lack sufficient information about the conflict and its cause, or when the problem will straighten itself out if given time. It is also a good approach to use if the situation is volatile and individuals need some time to regain composure. For example, one of two staff nurses who are becoming distressed about an issue might say, "You may be right, let's find a time to talk about it later." The issue may never be discussed later, or the parties involved in the disagreement may gain new understandings that change their perspectives.

Although appropriate at times, avoiding conflict is often preferred by people who are very uncomfortable with conflict situations, and it may not be the best approach. In a competitive society, individuals who will back away from a conflict can be taken advantage of. It is important to learn to advocate for yourself as well as for your clients. An example might be a situation in which both you and another nurse want to be off duty on Halloween evening so that you can participate in your children's trick-or-treat activities. Although the other nurse enjoyed that evening off last year, you again concede to her request because you do not want to deal with her comments and criticisms if you are awarded the evening off.

Smoothing or Accommodating

Smoothing or accommodating conflict involves trying to relieve feelings associated with conflict without solving the underlying problem. It may involve apologizing for something that is not one's fault, stating agreement with a position with which one does not truly agree, or taking action that one does not really support to stop the feelings of conflict from occurring. Similar to avoidance of the issue, smoothing or accommodating also may be referred to as surrendering to the conflict. In such situations, it is easier not to address the issue and to deal with feelings of anger than it is to deal with the conflict.

This approach may be used by individuals with a strong need to be liked, or those who are overly concerned with the welfare of others. They tend to take a self-sacrificing approach that will result in a peaceful environment. An individual who wishes to preserve harmony or build up social credits may employ this technique.

Smoothing or accommodating may be appropriate and the best approach if the conflict and anger that accompanies it disrupts the work situation or interferes with the immediate needs of the patients. In such situations, harmony and constancy are important. If the outcome does not matter to you, or if you obviously are wrong, this is a good approach. If you have little chance to win, or if this represents a situation in which you can lose the battle but win the war, it is appropriate. Consistently using this approach may make one feel "put upon" and as if you don't count in the organization.

Forcing the Issue or Competing

Competing or forcing the issue in a conflict situation means you are working exclusively for your own solution to the problem. You may have taken this approach because you believe you know more about the issues involved than others or when your values will allow no other compromise. Typically, individuals who use this approach are accustomed to being the winner and often fail to consider the needs and opinions of others. Thus, it can prevent good problem solving and innovative approaches. This would be considered a win–lose outcome—one person wins, others lose. It is an aggressive approach that could result in retaliation at another time. However, it might be the best approach if you observe a violation of ethical or legal standards.

Negotiating and Compromising

Compromising and negotiating involve give-and-take; one factor is balanced against another. It is the approach to the conflict seen in collective bargaining—one factor in the situation is balanced against another. It serves to minimize the losses for all parties while allowing each to realize some gains. It may be the approach of choice if the opposing goals are so incompatible that no resolution can be reached and discussion has stalled. It also would be appropriate if an immediate settlement to the issue were needed because of time constraints or other factors.

Problem Solving and Collaborating

Although problem solving or collaborating to achieve a mutually agreed-upon plan of action may be the most difficult to achieve, many believe this to be the best approach to conflict. It encourages participants in the conflict to work toward common goals and to work toward consensus. The process can be time-consuming and requires that all persons involved come to the table willing to examine and discuss issues openly and honestly. If effective in resolving the conflict, it is viewed as a win–win situation for everyone.

Personal Preparation for Conflict

If you find yourself in a conflict situation, try to be as prepared as possible to deal with the conditions at hand. This is often hard to do at the time the conflict occurs.

One of the best techniques is to practice for the situation. Rehearse what you will say. Think about the tone of your voice, the speed with which to talk, and your body language. Think positively about yourself. Be confident. Visualize what a successful interaction would be like.

When engaged in the confrontation, do not interrupt others. Give them an opportunity to express their position. When they talk, practice the good listening skills discussed earlier in this chapter. Insist that you are given the same courtesy of uninterrupted explanation. Politely saying, "Please let me finish" usually ensures that you can continue presenting your position.

Be clear and concise in presenting your point of view. Long, complicated presentations lose everyone's interest. Be assertive but considerate of others.

If you find that you are involved in conflict situations more frequently than most other individuals, a personal inventory is appropriate. Questions you should ask yourself might include the following:

- Do I have good relationships with most of my coworkers?
- How do I manage stress in other situations?
- Do I have the proper balance between work and relaxation?
- Do I feel competent in this situation?
- Do I hold personal biases that are interfering with my interactions with others?
- What else is going on in my life?

If after completing this inventory you find there are areas that give you concern, they can be addressed in an appropriate manner. If you are experiencing high levels of stress in any area of life, you may find yourself more easily in conflict with others and less able to manage conflict effectively. If there is a lack of opportunity for relaxation in your life, you can adjust your schedule so that you maximize the time you spend on things that result in leisure and rest. If you feel less than competent regarding the expectations of your job, some continuing education, reading, or research may be helpful. Seeking and working with a mentor may also bring positive results. If relationships with other coworkers or in your private life are lacking, seeking the help of a qualified counselor may be the best approach.

KEY CONCEPTS

- A team is a group of people working together for a common goal. Because of the diverse disciplines that are now involved in healthcare, the effective functioning of the healthcare team is critical to the provision of quality healthcare. Trust and respect of others are key ingredients in team function.

- Nurses have key roles on the team and have a number of roles other than that of provider of care. They may serve as an educator, a patient advocate, a counselor/coach, or a manager and leader for the nursing team. They also might work in nursing informatics or in nursing research.

- Because they fill key positions on the healthcare team, the relationship between nurses and physicians must be symbolized by mutual respect and consideration. Nurses can take positive actions to help assure that this occurs.

- Many leaders in healthcare are using team-building techniques to strengthen the functioning of their teams. Team building involves setting common goals, recognizing the contribution each person makes to the team, involving others in decision making, focusing on problems rather than on individuals associated with the problem, and sharing in accomplishments.

- As important as leading a team is being a good team member. Most new graduates begin in the role of team member. You need to be able to assess your abilities as a team member.

- The coaching role is being seen more frequently in healthcare. Rather than telling a younger nurse what to do, an individual serving as a coach helps him or her search for answers, providing necessary support, encouragement, and information.

- Motivation encompasses the sum of all the factors that cause an individual to do something. To motivate individuals, the leader must understand personal behaviors and role model those that are desired in others.

- In nursing, delegation is the process by which a nurse directs another person to perform nursing tasks and activities. Nurses remain accountable for all nursing care that is provided. It is important to follow the guidelines for effective delegation and know which aspects of care can never be delegated.

- The five rights of successful delegation include the right task, the right circumstances, the right person, the right direction and communication, and the right supervision and evaluation.

- Nurses cannot delegate aspects of care that require nursing judgment, including such activities as patient assessment.

- Change is inevitable in today's healthcare environment. Individuals tend to resist change, and leaders must become familiar with the steps that will facilitate the change process.

- A number of theories of change have been developed. Many of them describe processes to facilitate change, including helping others see the need for change, involving those who will be affected by the change in the process, and stabilizing the change once it is in place.

- Three major strategies for change include the empirical–rational strategy, the power–coercive strategy, and the normative–reeducative strategy. Each one might be the appropriate strategy to use in a particular situation.

- Changes often are led by a change agent who may come from within the organization or might be hired from outside to assist with the change. Sometimes groups or teams can serve as change agents.

- A number of activities facilitate change. Good communication is primary. In addition, the environment where change is to occur should be assessed, thinking and planning need to occur, the change must be implemented, and the process evaluated. Finally, the change should be standardized and refined in order for it to persist.

- As you experience change as a new employee, you can make the process more positive by learning all that you can about the anticipated changes, understanding the benefits, asking appropriate questions of the right individuals, and respectfully expressing any concerns you may have to the right people.

- Conflict occurs in all aspects of our lives; it can be intrapersonal, interpersonal, intergroup, or organizational.

- Filley (1975) has identified three possible outcomes of conflict: the lose–lose outcome, in which both parties leave the situation feeling defeated; the win–lose outcome, in which one party wins and the other loses; and the win–win outcome, in which both parties have positive feelings about the end results.

- Strategies for dealing with conflict include withdrawing or avoiding the conflict; smoothing, suppressing, or accommodating to the conflict; forcing, fighting, or competing; negotiating or compromising; and problem solving or collaborating. There is a proper time and circumstance for the use of each strategy.

- Conflict can have positive aspects. It can provide an impetus for change, it can energize individuals, it can help persons in different roles better understand one another, and it can facilitate communication.

- If you find yourself in conflict more than is desirable, a self-inventory can be helpful. Asking yourself a variety of questions may help identify the actions you will want to take.

RELEVANT WEB SITES

Web sites relevant to this chapter can be found at thePoint, accessed through *http://thePoint. lww.com/Ellis10e* and by entering the code found on the inside cover of your text.

REFERENCES

Abrahamson, E. (2004). *Change without pain*. Boston, MA: Harvard Business School Publishing.

American Nurses Association. (1997). *Attachment I: Definitions related to ANA 1992 position statements on unlicensed assistive personnel*. Kansas City, MO: Author.

Asprec, E. (1975). The process of change. *Supervisor Nurse, 6,* 15–24

Baggs, J. G., Ryan, S. A., Phelps, C. E., Richeson, J. F., & Johnson, J. E. (1992). The association between interdisciplinary collaboration and patient outcomes in a medical intensive care unit. *Heart Lung, 32*(1), 18–24.

Benne, K. D., Bennis, G., & Chin, R. (1976). Planned change in America. In W. G. Bennis, K. D. Benne, R. Chin, & K. E. Corey (Eds.), *The planning of change*. New York: Holt, Rinehart and Winston.

Filley, A. (1975). *Interpersonal Conflict Resolution*. Glenview, IL: Scott, Foresman.

Herzberg, F. (1966). *Works and the nature of man*. New York: World Publishing Co.

Herzberg, F., Mausner, B., & Snyderman, B. B. (1959). *The motivation to work*. New York: John Wiley.

Kupperschmidt, B. R. (2006). *Addressing Multigenerational conflict: Mutual respect and carefronting as strategy.* OJIN Retrieved January 9, 2011, from http://www.nursingworld.org/—type "multigenerational conflict" into the search box.

Larsen, E. (1999). The impact of physician-nurse interaction on patient care. *Holistic Nursing Practice, 3*(2), 38–46.

Lewin, K. (1951). *Field theory in social service: Selected theoretical papers.* New York: Harper Brothers.

Lippitt, R., Watson, J., & Westley, B. (1958). *The dynamics of planned change.* New York: Harcourt, Brace & World.

Martin, S. (2009). *Change agent definition.* Retrieved April 12, 2010, from http://www.askjim.biz/answers/change-agent-definition_3754.php

Maslow, A. (1954). *Motivation and personality.* New York: Harper & Row.

McClelland, D. (1953). *The achievement motive.* Norwalk, CT: Appleton-Century-Crofts.

McClelland, D. (1961). *The achieving society.* Princeton, NJ: Van Nostrand.

McGregor, D. (1966). *Leadership and motivation.* Cambridge, MA: MIT Press.

National Council of State Boards of Nursing. (1995). *Delegation: Concepts and decision-making process.* Chicago, IL: Author.

National Council of State Boards of Nursing. (2006). *Joint Statement on Delegation: American Nurses Association (ANA) and the National Council of State Boards of Nursing (NCSBN).* (2006). Retrieved January 9, 2011, from http://www.ncsbn.org/1056.htm

Nelson, G. A. (2008). Nurse-physician collaboration on medical-surgical units. *Medsurg Nursing, 17*(1), 35–40.

Osterman, T., Bertram, M., & Büssing, A. (2010). *A pilot study on the effects of a team building process on the perception of work environment in an integrative hospital for neurological rehabilitation.* Retrieved January 9, 2011, from http://www.biomedcentral.com/1472–6882/10/10

Perlman, D., & Takacs, G. J. (1990). The ten stages of change. *Nursing management, 212*(4), 33–38.

Rogers, E., & Shoemaker, F. (1971). *Communication of innovations: A cross cultural approach.* New York: Free Press.

Rosenstein, A. H. (2002). Nurse–physician relationships: Impact on nurse satisfaction and retention. *American Journal of Nursing, 102*(6), 26–34.

Schmalenberg, C., & Kramer, M. (2009). Nurse–physician relationships in hospitals: 20,000 nurses tell their story. *Critical Care Nurse, 29*(1), 74–83.

Senge, P. M. (1990). *The fifth discipline: The art and practice of the learning organization.* New York: Doubleday.

Sirota, T. (2007) Nurse/physician relationships: Improving or not. *Nursing, 37*(1) 52–56.

Smith, D. K. (1996). *Taking charge of change: Ten principles for managing people and performance.* Menlo Park, CA: Addison-Wesley.

Thomas, J. M., & Bennis, W. G. (1972). *The management of change and conflict.* Baltimore, MD. Penguin.

Whitworth, L., Kimsey-House, H., & Sandahl, P. (1998). *Co-active coaching: New skills for coaching people toward success in work and life.* Palo Alto, CA: Davis Black Publishing.

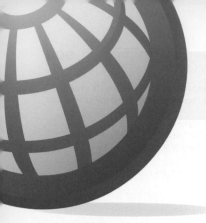

14

Facing the Challenges of Today's Workplace

KEY TERMS

Burnout	Novice to expert
Coaching	Occupational hazard
Discrimination	Preceptor
Ergonomics	Reality shock
Mentee	Sexual harassment
Mentor	Stereotypes

For many of you, graduating from a nursing program and becoming a registered nurse (RN) is the realization of a long-cherished goal. You have put a great deal of effort into preparing for this status, and now it is almost here! What you have viewed as an ideal state, freed from financial pressures that you have felt as a student and liberated from the tyranny of assignments and examinations, may prove to be quite different from what you expect. Let us consider some of the problems that may emerge as you make this transition from student to professional.

MOVING FROM "NOVICE TO EXPERT"

The path from **novice to expert** is a challenging one. Benner's (1984) classic research in this area provides a basis for an understanding of the process. Based on the work from Dreyfus and Dreyfus (1980), she examined nursing and described five stages through which an individual moves as a professional: from *novice* to *advanced beginner* to *competent* to *proficient* to *expert*. Table 14.1 presents characteristics of these skill levels.

The first role Benner identified is the *helping role*. This role encompasses planning and implementing all the basic nursing skills used to assist patients. The second, the *teaching–coaching role*, pertains to teaching patients and their families to manage their own health status and adaptations in living. The third, the *diagnostic and monitoring role,* relates to assessment and evaluation of the patient's health status and various needs. Responding to changing situations is rooted in critical thinking and a comprehensive knowledge base. While all of these roles differ between the novice and the expert category, it is in the fourth role of *responding to changing situations* that outsiders more clearly see the differences between the novice and the expert nurse. The fifth role of *administering and monitoring the therapeutic interventions and regimens* relates to the medical plan of care. The final role is the *leadership and management role* that all nurses must perform but differs for the nurse in each stage. All nurses in all stages must be concerned about quality improvement and ensuring the best healthcare practices for the patient, but expert nurses can influence changes for the system as well as changes for the individual patient.

Through interviews with nurses, Benner described the depth of nursing skills and abilities found in the expert nurse. This expertise is forged over time and results from personal experience and personal knowing. One of the challenges for beginning nurses is pressure to function as a competent, proficient, or even expert nurse without this background of growth. Competent in the Benner context reflects an ability to work independently and be responsible for decision making. This is different from the use of the term competent in many other contexts where competent means that you have the skills for your current state—that is you can

Table 14.1   **Benner's Levels of Function**

LEVEL	CHARACTERISTICS
1. Novice	No experience of the situations. Have context-free rules to guide behavior. Relatively inflexible.
2. Advanced beginner	Marginally acceptable performance. Have some experiences with real situations. Can identify "aspects of the situation" (p. 22). May formulate principles or guidelines for action.
3. Competent	Begins to see current situation in terms of long-range goals. Is able to prioritize among patients and base actions on conscious deliberate planning. May still lack speed and flexibility.
4. Proficient	Perceives situations as wholes rather than as a collection of parts. This perception is not thought out but is unconscious. Experience has given this nurse a "web of perspectives" (p. 28). Responds to nuances of the situation using maxims.
5. Expert	Has an intuitive grasp of the whole situation and does not rely on rules, guidelines, or maxims. Focuses immediately on the most critical elements of the situation. May have difficulty articulating the thought processes that resulted in decisions.

Benner, P. (1984). *From novice to expert: Excellence and power in clinical nursing practice.* Upper Saddle River, NJ: Prentice Hall.

be a "competent" novice. The transition from novice to advanced beginner to competent in Benner's categorization usually happens within the initial months of employment during an orientation period.

It is estimated that 30 to 40% of new graduates leave their first job within the first year (Kovner, Brewer, Fairchild, et al., 2007). These attrition rates are costly for hospitals and other healthcare organizations. Resources of the educational system are not well used when new graduates leave the profession soon after graduation. These writers suggest that employers should do more to manage this transition for new graduates. Strategies to support transition are being developed in many institutions. Some states have developed statewide initiatives to address this concern.

As you look for a first nursing position, learn about the mechanisms the employer has in place to facilitate your transition to the independent RN role. Is there an orientation program specially designed for new graduates? Will you have an individually assigned preceptor or mentor for support? How long will you be given support before being expected to function independently? If you feel you need more time to be independent, will the employer accommodate this need? As a new graduate, will you be expected to float to different units, or will you be helped to become competent in one area before being asked to go to another? Is there assistance with and support for continuing education for nurses to help you develop beyond the level of competent to proficient and expert? As you answer these questions, you will begin to develop a broader picture of the employer and be able to evaluate whether this job is a fit for your personal journey from novice to expert. This, along with personal preparation, may protect you from the impact of issues that lead to early retreat from nursing.

Critical Thinking Activity

Examine your own background and experience in light of the characteristics noted in Benner's levels of skill. In your analysis, identify areas where you might exhibit a particular level of skill. What do you believe is the general level of skill expected of the new graduate?

REALITY SHOCK

One problem confronted by the new graduate is the seeming impossibility of delivering quality care within the constraints of the system as it exists. You may feel powerless to effect any changes and be depressed over your lack of effectiveness in the situation. Marlene Kramer (1979) was the first to call the feelings that result from such a situation **reality shock**. She noted that the new graduate often experiences considerable psychological stress and that this may exacerbate the problem. The person undergoing such stress is less able to perceive the entire situation and to solve problems effectively (Fig. 14.1).

Effects of Reality Shock

The person experiencing reality shock may feel discouraged and depressed over the conditions of work. There may be anger toward the system, and this may result in diffused anger that erupts over situations that in other circumstances might be met with a calm demeanor.

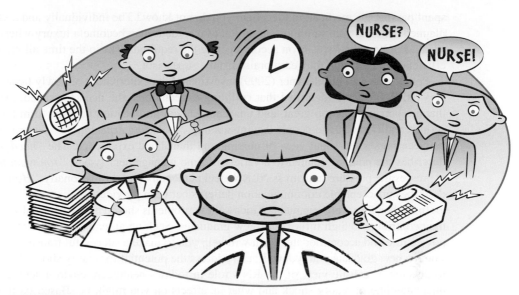

FIGURE 14.1 Some new graduates are disillusioned by the working conditions that they find on their first job.

In an attempt to cope, some push themselves to the limit, trying to provide ideal care and criticizing the system. This may result in their being labeled nonconformists and troublemakers. Still others give up their values and standards for care and reject ideals as impossibly unrealistic expectations that cannot be fulfilled in the real world. These persons simply mesh with the current framework and become part of the system. When reality shock occurs, some nurses begin to job hop or return to school, searching for the perfect place to practice perfect nursing as it was learned. Others become disillusioned and leave nursing altogether (Kramer, 1979).

Causes of Reality Shock

With all of the uncertain expectations and demands, the new graduate often feels caught in the middle. As a student, you may think that you are expected to learn a tremendous amount in an alarmingly short time. The expectations may seem high and in some ways unrealistic.

As a new graduate suddenly thrust into the real world, you may feel unsure of yourself without the security of the instructor's availability and the support of your fellow students. You may think that your education program did not adequately prepare you for what is expected of you. On one hand, you are expected to function like a nurse who has 10 years of experience, but on the other hand, your new ideas may not be considered because you have so little experience. You may become frustrated because you do not have time to provide the same type of care you gave as a student. For example, you may not have sufficient time to deal with a client's psychosocial problems or teaching needs.

As a student, you are taught that the good nurse never gives a medication without understanding its actions and side effects, and that evaluating the effectiveness of the drug is essential. As a staff nurse, you may find that the priority is getting the medications passed correctly and on time, and that there is little or no time to look up 15 new drugs. As for evaluation, that becomes a dream. How can you evaluate the subtle effects of a medication in the 2 minutes spent passing the medication to a client you do not know? The individually and meticulously planned care that was so important to you as a student may become a luxury when you are a graduate. Often the focus is on accomplishing the required tasks in the time allotted, and it is efficiency in tasks that may earn praise from a supervisor.

Pellico, Brewer, and Kovner (2009) investigated the experiences of newly licensed graduates (NLRNs). They identified that colliding expectations, the need for speed, expectations that are perceived as too great, and unacceptable communication patterns form the basis for serious reality shock and people leaving nursing. "*Colliding expectations*" describes conflicts between nurses' personal view of nursing and their lived experience. The "*need for speed*" describes the pressure related to a variety of time management issues. "*You want too much*" expresses the pressure and stress NLRNs feel personally and professionally. "*How dare you*" describes unacceptable communication patterns between providers."

In the healthcare environment of today, these problems should not be "normalized" because they contribute to high turnover of new graduates. Seeking an employer who recognizes the novice role and accommodates for it will help you to make a successful transition.

As a new graduate you, yourself, can address the potential for reality shock. You will need to develop a realistic view of the RN's role in today's healthcare environment and a better understanding of reality shock and what its effects on you might be. Based on this you can plan your own strategies to manage the issues that will confront you as a new graduate.

Finding Solutions for Reality Shock

It is possible to create a role for yourself that blends the ideal with the possible—one in which you do not give up ideals but see them as goals toward which you will move, however slowly. To do this, you need to be realistically prepared for the demands of the real world.

Self-Appraisal and Personal Development

One way of meeting the challenge is to assess yourself as you approach the end of your education program. Evaluate your own competencies in relationship to the common expectations of employers of new graduates that were discussed in Chapter 4.

After you have done a self-appraisal and gained information about prospective employers, analyze your own ability to function in accordance with an employer's expectations. If you identify any shortcomings, try to remedy them before graduation. If you identify a lack in certain technical skills, register for extra time in the nursing practice laboratory to increase your proficiency. You could even time yourself and work to increase speed as well as skill. Consult with your clinical instructor to arrange for experiences that would help you gain increased competence, especially in procedures with which you have had little experience. If you recognize that you consistently have difficulty functioning within a time frame, you might obtain employment in a hospital or other healthcare facility while still in school; this will give you more experience in organizing work within the time limits that the employer sees as reasonable.

Critical Thinking Activity

With a group of nursing students, develop personal strategies for managing reality shock. Discuss your rationale for any strategy you propose.

Evaluating Employers

It is helpful to understand what prospective employers in the community in which you plan to seek employment expect of a new graduate. You can gain this information by talking with experienced nurses, meeting with faculty, and contacting recent graduates who are currently employed. Try to get specific information. If you have a nursing student organization, setting up a forum for speakers from various agencies might be one avenue to gaining this insight. Once you apply for a position, you could explore this issue in an employment interview.

When you are selecting a place of employment, there are many factors to consider. While the specific position is important to you, there are aspects of the overall setting that will make a great deal of difference to your success. You are not as likely to experience severe stress if the employment setting is a good match for you. The professional practice environment makes a difference in the problems of reality shock and of burnout, which we will discuss.

Some hospitals attempt to help new graduates deal with reality shock by making orientation programs more comprehensive and by providing an experienced nurse to work as a preceptor to the new graduate (Scott, Engelke, & Swanson, 2008). Nurse internships or residencies in some settings have been created to provide a planned and organized transition time during which the new graduate participates in a formal program, including classes, seminars, and rotations to various units of the hospital (Dyes & Sherman, 2009). In some settings, the new graduate is required to be more self-directed in identifying needs and the ways that those might be met within the constraints of the system.

Some hospitals provide an opportunity for nursing students to work during the summer before the last year of their basic program to become familiar with the hospital and the nursing role. In this type of program, the nursing student may be employed in a role developed specifically for nursing students that includes a planned program that introduces the role of the RN. In other instances, nursing students work as nursing assistants, and the orientation to the nursing role in the agency depends on the initiative the individual takes. You may wish to inquire whether hospitals in your area have developed any of these or other programs to assist you when you are a new graduate.

Preceptors, Coaches, and Mentors

In nursing, many new graduates are assigned to a **preceptor** as part of their orientation process. A preceptor is an officially assigned role in which an experienced and capable employee assists with the orientation and development of a new graduate. Some of you may have experience with preceptors as part of your educational program. The preceptor usually has responsibility for supervising and evaluating the work of the preceptee. Some preceptors may see the role as primarily one of supervising, teaching, and evaluating in relationship to the specific job and do not see it as a broader role of encouraging professional development. Some preceptors develop personal relationships with new nurses. They act in ways described as mentoring (see below).

If you are fortunate enough to have a preceptor who becomes your mentor, you will have additional support and guidance from the beginning of your career. If your individual preceptor does not view the role that way, then you may wish to develop relationships with other experienced nurses who might provide a mentoring relationship.

Coaching is an informal teaching/helping relationship. Coaches are experienced nurses who focus on a specific aspect of growth and development such as helping a nurse to master a more advanced skill or to understand how to work within the organization. A coach may help individuals at all stages of their work life. Coaches may help an individual navigate the stressful aspects of the job by sharing tips on how to manage organizational challenges and by simply providing a listening ear.

A **mentor** is an individual who actively supports the overall professional development and growth of another person (referred to as the **mentee** or protégé). Within a professional field, the mentor is usually an experienced professional who develops a supportive relationship with someone with less experience in the profession and provides advice and emotional support for that person. Mentor–mentee relationships typically begin when an experienced senior nurse takes an interest in a nurse with beginning experience who is pursuing a similar professional pathway as the senior nurse. It often works best when it occurs spontaneously as a relationship develops between a junior and a senior employee within an organization.

The mentor usually assists the mentee with career and personal development and provides personal support, acceptance, and counseling. The mentor may sponsor the mentee and often facilitates that person's advancement within the organization by helping to establish networks and organizational know-how. Any plans for the development of the mentee need to be discussed and reviewed with periodic feedback and debriefing sessions. While the mentor may provide some direct assistance in learning the specific skills of the nursing role, more importantly, the mentor provides help in learning how to work effectively within the system. The mentor is a role model of effective practice.

A good mentor is an effective and experienced practitioner. Attributes that contribute to success for a mentor are a positive attitude, a caring approach toward others, and effective communication. Mentor training is provided by some employers and is available online (O'Keefe & Forrester, 2009). Mentees or protégés also have significant responsibilities in the relationship. The mentee must be willing to accept feedback, to try new ways of functioning, and to communicate with the mentor regarding what is helpful and what is not. Honesty and trust must lie at the heart of the relationship.

Mentor–mentee relationships change over time and may become more collegial. As you progress in your career, you may need a new mentor in a new setting or in regard to a new field of practice. When you become an experienced expert nurse you can become a mentor to others (Wroten & Waite, 2009).

Peer Support Groups

Understanding that you are not alone in your feelings of frustration in a new job is often helpful. It may be useful to form a peer support group of new graduates who meet regularly to discuss problems and concerns and seek solutions jointly. A peer support group is usually composed of new nurses at a particular facility and is often initiated by the new nurses themselves. The group meets regularly to share its experiences, offer support and advice, and help all the individuals to recognize that others are also experiencing stress during this time.

Some peer support groups are composed of individuals from a single graduating class who may be working in different settings. Although their settings differ, many of the individuals' concerns surrounding transition are similar, and their relationships with their educational program have created a bond that makes the group able to function effectively.

Personal Stress Management

Recognizing your own response to stress and identifying your personal stress management strategies will be significant. As a nursing student, you experienced stressful times and coped successfully or you would not have graduated. Remind yourself of your own successful coping and draw on the strategies you found successful in the past. As is always the case, personal health needs to be a part of those strategies. Attend to your diet, rest, and activity plan. Maintain time for family and friends in order to have balance in life. Life should never be all work.

When confronted with areas of practice in your work environment that you would like to see changed, weigh the importance of an issue. Use your energies wisely. The "politics of the possible" is important. Learn how the system in which you are employed functions and how to use that system for effective change. You are important to nursing, so it is essential that you neither burn yourself out nor abandon the quest for higher-quality nursing care. You should be able to continue to work toward improving nursing and bringing it closer to its ideals (see Chapter 13 for more information about change).

BURNOUT

Burnout is a form of chronic stress related to one's job. Burnout can occur to individuals in any occupation, and articles regarding burnout appear in the professional literature for almost all the helping or supporting professions.

This problem arises after you have been in practice for a period of time. It can be identified by feelings of hopelessness and powerlessness, and is accompanied by a decreased ability to function both on the job and in personal life. Burnout occurs more frequently in nurses who work in particularly stressful areas of nursing, such as critical care, oncology, or burn units. Some writers explore burnout as "compassion fatigue," relating it to the high stress of managing personal feelings in the face of overwhelming crises experienced by others. Burnout also occurs when staffing is inadequate or interpersonal relationships are strained. The downsizing of nursing staff and the rapid changes in the healthcare environment have contributed to burnout in some settings.

Symptoms of Burnout

Symptoms of burnout include both physical changes and psychological distress. The items found in the Maslach Burnout Inventory (Maslach, Leiter, & Schaufeli, 2009) provide an overview of symptoms that may occur in burnout. These include exhaustion and fatigue, frequent colds, headaches, backaches, and insomnia. General disinterest in the job and dreading going to work may occur. There may be changes in disposition, such as being quick to anger or exhibiting all emotions excessively. Individuals experience a decreased ability to solve problems and make decisions as burnout progresses. This frequently results in an unwillingness to face change and a tendency to block new ideas. There may be feelings of guilt, anger, and depression because one cannot meet the expectations for doing a "perfect job." Burnout begins gradually and is more effectively managed early in its onset.

In response to these feelings, some nurses quit their jobs and move on to other settings that may be outside the nursing profession. Others remain in their jobs but develop a personal shell that tends to separate them from real contact with clients and coworkers; they may become cynical about the possibility of anyone doing a good job and may function at a minimal level. A few become increasingly unable to function and find themselves in jeopardy of losing their positions.

Causes of Burnout

Many causes of burnout have been discussed in the literature. Prominent among them is the conflict between ideals and reality. Just as this is a problem for the new graduate, it is also a problem for the experienced nurse. These nurses believe they are responsible for all things to all people and often take on more responsibility, thus increasing their own stress level.

Another cause of burnout is the high level of stress that results from practicing nursing in areas that have high mortality rates. Continually investing oneself in clients who die can take a tremendous toll on personal resources. In addition, the demand for optimal functioning is constant.

Inadequately staffed institutions also may place great stress on nurses. The clients are in need of care, the nurse has the skills to provide the care, and yet the clients do not receive good care. The nurse typically tries to accomplish more, putting in overtime, skipping breaks and lunch, and running throughout the shift. Despite this effort, there is little job satisfaction because the things that are left undone or that are not done well seem to be more apparent than all the good that is accomplished.

Preventing and Managing Burnout

As an individual nurse, you can take actions to prevent burnout. These are the same general actions that are designed to control stress in any aspect of life and may help you if you believe that you are beginning to experience burnout.

Paying attention to your own physical health is an important preventive measure; this includes maintaining a balanced program of rest, nutrition, and exercise. Another important point is not to subject yourself to excessive changes over short periods of time, because changes increase stress. You may decide, for example, not to relocate your living setting (apartment or house) at the same time you change to a different shift. A period of wind-down or decompression after work will help you to avoid carrying the stress of the workplace into your private life; this period may involve physical exercise, reading, meditation, or any different activity. This may seem like a daydream to individuals who are working full-time, have responsibility for children, and perhaps also for aging parents. Yet, it is important that some personally rewarding activity be incorporated into the daily routine. The activity you choose should not create more demands and increase stress. An important resource is someone who is willing to listen while you express your feelings and talk about your problems. Sometimes this is a family member or personal friend, but it may be more appropriate for this to be a coworker or counselor.

Rotating out of a high-stress area, such as a burn unit or pediatric oncology, before you begin to experience burnout or when you first identify that you are beginning to burn out may allow you to rebuild resources and return to the job with enthusiasm. This can be done only if there is no stigma or blame attached to the need to rotate and if other nurses are available for replacement.

COMMUNICATION IN ACTION

Acting to Prevent Burnout

Linda Wilson returned to employment after maternity leave when her baby was 3 months old. A new critical care unit was being opened in the hospital and she eagerly accepted the invitation to work there. However, after 2 months on the 3 pm to 11 pm shift, she found she was burning out, due in part to understaffing, lots of overtime, and the critical nature of the patients for whom she cared. With the demands of the baby, she seldom got more than 4 to 5 hours sleep. She approached the supervisor of the unit and asked for an appointment to meet with him prior to beginning her shift. During their meeting Linda explained, "I am very appreciative of the opportunity to work in this unit. However, I think it was not the right time in my life to undertake such a challenge. With the demands of a new baby at home, I just do not have the energy this position demands. I get home late, often have trouble going to sleep, and the baby wakens during the night and is up early. I would like to request a transfer to a less intensive work unit." The supervisor was supportive of Linda and her request and agreed to follow through on the request for transfer.

In this communication, Linda did not blame others for the situation in which she found herself. She was honest and forthright in her explanations, and clear in her request.

Another strategy is to focus on those positive aspects of nursing that drew you to it initially. Cognitively reframing or restructuring one's thoughts about a situation to identify those parts that are positive and affirming and redirect nonproductive and self-damaging beliefs may ease stress and enhance coping (Luquette, 2007). In this case, you spend time identifying those situations where you made a difference, where you demonstrated both the art and science of nursing. You then are able to recognize when you are focusing on the problems in the situation and blaming yourself for them. Instead you refocus your attention on the fact that you did not create the situation, but that you are a positive force in that milieu.

The most effective prevention of burnout is an institution-wide stress-reduction effort to prevent burnout involving the nursing staff, supervisory personnel, the hospital administration, and other healthcare workers. The most important objective seems to be bringing burnout into the open and acknowledging the existence of the problems. This alone helps the individual nurse move away from the feelings of separation and alienation that often accompany burnout. Whatever the problems, they seem less frightening if they are defined as normal and if the individual nurse does not see himself or herself as the only person not performing as the perfect nurse. Investigate the resources that a prospective employer has to assist nurses in preventing burnout.

Employers can offer resources to prevent and manage burnout. Having adequate staff and support for taking days off and vacation time are all ways employers can help fight burnout. In client care areas that are known to be stressful, it is helpful to have a counselor available for nurses. Consulting with this counselor should be viewed by the staff as a positive step and not as an admission of some lack or fault. The counselor needs to be someone who understands the setting and who has the skills to assist people in coping with stress.

Another approach may be initiated by individual nurses but requires the cooperation of the institution; this includes establishing group discussions during which nurses can share feelings and specific concerns in an accepting atmosphere. This sharing may lead to concrete plans to reduce the stress created by the setting. For example, if one source of stress is conflicting orders between two sets of physicians involved in care, a plan might be developed whereby the nurses no longer take responsibility for the conflict but refer the problem to some authority within the medical hierarchy. This type of resolution is possible only when the whole healthcare team addresses the problem of burnout. However, it also requires that nurses give up trying to control everything for which they feel responsible.

Giving nurses more control over their own practice often decreases stress. Although more control is limited by the constraints of the setting, it could involve flexible scheduling, volunteering for specific assignments, and participating in committees that determine policies and procedures.

Critical Thinking Activity

Compare burnout with the stress response you have studied in relation to client care. Compare the strategies that you have taught clients with those suggested for preventing burnout. Discuss these with a classmate and see how many similarities you have.

WORKPLACE SAFETY AND HEALTH FOR NURSES

Nurses have expressed concern regarding safety in the working environment for many years. Employees have a right to expect their employers to provide the safest working environment possible. Some hospitals employ an occupational health nurse to examine the working environment, and use employment practices to promote health and safety on the job. Nurses themselves, however, often have been lax in recognizing on-the-job hazards and acting for self-protection; this can be likened to the response of those who continue to smoke despite their knowledge of the health hazards of smoking, or those who fail to wear seatbelts even though some state laws require it and statistics show fewer fatalities in automobile accidents when seatbelts are worn. Some people continue to do those things that they know are detrimental to their health and well-being. Unfortunately, nurses are no exception. Personal awareness and commitment to change by each nurse is essential to correcting **occupational hazards** and other problems in the work environment (Kupperschmidt, Kientz, Ward, et al., 2010).

Nurse Staffing Levels

As acuity levels in hospitals have risen, concerns about the nurse to patient ratio have become prominent. Inadequate staffing contributes to burnout because nurses are unable to meet all the needs of patients. An even more compelling concern regarding staffing involves the increased rate of errors when the staffing is inadequate.

Across the country nurses have begun to lobby for legislation that would control staffing levels. California was the first to pass such legislation. The results of this legislation are mixed in a situation in which there have been serious nursing shortages. Because of the wording in the law, both LPNs and RNs are included in "nurses" when calculating staffing ratios.

The American Nurses Association (ANA) has launched a major campaign titled *Safe Staffing Saves Lives (n.d.).* Research has demonstrated that inadequate staffing was a contributor in unanticipated events that resulted in patient death, injury, or permanent loss of function (Needleman, Buerhaus, Mattke, et al., 2002a). On the other hand, they found that when a higher proportion of hours of registered nursing care per day are available, there are positive patient outcomes and cost-savings to the system (Needleman, Buerhaus, Mattke, et al., 2002b). The ANA recommends that institutions be required to establish appropriate ratios at the unit level through negotiation rather than mandating absolute ratios for all settings. Other groups seek mandatory staffing levels through regulation or legislation.

In settings with limited staffing of RNs other problems emerge. There may be difficulty in obtaining RN coverage for anyone who leaves the units and nurses may work an entire shift without a break. Overtime becomes more common when there are too few nurses to accomplish the needed tasks during the shift. When facilities mandate that unit staff provide their own coverage for sick days and all shifts, nurses may end up working many extra shifts. As these demands increase, the problem of nurse fatigue increases. Research is demonstrating the relationship of nurse fatigue to errors (Ellis, 2008).

Infection as an Occupational Hazard

Transmission of infection is a major concern when caring for infected clients. The presence of resistant organisms causes extra concern and makes treatment difficult. All hospitals have an infection control officer, usually an RN, who has the expertise to guide the staff in planning appropriate infection control procedures. Staff in other settings may not have access to such an expert.

The hidden danger for nurses lies in those clients who have not been diagnosed as having an infection and for whom specific infection control measures have therefore not been prescribed. Universal precautions have been mandated by the Occupational Safety and Health Administration (OSHA) for use with clients in all settings to protect staff members from blood-borne pathogens. These precautions prevent the spread of HIV, hepatitis B, and other such blood-borne pathogens.

One of the first employer actions toward preventing blood-borne diseases was the provision of sharps containers wherever needles were used. Another important employer responsibility is the provision of a supply of gloves and protective eyewear for employee use. OSHA mandates these measures as part of universal precautions. However, not all cases of transmission of blood-borne pathogens can be prevented by universal precautions. Needlestick injuries—especially those with large-bore needles (eg, bone marrow aspiration needles)—continue to be the most frequent transmission source. Wearing gloves does not prevent these injuries (Fig. 14.2).

More attention is now being given to designing needles and other sharp devices in ways that prevent needlestick injuries. For example, a needle with a protective plastic housing is available for injections. Even if these needles are not handled properly, they are unlikely to injure the individual. Needleless IV connections are also available. Syringes are available that have a protective cover into which the needle retracts immediately after use. To participate knowledgeably in decisions regarding needle systems and devices, nurses need to seek information about what devices are available. OSHA does mandate that healthcare facilities have in place a plan to reduce the risk of needlestick injuries through using safe devices. The ANA has been active in workplace advocacy related to needlestick injuries and supports a Web site devoted to this topic (*http://needlestick.org*).

Blood-borne pathogens are not the only pathogens of concern in the healthcare environment. The Standard Precautions recommended by the Centers for Disease Control and

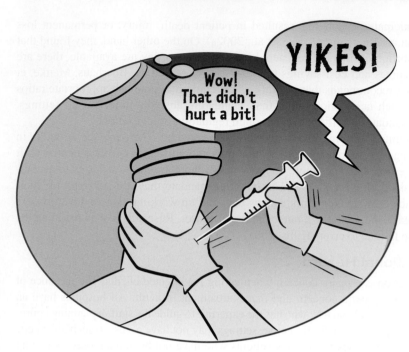

FIGURE 14.2 Needlestick injuries are a major concern in all healthcare environments.

Prevention (CDC) (Siegel, Rhinehart, Jackson, et al., 2007), often referred to as Body Substance Precautions, are used in all settings. These precautions protect clients and staff members from infections that might be transmitted by any body substance.

The incidence of tuberculosis (TB) is again on the rise, with drug-resistant strains of the organism appearing. Although rooms with special ventilation and special masks that are impervious to the TB organism are available, individuals with the disease may be in contact with healthcare providers long before they are clearly diagnosed. Should nurses in high-risk areas, such as the emergency room, wear special masks during all client contact, or is this unrealistic? These are important questions to consider.

Although the details of infection control are beyond the scope of this text, we remind you that you hold the key to protecting yourself in many ways. Healthcare workers often become lax in their attention to the use of gloves or eye protection because these measures are inconvenient. It is your responsibility to use the very best techniques for self-protection, including diligent attention to hand hygiene. Nurses must assume responsibility for their own protection by conscientiously carrying out appropriate measures at all times. Employers must be held accountable for providing the supplies and environment to make this possible.

Doing your own part in infection control also extends to maintaining your personal immunizations in order to not be a source of illness for patients or colleagues. During flu season, a healthy individual may carry a subclinical case of influenza and transmit it to vulnerable patients and all healthcare providers are urged to be immunized (CDC, 2009). Employers may pay for immunizations that will protect everyone in the healthcare environment.

Hazardous Chemical Agents

Anesthetic gases can increase the risk of fetal malformation and spontaneous abortion in pregnant women who are exposed to them on a regular basis. Standards exist for waste-gas retrieval systems and the allowable level of these gases in the air. Nurses working in operating rooms should seek information on the subject and expect hospitals to provide a safe work environment.

Chemotherapeutic agents used in the treatment of cancer are extremely toxic, and nurses who work in settings where such agents are prepared and administered should seek additional education regarding their administration, not only in relation to the client's safety but also in relation to personal safety. The employer is responsible for providing the equipment needed to maintain safety when handling these agents. In many settings, protocols now require the routine use of personal protective equipment when handling chemotherapeutic agents.

Contact with many medications, especially antibiotics, during preparation and administration may cause the nurse to develop sensitivity. This can create transitory problems (eg, a hand rash), and may be a threat if treatment for a serious infection is compromised later. Other medications are absorbed through the skin and may produce an undesirable effect. Nurses must take responsibility for their own safety regarding these agents. Nurses who understand these hazards handle all drugs with discretion and are careful not to expose themselves to these agents.

COMMUNICATION IN ACTION

Speaking up Regarding Unsafe Practice

Jose Morales, RN, worked in the medication administration area side-by-side with another RN. He noted that the RN spiked an antibiotic bag, hung the bag on a hanger, and proceeded to open the tubing to clear air but got fluid from the bag on the counter. Jose spoke up, "Hey, John, I don't mean to be overly critical, but I am concerned about antibiotics getting spilled around here. That contributes to the development of resistant organisms that are a danger to us as well as patients. Besides, you and I might get sensitized to that stuff. I learned a technique for backfilling from the primary bag so that there is never a danger of spilling. Are you familiar with that technique? I would be glad to show you."

Cleaning agents and disinfectants used in the hospital also may be hazardous if used improperly. Employers are now required by OSHA to maintain a list of all chemicals used in the work environment, along with information on their possible effects and the appropriate treatment if individuals are accidentally exposed to them. If you work with these agents, seek out this information, found in the Material Safety Data Sheets (MSDS), and be sure that you handle chemicals correctly.

Ergonomic Hazards in the Workplace

Ergonomics is the science of fitting a task to one's physical characteristics in order to enhance safety, efficiency, and well-being. When the task does not conform to one's physical characteristics, musculoskeletal stress and injuries may occur. Patient handling and transfer require the movement of a weight load beyond that which most human bodies are designed to manage. In addition, the healthcare setting often requires that patient movement and transfer be done in awkward positions and inadequate spaces. Thus, musculoskeletal disorders (MSD) are a common occupational hazard for nursing care staff (NIOSH, 2009).

Many employers have programs to prevent musculoskeletal injuries. Some institutions provide instruction in lifting, transfer, posture, body mechanics, and other back-saving strategies to help prevent injury. None of these strategies can protect an individual from repetitive stress injury from lifting more than is appropriate. Further, a patient is, by definition, unstable when being helped, and a sudden move or change in the patient can have a devastating effect on the caregiver. Mechanical lifting and transfer devices provide a means of moving clients without danger to staff members. More types of lifting and transfer devices are now available, and more employers are open to purchasing equipment to prevent these costly injuries.

The ANA, in cooperation with Johnson & Johnson, spearheaded a nationwide campaign titled "Handle With Care," aimed at safe patient transfer (ANA, 2004). In its materials titled "Safe Patient Handling" (*http://www.anasafepatienthandling.org/*), the ANA emphasized that that there is no safe way for caregivers to lift and transfer dependent patients. They advocated a no-lift policy, the use of mechanical devices for lifting and transfer, and the use of lift teams when lifting is essential. In its brochure, background statistics were highlighted to emphasize the importance of the problem, and specific suggestions for lifting strategies and approaches were provided (ANA, 2004). The ANA is also active in supporting the efforts of state constituent organizations to work for the enactment of safe patient handling state legislation which has now passed in several states. Many nursing programs are using materials from the ANA Toolkit regarding safe patient handling to teach students about this important issue.

An ergonomic concern that is growing for nurses relates to computer work stations. Those who work at computer work stations for long periods of time are subject to back, neck, wrist, and hand strain. While most nurses do not spend long periods of time at the computer, this is changing as nurses work in telephone care while sitting at computers and even spend long periods documenting care. When one individual uses the same computer station throughout the work day, that station can be adapted to the individual. However, in most nursing settings, the computer station is used by many people. Adjustability of the screen, keyboard, chair, and armrests becomes important in order to provide each person using it with an ergonomically safe work station. In many settings, computer work stations were added to an existing desk area. This may or may not serve the users well. Be alert to the problems that may occur; help yourself by maintaining correct posture and using the adjustments available; report concerns to the appropriate manager.

Be aware of the potential for musculoskeletal injury and examine your work habits. Some nurses feel that they must accomplish certain tasks even if the necessary assistance is not available and therefore carry out actions of danger to themselves. Nurses need to continue to work toward safer workplaces for all healthcare providers. They must learn to be assertive regarding their own safety (Fig. 14.3).

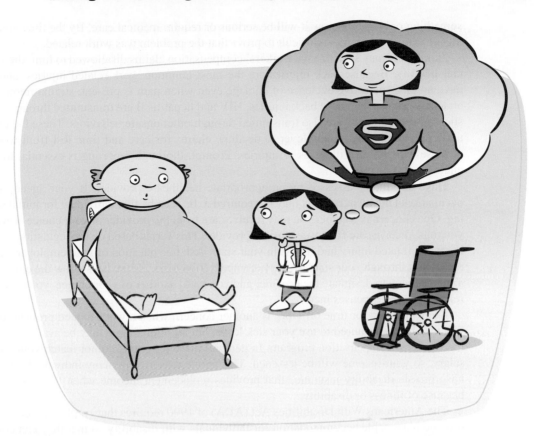

FIGURE 14.3 Nurses must become active in protecting themselves from musculoskeletal injuries.

Critical Thinking Activity

Research the occupational health program offered by a local employer of nurses. Evaluate that program in relation to health hazards in the workplace of which you are aware.

Workers' Compensation

If you believe that you have a work-related injury or illness, follow the policies and procedures prescribed by your facility or by state regulation. This includes reporting the injury as soon as possible after it happens. In most institutions, this is done on an incident report or quality assurance report. A common error is to delay reporting in the belief that you should report something only if you know it will be serious or require medical care. By the time you know this, it may be much more difficult to prove that the problem was work related.

Employers may seek to have workers' compensation claims disallowed to limit their financial liability. Because back injuries are the most common work-related injuries, and often have no clear objective evidence of damage even when pain is present, stigma frequently is attached to those who have back injuries. HIV and hepatitis B are transmitted through needle-stick injuries, but they are also transmitted through other unsafe behaviors. These factors may underlie attempts by an employer to disallow claims for care and time lost from work due to these work-related illnesses or injuries. Prompt, thorough reporting is essential to future claims.

Have any injury assessed by an appropriate healthcare provider. If your agency has an occupational health nurse, you may be required to be seen by that individual for initial screening. One concern is whether you may receive care from the provider of your choice or whether you must receive care from a designated provider. This varies based on the regulations governing work-related injury and illness in your state. Ask this question of your employer and then research it through your state workers' compensation office. If the laws allow the employer or a state agency to designate the provider and you go to another of your choice, you may not be reimbursed for expenses incurred.

Compensation for time off work is another concern when a work-related problem occurs; you usually are required to use your sick leave, but additional time may be available through the workers' compensation program. In general, these programs do not match your working salary, so your income will be lessened. This is one reason why many individuals choose to have private disability insurance that provides replacement income when they cannot work because of illness or disability.

The Americans With Disabilities Act (ADA) of 1990 requires that employers seek ways to provide reasonable accommodation for individuals with disability so that they can continue to work. This might include transferring an individual to a different position or modifying the work environment to provide a setting in which the individual can function. Employers have been known to refuse to make accommodations and to try to terminate an individual who has an ongoing disability. Those with work-related illness and disability do have legal rights within the system. Sometimes it requires considerable effort to sustain those rights. There are both state and federal resources to assist an individual who does not receive reasonable accommodation for disability. The US Department of Justice maintains a Web page with links to many different resources about upholding the provisions of the ADA (*www.usdoj. gov/crt/ada*).

Discrimination in Nursing

Discrimination relates to treating others differently based on **stereotypes** about groups of people. Discrimination may occur regarding racial or ethnic background, gender or sex, sexual orientation, and/or age.

Racial/Ethnic Discrimination

Racial and ethnic discrimination remain problems in society as a whole, and unfortunately healthcare systems are not immune to these problems. Although there are indications that nurses have moved into greater acceptance of all individuals in advance of some other portions of society, concerns about discrimination remain. Historically, the American Association of Colored Graduate Nurses united with the ANA in 1952, before the general civil rights movement in the United States. There have always been prominent nurses of color, such as the past president of the ANA (Beverly Malone) who is now the Chief Executive Officer of the National League for Nursing, former president of the National League for Nursing (Rhetaugh Dumas), and past president of Sigma Theta Tau (May Wykle), who are all African American women who have been leaders for all of nursing throughout their long and distinguished careers. They are just three of the many ethnic/racial minority nurses who have made significant contributions to nursing.

However, the number of minorities in nursing does not reflect the number of minorities in the general population. The 2008 Sample Survey of RNs (US Department of Health and Human Services [USDHHS, 2010]) reveals that 16.8% of nurses represent minority groups. This contrasts with a general population that had approximately 25% racial/ethnic minorities in 2000 (US Census Bureau, 2000) and an estimated 33% racial/ethnic minorities in 2008 (US Census Bureau, 2010). The 2010 census is expected to demonstrate a higher percentage of minority population when these data are released. This difference in the composition of the nursing profession and the general population may stem from many causes, but is of concern because a workforce that reflects the population is more likely to meet the healthcare needs of that population in a culturally sensitive manner. Some of the root causes of the lower participation of minorities in nursing have to do with access to education, support for high career goals, economic status, the image of nursing, institutionalized racism, and other general societal problems.

A survey of minority nurses published by the ANA indicated that many believe they have been adversely affected by discrimination in the nursing profession. Some concerns cited were the perception that others questioned their capabilities and that they were passed over for promotions. To combat these issues as well as to serve as a voice for care for ethnic minority patients, several organizations for ethnic nurses have joined together to create the National Coalition of Ethnic Minority Nurses Associations (*http://www.ncemna.org/*).

All nurses are challenged to examine this situation and be a part of the solution. All of us need to recognize and welcome diversity in the nursing profession. We need to acknowledge that a diversity of views and life experiences will enrich nursing as a profession and support excellence in patient care. When we see discrimination occur, whether in education or in the workplace, we each need to speak up as agents for change. The National Student Nurses' Association has supported a program called Breakthrough to Nursing, in which nursing students mentor minority individuals in nursing education. These efforts and similar ones help nursing to move forward as a profession that welcomes and provides opportunities for all.

Discrimination Against Men

Men in nursing also have expressed concern about discrimination. Their concern is related to being allowed to practice in all areas of nursing and being accepted within the profession. As reported by Nelson and Belcher (2006), this is not an issue of the past; men still continue to feel discriminated against while in nursing school as well as after graduation. Some report having been called names such as "jerk" or "idiot" and having been denied promotion due to their gender.

Antimale sexism of nurses in the United States was brought to the forefront by the research of Kus (1985), who pointed out that society stereotypes men just as feminists have criticized that it stereotypes women. He made a strong case for the importance of nurses examining the stereotypes they hold about men. Stereotypes narrow our thinking and interfere with people being able to develop to their fullest potential. It is important for women in nursing to examine their own behavior and identify whether they have been guilty of perpetuating outmoded stereotypes of the nurse and supporting a type of discrimination toward men that they would fight to eliminate for women.

Stereotyping may have contributed to the low percentage of men in the nursing profession but changes in society are occurring. According to the 2008 Sample Survey of Registered Nurses (USDHHS, 2010), women outnumber men by 15:1 among all nurses; however, among those who became RNs after 1990, 10% are men.

In some facilities or areas, men are not allowed to care for women clients, or if they are allowed to care for women, restrictions are placed on them in terms of obtaining consent for care from each client. Those who support the limitations on the practice of men in nursing state that it is a matter of providing for the modesty and privacy of female clients. The argument is made that clients do not have free choice of a nurse but, rather, are assigned a nurse for care, and therefore restrictions are appropriate.

In an interview, Luther Christman, PhD, RN, discussed the discrimination that he encountered throughout a long and prestigious career in nursing. His career began with his graduation from a hospital-based diploma program in 1939 and extended through doctoral studies and a joint position as dean of Rush University and vice president of nursing for Rush-Presbyterian-St. Luke's Medical Center in Chicago. He identified overt acts that excluded him from positions and covert acts that tried to undermine his influence. He identified this as being an issue of power and control just as is sex discrimination against women (Sullivan, 2002).

Those who oppose limitations on the practice of men in nursing state that, as a professional, a nurse (whether a man or woman) should always consider the privacy and modesty of a client of either gender. This can be done without excluding anyone from providing care in any area. By careful assessment, the nurse can determine the true needs of the client and plan for appropriate avenues to deliver that care. Further, the point has been made that male physicians have not been excluded from any branch of medicine and this has not created problems. The client does not always choose physicians, either. Resident physicians are assigned, referrals are made to specialty physicians, and many group plans designate a physician to provide care. Female nurses care for male clients in all situations. This has been accepted because women are seen in a nurturing, mothering role that the public associates with nursing.

The American Assembly for Men in Nursing provides a forum for the concerns of men in nursing and those who are concerned about the problems of sex discrimination. This organization seeks to educate people and opposes any limitations on opportunities available to men. A specialty journal for men titled *Men in Nursing* has begun publication. Further information can be found on its Web site *http://aamn.org/*.

Critical Thinking Activity

Review the advertisements for nursing positions in three current journals and analyze them for gender bias.

Sexual Harassment

Sexual harassment, disruptive behavior, and violence are often discussed together because they may be rooted in the same issues of the abuse of power. Disruptive behavior and violence are discussed below.

Sexual harassment is grouped into two sets of behavior. The first is the creation of a hostile work environment through behavior of a sexual nature. This type of sexual harassment may take the form of comments about an individual's body, persistent unwanted attempts to initiate a personal relationship, the ongoing use of suggestive or obscene language, unwanted touching, or direct sexual advances. Another type of sexual harassment is called "quid pro quo." This involves the explicit offer of job-related benefits (working conditions, salary, privileges, or even simply the benefit of remaining employed) in return for sexual favors (Roberts & Mann, n.d.).

Both men and women may be the objects of sexual harassment. Because nurses are involved with personal care of individuals of the opposite sex, there is sometimes the unspoken assumption that nurses will not be offended by sexual comments, jokes, or innuendo.

Sexual harassment was the subject of a position paper by the ANA (1993), as nurses began to voice their concerns about its presence in nursing. This position paper provided background on the costs of the problem and identified areas of redress for nurses who were subjected to sexual harassment.

Harassers in the healthcare workplace may be clients, coworkers, or physicians. The general data show that sexual harassment is a demonstration of personal power over others. Traditionally, physicians have had the most power in healthcare environments and are the group most often identified as harassers. While recognizing the problem, it is important not to stereotype physicians, because the majority of physicians are professional and appropriate in their relationships.

Individuals should take steps to stop sexual harassment by giving clear, direct verbal messages indicating that the behavior in question is unwanted, unpleasant, and must stop. Sometimes this action alone stops inappropriate behavior. If clear, direct messages are not successful, the individual then should report the matter in writing to an immediate supervisor. Any individual who believes that he or she has been the victim of sexual harassment should keep personal records of the behavior and of all attempts to stop the behavior in question.

Most organizations and agencies have an individual designated to deal with issues related to sexual harassment. If you encounter problem behavior, discuss your concerns with this person. If you belong to a collective bargaining group, that group can serve as a resource to assist you. Unfortunately, some employers do not respond appropriately to sexual harassment. In some instances, it may be necessary to seek independent legal counsel familiar with workplace legal issues to force resolution of the problem.

Employers are legally and ethically responsible for having clear policies that prohibit sexual harassment, and for providing an appropriate work environment. If an employer fails to respond appropriately, the employer may be legally liable. These policies should be publicized so that everyone is aware of them. The courts support the responsibility of the employer to maintain a work environment free of sexual harassment (Equal Employment Opportunity Commission [EEOC], n.d.).

COMMUNICATION   IN   ACTION

A Clear Message About Sexual Harassment

Jean Wilson, RN, was new to the medical center where she worked. While sitting at the desk by herself in the evening, a male resident physician sat down beside her. He draped his arm around her shoulders, put his face close to hers and said, "Hi there, sweetie! How's it going for the prettiest nurse on 3-Southwest?" Jean was taken aback and very uncomfortable. She immediately stood and said, "We are virtual strangers. I don't like your touching me in that way or calling me 'Sweetie.' It is inappropriate. Don't do that again." He then said, "Hey, hey—don't get so upset. I was just being friendly." She replied, "We're not friends, we are colleagues, and that does not include touching me and calling me names like 'Sweetie.' " He muttered to himself and walked away. Jean felt nervous but glad she had stood her ground.

Disruptive Behavior

Disruptive behavior which includes incivility, verbal abuse, and bullying may occur in any setting (Scott, n.d.). In efforts to increase retention of nurses, hospitals have begun asking why nurses leave specific hospitals and nursing altogether. An important factor is the extent to which nurses see themselves as disrespected and verbally abused in the workplace (Rocker, 2008). The most frequently cited type of disruptive behavior was verbal abuse such as yelling or raised voices, disrespect, condescension, berating colleagues, berating patients, and use of abusive language (Longo, 2010). Nonverbal behaviors such as eye-rolling, giving a "cold shoulder", instituting the "silent treatment", and passive dismissal may be as distressing to the victim as verbal abuse (Scott, n.d.).

In the past, these behaviors often were tolerated from physicians because other health professionals knew that they did not have the power to change them. Disrespectful behavior has been identified by the Institute for Safe Medication Practices (2009) as contributing to errors in healthcare. The person who fears being the subject of verbal abuse may delay communicating about a problem. The person who feels free to be disrespectful of a colleague may carry that disrespect into ignoring concerns about the patient.

While disruptive behavior may occur from a person in a more powerful position, not all verbal abuse is vertical, moving from more powerful to less powerful. Some disruptive behavior is horizontal or lateral—nurses verbally abusing one another, saying things to one another that would be clearly inappropriate if said to a patient. Verbal abuse may also come from patients who become demanding.

Why does disruptive behavior continue? There are many contributing factors including both individual characteristics and attributes of the work system (Washington State Department of Labor, 2011). The bottom line must be that regardless of why it happens, disruptive behaviors must be stopped.

Employers have a duty to create a safe and effective working environment. Establishing a culture of civility toward one another and a zero tolerance policy toward disruptive behavior are steps that agencies must take (Longo, 2010). When such policies are established, education of all staff will be needed to underscore the components of civil and respectful behavior and to sensitize people to the problem. Everyone can be encouraged to be part of the solution. Familiarize yourself with your employer's policies; there may be policies regarding collegial behaviors and reporting mechanisms for disruptive behavior.

Scott (n.d.) suggests the following general strategies to establish a more equitable workplace initially. Nurses must assess themselves and identify their own feelings about self-worth. They must recognize their own potential for verbal abuse toward others and deal ethically with one another. She suggests that nurses must be willing to engage rather than avoid conflict when disruptive behaviors occur. The only person who benefits from silence and avoidance is the disruptor. Specific actions a nurse should take regarding disruptive behaviors are similar to those suggested above for sexual harassment. Address the behavior at the time it occurs in a clear, calm manner. Describe the behavior and its effect on you and your ability to function. Ask for that behavior to stop. Longo (2010) suggests that confronting an individual in private may yield better results. When personal efforts are not successful, you should talk with your manager about the situation. Managers also have responsibilities to work with disruptive behaviors. Making a plan and taking action are essential. The aggressor should be confronted and formal written complaints filed when appropriate. Legal action may be needed. Keep good personal records with details of the incident, the time, the circumstances, and a listing of any witnesses. Nurses need not remain powerless regarding situations of workplace abuse.

Nurses must work together to not succumb to intimidation. Some hospitals have initiated what they are calling a code white, which is a signal for others to come and be observers when an individual begins any type of verbal abuse. This verbal abuse might consist of insults, a personal attack, a temper tantrum, or a tirade. These people are witnesses and provide emotional support to the recipient of abuse. Administrators and other physicians must also learn not to turn their backs to abuse occurring in the environment. They have both ethical and legal (in the case of administrators) responsibilities for the workplace.

Violence in the Workplace

Most nursing students think of hospitals as places where victims of violence are helped. Rarely do they think of themselves as potential victims of violence in their own workplace. Many nonfatal workplace assaults happen in health and social services facilities. The majority of these are assaults by clients on nursing staff, and more client assaults occur in psychiatric mental health settings than in other settings. Assaults on staff members by visitors and outsiders also occur; most of these take place in emergency rooms. Healthcare workplace violence is not confined to industrialized societies. Violence is also very costly when costs of treatment, lost work time, and even loss of an educated professional to healthcare are considered.

OSHA has issued guidelines for use by facilities trying to establish a safer workplace. These are not enforceable rules but may represent what is termed the "General Duty" clause (Section 5(a)(1) in the OSHA Act [OSHA, 1970]). The guidelines call for clear programs designed to protect workers. These programs would include an assessment and analysis of the workplace for hazards and a plan for prevention of problems.

One form of prevention is to train employees in the management of hostile and violent behavior. Ways of identifying hostile and assaultive clients should be developed so that staff can be warned to take extra personal safety precautions.

Other important environmental safeguards include the use of such devices as metal detectors, panic buttons, and bulletproof glass, where appropriate. Adequate staff to manage potentially violent behavior is of particular concern in psychiatric/mental health settings. The addition of security personnel is important in some environments. There should be an attitude throughout the institution of zero tolerance for abusive or assaultive behavior.

In addition to preventing and managing problem situations, there should be clear guidelines for reporting both verbal and physical abuse and following through on all complaints. Healthcare institutions should work with law enforcement professionals when abusive or assaultive behavior occurs to ensure that legal procedures are carried out correctly.

Those who report incidents should receive support and assistance and be assured that there will be no reprisals or blaming. Some nurses have been reluctant to report verbal and physical abuse or assault because of personal and institutional beliefs that healthcare employees should be able to handle these behaviors independently. Another common belief in healthcare environments is that all behavior has meaning for the individual and that employees should accept inappropriate behaviors on the part of clients. Social constraints and adverse consequences related to inappropriate behavior are a valuable ally in redirecting the behaviors of those who are cognitively impaired, mentally ill, or developmentally delayed. Nurses need support from their work environments in accessing these avenues to protect themselves.

Critical Thinking Activity

Formulate an appropriate response to experiencing verbal abuse in the workplace. Include specific statements you would use and each step you would take if the verbal abuse occurred again.

KEY CONCEPTS

- The process of moving from novice to expert has been divided into five stages: novice, advanced beginner, competent, proficient, and expert.
- Reality shock occurs when an idealistic new graduate enters the real world of practice and has difficulty with the expectations and demands found there. You can prepare for the stress created by this transition through attending to your own expectations and developing personal strategies for coping including self-appraisal; evaluating employers; seeking mentors, preceptors, or coaches; joining a peer support group; and using personal stress management strategies.
- Burnout is a stress response experienced by nurses and others who work in occupations that make many emotional demands. Burnout may be alleviated by planned actions. In some instances, it may be necessary to change job settings when stress accumulates.

- Occupational safety and health are special concerns for nurses because of the infectious nature of the illnesses with which they come in contact, the toxicity of some chemicals in the nursing environment, and the potential for musculoskeletal injury and violence.
- Nurses who experience a work-related injury must carefully follow all relevant rules and regulations for reporting the injury, completing appropriate forms, and seeking care to ensure that they receive assistance for any medical care and lost wages.
- Nurses may see discrimination in the workplace manifested as racial/ethnic discrimination, wage discrimination against women, and job opportunity discrimination against men.
- Sexual harassment in the workplace is illegal. Understanding how to defend oneself against sexual harassment provides a greater feeling of personal power and control in the situation.

● Disruptive behavior contributes to patient safety concerns as well as to an aversive workplace where individuals decide to leave nursing. Administrative authorities should act to stop all types of disruptive behavior, but nurses working collectively can also act to decrease the impact of disruptive behavior.

● Violence in the workplace is found in healthcare settings as well as the rest of society. Nurses working individually and collectively can develop strategies to combat this serious concern.

RELEVANT WEB SITES

Web sites relevant to this chapter can be found at **thePoint** accessed through *http://thePoint. lww.com/Ellis10e* and by entering the code found on the inside cover of your text.

REFERENCES

American Nurses Association. (1993). *Position statement: Sexual harassment.* Retrieved March 23, 2010, from http://www.nursingworld.org/harassmentps.aspx

American Nurses Association. (2004). *Handle with care.* Retrieved March 22, 2010, from http://www.nursingworld.org/MainMenuCategories/OccupationalandEnvironmental/occupationalhealth/handlewithcare/hwc.aspx

American Nurses Association. (n.d.). *Safe staffing saves lives.* Retrieved March 13, 2010, from http://www.safestaffingsaveslives.org

Benner, P. (1984). *From novice to expert: Excellence and power in clinical nursing practice.* Commemorative edition (2001). Upper Saddle River, NJ: Prentice Hall.

Centers for Disease Control and Prevention (CDC). (2009). *Prevention and control of seasonal influenza with vaccines: Recommendations of the advisory committee on immunization practices (ACIP), MMWR* July 24, 2009/58(Early Release), 1–52 (2010). Retrieved March 29, 2010, from http://www.cdc.gov/flu/professionals/acip/

Dreyfus, S. E., & Dreyfus, H. L. (1980). *A five-stage model of the mental activities involved in directed skill acquisition.* Unpublished report supported by the Air Force Office of Scientific Research (AFSC), USAF (Contract F49620-79-C-0063), University of California at Berkeley, 1980 (as reported in P. Benner [1984], *From Novice to Expert,* Upper Saddle River, NJ: Prentice Hall).

Dyes, S. M., & Sherman, R.O. (2009). The first year of practice: New graduate nurses' transition and learning needs. *Journal Continuing Education in Nursing, 40*(9), 403–410.

Ellis, J. R. (2008). *Quality of care, nurses' work schedules, and fatigue: A white paper.* Seattle, WA: Washington State Nurses Association. Retrieved March 20, 2010, from http://www.wsna.org/Topics/Fatigue/

Equal Employment Opportunity Commission (EEOC). (n.d.). *Sexual harassment.* Retrieved March 23, 2010, from www.eeoc.gov/eeoc/publications/fs-sex.cfm

Institute for Safe Medication Practices. (2009). *Results from the ISMP survey on workplace intimidation.* Retrieved March 29, 2009, from www.ismp.org/Survey/surveyResults?survey0311.asp

Kovner, C. T., Brewer, C. S., Fairchild, S., Poornima, S., Kim, H., & Djukic, M. (2007). Newly licensed RNs' characteristics, work attitudes, and intentions to work. *American Journal of Nursing, 107*(9), 58–70.

Kramer, M., (1979). *Reality shock.* St. Louis, MO: CV Mosby.

Kupperschmidt, B., Kientz, E., Ward, J., Reinholz, B. (2010, January 31), A healthy work environment: It begins with you, *OJIN: The Online Journal of Issues in Nursing, 15*(1), Manuscript 3. DOI: 10.3912/OJIN.Vol15No01Man03, Retrieved March 19, 2010, from www.nursingworld.org/MainMenuCategories/ANAMarketplace/ANAPeriodicals/OJIN.aspx

Kus, R. J. (1985). Stages of coming out: An ethnographic approach. *Western Journal of Nursing Research, 7*(2), 177–194.

Longo, J. (2010 January 31). Combating disruptive behaviors: Strategies to promote a healthy work environment. *OJIN The Online Journal of Issues in Nursing 15*(1), Manuscript 5. DOI: 10.3912/OJIN.Vol15No01Man05. Retrieved March 29, 2010, from www.nursingworld.org/MainMenuCategories/ANAMarketplace/ ANAPeriodicals/OJIN/TableofContents/Vol152010/No1Jan2010.aspx

Luquette, J. (2007). Stress, compassion fatigue, and burnout: Effective self-care techniques for oncology nurses. *Oncology Nursing Forum 34*(2), 490–492.

Maslach, C., Leiter, M. P., & Schaufeli, W. B. (2009). Measuring burnout. In C. L. Cooper & S. Cartwright (Eds.), The Oxford handbook of organizational well-being (86-108). Oxford UK: Oxford University Press.

National Institute for Occupational Safety and Health (NIOSH). (2009). *Safe patient handling training for schools of nursing.* Publication No.: 2009-127. Retrieved March 23, 2010, from www.cdc.gov/niosh/docs/2009-127/

Needleman, J., Buerhaus, P., Mattke, S., Stewart, M., & Zelevinsky, K. (2002a). Nurse-staffing levels and the quality of care in hospitals. *New England Journal of Medicine, 346*(22), 1715–1722.

Needleman, J., Buerhaus, P., Mattke, S., Stewart, M., & Zelevinsky, K. (2002b). Nurse staffing and quality of care in hospitals in the United States. *Policy Politics Nursing Practice 3*(4), 306–308.

Nelson, R. & Behcher, D. (2006) Men in nursing: Still too few. *American Journal of Nursing, 106*(2), 25–26.

O'Keefe, T., & Forrester, D.A., (2009 July–September). A successful online mentoring program for nurses. *Nursing Administration Quarterly. 33*(3), 245–50.

Pellico, H., Brewer, C. S., & Kovner, C.T. (2009 July). What newly licensed registered nurses have to say about their first experiences. *Nursing Outlook, 57*(4) 194–203.

Roberts, B. S., & Mann, R. A. (n.d.). *Sexual harassment in the workplace: A primer.* Retrieved March 21, 2010, from www3.uakron.edu/lawrev/robert1.html

Rocker, C. (2008 August 29). Addressing nurse-to-nurse bullying to promote nurse retention. *OJIN: The Online Journal of Issues in Nursing*; *13*(3). Retrieved March 22, 2010, from www.nursingworld.org/ MainMenuCategories/ANAMarketplace/ANAPeriodicals/OJIN/TableofContents/vol132008/No3Sept08/ ArticlePreviousTopic/NursetoNurseBullying.aspx

Scott, D. (n.d.). *10 tips for addressing disruptive behavior at work.* Center for the American Nurse, Webinar. Retrieved from www.centerforamericannurses.org/displaycommon.cfm?an=1&subarticlenbr=195

Scott, E. S., Engelke, M. K., Swanson, M. (2008 May). New graduate nurse transitioning: Necessary or nice? *Applied Nursing Research, 21*(2), 75–83.

Siegel, J. D., Rhinehart, E., Jackson, M., Chiarello, L., & the Healthcare Infection Control Practices Advisory Committee [HICPAC]. (2007). *Guideline for isolation precautions: Preventing transmission of infectious agents in healthcare settings.* Centers for Disease Control and Prevention. Retrieved March 29, 2010, from http://www. cdc.gov/hicpac/2007IP/2007isolationPrecautions.html

Sullivan, E. (2002). In a women's world. *Reflections on Nursing Leadership, 28*(3), 10–17.

US Census Bureau. (2000). Population by race and Hispanic origin 2000. *Census 2000 (Redistricting Public Law 94–171) Summary file Tbls PL1 and PL2.* Retrieved December 28, 2010, from http://www.census.gov/ prod/2001pubs/c2kbr01-1.pdf

US Census Bureau. (2010). *Minority census participation.* Retrieved December 28, 2010, from http://2010.census. gov/mediacenter/awareness/minority-census.php

US Department of Health and Human Services (USDHHS), Health Resources and Services Administration. (2010). *The registered nurse population: Initial findings from the 2008 national sample survey of registered nurses.* Retrieved March 29, 2010, from http://bhpr.hrsa.gov/healthworkforce/rnsurvey/initialfindings2008.pdf

United States Department of Labor. Occupational Health and Safety Administration (OSHA). (1970). *Occupational Health and Safety Act (1970) Section 5 Duties.* Retrieved December 28, 2010, from http://www.osha.gov/pls/ oshaweb/owadisp.show_document?p_table=OSHACT&p_id=3359

Washington State Dept of Labor, (April, 2011), *Workplace bullying and disruptive behavior: What everyone needs to know.* Retrieved April 24, 2011 from www.lni.wa.gov/safety/research/files/bullying.pdf

Wroten, S. J., & Waite, R. (2009 Fall). A call to action: Mentoring within the nursing profession—a wonderful gift to give and share, *ABNF Journal, 20*(4), 106–108.

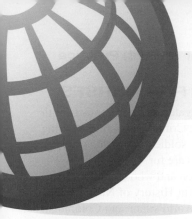

15

Valuing the Political Process

olitics is the way in which people in any society try to influence decision making and the allocation of resources (money, time, and personnel). Because resources are limited, it is necessary to make choices regarding their use. There is no perfect process for making optimum choices, because whenever one valuable option is chosen, some other option must be left out. Politics is a part of every organization and a part of government at every level. In a democratic society, all individuals can choose to be involved at some level in this decision-making process. This chapter presents the political process, discusses some of the current issues regarding political decisions, and describes how nurses can play a role in the political arena and in nursing organizations.

RELEVANCE OF THE POLITICAL PROCESS FOR NURSES

Nurses always have been involved in politics. Florence Nightingale used her contacts with powerful men in government to obtain support for traveling to the Crimea, including securing the supplies and the personnel she needed to care for wounded soldiers (Bostridge, 2008). Hannah Ropes was able to fight incompetence and obtain decent care for wounded Civil War soldiers because she understood who was influential in Washington and who would be receptive to her efforts on the soldiers' behalf (American Association for History of Nursing, Inc., 2007). Isabel Hampton used the buildup and excitement of the World's Fair and Columbian Exposition of 1893 to bring together nurse leaders to form the first nursing organization (ANA, 1996).

Modern times are no different. With many voices competing to be heard in the decision-making circles of any nation, the person who understands power and politics is the one most likely to obtain the resources needed to accomplish desired ends.

Decisions are made at federal, state, and local levels of government and with each health-care agency. These decisions may be legislated or made by administrative bodies. Within organizations, these questions are answered by committees, managers, and governing boards.

Your practice as a nurse is controlled by a wide variety of governmental decisions. One of the most basic is the Nurse Practice Act of your state or province as discussed in Chapter 3. All of the philosophic discussions about the role of the nurse must return to the reality of the nurse's role as legally defined in the state's practice act. Do you care what that role is now or what changes are made in it? Does it make any difference to you what education that law requires, or if that law requires continuing education? Answering "yes" to any of these questions emphasizes the relevance of the political process for you.

Knowing where the decision making occurs, who makes the decision, and being familiar with how you can influence that process is critical. Each governmental entity, agency, and organization has its own mechanism for operating. However, they share many similarities that can help you plan your activities.

Critical Thinking Activity

Identify a current healthcare issue in your state or province. Investigate that issue and form a position that you can support with data. Examine your position for personal biases.

INFLUENCING THE POLITICAL PROCESS

You can have an effect on such things as what healthcare legislation is submitted, the content of the legislation, and what legislation is passed. However, this does not happen without effort and action. As a result of a variety of societal factors, historically, women have been less active in politics than men. Gradually, women are assuming a more active role in politics: More are being appointed to the high offices within the government, more are running for and being elected to office, more work with policy-making bodies, and more vote. Because more than 83% of nurses are women (USDHHS, 2010), this changing social climate is important to

DISPLAY 15.1 Influencing the Political Process

- Become informed through a variety of sources.
- Vote for candidates or ballot issues that reflect your concerns.
- Vote for officers within professional or political organizations.
- Express your opinions through letters or in public forums.
- Communicate directly with legislators and public officials.
- Work for or contribute to nonlobbying nursing organizations or political action committees.
- Work for or contribute to candidates who represent your views.
- Testify before decision-making bodies.

nursing. All women, and women who are nurses in particular, have demonstrated increasing political awareness.

Each person must determine his or her own level of personal involvement, but there is, in the broad realm of the political process, room for everyone to find a suitable role. Some of these ways are outlined here and in Display 15.1.

Becoming Informed

To become informed about legislation and healthcare, you need to learn about the sources of information available. Each source of information is valuable to you but should be weighed based on its known biases. Even the most objective-sounding report can be biased, not only in what is reported but also in what is not reported. Identifying the groups that support or oppose a particular viewpoint might help you to recognize bias. Determine whether a group and its members would tend to gain or lose personally by the passage of proposed legislation. Are special interest groups voicing an opinion? When biases are evident, it is advisable to obtain information from groups with divergent viewpoints. Decisions based on firm factual data are more likely to benefit the entire group, organization, or society as a whole.

Once you are informed about the current issues in legislation or in an organization, you are better prepared to form personal opinions about them and to try to influence the outcome of the political process. A wide variety of resources are available.

News Media

The daily newspaper, weekly newsmagazine, and online news reports can be excellent sources of information about significant legislation being proposed, about controversial issues, or about an issue that has attracted widespread interest.

Television and radio news reports are usually quite brief and give only an overview of a particular piece of legislation being introduced. This overview may be helpful in alerting you to something that you will want to study more intensively. Often radio commentators speak from a particular viewpoint or bias. Remember to weigh information in light of that viewpoint and seek information more broadly. Some television programs, such as those on public television, do discuss issues in depth with commentators who hold different positions on an issue. These programs usually make an attempt to present both sides of any issue.

Specialized Publications

Voters' pamphlets are prepared by many governmental jurisdictions. These pamphlets may introduce each candidate for office and contain a brief candidate statement regarding their platform. Endorsements by groups often are included to help the reader better understand the position taken by the candidate. When issues are on the ballot, both a "pro" statement and a "con" statement are provided. The individuals and groups supporting each position may be identified.

Professional journals usually devote some space to current legislative issues. This is done routinely in *American Journal of Nursing* and *The American Nurse* in the United States and in *Canadian Nurse* in Canada. When major issues are being debated, other nursing periodicals often contain articles of interest. The journals of other healthcare professions also may carry information regarding current nursing issues. Web sites such as the ANA's *www.nursingworld. com* will usually have pages devoted to any major healthcare issue. Newsletters and journals of organizations that have a political focus provide information on what they see as current issues. These organizations include consumer groups such as Common Cause, political groups such as the Young Democrats and Young Republicans, and nonpartisan groups such as the League of Women Voters. Magazines directed to special interest groups, such as *AARP The Magazine* for those over the age of 50, carry articles related to political issues that would be of particular interest to that group.

Copies of legislation are usually available through your congressional representatives (for federal matters) and your state or provincial representatives (for state/provincial matters). They also are available online at your legislature's Web site. Along with copies of the legislation, a legislator may send other informational material. Government agencies affected by proposed legislation also may provide information about the legislation's potential effects, although they are not allowed to try to influence legislation. You will find it helpful to understand the process of how a bill becomes a law to recognize where and when communication with a legislator might influence the process. Project Vote Smart (2010) provides an overview of this process that you might wish to review (*http://www.votesmart.org/resource_govt101_02.php.*)

Online Resources

Online resources are an increasingly useful source of information. Some common ones were mentioned in the discussion above. In addition, there are specialized sites that may be useful to you.

Federal legislation can be found at *http://thomas.loc.gov/*, a site maintained in the public interest by Congress. In most states, the text of bills being introduced is available on a governmental Web site, where you can read the bill on the computer or print the document to read. You can access state sites by going to *www.loc.gov/rr/news/stategov/stategov.html*.

Nursing and healthcare organizations that maintain Web sites often have a site devoted to political issues affecting members of the organization or relevant issues that affect healthcare. The American Nurses Association (ANA), for example, maintains a legislative Web site at *http://nursingworld.org/gova/*. Many news organizations (television stations, newspapers, and magazines) maintain Web sites with information on current issues. Project Vote Smart provides data on candidates and issues for both federal and state elections. Any of these sites may provide links to still more sites that provide useful information. There are also individuals and organizations that maintain Web sites with information and opinion. Investigating bias in these resources is critical and requires careful analysis.

Organizational Meetings

Nursing organizations and other health-related organizations, as well as community groups, sometimes hold open meetings to present and discuss legislative issues. Often, knowledgeable speakers can help you to understand what is being proposed and the potential effects of a proposal. These organizations also may sponsor e-mail networks to get out information on important pending legislation. Nursing organizations can be excellent sources of information because they often are in touch with legislators and legislative staff.

▶ ## *EXAMPLE*

Seeking Information About a Political Concern

Jeff Whitmore was a registered nurse (RN) in a long-term care facility. One day, another nurse asked, "Do you know what this new change in the Medicare regulations will mean for us?" He replied, "I am not even sure what those changes are. I'll have to check on it." Once home, he went onto the Internet and began searching. He looked at the Web site for Medicare to see whether there was an announcement of changes in regulations. After reading the section on "Spotlight" (Centers for Medicare & Medicaid Services [n.d.]) that gave an overview of the changes, he then began looking for articles and other people's views of what was happening. He checked *http://nursingworld.org* to see if the ANA had information available. He thought some more and decided that organizations associated with nursing homes and long-term care might have information of value. After spending an hour researching the new regulations, he felt that he understood them enough to discuss them with his colleague and began to form an opinion on what it might mean for their facility.

Voting

Your individual vote on a ballot issue is significant. Recent major elections in the United States have demonstrated how important every vote can be. According to the US Census Bureau Survey of Voting and Registration (2009), in the 2008 elections, only 64.9% of those eligible to vote were registered to vote and only 58.2% of those eligible to vote actually voted. Nurses, as a group, are thought to vote in higher percentages than the general population, which may relate to a higher educational level among nurses. Although you cannot vote directly on legislative issues, you can vote for candidates whose positions you support on initiatives and referendums and who share your values. Absentee ballots are always available for those who cannot be present at their polling place on the day of an election. These ballots must be requested well in advance of the election, however. In many jurisdictions, you may elect to always vote by mail; in some, it is the only option.

Voting for officers in organizations may be ignored by a large majority of members. They look at the ballot, are unfamiliar with those running for office, and therefore do not vote. Most organizations do make an attempt to introduce members to the various candidates. If you do not know the candidates, you can seek information about them by reading their prepared statements of position and learning about their previous activities. Those elected to office usually determine the direction and priorities of an organization. If you are contributing your dues dollars, you want to have a voice in choosing those who are entrusted with making the decisions.

Shaping Public Opinion

Public opinion does influence the actions of legislators and regulatory bodies. As an RN, you can help to shape public opinion; your judgment about matters that affect healthcare can help others make their own decisions. Share the knowledge you have gained through your personal experience and research. Do not be afraid to state your own position, although you must be prepared to support your position with evidence if you want to be considered a thoughtful healthcare professional. Certainly, you will not want to make every social occasion an opportunity to share political positions, but do take advantage of opportunities that arise to present your concerns to others (Fig. 15.1).

COMMUNICATION IN ACTION

Carlos Romano was having coffee with a group of friends, and the new legislation regarding healthcare became a topic of discussion. One member of the group commented, "Well, that will take care of all the concern for staffing and funding the free clinics I have been reading about." Carlos volunteered as an RN at a local clinic. He responded, "While the President has signed the healthcare legislation, it is important to remember that implementation starts in 2014 and will be fully enacted in 2019. According to the Congressional Budget Office, there will still be 23 million uninsured in 2019 after full implementation of the Healthcare Reform Legislation. I believe there will continue to be a genuine need for free clinics for those who have no other access to healthcare.

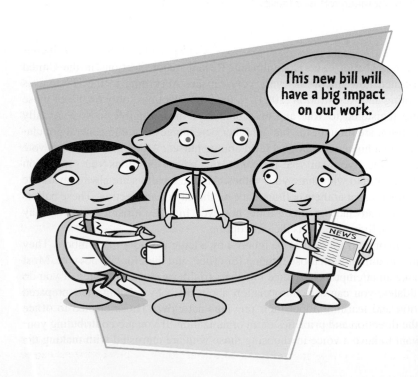

FIGURE 15.1 Sharing your opinions is one avenue of political involvement.

DISPLAY 15.2   Writing Letters to the Editor

• Carefully follow the instructions provided by the publication for letters to the editor. These usually will refer to length, signature, address, and telephone number. Typically, letters should be short and to the point, about 200 to 300 words.
• Clearly present your opinion with well-reasoned arguments. Make only one point per letter.
• Including personal experiences that illustrate healthcare concerns can be useful; however, be careful that healthcare examples do not violate the confidentiality of clients or divulge confidential information regarding your employer.
• Use a direct but respectful tone. Avoid personal attacks on others.
• Include your name, address, and phone number as well as your nursing credentials after your name.
• If responding to a particular article, give the title of the article and include the date of publication in parentheses.

Another means of shaping public opinion is by writing a letter to the editor of a newspaper or newsmagazine. Editorial letters are read by many people. The suggestions in Display 15.2 will maximize your chances of appearing in print.

Within an organization, you may also influence opinion and action by clearly presenting reasoned arguments. You can discuss issues with other members and present your opinion at meetings. Remember that a viewpoint supported by strong, reasoned judgment, facts, and rationale will be better received than a simple statement of opinion.

Communicating With Legislators and Officials

Legislators are affected by the views of their constituents. The legislator's staff reviews incoming letters, tabulates views, and directs letters with significant opinions or information to the legislator for individual consideration. Although some groups encourage members to sign form letters or postcards, personal letters have a greater impact.

A carefully written personal letter reflecting thoughtful and informed opinions on an issue will receive the most attention from any governmental person or department. As an RN, your expertise can provide a valuable viewpoint. Identify yourself as an RN in your letter and outline why you are concerned about the issue in question. Legislators often appreciate personal anecdotes from your practice (with patient/family privacy protected, of course) that underscore your point. The names and addresses of your congressional representatives are available on the Senate and House Web sites. Go to *www.firstgov.gov* and link to the House or Senate. These sites also explain who serves on which committees. Canada maintains a similar site at *http://canada.gc.ca/main_e.html*. The names and contact information for your individual state representatives also are linked online from the ANA Government Affairs page *http://nursingworld.org/gova*. Additional information about effective communication with legislators also is provided by the ANA from this same Web site. The Canadian Nurses Association maintains a similar Web site at *www.cna-nurses.ca/CNA/issues/matters/default_e.aspx*. Information about provincial officials is available on the Web site of each individual province.

Concern regarding the rules and regulations of a specific department of government can be addressed to the officials of that department. Communication from concerned citizens can be as important to them as it is to legislators. To be most effective, letters addressed to officials should reflect the same care and professional viewpoint as those addressed to legislators.

Many governmental agencies, both legislative and regulatory, accept letters in the form of e-mail. E-mail has the advantage of being extremely timely. However, be aware of the rules for Internet usage at your facility. Although you may have e-mail access at your place of work, your employer may not allow you to use it for political activity. If you are employed by a government entity, such as a public health department, the law prohibits you from using governmental resources such as e-mail for political activity.

An e-mail message should be composed as carefully as a letter. One important point is to include your full name and home address in your message. Staff members review the address, forwarding only those messages that are personally identifiable and noting those from a congressperson's district. Do remember that e-mail is public. Do not state things in an e-mail that would make you feel uncomfortable to present in public. See Display 15.3 for an example.

You may make a telephone call to a legislator's office. Staff members keep a record of all calls, and the positions of callers are noted. To call a member of Congress, contact the US Capitol Switchboard at (202) 224-3121 and ask for the individual's office. In some states, a toll-free number is maintained for calls to state legislators during the legislative session. You will be asked to leave a message. Be sure to identify yourself fully, including both your name and address. State the bill or issue about which you are calling and clearly state your position.

Visiting congressional or state representatives also is an effective means of expressing your concerns. One of the best ways to arrange to speak with congressional representatives and senators is to contact their local offices. Through these offices, you may receive assistance in arranging your visit. Staff members may help you to arrange other interesting and valuable activities, such as attending committee hearings, taking tours, and observing Congress

 DISPLAY 15.3   A Carefully Written E-mail

Subject: House Bill 1458 Safe Patient Handling

Dear Representative Smith:

As an RN constituent in your legislative district, I urge you to support passage of this important legislation. As a nurse in a hospital, I am familiar with the care needs of dependent individuals. Unfortunately, the current solution to care has been to urge care providers to lift and move patients, resulting in injuries, lost work, and even lost careers for the caregivers. I personally know two RNs who have become unable to work as nurses after sustaining back injuries in moving incapacitated patients. In addition to the human cost, the community cannot sustain the loss of needed RNs when there is such a shortage. There are now many effective lifting and transfer devices available for purchase. This legislation will provide the impetus for healthcare agencies to purchase them and implement their use. Thank you for your attention to this important matter.

Mary K. Winslow, RN
2314 12th Ave.
Seattle, WA 98201
Phone: (206) 981-1234

in session. Make appointments well in advance, as representatives and senators have busy schedules. If your time is limited, you may have to modify your expectations and meet with a staff member who will relay your concerns. Plan carefully for your visit; it is helpful to write out concerns and questions. Be sure to leave time for answers to the questions that you pose. Even when you disagree with the position taken by your legislator, be polite and present your concerns calmly. Rudeness could result in the legislator's unwillingness to listen to what you have to say.

Some legislators hold public meetings (often referred to as "town hall" meetings) in their legislative districts for the purpose of hearing from their constituents. These meetings can be both an opportunity to learn about issues and the legislator's current position and to give input regarding issues of concern to you. If you bring written materials to support your viewpoint, these may be given to the legislator and further reinforce your position. These same activities may be useful in working within an organization. Those elected to office do not know the views of members unless communication occurs. For communication to be effective, you must know when and where boards meet, how to get information to board members, and the names of those responsible for specific aspects of the organization's operations.

Critical Thinking Activity

Identify a current political issue about which you feel strongly. Write a letter or an e-mail to a governmental official (local, state, or federal) that provides a sound rationale in support of your position. Ask someone else to review it for you and then send it.

Group Action

The political process in the nursing profession takes many forms. Nurses can be involved as individuals, but they are far more effective when they work in groups. Because nursing is the largest single healthcare occupation, nurses have many votes. For this reason, legislators pay attention to positions held by groups of nurses.

Nonlobbying Nursing Organization Efforts

Most traditional nursing organizations are nonprofit groups and therefore are limited in their political activity. The major role of nonprofit groups in politics involves testifying to facts, organizational positions, and concerns in the healthcare arena. The ANA has an office in Washington, DC, and tries to keep the nursing profession informed about legislative matters of importance in healthcare. The ANA also provides experts in the nursing profession who testify before congressional and regulatory groups about proposed legislation.

The **Tri-Council for Nursing** is a collaborative effort of four organizations: the ANA, the National League for Nursing (NLN), the American Organization of Nurse Executives (AONE), and the American Association of Colleges of Nursing (AACN) in support of nursing practice, education, and research. By working collaboratively, these organizations have strengthened the voice of nursing and its visibility in Washington, DC. This coalition has become the trusted representation for nursing. Legislators rely on the information it provides and recognize it as a united voice for the nursing profession.

The ANA organized the **Nurses Strategic Action Team (N-STAT)** to provide nurses with a means to mobilize quickly to influence legislative policy. This organization promotes grassroots involvement in legislative issues, meets with members of Congress, and organizes letter-writing and telephone campaigns. Interested nurses can sign up to be a part of N-STAT on the *http://nursingworld.org* Web site. Those registered with N-STAT receive a message about an issue of importance along with information and resources on how to contact legislators. N-STAT includes thousands of nurses. You can imagine that receiving thousands of letters about a single topic might get the attention of a legislator.

Another effort by the ANA to inform nurses about legislative issues is *Capitol Update*, an online legislative newsletter for nurses found at *www.capitolupdate.org*. This publication brings the latest in legislative concerns to your attention on a regular basis throughout the year.

Many specialty nursing organizations have a political action interest as well. Their Web sites and publications often provide information about issues of concern, and the organization may provide expert testimony for legislators.

Most state and district nurses' associations have legislative committees that monitor legislative and regulatory actions in their areas. They may provide educational events for nurses regarding current issues and testify at hearings concerning health-related issues. They also may seek to mobilize letter-writing or telephone campaigns.

Political Action Committees

Lobbying is the process of attempting to influence legislators to take a particular action. The law differentiates lobbying from providing general information and places restrictions on who can lobby. Nonprofit groups such as the ANA can provide information but cannot take direct action on behalf of specific candidates or partisan issues. To take a more active role in seeking the passage of desired legislation, the defeat of undesired measures, and the election of particular candidates, groups form organizations called **political action committees (PACs)**. These organizations are registered as political action groups and are free to try to affect the political process. They are not considered nonprofit organizations because their funds are used for political purposes; therefore, donations to them are not tax deductible (Fig. 15.2).

The ANA political action organization is titled the ANA-Political Action Committee (ANA-PAC). ANA-PAC actually lobbies for the passage or defeat of bills and supports candidates for public office. Since the 1976 federal elections, ANA-PAC has raised funds to support candidates for the Senate and the House of Representatives based on their expressed and demonstrated stands on key health issues, such as funding for nursing and biomedical research, funding for nursing education, and third-party reimbursement for nurses. Not all candidates endorsed by ANA-PAC were supported financially because of the limited funds available. Candidates' successes are attributable to many factors, but the effect of nursing support has been demonstrated. Many state nursing associations also have political action organizations. These groups serve the same function on the state level as ANA-PAC does on the national level. Many candidates actively seek the endorsement of nursing organizations that are perceived as influential with voters.

Although these nursing political action groups have not grown rapidly, growth has been steady. In addition, nurses are gaining more sophistication in their approach to the political process. The power of nurses in the political sphere is increasing.

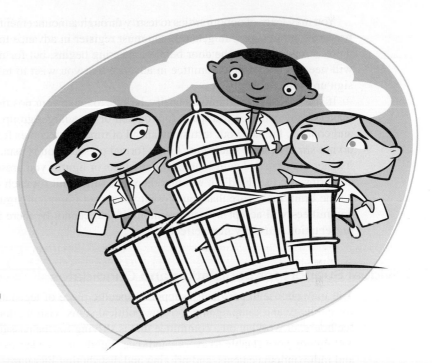

FIGURE 15.2 Nurses may lobby to get desired legislation passed by visiting legislators, by presenting information and arguments about the bill, and by writing letters.

 Critical Thinking Activity

Locate your state nurses' association Web site. Identify the issues that the organization believes are important to nurses in the state. Investigate those issues and identify ways you could support one of the issues presented.

Other Politically Important Groups

Many organizations, in addition to those specifically related to nursing, are concerned about health and social issues. Some are official lobbying groups; others provide information resources. Groups such as Common Cause (a consumer lobbying group), AARP, the League of Women Voters, and even church organizations often act to affect the political process. You may support these groups by donating money for their needs or by being actively involved in their work.

Testifying for Decision-Making Bodies

Many decisions affecting nursing and healthcare are made by committees and commissions at various levels of government. These decision-making bodies often hold hearings to gather information before decisions are made. As a nurse, your testimony may have particular value in certain areas of healthcare. A nurse may testify either as an official representative of an organization or as an independent individual.

You may learn of opportunities to testify through announcements in the newspaper and professional publications. In general, you must register in advance to testify. In some instances, there is registration at the door before a meeting begins, but for more formal situations, you will need to notify the committee in advance that you wish to testify. Increasingly, you can sign up online to testify.

If you have an opportunity to testify, be sure to make your position clear so that the decision makers know whether you speak for yourself or for a larger group. Keep your testimony brief and concise. Prepare your testimony ahead of time (with copies for committee members), but do not simply read a statement. A less-formal presentation is usually more interesting for the listener. Be prepared with sources for any facts or figures you present and explain any technical terms you use. Find out whether there is a time limit for each testimony. If you are given a time limit, make sure that you present your most important arguments and facts first. Most committees will accept written testimony if you cannot be there in person, but the personal presentation is usually more effective.

Individual Support for Legislation and Candidates

You may choose to personally support a specific piece of legislation by contributing money for publicity and campaigning, posting political signs, visiting door-to-door, sponsoring coffee hours, or working on a committee that is striving for the passage of a proposal. Both time and money are valuable to every candidate. Funds are needed for newspaper ads, television and radio announcements, and printing and distributing literature. Workers may be needed to perform secretarial tasks, contact people in a door-to-door campaign, and speak on behalf of the issue.

Supporting a candidate for public office is accomplished in the same way. In our political system, the reality is that those who have actively supported a candidate during an election campaign are listened to more closely when decisions are being made. Working for a candidate is one way to make your view known. It is also an excellent way to gain firsthand knowledge of the political process.

▶ *EXAMPLE*

Working in a Political Campaign

Inge Helgeson was an RN working in a community health center that provided healthcare on a sliding scale fee for homeless, unemployed, and low-income residents of their service area. She was distressed when she learned that one of the two candidates for county executive had announced that there was really no need for such health services and they should be cut back as a budgetary reduction. The opposing candidate, however, made a strong proposal for strengthening the role of the community health clinics. Inge decided to call the candidate who was supporting community health and volunteer to work on the campaign. She spent one evening a week on a phone bank. She called residents, explained the issues, and asked for their vote for her candidate. When it was time for the election, she said to a colleague at work, "For the first time I feel as if I am really doing something about the problem, not just watching while others do all the work."

Working in Policy-Making Agencies

Nurses have been appointed to major administrative positions in state and federal health agencies and to the staffs of several senators and representatives. In these roles, they have major policy-making responsibilities. Knowledgeable nurses may be appointed to task forces that study healthcare concerns and recommend regulatory or legislative action. The Robert Wood Johnson Foundation has provided 1-year fellowships for nurses to study policy in Washington, DC. Nurses who complete these fellowships have the skills and abilities to be effective in influencing healthcare policy. All of this points to nurses having a promising future in the health policy arena.

Seeking Election to an Office

Those elected or appointed to an office, whether in a local nursing organization or the US Congress, have the power to affect outcomes considerably. Leaders in nursing organizations help to shape the direction and efforts of those organizations. Legislators have power to affect significant regulations and spending plans. Nurses in several states have been effective in shaping health policy by being elected to office as members of their state legislatures. Eddie Bernice Johnson, elected as a congresswoman from Texas in 1994, was the first nurse to hold an elective federal office and still serves in that role. Three nurses were elected to the 111th US Congress, 2009. As women in general become more politically visible, nursing as a whole feels the impact.

Limitations on Your Political Activity

If you are an employee of any government agency, such as a public health department or the Veterans Administration, your political activity is subject to restrictions that do not apply to the general public. Restrictions applying to federal government employees are defined in the **Hatch Act** (5 USCA 7324) revision of 1993 (Hatch Act, 1993). Prohibited activities are mainly those that have to do with supporting a particular political party by being an officer or party spokesperson. The Hatch Act also prohibits any political activity on the part of a government employee, on behalf of a party, or in support of legislation, that could be construed as representing his or her government agency.

The Hatch Act does not interfere with a private citizen's right to support parties and candidates financially, to join political parties, to work for or against measures that will appear on a ballot, or to participate in nonpartisan (ie, not connected with a political party) elections as a candidate.

Each state has its own version of the Hatch Act. If you are employed by a government agency of any kind, investigate the limitations that your employment may place on your political activity.

THE FEDERAL GOVERNMENT'S ROLE IN HEALTHCARE

Federal legislation affects nursing and healthcare in important ways. If you understand key concepts of the federal government's involvement in healthcare and how federal legislation affects healthcare delivery, you will be more effective in the political arena.

Federal Agencies Related to Healthcare

The federal government operates in the healthcare field in complex ways. Literally, dozens of federal agencies are involved with healthcare in some way. The **Department of Health and Human Services (DHHS)** is a cabinet-level administrative unit of the federal government with four major service divisions and many different sections. The Public Health Service, which includes the Centers for Disease Control and Prevention (CDC), is one agency with which you should already be familiar. The National Institutes of Health (NIH), the Food and Drug Administration, the Health Resources Administration, and the Center for Medical & Medicare Services (CMS) are all part of DHHS. This agency has tremendous impact through its rules and regulations and the projects it funds.

The Federal Budget Process

Because funding is a driving force in all decision making, you will find it useful to understand something of the federal budget process. The availability of government funding for each federal program depends on two legislative actions: the **authorization act** (which outlines the actions to be taken) and the **appropriations act** (which provides the funding). Both the House and the Senate pass a budget appropriations act. Then a joint House and Senate committee meets to achieve a compromise that both will accept. The final result is called the **Omnibus Budget Reconciliation Act (OBRA)**, and it includes the compromises the budget committee has worked out between the House and Senate versions of the budget. Each budget act—for example, OBRA 2004—is identified by the year in the title. This is sometimes confusing because two monetary amounts, the authorized amount and the final budgeted (or appropriated) amount, may be reported in connection with the same act.

The budget act also may place restrictions on the people and organizations receiving federal funds. It is under this authority that the federal government sets standards for nursing homes that receive reimbursement through Medicaid and Medicare. The rules and regulations for nursing homes, called the **conditions of participation (COPs)**, included in OBRA 1987, were extensive and included such issues as restraint reduction, nursing assistant training, and resident privacy. These rules and regulations did not take effect until October 1, 1990. This allowed the affected organizations to begin the process of change to meet the new requirements. COPs for Medicare continue to have great effects on healthcare systems as they are revised.

Historically, a third factor has affected the amount of money available for a specific federal program: the participation of the executive branch of government in decisions regarding how and when available funds will be spent. If money that has been authorized and appropriated has not been spent by the end of a budget period, it is lost. This money then must be reauthorized and reappropriated. The executive branch has used this mechanism to withdraw support for programs it opposes.

Funding for Nursing Education and Research

Beginning in 1964, the federal government provided funding to support nursing education through the Nurse Training Act, later called the Nurse Education Act, signed by President Bush in 2002 as the Nurse Reinvestment Act. The most recent is the American Recovery and Reinvestment Act of 2009 that included funds for nursing. In the 1960s and early 1970s, the funding was generous and included money for buildings, classroom renovation, equipment, faculty education and development, and student scholarships and traineeships. The current nurse shortage has once again resulted in political pressure by nursing organizations for increased funds for nursing education.

A major advance for nursing research in the 1980s was the addition of a National Institute for Nursing Research (NINR) to the other major divisions of the NIH. It is now a major financial source of nursing research dollars. Nursing groups continue to lobby for increases in the appropriation for the NINR. However, even the existence of the NINR is not guaranteed. Proposals for reorganizing the work and research conducted in all areas of healthcare have included the elimination of many specialty institutes and a different method of focusing research. Many nurses view this proposal with alarm because nursing research does not claim the high profile of disease-specific research.

Occupational Safety and Health

The **Occupational Safety and Health Act (OSHA)** mandates actions and prescribes safety equipment to improve the health and safety of the working environment. Many people think the rules and regulations created by OSHA are too cumbersome. Nevertheless, concern for the safety of the working person is of considerable importance to nurses. Occupational injuries create major health problems for the adult population. They are costly not only in terms of health and personal loss but also in terms of lost productivity. Nurses also are affected by the provisions of OSHA in their own work environments. They, too, are subject to injury and accident on the job. The safety concerns of nurses in the workplace are discussed in Chapter 14.

Nurses in occupational health nursing are involved in OSHA through educating workers about job safety. In some situations, using safety precautions may be time-consuming and physically uncomfortable, and workers may be tempted to ignore them. Nurses may be able to curb this by helping workers understand the importance of following health and safety regulations. Occupational health nurses also assist management in planning to make the environment safe and in establishing appropriate procedures for treating injuries. OSHA regulations have required healthcare employers to provide the equipment, supplies, immunizations, and education to enable the implementation of CDC recommendations for universal precautions.

There is a "general duty" clause in the OSHA regulations stating that employers "must provide each employee a place of employment which is free from recognized hazards that are causing or likely to cause death or serious physical harm to his employees" (OSHA, Section 5A, 2004). Under this clause, if the hazard is recognized, if it can cause serious harm, and if there are reasonable methods to avoid that hazard, the employer may be cited for failure to maintain safety. This general duty clause is now being directed toward healthcare workplace concerns such as repetitive strain injuries and infection.

OSHA has been investigating the effects of repetitive strain injuries, among which are back injuries in healthcare workers. In 2003, the ANA launched "Handle With Care", a campaign focusing on solutions to the problem of musculoskeletal injuries among caregivers. Since that time, some states have passed legislation regarding safe patient handling in hospitals and nursing homes. Manufacturers are providing a greater variety of lifting and moving equipment, and many facilities are developing policies that promote greater safety in patient handling. In 2009, the National Institute for Occupational Safety and Health released a booklet titled *Safe Patient Handling Training for Schools of Nursing* (NIOSH, 2009a) and subsequently provided an online module *Safe Patient Handling and Movement* (NIOSH, 2009b) for teaching safe patient handling. The ANA supports all of these different efforts with information and resources (*http://nursingworld.org/handlewithcare*).

Another occupational concern to nurses that was politically addressed was needlestick injuries. Based on control of blood-borne pathogens, the FY1999 appropriations bill required employers to record all injuries from potentially contaminated needles and other sharp instruments, and in 2000, legislation was passed to require hospitals to provide safer devices to prevent injury (NIOSH, 1999).

Another safety concern of healthcare workers is violence in the workplace NIOSH (2002). Nurses in psychiatric settings have long recognized the hazards they face in working with aggressive, violent, and sometimes out-of-control clients. Emergency rooms are sites where the violence of society spills over into the healthcare setting. Even obstetric units may encounter violence by family members. Nurses are asking that OSHA mandate healthcare workplaces to provide safety from violence. See Chapter 14 for a further discussion of violence in the workplace.

COMMUNICATION IN ACTION

Mobilizing Support for Safety Measures in the Workplace

Irma Gunderson was an RN in the emergency room of a large urban hospital. There had been several instances when friends of patients had become belligerent and threatening to the staff, but there were no plans in place for managing staff safety. Irma began talking with her nurse manager. She said, "I was here the two evenings when those visitors threatened doctors, nurses, and others on the staff. I believe that we need to develop policies of how to manage such instances." Her manager replied, "What is the problem? I wasn't here those evenings, but I think the staff did fine—no one was hurt and the patient was cared for." Irma then said, "I was really afraid, and it is affecting my work. I have talked to some of the others on the evening shift and some of them even have nightmares. Millie the receptionist said she is going to ask for a transfer because she doesn't want to be here the next time it happens. We don't have a clear plan of how to call security, what people are supposed to do, and what our rights are in terms of protecting ourselves." The manager said, "No one else has said anything." Irma said, "I think they believe that nothing can be done. I have done some reading and I have learned that other hospitals have extensive plans in place. Could we get a committee together to investigate some of those and make some recommendations?" The manager said, "I appreciate your talking with me. I will talk with the management team tomorrow and maybe we can get something started here." By speaking directly to the person in charge who had the authority to initiate change, by having specific instances and concerns, Irma had facilitated improving the workplace climate.

Nursing Home Regulations

OBRA 1987 contained regulations that for the first time mandated a national standard for quality of care in nursing homes receiving federal money through Medicare or Medicaid with the provisions of this act set to take effect in October 1990. Because some of the requirements required additional time for implementation, some of the provisions of OBRA 1987 took effect as late as 1994. Despite earlier concerns, it is now clear that these regulations have positively affected the care environment in nursing homes. The use of restraints has decreased, resident rights are more effectively supported, and basic care needs are identified and met.

THE STATE GOVERNMENT'S ROLE IN HEALTHCARE

Many issues that vitally affect the healthcare arena are decided at the state level. Because the healthcare issues in each state are different, only some general areas of concern are outlined here.

State Agencies and Healthcare

State institutions range from those that care for the mentally retarded and the mentally ill to penal systems and institutions of higher education. Healthcare is a consideration in all of these settings. When budgets are planned, topics as diverse as immunization and contraception may be part of the debate. Nurses often can advocate for those who are unable to speak for themselves about their own healthcare needs. Sometimes nurses who work in state institutions are unable to deliver quality care because of severe budgetary deficiencies. All nurses can support efforts to provide quality healthcare in such settings.

State Legislative Concerns

Some of the major workplace concerns of nurses are emerging as topics of state legislation. The passage of any revision to the nurse practice act is an important state-level issue for nurses. See Chapter 3 for a discussion of nurse practice acts. The ANA has identified nine major state-level legislative issues of importance to nurses (see Display 15.4). In some states, legislation has already been passed regarding some of these issues.

Concerns about the nurse's vulnerability when unsafe care is part of an institution's practice have led to efforts toward achieving whistleblower protection through legislation. Whistleblowing was discussed in Chapter 8. The state of New Jersey was the first to pass legislation that protects from retaliation healthcare employees who refuse to participate in or who report unsafe practices. A major whistleblowing event took place in Texas in 2009. While the nurse involved was acquitted of both civil and criminal charges, the case raised many issues including job loss and the cost of self-defense subsequent to whistleblowing and renewed calls for protective legislation (Lowes, 2010).

Many of the state-level issues, such as prohibition of mandatory overtime, nursing staffing systems and ratios, and safety in the workplace, relate to increasing workplace satisfaction.

 DISPLAY 15.4 **State-Level Legislative Concerns Identified by ANA**

- Prohibition of mandatory overtime
- Nurse staffing systems and ratios
- Nursing workforce data collection
- Nursing education incentives
- Ergonomics
- Needlestick injury prevention
- Nursing quality indicators
- Violence in the workplace
- Whistleblower protection

Improving working conditions is an important aspect of addressing the nursing shortage. These issues are discussed in greater detail in Chapter 14.

LOCAL POLITICAL CONCERNS

In most communities, budgets for public health departments, school nurses, and so forth are developed over a period of several months. Hearings are often held, at which members of the public may ask questions and address issues. Nurses often have found that involvement at this planning stage is most rewarding. Determining priorities for healthcare is essential, and nurses can speak with authority on these matters. Nurses actually employed in a public department undergoing review may be limited in making their views known because of regulations governing their action in the political sphere. For this reason, it is significant that nurses outside of government institutions recognize the importance of community health. It is not only the practice of the public health nurse that is affected by the priorities of the agency. For example, a nurse who is employed in a hospital may wish to refer a discharged patient to a public health nurse for follow-up, only to find that, owing to changes in the ordering of priorities, home visits for the identified purpose are no longer being made.

In many communities, decisions about the allocation of federal money are made at the local level. Recent congressional actions have leaned toward enhancing state and local control through creating large block grants where priorities would be decided locally. Support for alternative healthcare centers, blood pressure screening, and senior citizen centers may depend on whether those who are knowledgeable about the benefits of these services are willing to voice their advocacy in local decision-making bodies.

FEDERAL HEALTHCARE REFORM LEGISLATION

Financing healthcare for all citizens has been the focus of many efforts for healthcare reform going back as far as the Franklin Roosevelt administration during World War II. In 1968, legislation instituted Medicare and provided health insurance for those over 65 years, the disabled, and special groups. Many saw this as the beginning of a drive toward universal healthcare. Through many administrations and congresses, the subject of healthcare reform continued to be raised and continued to be set aside.

In the 2010 landmark and controversial federal legislation, the Quality and Affordable Care Act was passed that began the process of providing health coverage for all legal residents of the United States. The DHHS has developed a Web site *www.healthreform.gov* to provide information about the contents of this legislation (DHHS, 2010.) While including many reforms to healthcare insurance and how it is administered and made available, the legislation also makes changes in both Medicare and Medicaid to increase availability and affordability within these two programs.

The new law provides opportunities for nurses and nursing. Funding for nursing workforce development was reauthorized, and there are incentives for nurses to seek advanced education. Nursing faculty in associate and baccalaureate programs will be eligible for support to continue their education. The law supports, among other provisions, an increased scope of practice, encouraging the expansion of nurse-run clinics, home visits for high-risk populations, and increasing reimbursement for nurse midwives (Robert Wood Johnson Foundation, 2010.)

Funding of these changes has been controversial as well. Some changes will be funded through eliminating waste and fraud in Medicare and other government health programs.

There will be changes in reimbursement policies. There will be increased costs for individuals and insurers through taxes and through mandates for coverage. More employers will be required to offer healthcare benefits. The legislation will be implemented in a gradual manner from 2010 to 2019 (Kaiser Commission, 2010).

Most people expect that this endeavor will require modification and compromise as implementation proceeds. There will always be some people not covered by the provisions established in this legislation. Costs will be a major concern. Nevertheless, the precedent has been established that healthcare should move into the realm of rights for all and out of the realm of privilege.

Critical Thinking Activity

Identify an aspect of the healthcare reform legislation that concerns you. Analyze the various proposals currently before Congress or your state legislature regarding that specific concern. Rank the proposals in order of your preference, providing rationales for your decision making. In a small group, hold a discussion in which you share your analysis of the various proposals.

THE DEVELOPMENT OF NURSING ORGANIZATIONS

Nursing organizations have political processes similar to those in found in governmental institutions. What is the role of the organization and how should its resources be spent? Where is authority for decision making? How can individual members affect decision making? What is the individual's role as a nurse in the organization?

When you first learn about the great number of nursing and nursing-related organizations, it may seem confusing, and their purposes and functions may seem duplicative. Here we will try to clarify some of that information.

Understanding the genesis of nursing organizations can help you to understand their current focus and activities. By the end of the 19th century, changes were accomplished most effectively through organizations. Nursing pioneers saw this as an opportunity to bring about transformation in nursing practice and nursing education and began forming nursing organizations.

Nursing Organizations in England

In England, the establishment of an organization for nursing was driven by the energies of Mrs. Bedford Fenwick (Ethel Gordon Manson), a prominent leader who, in 1887, campaigned for nurse registration. She believed that standards were necessary to improve nursing. Although her ideas for nurse registration were not well accepted, she founded the British Nurses' Association in 1888. It grew rapidly to 1,000 members by the end of the first year. It later became the Royal British Nurses' Association.

The American Society of Superintendents of Training Schools for Nurses

In 1893, the World's Fair and Columbian Exposition was held in Chicago to celebrate the 400th anniversary of Columbus' arrival in the United States. The Fair provided the meeting place for many professions and artisans. The first nurses' meeting was held in the Hall of

Columbus June 15–17, 1893, as part of the International Congress of Charities, Corrections, and Philanthropy. The nursing meeting was chaired by Isabel Hampton and was attended by American and Canadian nurses. Attendees included such individuals as Lavinia Dock—suffragist, nurse activist, historian, and educator—who spoke about the relation of training schools to hospitals. An address sent by Florence Nightingale was presented to the group. The papers presented were later compiled in a publication, *Nursing the Sick, 1893*. The day after the meeting, Isabel Hampton arranged a meeting of a small group of leaders to discuss the possibility of starting a nursing organization. This meeting resulted in the formation in 1896 of the American Society of Superintendents of Training Schools for Nurses, so named because most of the attendees were directors of nursing schools and the membership was restricted to those nurses associated with nurse training. Concern for the standards of nursing education was primary, and a committee to study nursing education was quickly appointed. In 1907, the Canadian members formed their own organization, the Canadian Society of Superintendents of Training Schools. The American organization changed its name in 1912 to the NLN Education (Donahue, 1996, p. 326).

In 1952, the NLN Education became the NLN when six organizations merged into one. The organizations involved in the merger were the National Organization for Public Health Nursing (est. 1912), the Association of Collegiate Schools of Nursing (est. 1933), the Joint Committee on Practical Nurses and Auxiliary Workers in Nursing Services (est. 1945), the Joint Committee on Careers in Nursing (est. 1946), the National Committee for the Improvement of Nursing Services (est. 1949), and the National Nursing Accrediting Service (est. 1949).

Nurses' Associated Alumnae of the United States and Canada

As the number of nurses increased throughout the United States and hospitals formed individual alumnae groups, the need arose for an organization of trained nurses. At the third meeting of the American Society of Superintendents of Training Schools in 1896, a committee prepared a constitution and bylaws for such an organization with the delegates representing the various alumnae associations. The constitution was accepted a year later, and the Nurses' Associated Alumnae of the United States and Canada was formed. The first president was Isabel Hampton Robb. The group had three purposes:

1. To establish and maintain a code of ethics
2. To elevate the standards of nursing education
3. To promote the usefulness and honor, the financial and other interests of the nursing profession (ANA, 1996, p. 2)

When it was discovered that New York law would not permit foreign membership in an incorporated association, the words "and Canada" were dropped from the title in 1901, and Canadian participation was prohibited. In 1911, the name of the organization in the United States became the ANA.

The Provisional Organization of the Canadian National Association of Trained Nurses was formed in 1908, and renamed the Canadian Nurses Association in 1924. This group also had as its primary concerns the education of nursing students, the improvement of nursing care, the amelioration of conditions for nurses, and state registration of nurses to protect the public.

NURSING ORGANIZATIONS OF TODAY

The existence of a large number of diverse organizations for nurses is, in many ways, a reflection of nursing itself. The profession offers a wide variety of employment opportunities to its members, with distinct and varied contributions and interests in healthcare. When nurses become committed to a particular specialty group, they have a tendency to want to advance the purposes and interests of the people working in that area. For example, operating room nurses have more in common with other operating room nurses, in terms of interests and concerns, than they have with nurses working in hospice care. Likewise, nurses involved in hospice care would probably prefer to share concerns with one another than to discuss them with critical care nurses. With more than 3.1 million nurses in the United States (HRSA, 2010), it is understandable that there are many different areas of nursing interest, and therefore many different nursing organizations.

The formation of so many nursing organizations has resulted in concern regarding the overlapping of function and interrelationships among some of the organizations. Unfortunately, there has been a spirit of competition rather than cooperation among these groups in the past. Because nurses traditionally have not had high incomes, joining more than one organization has not been a desirable option for economic as well as philosophic reasons. Different nursing organizations can be found listed on the World Wide Web at *http://nursingworld.org/rnindex*. The links provided at this Web site can help you to research individual organizations that may be of interest to you. As you review that list, you can understand why some critics suggest that nursing has too many organizations working in too many different directions.

Nursing organizations recently have made a concerted effort to promote cooperation. Nurses are better informed about the various organizations and receive better salaries than in the past. However, these facts have not resulted in significantly greater participation by professional nurses in their organizations. Some people specifically do not join because of philosophic differences, but many nurses seem to be apathetic and do not recognize the importance of nurses acting together. Some, because they are combining a job with family and home responsibilities, feel they do not have the time or energy to become involved. Nurses need to recognize the potential for power that they possess as a group. As the nation moves toward healthcare reform, this has never been a more critical issue.

The International Council of Nurses

The International Council of Nurses (ICN), the oldest of all international nursing organizations, was formed in 1899. Founded by Mrs. Bedford Fenwick, it held its first meeting in Buffalo, New York, at the World Exposition in 1901. Mrs. Fenwick was the first president of the organization. The membership originally was composed of self-governing national nurses' associations rather than individual members, although, until 1904, individual members could belong because few countries had organized nursing associations. Its purpose was to encourage communication among nurses of all nations and to provide opportunities for nurses from all over the world to meet and discuss concerns about the profession and about patient care. At the present time, the ICN meets every 4 years.

The ICN is the international organization for professional nursing, with membership consisting of national nursing organizations. The ANA, as a constituent member of the ICN, sends delegates to its convention and participates in its activities. The ICN is interested in healthcare in general and nursing care in particular throughout the world. It works with the United Nations, when appropriate, and with other international health-related groups, such as the International Red Cross.

The ICN concerns itself with such issues as the social and economic welfare of nurses, the role of the nurse in healthcare, and the roles of national nursing organizations throughout the world and their relationships to their governing bodies. The primary governing body of the organization is the Council of National Representatives, which meets biennially.

The ICN has representatives from more than 120 national nurses' organizations. The Council of National Representatives governs the organization, which consists of all the presidents of the member organizations. Activities of the organization are carried out by its Board of Directors, the officers, volunteer nurse members of constituent organizations, and employed staff, including an executive director. The ICN maintains headquarters in Geneva, Switzerland.

Every 4 years, a quadrennial congress is held. This meeting is open to all nurses and to delegates from the national organizations. Concerns addressed at recent congresses focused on such issues as career ladders, educational standards, research, human rights, and nursing's role in the planning of a national health policy. Current major efforts lie in the areas of international nurse migration, nursing regulation, and an innovations database. Information about all of these efforts may be found on the ICN Web site *www.icn.ch*.

American Nurses Association

The ANA has been identified as the professional organization for all RNs. As such, it has always had as its primary interest the concerns of the nurses it represents. Throughout history, the organization has been active in issues relating to nursing education (see Chapter 2), licensure (see Chapter 3), collective bargaining (see Chapter 5), and a host of other concerns facing nurses and nursing. The ANA is referred to many times throughout this book. As a professional association, it has been involved in all the issues that nursing has confronted.

Membership

The ANA membership comprises 49 state nurses' associations and the three territorial constituent units. In most cases, the individual nurse belongs to the ANA through the SNA. Since the organization has been restructured, individuals may now join the ANA directly. There are also opportunities for affiliate memberships.

While the reported supply of RNs is 3.1 million (HRSA, 2010), the membership in the constituent associations of the ANA is a fraction of that (*http://nursingworld.org*). Those who do participate are often the leaders in the nursing profession. Individuals who do not join give a variety of reasons, such as cost, a lack of time to participate in activities, and a lack of interest in the issues put forth. Some nurses do not join because they do not agree with the position of the ANA on major issues such as collective bargaining, nursing education, and political involvement.

Strategic Imperatives

The ANA has identified a set of strategic imperatives that structure its efforts. These include championing professional practice and excellence, formulating healthcare and public policy as they affect the profession and the public, providing accurate and comprehensive health policy information based on knowledge from research, advocating for nurses in the workforce and through workplace rights, facilitating unification and advancement of the profession, and improving its own organizational structure and resources. In order to work on these, the ANA has a wide-ranging set of activities. For the most comprehensive and up-to-date information, go to *www.nursingworld.org* and examine the information under each of the main menu headings. An overview is provided below (American Nurses Association [ANA], 2010).

The ANA supports work on policies related to the profession as a whole, such as the Code of Ethics for Nurses (ANA, 2001). The ANA also supports research on topics related to the profession itself. By serving as the coordinating body for the various affiliate organizations, the ANA helps to ensure its ongoing effectiveness. In its efforts to support the profession of nursing, the ANA has developed the Bill of Rights for Registered Nurses. This tool addresses the workplace environment needed for effective nursing practice. While not a legal document, this Bill of Rights serves as a guide to nurses as they seek to influence policy in organizations where they are employed (see Display 15.5). A discussion of how this Bill of Rights might be used and the foundations underlying the rights are available on the ANA Web site (*http://www. nursingworld.org/EspeciallyForYou/staffnurses/FAQs.aspx.*).

The ANA researches and promotes information on a variety of workplace issues for nurses especially those relating to occupational health for nurses. Some of the major issues currently being promoted were discussed previously.

The ANA is extensively involved in legislative activity and healthcare policy. The organization often represents the profession in testimony before Congress on numerous issues affecting nursing. The need to be geographically closer to legislators to have greater participation in legislative and policy efforts was the major reason for the relocation of the ANA offices to Washington, DC, in 1992. The organization provides testimony for or against legislation

DISPLAY 15.5 **American Nurses Association's Bill of Rights for Registered Nurses**

1. Nurses have the right to practice in a manner that fulfills their obligations to society and to those who receive nursing care.
2. Nurses have the right to practice in environments that allow them to act in accordance with professional standards and legally authorized scopes of practice.
3. Nurses have the right to a work environment that supports and facilitates ethical practice, in accordance with the *Code of Ethics for Nurses with Interpretive Statements.*
4. Nurses have the right to freely and openly advocate for themselves and their patients, without fear of retribution.
5. Nurses have the right to fair compensation for their work, consistent with their knowledge, experience, and professional responsibilities.
6. Nurses have the right to a work environment that is safe for themselves and for their patients.
7. Nurses have the right to negotiate the conditions of their employment, either as individuals or collectively, in all practice settings.

Adopted by the ANA Board of Directors June 26, 2001. *http://www.nursingworld.org/EspeciallyForYou/staffnurses/ FAQs.aspx.*

that will affect the profession, either directly or indirectly; legislative topics include funds for nursing education, collective bargaining issues, concerns for higher education, and human rights issues. It also testifies on health-related policy issues affecting the general public, such as the quality of care in nursing homes and healthcare reform. A newsletter, *Capitol Update*, (mentioned earlier) is distributed via the Internet.

Through its educational services, the ANA produces and distributes a wide variety of nursing materials, such as journals, films, and monographs. Reports of committees and commissions and special studies supported by the ANA also are published. The ANA also publishes many pamphlets and informational resources of value to nurses. A complete list of publications is available at the ANA Web site and in print from the organization. The ANA Web site continues to expand the content available and now includes the *Online Journal of Issues in Nursing*, and the many documents and position statements produced by the ANA. *American Nurse Today* is the official publication of the ANA; official announcements of ANA business are published in this journal. ANA also publishes a newspaper, *American Nurse,* that contains current news relevant to nursing and healthcare, editorials, letters, and classified advertisements.

In addition to its activities on behalf of the profession as a whole, the ANA provides direct services to members. These services include online continuing education, access to a group professional liability insurance plan, and group insurance for health, disability, and accident coverage. The ANA also provides access to group travel arrangements and a variety of purchasing discounts.

American Nurses Credentialing Center

The ANA in collaboration with specialty nursing organizations established the American Nurses Credentialing Center (ANCC) as an autonomous organization to manage the process of specialty credentialing. The ANCC also operates the magnet hospital recognition program for hospitals that demonstrate excellence in nursing practice and the environment for nursing. The ANCC remains an affiliated organization for the ANA.

American Nurses Foundation

In 1955, the ANA established the American Nurses Foundation (ANF), an affiliate of the ANA, as a tax-exempt, nonprofit corporation for the purpose of supporting research related to nursing. It is independently financed and self-governing. Its board of trustees is composed of members of the board of directors of the ANA, other nurse members, and nonnurse members from other health-related fields and from the public. To accomplish its varied objectives, the ANF solicits gifts and contributions from individuals and organizations. These gifts are tax deductible.

The ANF maintains a three-pronged approach to supporting research. The first objective is to conduct policy analyses to provide nursing leaders and public-policy makers with the information they need for decision making. The second objective is related to developing nurse scholars, individuals who engage in study of such areas as journalism and public policy. Support is directed toward independent study, research, and doctoral and postdoctoral work for these nurse scholars. The third objective is to facilitate the research and educational activities of ANA. This includes providing consultation and funding for groups in the ANA that wish to initiate projects.

American Academy of Nursing

The ANA established the American Academy of Nursing (AAN) in 1973 as an honorary association in the ANA. The ANA's board of directors chose the original members. The AAN is now an independent organization that is an affiliate of ANA, and new members are selected by those currently in the AAN. Those elected to the AAN are considered fellows and may use the title Fellow of the American Academy of Nursing (FAAN). The purpose of this organization is to recognize nurses who have made significant contributions to the profession of nursing.

National League for Nursing

The mission for the NLN states, "The National League for Nursing promotes excellence in nursing education to build a strong and diverse nursing workforce" (NLN, 2010). The goals of the organization focus on four areas: (1) being a leader in nursing education, (2) commitment to members, (3) acting as a champion for nurse educators, and (4) advancing the science of nursing education.

Membership

The NLN offers membership to individuals and agencies. It is unique among nursing organizations in that it also offers membership and participation to consumers, nonnursing members of healthcare teams, and institutions concerned with nursing service and nursing education.

Activities and Services

The NLN works in a complementary, rather than competitive, manner with the ANA. Whereas the ANA speaks as the official voice of nurses, the NLN seeks to unite the interests of nursing with those of the community in support of excellence in nursing education.

The NLN sponsors continuing education workshops and conferences related to nursing education throughout the country, often repeating a workshop in different locations to spare participants the expense of travel. Subjects are determined in consultation with members and are geared to current needs and interests. Curriculum, research, accreditation, testing and evaluation, student recruitment and retention, political awareness and healthcare legislation, and a nurse executive series are regular subjects for continuing education. The constituent leagues, which are grouped by regional assemblies, also offer workshops designed to meet the interests of particular areas of the country.

Through its journal, *Nursing Education Perspectives*, and a newsletter, *NLN Update* (both available on the Web), members are kept informed about current issues. *Reflection and Dialogue* is a Web publication that presents timely information regarding major topics such as the doctor of nursing practice (DNP) degree. Sometimes NLN spokespersons offer testimony on legislation or rulings significant to the organization. The NLN publishes many texts and references about curriculum, ethics, public policy, nursing administration, long-term care, and other topics of interest to nursing. It also produces educational videos.

The Centers for Excellence (nursing programs designated for their achievements), and documents such as *Hallmarks of Excellence in Nursing Education* and *Resources for Excellence* are all part of the Excellence Initiatives. Another excellence initiative, the Academy of Nursing Education honors nurses who have made significant contributions in nursing education. Members use the title Academy of Nursing Education Fellow (ANEF).

The NLN has developed a certification program for nurse educators. This includes educational materials and a testing program that recognizes those who meet these high standards for certification.

NLN serves as a resource for data regarding nursing education such as enrollments, admissions, and graduations. Other data such as the numbers of men and minorities in schools of nursing and faculty shortages also are gathered through their annual surveys of nursing programs.

Through its testing service, the NLN produces standardized assessment tests to be used in the nursing program admission process, achievement tests for various levels in a program that can be used by a program for evaluation, the NLN mobility examinations (which are used to provide advanced placement credit), and diagnostic examinations for those preparing for the National Council Licensure Examination, or NCLEX.

Accrediting Organizations

The National League for Nursing Accrediting Commission (NLNAC) and the Commission on Collegiate Nursing Education (CCNE) are the two nursing organizations that accredit nursing education programs. These two organizations were discussed in detail in Chapter 3 (Fig. 15.3).

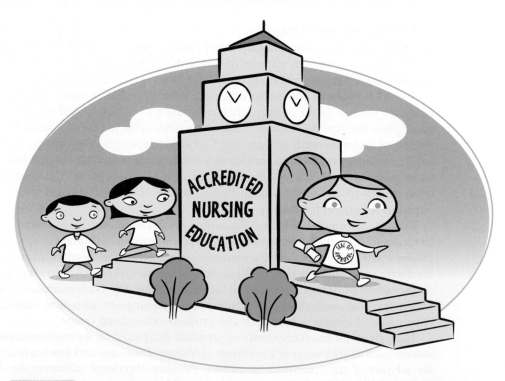

FIGURE 15.3 Accreditation is designed to help ensure that the desired outcomes of education are achieved.

American Association of Colleges of Nursing

The AACN was formed to assist baccalaureate and higher degree schools of nursing in working cooperatively to improve higher education for professional nursing. Membership is limited to programs that offer a baccalaureate degree or higher in nursing, with an upper-division nursing major, and that are part of a regionally accredited college or university. The AACN focuses on the quality of nursing education in baccalaureate and higher degree programs and support and assistance to deans and programs in providing excellence in education. The organization also provides data regarding these programs and is active in public advocacy for nursing and nursing education both independently and through the Tri-Council.

National Council of State Boards of Nursing

Although it is not a nursing organization like those previously discussed, our discussion would not be complete without mention of the National Council of State Boards of Nursing, Inc. (NCSBN). This organization was formed in 1978 to replace the Council of State Boards that had been part of the ANA. The purpose of this organization is to provide a forum for the legal regulatory bodies (whatever their particular state titles might be) of all states, the District of Columbia, and US territories to act together in the regulation of nursing practice for the protection of the public. There is one delegate to this council from each state agency. The actions of this council are particularly important because its membership represents the legal authority for the control of nursing education and nursing practice.

Although each state agency must operate within its own laws, it does have authority to establish many specific rules and regulations. Working together, the state boards hope to promote uniform standards for the nursing profession. One of the agenda items they have addressed is the development of a Model Nurse Practice Act, which serves to guide states as they work on licensure laws. Much energy has gone into the development, validation, and establishment of computerized testing for the licensing examination for both registered (NCLEX-RN) and practical (NCLEX-PN) nursing. Currently, the organization is addressing the issues related to approving and licensing advanced practice nurses and the concerns associated with multistate practice.

Organizations Representing Licensed Practical Nurses

Two nursing organizations are concerned primarily with advancing the interests of licensed practical (vocational) nurses (LPN). These two organizations are the National Federation of Licensed Practical Nurses (NFLPN) and the National Association for Practical Nurse Education and Service (NAPNES).

The NFLPN is the professional organization for LPNs. Founded in 1949, its membership is limited to LPNs and students in practical nursing programs. This organization has developed a set of practice standards for the LPN and, through the NFLPN Educational Foundation, offers an IV Therapy and Gerontology Certification by exam program for LPNs possessing the knowledge and skills necessary to complete patient care tasks associated with these specialties. State and local groups of the NFLPN are active in educational issues affecting the LPN and have supported the associate degree as the appropriate educational preparation for the responsibilities of the LPN in the current healthcare system. Further information is available on the NFLPN Web site, *http://nflpn.org*.

The NAPNES was organized as the Association of Practical Nurse Schools in 1941. Its purpose was to address the needs of practical nursing education. The name was changed in 1942 to the National Association for Practical Nurse Education; in 1959, it added "and Service" to that title. The official publication of the organization is *The Journal of Practical Nursing*, which has been published since 1951. Membership is open to LPNs, practical/vocational nursing students, faculty, directors, physicians, organizations, the lay community, and other individuals who are interested in promoting the professional practice and education of practical nurses. It was the first organization to provide accreditation for practical nursing programs, although that role now rests with the NLNAC. You can learn more about NAPNES and their three councils at *www.napnes.org*.

NANDA-I

In 2002, NANDA, originally established in 1982 as the North American Nursing Diagnosis Association, became NANDA-International (NANDA-I) to reflect the increasing worldwide interest in the field of nursing diagnosis terminology. It is open to individuals as well as group members. The purpose of this group is to work toward uniform terminology and definitions to be used in nursing diagnosis and to share ideas and information regarding this topic. The general outline of the taxonomy (classification system) was established by a group of nursing theorists and then accepted by the organization. NANDA-I is organized into a taxonomy that includes 13 domains (categories) of nursing practice: Health Promotion, Nutrition, Elimination and Exchange, Activity/Rest, Perception/Cognition, Self-Perception, Role Relationships, Sexuality, Coping/Stress Tolerance, Life Principles, Safety/Protection, Comfort, and Growth/ Development. Nursing diagnoses are clustered under each of these domains. Members identify and research problems nurses manage, prepare documentation, and submit these to NANDA-I to be included in the consideration process. Committees then review the problems. Those that meet the basic criteria for nursing diagnoses are submitted to the membership. For each problem, defining characteristics are identified, conditions that form the etiology or are related to the development of the diagnosis are identified, and a place in the classification is established. An international convention held every 2 years is the final forum for the debate and discussion of proposed new nursing diagnoses. Two publications—*The International Journal of Nursing Terminologies and Classification* and *Nursing Diagnoses and Classifications*—are used to disseminate the work of the organization. See the Web site at *www.nanda.org*. More recently, this organization is coordinating its work with those working on the Nursing Interventions Classification and the Nursing Outcomes Classification to fulfill the goal of a coordinated system of nursing terminology.

American Organization of Nurse Executives

According to their Web site, AONE is the "national professional organizations for nurses who design, facilitate, and manage care" (*www.aha.org/resources/AboutAone.html*). This organization provides the forum for nurses with managerial and executive responsibility to work collaboratively both with other nurses in similar roles and through the organization with other organizations. AONE is one of the members of the Tri-Council for Nursing, which serves as an information resource for legislative and governmental personnel.

Sigma Theta Tau

Sigma Theta Tau is an international organization established in collegiate schools of nursing to recognize those with superior ability and leadership potential, and those who have made important contributions to nursing. Candidates may be asked to join during the senior year of a baccalaureate program, or any time thereafter. Sigma Theta Tau has established a nursing library at its headquarters in Indianapolis that has reference abilities to support advanced scholarship; the organization also provides two print journals *Journal of Nursing Scholarship* and *Reflections on Nursing Leadership* (which is also available online). Local chapters may maintain funds to support individual research projects, hold research conferences, and recognize those who have made significant contributions to nursing.

Tri-Council for Nursing

Mentioned several times above, the Tri-Council for Nursing is a joint effort of the ANA, the NLN, AONE, and the AACN to work collaboratively in presenting a unified voice for nursing in the policy arena. Addressing the three major areas of education, practice, and research, the Tri-Council establishes positions on health issues, proposed legislation, and regulations. When individuals represent the Tri-Council while testifying before decision-making groups, they have great credibility in regard to the issues.

Clinical Organizations

Some of the earliest specialty organizations were related to specific clinical practice areas of nursing. A major focus of these organizations now is continuing education related to a particular nursing specialty. Most groups also have some mechanisms, such as certification, for recognizing achievement in the field. One of the earliest specialty organizations, founded in 1941, was the American Association of Nurse Anesthetists, a group of approximately 40,000 members (American Association of Nurse Anesthetists, 2010).

Specialty organizations also include groups that began as auxiliaries to specialty physicians' organizations, such as the Association of Women's Health, Obstetric and Neonatal Nurses. This organization was started for nurses affiliated with physicians who were "fellows" of the American College of Obstetricians and Gynecologists. As more members joined and nurses became more active, groups such as this one became autonomous. Most specialty organizations, such as the Critical Care Nurses Association, began as nurses sought forums to exchange information and obtain education in their specialty.

The Nursing Organizations Alliance (The Alliance) was formed in 2001 when two long-standing coalitions of nursing organizations, the National Federation for Specialty Nursing Organizations (NFSNO) and the Nursing Organizations Liaison Forum (NOLF), united. The purpose of the Alliance is to provide a forum for identification, education and collaboration building on issues of common interest to the specialty organizations to advance the nursing profession (*www.nursing-alliance.org/content.cfm/id/about_us*).

The National Alliance of Nurse Practitioners was organized in 1986. Its purpose is to promote the healthcare of the nation by promoting the visibility, viability, and unity of nurse practitioners. Its activities focus on advancing the role of the nurse practitioner in the healthcare delivery system. Issues related to the reimbursement of nurse practitioners are of major concern to this organization.

Groups Related to Ethnic Origin

As the movement for self-determination and preservation of identity arose within ethnic groups in the United States, nurses within various ethnic groups began to unite to achieve a greater voice in healthcare. Some ethnic groups are nationally organized; others are organized on a more local level. As these groups have become stronger and more organized, their interests have included the recruitment and support of nursing students from the particular ethnic groups they represent. These ethnic groups also encourage their members to become more politically involved in nursing and nursing leadership.

Religious Organizations

The National Council of Catholic Nurses and the Nurses' Christian Fellowship (primarily a nondenominational Protestant group) were organized to assist nurses in sharing concerns and integrating their work and their religious beliefs. These two organizations place special emphasis on meeting a patient's spiritual needs and on dealing with ethical issues.

National Student Nurses Association

The National Student Nurses Association (NSNA), started in 1952, is a professional organization for students in schools of nursing. Although it works with the ANA, it is a fully independent organization, run and financed by nursing students. It sponsors its own annual convention.

Although the NSNA is an autonomous organization, it has close ties with the ANA. Members of the NSNA serve on selected committees in the ANA, speak to the House of Delegates at the ANA convention to provide a student viewpoint, and work together with the ANA regarding current issues.

Each state has a nursing student association that operates in the same relationship to the state professional organization as the NSNA does to the ANA. State conventions and workshops are held in many states. State issues are addressed by the state association in the same way that national issues are addressed by the NSNA. Local nursing student organizations may or may not exist in individual schools of nursing. These local organizations may be closely tied to the state and national groups, or they may be independent. It is possible for an individual student to join the state and national student nurses' organizations even if no local counterpart exists.

A major project of the NSNA is "Breakthrough into Nursing," organized in 1965. This project is designed to recruit and maintain the enrollment of minorities in schools of nursing through mentoring and to create a respect for the differences and similarities between people. The project has enlisted nursing students to speak to minority teenagers to interest them in nursing early in their scholastic careers, and to act as preceptors and tutors to increase the retention of minority students when they enroll in schools of nursing. Other activities are directed at the image of nursing and disaster planning. They publish a magazine titled *Imprint* and *NSNA eNews,* an electronic newsletter.

The NSNA often is asked to testify before congressional committees when issues relevant to nursing education are being considered. In this role, the organization becomes the public voice for all nursing students.

The NSNA has developed a series of documents that support the role of the nursing student. These include a Code of Ethics for Students: Part I Code of professional conduct, Code of Ethics for Students: Part II Code of academic and clinical conduct, and the Bill of Rights and Responsibilities for Students of Nursing. These documents are all available from the NSNA Web site (www.nsna.org).

Educational and Research Organizations

Since the 1960s, there has been a great deal of change and development in nursing education as it has moved from the hospital into the educational setting. During this time, there has been an increased emphasis on educational methods, curriculum development, and research.

In several major geographic regions of the United States, education organizations extending membership to schools of nursing, members of the state boards of nursing, and other interested individuals were developed to promote interstate and interinstitutional cooperation in seeking ways to improve nursing education and scholarship. These organizations are the Western Institute of Nursing, the Council on Collegiate Education for Nursing of the Southern Regional Education Board, the New England Organization for Nursing, the Midwest Alliance in Nursing, and the Mid-Atlantic Regional Nursing Association.

The National Organization for the Advancement of Associate Degree Nursing (N-OADN), founded in 1984, is dedicated to enhancing the quality of Associate Degree nursing education, strengthening the professional role of the Associate Degree nurse, and protecting the future of Associate Degree nursing in the midst of healthcare changes. N-OADN publishes a quarterly journal *Teaching and Learning in Nursing*. Membership is open to individuals, states, agencies, and organizations.

Miscellaneous Organizations

The American Assembly for Men in Nursing was formed by those who believed that, as a minority in the profession, men needed to speak about issues with a united voice. The membership has expanded to include women who are concerned about gender issues in nursing. The organization has addressed the issue of discrimination toward men in nursing and seeks to present nursing as a profession in which both men and women can contribute and excel. In March 2006, *Men in Nursing*, the first journal to address issues and concerns facing the growing number of men who have chosen nursing as a career, was published.

Nurses House, Inc. provides assistance for nurses in need. It originated from a bequest in 1922 from Emily Bourne, who donated $300,000 to establish a country home where nurses might find needed rest. As the need for this residence decreased, supporters of this endeavor sold the estate and invested the proceeds. Income from the investment and funds donated by nurses (and friends of nurses) are used to provide guidance and counseling for nurses with emotional and chemical dependency problems, encouragement to homebound nurses, and temporary financial assistance to nurses who are ill, convalescing, or unemployed. Nurses House seeks members and donations to assist in continuing these activities.

The Gay Nurses' Alliance was an outgrowth of the movement of homosexual individuals to be accepted without having to disguise their sexual orientation. This group primarily has focused on the issue of gay rights. They also provide a forum for gay individuals to address the difficulties they may face in the nursing profession.

Critical Thinking Activity

As a new graduate, assume you have $400 per year to spend on membership in a nursing organization. In trying to decide which organization to join, how would you go about learning the focus of several groups that have attracted your interest? What process could you use to ensure that you are joining the group that best serves your needs? Which organization would you join? Provide a clear rationale based on both economic and professional reasons for your choice.

KEY CONCEPTS

- Because scarce resources are allocated through the political process, nurses will find that understanding this process is essential to influencing the healthcare system.

- Each nurse has many opportunities to affect the political process. This can be done simply by keeping informed, voting, or trying to shape public opinion. Communicating with legislators and officials can be done individually or as part of a group. Testifying presents issues of importance, and individual support can be given to those running for office. You may even decide to run for a public office.

- The federal government is active in healthcare through many existing agencies in the HHS and in other branches of government. The federal budget process affects the healthcare services available through the many legislative acts affecting healthcare such as Medicare, for the elderly and certain disabled individuals, and Medicaid, for the poor.

- A political process is part of any large organization, and nursing organizations are no exception. Understanding the political process can help you participate more effectively in a large organization.

- The variety of organizations in nursing is often confusing to the new nursing graduate and to the public. These organizations represent the nursing profession as a whole, as well as special interest groups within nursing.

- The ANA, whose membership is open to RNs through their state constituencies, provides the voice of professional nursing. Actions of the ANA are directed toward nursing practice issues, economic welfare of nurses, and broader issues of healthcare.

- Another major nursing organization is the NLN, which, historically, has championed better nursing education. Membership is open to individuals and agencies interested in nursing.

- The NLNAC and CCNE provide for the accreditation of nursing programs throughout the United States.

- The NCSBN coordinates the development of the licensure examinations used for both practical nurses and RNs. It also coordinates and supports the development of common licensure standards, licensure agreements between states, and an examination for certifying nursing assistants.

- Two nursing organizations exist expressly to serve the needs of LPNs. These groups are the NFLPN and the NAPNES.

- Organizations also exist that represent specialty groups in nursing. Members usually are drawn together by their common interests and concerns. A very active and prominent organization is the AONE representing nurse administrators. Some of the specialty organizations provide continuing education and, in some instances, certification.

- Some organizations, such as Sigma Theta Tau, are honorary in their focus. These groups strive to bring recognition to nurses and nursing.
- The NSNA addresses the interests and needs of nursing students. As a fully autonomous organization, NSNA membership is open to nursing students only.

- A wide variety of other organizations meet the special needs of their membership. This may relate to social interests, ethnic background, or other common denominators.

RELEVANT WEB SITES

Web sites relevant to this chapter can be found at thePoint ※ accessed through *http://thePoint. lww.com/Ellis10e* and by entering the code found on the inside cover of your text.

REFERENCES

American Association for History of Nursing. (2007). *Hannah A. Ropes*. Retrieved January 19, 2011, from www.aahn.org/gravesites/ropes.html

American Association of Nurse Anesthetists. (2010). *Certified registered nurse anesthetists at a glance*. Retrieved January 19, 2011, from www.aana.com/ataglance.aspx

American Nurses Association. (1996). *In the beginning*. Retrieved January 19, 2011, from www.nursingworld.org/FunctionalMenuCategories/AboutANA/WhoWeAre/History.aspx

American Nurses Association. (2001). *Code of ethics for nurses with interpretive statements*. Washington, DC: ANA Publications. Retrieved January 20, 2011, from www.nursingworld.org/MainMenuCategories/EthicsStandards/CodeofEthicsforNurses.aspx

American Nurses Association. (2009). *Bill of rights FAQs*. Retrieved January 18, 2011, from http://www.nursingworld.org/EspeciallyForYou/staffnurses/FAQs.aspx

American Nurses Association. (2010). *Hill basics*. Retrieved January 19, 2011, from www.nursingworld.org/MainMenuCategories/ANAPoliticalPower/Federal/ToolKit/VisitingCapitolHill.aspx.

American Nurses Association. (2010). *2009 annual report*. Retrieved January 19, 2011, from www.nursingworld.org/FunctionalMenuCategories/AboutANA/ANA-2009-Annual-Report.aspx

Bostridge, M. (2008). *Florence Nightingale: The woman and her legend*. London: Penguin-Viking.

Centers for Medicare & Medicaid Services. (n.d.). *Spotlight quarterly: What's new*. Retrieved January 20, 2011, from www.cms.gov/QuarterlyProviderUpdates/02_Spotlight.asp

Department of Health and Human Services. (2010). *Health reform and the department of health and human services*. Retrieved January 19, 2011, from www.healthcare.gov/

Donahue, M. P. (1996). *Nursing: The finest art* (2nd ed.). St. Louis, MO: CV Mosby.

Hatch Act. (1993). Retrieved January 19, 2011, from www.osc.gov/hatchact.htm

Health Resources and Services Administration (HRSA). (2010). *National sample survey of registered nurses, March 2008: Preliminary findings*. Retrieved January 19, 2011, from http://bhpr.hrsa.gov/healthworkforce/rnsurvey/2008/

Kaiser Commission on Medicaid and the Uninsured and the Health Care Marketplace Project. (2010). *Health reform implementation timeline*. Publication Number: 8060 Publish Date: 2010-04-27. Retrieved January 19, 2011, from www.kff.org/healthreform/8060.cfm

Lowes, R. (2010). Whistleblowing nurses case highlights need for more open quality-of-care culture. *Medscape Medical News,* March 3. Retrieved January 20, 2011, from www.medscape.com/viewarticle/717867

National Institutes for Occupational Safety and Health. (1999). *NIOSH alert: preventing needlestick injuries in healthcare settings.* Pub #2000-108, Retrieved January 19, 2011, from www.cdc.gov/niosh/docs/2000-108/

National Institutes for Occupational Safety and Health. (2002). *Violence: Occupational Hazards in Hospitals.* Publication 2002-101. Retrieved January 16, 2011, from www.cdc.gov/niosh/docs/2002-101/

National Institutes for Occupational Safety and Health. (2009a). *Safe Patient Handling and Movement,* Web based training. Retrieved January 19, 2011, from www.cdc.gov/niosh/docs/2009-127/

National Institutes for Occupational Safety and Health. (2009b). *Safe Patient Handling Training for Schools of Nursing.* DHHS (NIOSH) Publication No. 2009-127. Retrieved January 18, 2011, from www.cdc.gov/niosh/docs/2009-127/

National League for Nursing. (2010). *Our mission.* Retrieved January 12, 2011, from www.nln.org/aboutnln/our-mission.htm

Occupational Health and Safety Act. (2004). *Public law 91–596, 84 STAT.* 1590, 91st Congress, S.2193, December 29, 1970, as amended through January 1, 2004 Retrieved January 15, 2011, from www.osha.gov/pls/oshaweb/owadisp.show_document?p_table=OSHACT&p_id=2743

Project Vote Smart (2010). *How a bill becomes a law.* Retrieved January 19, 2011, from www.votesmart.org/resource_govt101_02.php

Robert Wood Johnson Foundation. (2010). *Health care overhaul means more opportunities and demand for nurses.* Retrieved January 10, 2011, from www.rwjf.org/healthreform/product.jsp?id=62128

US Census Bureau. (2009). *Survey of voting and registration, table 1 reported voting and registration.* Retrieved December 29, 2010, from www.census.gov/hhes/www/socdemo/voting/publications/p20/2008/tables.html

US Department of Health and Human Services (USDHHS), Health Resources and Services Administration. (2010). *The registered nurse population: initial findings from the 2008 national sample survey of registered nurses.* Retrieved January 20, 2011, from http://bhpr.hrsa.gov/healthworkforce/rnsurvey/2008/

See the following regular publications for current information:
American Journal of Nursing. New York City, NY: Lippincott Williams & Wilkins.
American Nurse Today. Kansas City, MO: American Nurses Association (a bimonthly journal).
The American Nurse. Kansas City, MO: American Nurses Association (a bimonthly newspaper).

See also the official publication of your state nurses association.

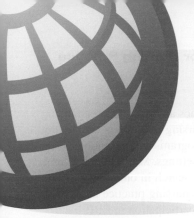

16

Applying Research and Technology to Nursing Practice

LEARNING OUTCOMES

After completing this chapter, you should be able to:

1. Construct an effective strategy for evaluating information resources.
2. Discuss the value of the research in nursing.
3. Describe the role of the staff nurse in nursing research.
4. Explain the term "evidence-based practice" (EBP) and its application to nursing.
5. List the types of evidence that may be used for EBP, moving from the most reliable to the least reliable.
6. Outline a process for establishing an evidence-based nursing practice in an institutional setting or in your own personal practice.
7. Analyze the role of technology in nursing.
8. Assess your own competence in the realm of nursing technology.

KEY TERMS

Clinical significance	Population
Computerized provider order entry (CPOE)	Probability
Control group	Qualitative research
eICU	Quantitative research
Evidence-based practice (EBP)	Randomized controlled trial (RCT)
Informatics	Reliability
Institutional review board (IRB)	Sample
Level of significance	Validity
Participant/subject	

As you look toward the future, you may find it hard to imagine what nursing will be like. What new insights will nursing research bring? What expectations for practice responsibilities will rest with each nurse? How will evidence-based practice (EBP) change nursing? What technology will be a part of nursing practice? These factors are shaping nursing as you will practice it.

VALUING NURSING RESEARCH

If you are in a baccalaureate nursing program, a course in statistics and one in understanding nursing research are usually requirements. While a course in nursing research is usually not an essential part of associate degree (AD) education, more AD programs are presenting a brief introduction to research as the emphasis on EBP increases in all settings. Many students come to AD nursing having taken courses related to statistics and/or research in other fields. Here, we provide a brief overview of the development of research for nursing practice along with some basic concepts and information to guide your reading and participation in EBP.

The Development of Nursing Research

Nursing research essentially began after World War II, when academic nursing programs expanded rapidly. Nurses began obtaining graduate degrees and learning how to conduct research. *Nursing Research*, which began in 1951, was the first nursing publication to focus on research. Gradually more journals, in the United States, the United Kingdom, and Canada, began to focus on nursing research. Table 16.1 provides an overview of the nursing research journals available and the dates they were first published. In addition to the journals, whose total content is research, many other nursing journals devote a significant number of their pages to research along with articles related to policy and current practice descriptions. This increase in nursing research publication has been a reflection of the increasing emphasis of the profession on scholarly work and the growing number of nurses academically prepared to conduct effective research.

For many individuals, a key landmark along the path toward a research-based profession was the authorization of the National Center for Nursing Research (NCNR) in 1986 (National Institute of Nursing Research [NINR], n.d.). Prior to this, nursing research was found in a variety of federal endeavors, such as the Division of Nursing within the Office of the Surgeon General and the various sections with the National Institutes of Health (NIH). While the NCNR was an important milestone for nursing research, it did not have the prestige or

Table 16.1   **Initial Publication Dates for Nursing Research Journals**

YEAR OF FIRST PUBLICATION	RESEARCH JOURNAL
1951	*Nursing Research*
1968	*Journal of Nursing Scholarship: International* (Sigma Theta Tau)
1969	*Canadian Journal of Nursing Research*
1976	*Journal of Advanced Nursing* (UK)
1979	*Western Journal of Nursing Research*
1988	*Applied Nursing Research*
1991	*Clinical Nursing Research* (Canadian editors)
1992	*Nurse Researcher: The International Journal of Research Methodology in Nursing and Health Care* (UK)
1993	*Online Journal of Knowledge Synthesis for Nursing*
1995	*International Journal of Psychiatric Nursing Research*
1995	*Journal of Nursing Research* (UK)
1998	*Evidence Based Nursing Online Journal* (UK)
2000	*BMC Nursing Online* (UK)
2000	*Southern Online Journal Of Nursing Research: Electronic Publication Of Research* (http://snrs.org/publications/journal.html)
2004	*World Views on Evidence Based Nursing* (www.blackwell-synergy.com/links/toc/wvn/1/1)

DISPLAY 16.1 Steps of the Traditional Nursing Research Process

- Developing the research question
- Reviewing the literature
- Developing the hypothesis
- Designing the study
- Carrying out the study
- Analyzing the data
- Identifying concerns about the study
- Drawing conclusions and applications
- Identifying future research needed

funding that was provided for the NIH. Based on an increasing recognition of the importance of nursing research, the NCNR was changed into a full-fledged NINR within the NIH in 1993 and celebrated its 25th anniversary in October 2010 (NINR, n.d.).

An Overview of the Nursing Research Process

A research study begins with one unanswered question. Literature is reviewed thoroughly to determine what is already known about the question. The question is then refined based on the knowledge available and identified *variables* (things in the setting that vary or change) and questions about how they are interrelated. In a traditional research study, a *hypothesis* (statement of the expected relationships) is established. A research study is designed to gather information that will help to answer the question. The study is carefully carried out, and the information collected is analyzed. Then the researcher reaches a conclusion about what has been learned from the study, discusses the application of the study to nursing, any concerns with the study are presented, and identifies further research needed (see Display 16.1).

Individuals within an institution who have research expertise are appointed to review research proposals and assure that they conform to standardized guidelines. This group is usually titled the **institutional review board (IRB)**, and it oversees the entire research process in any organization. The IRB determines whether the question is appropriate, the means of study fit the question, the study is ethical, and most especially, the rights of any subjects or participants are protected (see discussion of participants below). No research is allowed in an institution that has not been approved by the institution's review board. For research that occurs outside of institutions, private organizations serve as review boards to ensure the protection of the public.

While this greatly oversimplifies the research process, it provides a foundation to help you understand some of the important concepts and terms in nursing research we are about to discuss.

Basic Research Terminology

The *independent variable* in a research study can be controlled by the researcher and is applied, or manipulated, to determine its effect on the *dependent variable*. The dependent variable is the phenomenon being studied. In healthcare, the dependent variable is usually a health problem of some kind.

Validity refers to the ability of the research methods to actually measure or accurately describe the variables in the study. A physical measure, such as blood pressure, is usually thought of as valid. However, the device used for measuring the blood pressure must be checked for accuracy in order for the measure to be valid. Questionnaires must also be examined for validity. For example, a questionnaire that purports to measure depression (such as by numbering severity using a scale of 1 to 10 or by using words indicating severity: none, mild, moderate, and severe) must have evidence that it really is measuring depression and not some other related phenomenon. The concern also arises that a questionnaire may be valid in one group (such as college-educated students on whom it was tested) and not valid in another group (such as clients with limited education who may not understand the terminology used in the questionnaire). There are many different processes for establishing validity in the setting in which the research is conducted. An important role of the researcher is demonstrating the validity of the research method.

Reliability refers to the ability of the research instrument or tool consistently to yield the same results over repeated testing periods. Again, there are multiple methods for establishing the reliability of any instrument, and the researcher must establish the reliability of any instrument used. Reliability and validity are closely related and often are discussed together.

In a study, the **population** is the entire group of people affected by the problem under scrutiny. The **sample** is that group of people who will actually be studied. How representative the sample is of the entire population is one factor affecting whether the study will be useful. Selecting a *random sample* involves some type of nonbiased approach to selecting the individuals from the population that ensures that all persons in the population have an equal and independent chance of being chosen to be sampled. The use of a random sample increases the likelihood that the sample adequately represents the population. This often is not possible, and a *convenience sample* (a group that may be conveniently accessed) is used. The **participant** or **subject** is the individual person in the sample. Although the term "subject" has been traditionally used, many people now encourage the use of the term "participant" to emphasize the choice that is made to be in the study and the important partnership that occurs.

At least two groups of participants are usually formed. One group is considered the **control group**, sometimes also referred to as the comparison group. The control group will not receive any special treatment or procedure being studied. The *experimental group*, however, will receive the new treatment or procedure. Sometimes there are multiple experimental groups to test different treatments, but one group continues to be the control group that demonstrates the outcome if no treatment is given. In some instances, having no treatment is not possible. In such cases, two or more treatments might be compared. For example, if the focus of the study was the effectiveness of treatments of pressure ulcers, it would be unethical to not treat a pressure ulcer at all. Therefore, the study might compare different methods of treatment to determine the most effective one. Assigning individuals to the groups using a random method may be done even if the sample selected is not random.

An essential part of any research study is the provision for informed consent of the participants. Informed consent for research has the same attributes as informed consent for medical treatment. The individual must be informed of both potential risks and potential benefits of participating. The researcher must disclose that the participant may or may not receive the treatment under consideration. As part of the consent process, any restrictions on other types of healthcare that may occur while in the study must also be disclosed. Participation must be voluntary, with no adverse consequences occurring if subjects choose not to participate. Further, participants must be informed of their right to withdraw from the study at any time without needing a reason for doing so.

Quantitative Research

Quantitative research refers to a study in which items can be counted or measured and statistics can be used to analyze the results. There are many types of quantitative studies, but in experimental research, in which a new or different treatment is given to a sample group, it is important to demonstrate in an objective way the effectiveness of the treatment being studied.

The Randomized Controlled Trial

The type of experimental research emphasized most often in medicine is the double-blind, randomized controlled trial, often referred to more simply as the **randomized controlled trial (RCT)**. Double-blind means that neither the participant receiving the treatment nor the person administering the treatment knows whether the participant is receiving the real or active treatment or a placebo. Randomized indicates that the participants are assigned to either the treatment group or the control group by some type of random process. Controlled, as we have discussed, means that there is both a treatment group and a group that does not receive the treatment (Fig 16.1).

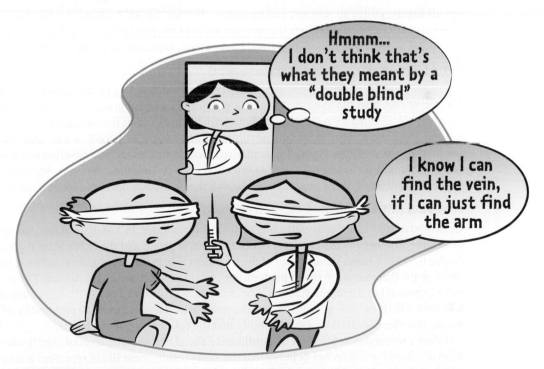

FIGURE 16.1 Double-blind random controlled trials are often not possible when researching nursing care.

▶ *EXAMPLE*

A Double-Blind Randomized Controlled Trial

Pharmaceutical Company X is testing a new medication for joint pain. People asked to participate in the research study are informed about the study in detail, and are told that there will be a random control group that will not receive any actual medication. Those agreeing to participate are told not to take any other medication for joint pain during the study. The researcher uses a random number table to assign the individuals to the two groups: one that receives the new medication and one that will not. Those not receiving the medication will receive an identical tablet that is an inert substance (a placebo). The knowledge of which persons are receiving the active medication is not shared with either the participants themselves or with those who distribute the medications to the patients. All participants are evaluated for joint pain on a regular schedule using the same pain assessment tools. Those assessing the participants do not know who has received the active medication. At the end of the trial, the pain scores over time will be analyzed statistically to determine whether the new medication had a significant effect on joint pain.

RCT research is valued for determining appropriate medical care. Although this might be the best evidence for choosing a medical therapy or drug, even within medicine this emphasis is narrow. RCTs often cannot be used for testing nursing actions. One cannot hide from a patient that he or she is receiving extra or different nursing care. Nursing activities such as special education, spending time on psychosocial interactions, or even monitoring more frequently are all highly visible to patients and providers. Further, an RCT would not be able to accurately capture individual settings for care, the skills of the practitioners, or the attributes of the individual patient, which include cultural background, expectations, preferences, and abilities.

Other Types of Quantitative Research

There are a variety of other types of quantitative research that may be more useful for nursing. It is sometimes possible to have a treatment group and a control group to be studied that occur naturally (ie, existing by nature and without artificial aid), rather than assigned as randomized groups. Research may be done by studying the same sample of people across time—called a longitudinal study. Other types of quantitative research studies include descriptive studies that collect naturally occurring data such as infection rates or complication rates. Methodological research is another type of quantitative research that is used to develop research instruments.

Analysis of Quantitative Research

Quantitative studies are analyzed using statistical techniques. In a statistical test, the aim is to determine whether any difference between the control group and the experimental group may be due to chance rather than a result of the treatment. There are many statistical tests, but most result in the determination of the **probability** of the result occurring by chance. The probability is expressed as a decimal fraction. For example, a probability of <0.10 means that there is less than a 0.10 or 10% possibility that the result was due to chance. A probability of <0.01 means that there is <0.01 or 1% possibility that the result was due to chance.

Often a researcher sets a **level of significance** ahead of time. The level of significance is the level at which the researcher believes that the study results most likely represent a nonchance event. A level of significance of <0.01 (less than a 1% probability that the result is due to chance) is commonly used. A result that meets the appropriate level of significance is often referred to as a "significant" result.

Statistical significance is not the same as **clinical significance**. Clinical significance relates to having an effect on actual patient outcomes. While the effect of the treatment might have made a change that is statistically significant, this change may not make a difference in the outcome for the patient and thus will not be clinically significant.

Qualitative Research

Qualitative research, frequently used to gain greater understanding of the experience of the patient and family, involves studying phenomena as they naturally occur. By doing this, the researcher achieves a "more comprehensive, contextual understanding of the topic in question" (Ellis & Hartley, 2009, p. 490) and may help the nurse to identify areas to explore with the client and family. This type of research may include interviews, lengthy observations, and detailed case histories. Analysis of qualitative research attempts to find themes within the data.

Types of Qualitative Research

Specific types of qualitative research include phenomenology, ethnography, case studies, and life histories.

In phenomenology, extensive and unstructured interviews are conducted with a limited number of participants. The goal is to identify the themes and patterns within their discussions. Phenomenology frequently results in extensive descriptive discussions of the "lived experience" of persons with a certain health concern. Understanding what patients experience helps the nurse to focus communication and support strategies to address important areas of life.

Case studies and life histories provide detailed information about a single individual. These may serve as an example that will present the various concerns and potential health professional responses. Case studies help the reader to see the specific and particular circumstances of the individual more clearly and then apply that same comprehensive inquiry to their patients. A life history helps the nurse to understand how a health problem might fit into an entire life.

Analysis of Qualitative Research

Analysis of qualitative research differs from analysis of quantitative research. No statistical tests are used, and there is no effort made to try to determine probability in regard to the information.

The analysis of the data gathered in a qualitative study involves an extensive immersion of the researcher into the data to begin to detect themes and patterns. The report is usually a lengthy narrative discussion with the liberal use of quotations from the data to illustrate the topic being presented. Some qualitative research results in the development of conceptual models of relationships. The results of a qualitative research study enable the reader to gain increased depth of understanding about the research topic.

A Staff Nurse's Role in the Research Process

For the results of nursing research to be successful, it must be carried out by an individual who has the educational background to thoroughly understand and direct the process. This may be a nurse with a master's degree; but for large studies, for funded research, and in large institutions, the principal researcher is usually a nurse with a doctorate. The research itself is most often conducted by a team that includes individuals who provide the treatment (if this is a part of the research design), those who collect the data, and specialists in statistics who assist with data analysis. The staff nurse may fulfill a treatment role or a data collection role in this process.

A major role for staff nurses is to identify questions or problems. Within an institution, there may be a specific method for a staff nurse to communicate questions to an individual or a committee that might plan research. If you believe a topic should be studied, do not be concerned if your question is not clearly formulated. Any question will need refinement and reconsideration as it goes through the process. Your question may just be the beginning of gathering important information.

Another role of the staff nurse is to guard the welfare of the patients for whom he or she cares. This means asking questions to be sure the research proposed has gone through the appropriate institutional processes before agreeing to participate as a data gatherer or the nurse providing the research intervention. There should be a formal consent process that is clear to the participants. Just as the staff nurse is not responsible for medical consent, the staff nurse is not responsible for research consent. If patients who have agreed to participate exhibit ambivalence or uncertainty about participating, do not try to convince them to participate. Ask the person from the research team who is managing consents to speak with concerned patients about the study. Patients do have the freedom to withdraw from a research study at any time. Additionally, nurses need to be sure that effective care can be provided to the patient. For example, they need to be able to assess for possible side effects or adverse reactions. Protocols for managing such side effects must be in place for patient protection.

COMMUNICATION IN ACTION

A Staff Nurse's Concern About Consent

Isabel Andretti was a staff nurse on the oncology unit at a large hospital where a double-blind controlled trial of a new medication was being researched. The researcher had talked with the potential participants and obtained consent. When Isabel went in to administer the first dose of the study medication to Mrs. Wilson, Mrs. Wilson asked, "Can you explain what this research thing is all about? I didn't understand half of what that woman said when she was here." Isabel said, "Tell me what you do know." Mrs. Wilson explained, "Well, I am going to get this new medicine, but I wonder if it is dangerous. Do you think it is?" Isabel then said, "That is a good question, and you should have an answer before we start this. The best person to explain this is the researcher in charge of this project. We will wait to give you this medication until she has talked with you again and you have made your decision about participating. We don't want you to agree to something you don't understand." Isabel immediately left the room and called the researcher. She explained to the researcher, "Mrs. Wilson, who signed the consent forms for the research project, just said that she did not understand what this was all about. She did not seem to understand that she might be receiving a placebo rather than the new medication, and she was concerned about whether the medication she would receive was dangerous. I know that you talked with her before, but she seems not to have been able to process the information. I am holding the first dose that was due to be given until you are able to talk with her again. When do you think you might be able to discuss her concerns with her?"

Using research in practice is perhaps the most important role of the staff nurse. The process of using research in practice is discussed below as part of evidence-based nursing.

EVIDENCE-BASED PRACTICE IN NURSING

One major thrust for the future of nursing revolves around the development of **evidence-based practice (EBP)**. EBP first began in medicine and is expanding to all of healthcare. EBP in nursing is being instituted in many healthcare organizations. All nurses need to develop a "spirit of inquiry" in regard to their practice and incorporate evidence into all that they do (Melnyk, Fineout-Overholt, Stillwell, et al., 2009).

Establishing a Definition of Evidence-Based Nursing

A variety of definitions of evidence-based nursing have been proposed. "EBP is a problem-solving approach to the delivery of healthcare that integrates the best evidence from studies and patient care data with clinician expertise and patient preferences and values" (Fineout-Overholt, Melnyk, Stillwell, et al., 2010). This definition provides an excellent foundation both for the individual nurse and for the institution to establish evidence-based nursing practice.

Let us examine this definition carefully. The major focus is on problem solving. Nurses are accountable for decisions, and they need to base those decisions on supporting evidence, not custom or habit. Another significant part of this definition is the emphasis on clinical nursing expertise. The expertise of nurses in applying information to the care of specific patients is essential. Nurses have an obligation to continually work to improve their own knowledge base and ability to identify appropriate applications of information to specific patient situations. An important aspect found in this definition is the autonomy of the client. This supports views set forth by Melnyk (2004), who suggests that patient values and preferences should always be added to any discussion of the use of EBP. Although the definition states "patient," this can be expanded to consider the client, whether that is the individual, family, or community.

An issue not included in this definition is the consideration of the available resources. This would include both human and material resources and is strongly related to the cost-effectiveness of an intervention. Cost-effectiveness constrains decisions that individual patients make, as well as the decisions made by healthcare providers. The individual patient may decide that the marginal difference between a new brand-name wound therapy and the older therapy is not worth several hundreds of dollars a month in costs. A system itself may reject providing certain high-cost options that demonstrate marginal improvement in outcomes. The human resources needed for implementation of some therapies may critically change the cost-effectiveness data. For example, some expensive wound management products may so significantly reduce nursing time and shorten the days of hospitalization that they are, in fact, still cost-effective. Thus considering cost-effectiveness is critical for nursing.

DISPLAY 16.2 Commonly Used Rating System for the Hierarchy Of Evidence

Level I: Evidence from a systematic review or meta-analysis of all relevant randomized controlled trails
             (RCTs), or evidence-based clinical practice guidelines based on systematic reviews of RCTs.

Level II: Evidence obtained from at least one well-designed RCT.

Level III: Evidence obtained from well-designed controlled trials without randomization.

Level IV: Evidence from well-designed case-control and cohort studies. Some infection control studies or
             quality assurance studies may fall into this category.

Level V: Evidence from systematic reviews of descriptive and qualitative studies. This would include
             multiple retrospective or chart reviews, quality assurance reviews, or infection control reviews
             that provide descriptive information.

Level VI: Evidence from a single descriptive or qualitative study. This would include a single retrospec-
             tive or chart review, quality assurance review, or infection control review that provides descrip-
             tive information.

Level VII: Evidence from the opinion of authorities and/or reports of expert committees.

From Melnyk, B. M. and Fineout-Overholt, E. (2005). *Evidence based practice in nursing & healthcare. A guide to
best practices* (2nd ed.) Philadelphia, PA: Lippincott Williams & Wilkins.

Determining Adequate Evidence

This brings us to the question of what constitutes adequate evidence upon which to base
practice. Melnyk and Fineout-Overholt (2005) provide a rating system for examining the
hierarchy of evidence that might be used as a basis for evidence-based nursing practice
(see Display 16.2). RCTs stand at the top of this list, with types of research studies encompassing the first four levels of evidence. Qualitative studies and single descriptive studies,
as well as reports of expert committees, are included at the end of the list. Qualitative
studies are often used in nursing because they are more likely to reveal the patient's
perception of the problem or of the intervention. This attention to patient preferences is
impossible in the RCT.

While the Melnyk and Fineout-Overholt list (2005) provides a good starting point, nursing generally relies on a broader array of evidence for determining the best practice for a
nursing situation. Display 16.3 provides a list of the types of evidence commonly used to
support nursing practice. Although they are in an approximate order of reliability, there is not
a clear-cut hierarchy. Research reports (the first on the list) include all the types of research
that are listed in Display 16.2 as levels I to VI. Retrospective or concurrent chart reviews,
quality improvement, risk management, and benchmarking data are all site specific and useful to nurses.

Guidelines for practice developed by groups of experts based upon the best available evidence are a useful tool for EBP. These panels of experts—whether international, national, or
local—use a variety of evidence and information resources as they seek to determine best practices. Their guidelines may be an excellent source for nursing decision making. The Agency
for Healthcare Research and Quality (AHRQ) convenes expert panels to develop guidelines
for some situations of common concern. It also maintains a clearinghouse of guidelines that

DISPLAY 16.3   Sources Used for Evidence-Based Nursing Practice

1. Research reports of all types
2. Retrospective or concurrent chart reviews
3. Quality improvement, risk management, and benchmarking data
4. International, national, and local standards or guidelines developed by expert panels evaluating a variety of information resources
5. Infection control data
6. Pathophysiology information
7. Cost-effectiveness analysis
8. Patient preferences
9. Clinical expertise of individuals

have been developed by other authoritative groups. These guidelines may be accessed on AHRQ's Web site at *www.ahrq.gov* and are an excellent resource for staff nurses seeking to use EBP.

Infection control data provides an important foundation for nursing decision making as well. For example, the infection control data of an individual setting may be stronger evidence for the effectiveness of a certain practice than a research study conducted in a very different setting. The infection control data reflect this individual setting with its providers, patient population, and physical setup. In the same way, quality improvement data may help an institution to target its own processes in a way that a RCT might not.

The difference between the evidence supplied in a RCT and that found in a real-life situation may be subtle but very real and important. Real-life situations lack the controls of research studies. Both patients and healthcare settings are more varied than typical research subjects and settings. Patients often have multiple health problems and confounding interactions that make their situations unique. Issues such as the patient's view of quality of life profoundly affect decisions about appropriate healthcare. Healthcare settings have differing resources, both material and human.

Nurses must also face the reality that there is *no* research evidence regarding some aspects of nursing practice. One cannot just delay making decisions and withhold care until data are forthcoming. That is why the list in Display 16.3 also contains the use of basic scientific information in regard to pathophysiology. However, this also highlights the need to remain open and actively seeking evidence for practice. Sometimes what seemed very appropriate when reasoned out from a pathophysiological basis turns out not to be the best action.

Patient values and preferences are unique to each patient situation, although there may be trends across patient populations treated in some settings. An understanding of these values and preferences may guide decisions about what interventions to investigate. In some situations, patient preferences may rise to the top of the list of appropriate evidence when a decision must be made and may outweigh all other evidence.

▶ *EXAMPLE*

Ensuring the Inclusion of Patient Preference in Evidence-Based Practice

A meeting was scheduled between Mildred (a 78-year-old woman diagnosed with multiple myeloma), her oncologist, her husband of 54 years, her family physician, and her primary nurse, after Mildred failed to respond to the chemotherapy initially prescribed. At this meeting, the oncologist presented the option of a stem cell transplant. He explained that the statistics for successful treatment were not excellent, but that this was the only option left. He then presented the risks, side effects, and benefits of the proposed treatment, along with a detailed analysis of the information. He emphasized that she had good health before this diagnosis and no coexisting health problems, which would help the situation. Her insurance company had been contacted and it would fund this care. To everyone's surprise, Mrs. Ogilvie said, "No, I really don't want to go through anymore treatment. I have had enough." She was then given more reasons why this was a good treatment option and the evidence for possible success was presented more strongly. The oncologist asked her husband to help convince her that she should have this treatment. Mrs. Ogilvie turned to her husband and said, "Dan, help me. I cannot do this." Her husband turned to the oncologist and said, "I don't want to lose her, but I can't ask her to do what she doesn't want to do." The oncologist began again to discuss the treatment. When he had completed his statement, the primary nurse spoke up. "I think that Mrs. Ogilvie has clearly told us what she wants. I think they both understand the consequences that you have so clearly explained. Perhaps now is the time to give them privacy so they can talk about the situation together." This nurse recognized that the patient's decision and values were going to be the determining factor and was supporting their autonomy in decision making.

The expertise of the staff is also a factor in determining the most appropriate practice. Expert staff members may attend conferences, read widely, and access resources that they may use when problem solving in regard to appropriate nursing interventions. Additionally, the expertise of the staff is a factor in deciding whether certain types of actions can be implemented.

When looking for evidence, many believe this to be an entirely scientific inquiry. However, there may be competing interests involved as well as simply the evidence. The evidence is rarely so clear that there is no room for differences of opinion in regard to the meaning of the evidence. When decisions involve competing values such as safety, quality of life, length of life, or cost, the process of determining the appropriate path becomes complex. Managed care organizations, insurance providers, and hospitals may make some decisions based on their own best interests more than those of the client. Nurses need to be aware of these political factors and recognize that adopting a new EBP may require astute attention to the politics of the setting.

The Evidence-Based Practice Process

Many different models for evidence-based nursing practice have been developed. One of the first was the project at the University of Minnesota in the late 1970s, which was designed

DISPLAY 16.4 The Five A's of the Evidence-Based Practice Process

Ask: Convert information needs from practice into focused, structured questions.
Acquire: Use the focused questions as a basis for literature searching in order to identify relevant external
           evidence from research and to identify relevant internal data from quality improvement, risk
           management, or infection control data.
Analyze: Critically analyze the evidence found for validity and the ability to generalize it.
Apply: Use the best available evidence alongside clinical expertise, the patient's perspective, and
           knowledge of available resources to plan care.
Assess: Evaluate performance through a process of self-reflection, audit, or peer assessment.

Adapted from University of North Carolina. (n.d.). *Evidence Based Nursing*. [On-line]. *http://www.hsl.unc.edu/
services/tutorials/ebn/practice.htm*. Retrieved July 28, 2010 and from Flemming, K. (1998) Asking answerable
questions. *Evidence Based Nursing, 1*(2), 36–37.

to encourage the translation of nursing research into practice. Later in the 1980s, the Stetler
Model of Research Utilization was developed as a process for the individual to incorporate
research into practice. The Iowa Model of Research in Practice, developed in the 1990s, grew
out of the quality improvement process and was designed for institutions moving toward EBP.
That model has been broadened into the Iowa Model of Evidence-Based Practice to Promote
Quality Care (Titler, Kleiber, Rakel, et al., 2001). At the University of North Carolina (UNC),
a simple rubric of "5 As" has been established to stimulate individuals to adopt EBP. The steps
in this rubric are "Ask, Acquire, Analyze (or Appraise), Apply, and Assess" (UNC, n.d.). See
Display 16.4. They relate these words to a process first described by Flemming in 1998.

All of these models describe the same phenomenon but use different language and may be
divided into different steps; all are useful. For the beginner, the UNC model is easy to understand and follow. You may use this process to improve your own practice, but, more important,
a group of nurses may use it to establish an EBP protocol or procedure. The use of the UNC
model is described below.

Asking Appropriate Questions

The first step, "Ask," involves developing a clear, focused question. This is essential to obtaining the information needed for decision making. Thompson, Cullum, McCaughan, et al.
(2004) identified a variety of decision-making questions that often face nurses. The effectiveness of the intervention may be the one that is thought of most often. Other questions
relate to the timing of the intervention and to referral patterns. Questions regarding assessment
strategies are important. Which assessments provide clinically relevant data and which are
merely custom? How frequently should assessments be done? Another category of questions
are those that relate to communication and teaching strategies. Nurses must continually strive
to find the most effective ways to communicate with and teach clients in order to achieve the
desired outcomes.

Vague questions about "best care for [any given health problem]" are seldom helpful.
The question should be framed to address a specific clinical problem in order to facilitate the literature search but at the same time remain focused on the patient or the patient
population.

Flemming (1998) suggested that a good question has three parts: the *situation*, the *intervention/action* under consideration, and the *desired outcome*. The situation might be for an individual patient or for a group of patients. The intervention might be one that will resolve the problem or an action that would enable early detection of a problem. The desired outcome focuses on the end result to be achieved such as decreased infection rate or decreased occurrence of some complication due to early detection of an incipient problem.

A more extensive approach to a question is based on the acronym PICOT—patient situation, intervention under consideration, comparison (possible other interventions that might be used), outcome, and time frame (Stillwell, Fineout-Overholt, Melnyk, et al., 2010a). Thus the question encourages the comparison of various possible interventions when those are known and includes the time needed to accomplish the desired outcome as an important aspect. Here, we provide an example using the simpler three-part question.

► **EXAMPLE**

Developing a Question Regarding Nursing Practice

A staff nurse frequently cared for patients with long-term central intravenous (IV) catheters. All the patients with long-term central line catheters became her "population" of interest. The nurse had read about several approaches to caring for these catheters. One of the complications she had observed was catheter-related septicemia. The results of these serious infections were often life threatening. The interventions of interest were the various ones that had been presented in the literature for catheter care. The outcome of concern was the incidence of catheter-related infection. The question might be stated as, "In hospitalized individuals with a long-term central venous catheter in place (*situation*), what is the most effective protocol for catheter care (*intervention*) to decrease the incidence of catheter associated blood stream infections (*desired outcome*)?"

Acquiring Information for Decision Making

The next step is to "Acquire" information related to the concern. This requires a systematic review of the literature in your search for scientific evidence to answer the question. You need to be able to access and effectively use information resources in order to gather the needed data. The information might include research studies, practice guidelines produced by authoritative bodies, infection control data from one's own institution, benchmarking data regarding infection of central venous catheters from other institutions, information on processes used in other settings along with their infection control data, and costs (both human and material) of processes that are suggested. Original studies; syntheses of studies, such as those available from agencies such as the Cochrane Review; evidence-based journal articles; and computerized data support systems may all be appropriate sources of information. Gathering all this information may require the collaboration from many people and consultation with a reference librarian and those responsible for budgeting for supplies. A team approach often is set up to include relevant contributors to the data-gathering process. Accessing information for practice is discussed later in this chapter.

Analyzing Information for Application

After the information is acquired, it's time for "Analysis." Analysis of a whole group of research studies is challenging. Often a clinical nurse specialist or other advanced practice nurse takes the lead in analyzing the research data. The reader must check that the research studied is valid, relevant, and can appropriately be applied to the given situation. Analysis does not end with traditional analysis of the research studies. There must be an integrative approach in which all the data are examined in relationship to other data. Consider resources, your own patient population, and how this might fit with patient preferences. The analysis results in a decision about a course of action. Again, a group discussion to analyze the data may be most productive. One result of analysis may be that no change is warranted. If that is the case, the analysis and report need to be written so that it can be accessed by others at a later time if a change is again contemplated.

Applying New Information

When the analysis has been completed and it has identified a need for a change in practice, preparations are made to "Apply" the new information. A protocol or procedure must be developed or adopted and a plan for implementation is needed. Will this plan be implemented for the entire facility, for a particular unit or units, or as a pilot project in one area with a decision about the entire facility made after results of the pilot are completed? How and when will this change in practice be introduced? What steps will be taken to ensure that the patient's values and desires are considered? Are resources available? The application of a new intervention needs the thoughtful use of information related to change and its implementation (see Chapter 13). After this careful and thorough planning process, the intervention is initiated.

Assessing Outcomes of New Practices

Introducing the change by itself is not enough, however. The next step is to "Assess" the change using the quality improvement process in place in the institution. A detailed plan for assessing outcomes must be established and carried out. Documentation of all outcomes is essential to making decisions about the intervention. Assessment may involve assessing the response of a single patient or of a group of patients. Is the desired outcome being achieved? What are the strengths as well as the drawbacks of the change in practice? What would be the challenges of expanding this change? Are nurses committed to the change in practice? Does the practice need modification or more education of staff to increase compliance with implementation?

Using Infection Control and Quality Improvement Data to Improve Care

In addition to specific questions that arise to care providers, most healthcare agencies are involved in processes of quality improvement. As part of these processes, ongoing data are collected and analyzed for problems or opportunities for improvement. Below, you will see an example of the use of infection control data for identifying a problem that is then solved through the EBP framework.

▶ *EXAMPLE*

Example of the Use of Infection Control Data for Evidence-Based Nursing

The manager of an intensive care unit (ICU) was contacted by the infection control nurse of the hospital about the series of urinary tract infections that had been identified in patients in that unit. All had had the same strain of *Serratia* as the infective agent, and one patient in the unit was currently infected. A committee was appointed to review data and make recommendations. The question was "In this ICU population, what actions will prevent these recurring serratia urinary tract infections?" The committee identified that all patients with serratia UTIs had indwelling urinary catheters and all had been in the same "pod" in the ICU. There were no infections among the patients who had been having hourly urine measurements performed by the staff RN. All staff members were interviewed in regard to care practices for patients with catheters. One interviewer talked with a nursing assistant who worked nights. This nursing assistant explained that he was responsible for emptying the urinary drainage bags when intake and output were measured at the end of the shift. When asked specifically about his technique, he revealed that he would commonly obtain one measuring container and use it as he moved from patient to patient. Identifying this as a deviation from the standard protocol for the unit, all measuring containers were immediately removed for cultures and replaced with clean ones. Education in using a measuring container for only one patient was provided along with the rationale for that action. Subsequent results revealed that the container for the infected patient cultured positive for the *Serratia*. Using this container could easily have transmitted the organism to another patient's catheter, and the infectious agent could be spread from patient to patient in this manner.

Using quality improvement processes requires that there be ongoing data collection regarding outcomes. When outcomes are known, then addressing areas for possible improvement in outcomes becomes possible. For example, if data collection reveals that the length of stay for a knee replacement varies from 3 to 6 days, the question might be raised as to how care processes might be improved to move toward a 3-day stay for the majority of patients. The process involved in making any changes would be the EBP described above.

Individual Accountability for Evidence-Based Practice

While this discussion has focused on the EBP process for an institution as a whole, individual nurses also have accountability for EBP. Nurses are obligated to adhere to evidenced-based guidelines developed by the institution. Nurses increasingly find the expectation that they must be critical decision makers in their own practice as well. This requires an ongoing commitment to asking questions and choosing paths.

The nurse as an employee, not an independent practitioner, has an obligation to identify how a change in personal practice will affect others and the system. Part of applying a new nursing intervention or assessment process may involve consulting with others, especially with the nurse manager. What may be needed is for the individual nurse to become the change agent to affect the practice within the system? (See Chapter 13 on leading change.)

Barriers to Evidence-Based Nursing Practice

Although the production of nursing research has grown, the use of nursing research as well as other types of evidence to inform practice has not moved forward as quickly as some nursing leaders would like. This has its roots in many different issues.

Access to Information Resources

Factors affecting nurses are the availability of information resources and the access to search capabilities. Many people mistakenly believe that all needed information is available without charge online. While many government sources of information, such as guidelines through the AHRQ and the Medline database, are available at no charge, the majority of databases that provide full-text articles require subscriptions for online access. Subscribing to one or more journals in your field provides some information for practice, but most nurses will find that they need the resources of a good library to find and retrieve all the information they need.

Academic medical centers may have a wide array of resources; however, there are many hospitals and other employment settings with limited access. The libraries in smaller hospitals have historically focused on supporting medical practice rather than nursing practice. Some hospitals and nursing homes have blocked any Internet access in order to deter inappropriate use and create a stronger firewall against unauthorized entry into their own computer system. The side effect of this action is decreased access to online resources for staff.

Lack of Time for Seeking Information Resources

Within most employment settings for nurses, there is no time in the workday to seek new information for practice. While general reading in one's field may be appropriately expected to occur on one's own time, seeking specific information regarding a patient currently receiving care or for establishing a policy or protocol would seem appropriate to the workplace. Integrating this need into a very busy workplace is a challenge. In facilities committed to EBP, individuals may be afforded time to meet in committees and to work on questions that need to be answered.

Lack of Background in Understanding and Valuing Research

Another issue that may affect the utilization of all types of evidence is the fact that the largest number of currently practicing nurses received their nursing education in an AD or diploma program in which the research process was not emphasized. Without an academic background in research understanding and utilization, these nurses may find it challenging to effectively interpret research results and weigh that research against other evidence. This suggests that having nurses work in teams to evaluate evidence for practice might alleviate this concern as those with greater knowledge and expertise in research evaluation take a leadership role. Baccalaureate- and master's-prepared nurses who have a more in-depth background can be effective leaders for this process.

An ongoing concern is whether nurses are committed to supporting the use of research and other evidence to improve their practice. If nurses do not value and support the development of nursing research in their own settings, nursing as a profession will be hampered in its growth (Fig. 16.2).

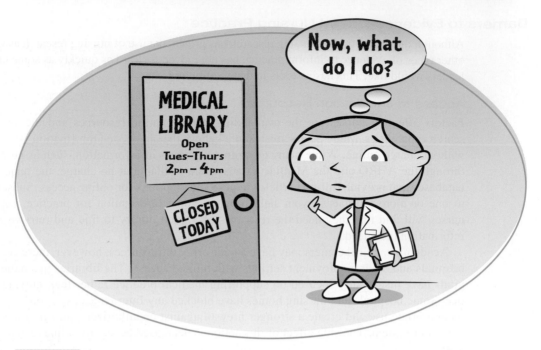

FIGURE 16.2 The lack of resources may be a barrier to evidence-based nursing practice.

Critical Thinking Activity

In the facility in which you have clinical experience, research the resources available for EBP. Is there a library? What resources for nursing in terms of databases, references, journals, and so forth are available? Can a nurse access the Internet? If so, what are the rules or restrictions? Does the institution have a committee or committees that have responsibilities in terms of evidence-based nursing practice? Are there nurse specialists who provide support and guidance for EBP? Analyze the resources and try to determine whether the resources are sufficient to meet the needs of the nursing staff for evidence-based nursing practice.

ACCESSING RESOURCES FOR EVIDENCE-BASED PRACTICE

With the rapid changes occurring in healthcare, all providers find themselves needing to access the most current information about specific illnesses, medications, and other treatments. Providers need strategies for finding information. Additionally, they need to be able to evaluate the information retrieved.

Strategies for Finding Information

When all bibliographic databases were in print form, the information lagged behind publication by many months. Additionally, searching databases was cumbersome and missing important information was not uncommon. With the computerization of databases, the search function provides flexibility in the language used and the combination of terms that can be entered. This sets the framework for specifically targeted searches of the healthcare literature. Many nursing programs require that students learn to use bibliographic references to support their education, an important skill that will continue throughout your career.

The most comprehensive database is Medline, a resource of the National Library of Medicine (NLM), which may be searched through the PubMed search site. PubMed provides a thesaurus of specific terms that are used by the NLM librarians to index articles into relevant categories within the Medline database. Additionally, the Medline database can be searched in terms of key words that might appear in the title or in the abstract or even within the article itself. PubMed searches are free and available online. After the search has enabled the identification of appropriate references, a source for those references is needed. The NLM operates a document retrieval service in which specific articles may be photocopied (for a charge) and mailed to a library that subscribes to the service. PubMed may also be used to identify resources and then the specific documents may be sought in a hospital, college, or medical center library.

There are several databases that include health-related publications to which libraries may subscribe. Access to these databases is restricted to those belonging to the agencies that subscribe to them, such as students and faculty of college and university libraries and employees of institutional subscribers. Many of these databases provide abstracts and some full-text articles (Fig. 16.3).

The Cumulative Index of Nursing and Allied Health Literature (CINAHL) available through Ebsco Host is a bibliographic resource focused on nursing and allied health. Nursing content can be searched using nursing-related terms as well as broader health-related terms. The thesaurus for CINAHL includes nursing diagnoses and steps of the nursing process as well as terms related to common nursing interventions. CINAHL is available by subscription only and may be included in a library's subscription base. Some indexed articles (but not all) are available from the CINAHL with full-text subscription.

Cochrane Library is a database of systematic reviews available online (see discussion of systematic reviews below). It includes four databases: the Cochrane Database of Systematic Reviews, the Database of Abstracts of Reviews of Effectiveness, the Cochrane Controlled Trials Register, and the Cochrane Review Methodology Database.

Online journals are indexed in databases along side print journals, but many online journals are also accessible through Internet search engines such as Google and Yahoo Search. Online journals may require a paid subscription to access full-text articles. These Internet search engines may also reveal government and organization recommendations or standards, papers, conference proceedings, reports, and other resources that are available online.

After you choose a database to search, you will need to formulate your search strategy. The help of a librarian is invaluable in this process. A knowledgeable librarian will direct you toward the various indexed terms and categories that will tend to retrieve more specifically targeted results. While key words are useful, they often return many references that

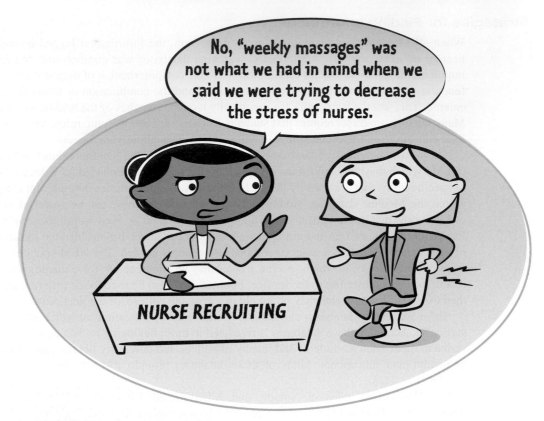

FIGURE 16.3 Improving the work environment for nurses has been identified as a key component in addressing the nursing shortage.

do not relate to your needs. Additionally, terms can be combined using connectors such as *and, or,* and *not.* Using such terms as *"clinical guidelines," "systematic review,"* or *"meta-analysis"* will return articles that provide a broad base of information (Twibell, Siela, Rook, et al., 2010). A search may be limited to English language, a specified range of dates, populations studied, and others. These are usually available under an "advanced search" tab. For a helpful step-by-step example, see Stillwell, Fineout-Overholt, Melnyk, et al. (2010b).

 ## Critical Thinking Activity

Identify a nursing diagnosis with which you are not familiar. Using PubMed online, seek information on the nursing care needs of individuals with that particular nursing diagnosis. After using PubMed use whatever databases (choose CINAHL if available) are in your school library to seek references about that topic. Then use an Internet search engine such as Google, MSN Search, or Yahoo Search to look up the same nursing diagnosis. Compare the resources you found from each of the different search techniques.

DISPLAY 16.5   Key Strategies for Evaluating Information Resources

1. Source of information:
  • Who controls the journal or Web site?
  • Is it peer reviewed?
2. The author or authors:
  • Are the authors or editors apparent in the resource?
  • What are the credentials of the authors or editors?
  • What are the affiliations of the authors or editors?
  • Who funded their research?
3. Context of the resource:
  • How closely does the resource speak to your situation or need?
  • Where was the provided information obtained? Consider the various sources for evidence-based care.
4. Consensus of multiple resources:
  • Are there other resources that agree with this one?
  • Is this resource suggesting actions that are outside the generally accepted standard?
5. Comparison of new information with previous information:
  • What are the differences from what you previously understood?
  • Are differences explained so that you can understand them?

Evaluating Information Retrieved

Regardless of the resource used for accessing data, critical judgment regarding the reliability and validity of information retrieved is essential. You will need to ask a series of questions about the source and content of the material you have accessed. These same questions may be taught to patients who are often researching information about their health conditions using online references (Display 16.5).

The first question to ask is about the source of the information. If this is a journal, who publishes it? It may be a nursing or medical organization, an independent party, or a pharmaceutical company. What are the credentials of the individuals on the editorial board? Do you recognize any of the names? If this is a Web site, who controls the content on this site? Is it identified by a date? By an author? Examine the policies regarding publication. There is often a page or section of a Web site designed to give information to potential authors or contributors. This may provide you with information about how content is reviewed. Is there a process in which appropriate professionals peer-review any manuscript before publication? Individuals are eligible to be peer reviewers when they have both subject matter expertise and an understanding of research. The journal selects appropriate peer reviewers, who read and critique the article and make recommendations as to whether it should be published. Peer review strengthens the reliability of the content. Consider the potential accuracy of the material and whether the source might be biased.

Look at the biographical material on the authors. What are their credentials for writing? If this is a report of a clinical practice in a particular institution, what is the author's role in that institution? If it is a research report, what are the author's credentials for research? Who funded the research?

As you read the material, consider the content from different perspectives. Consider how closely the basis of the report matches your situation or need. For example, a protocol used in a major medical center may be unrealistic for a small community hospital with fewer resources. Interventions that work well with a college-educated population may not work well for a low-income, low-educational-level group. An intervention that has limited study may be useful for an individual patient for whom the standard interventions are not being successful. However, this same intervention might be inappropriate as a standard of care. Is the information anecdotal only or was there a planned method of measuring outcomes and results that are being reported?

When using references for practice, you will find it useful to look for multiple references. What worked in one small study may have been unsuccessful when a similar study was done. What might have contributed to this disparity in outcomes? If multiple sources all achieved the same outcome or made the same recommendation, this strengthens the recommendation. Consider how the recommendations fit in with prior standards of practice. While new standards will emerge, changing dramatically from known standards requires a higher level of proof than would be required when making a minor change.

For some problems, a systematic review may be available from a source such as the Cochrane Review or in an article. A systematic review examines a broad spectrum of research regarding a specific problem. The review presents the strengths and weaknesses of the various research studies and then provides an analysis of the meaning of all of them combined. Often this review is done by an expert panel providing excellent information on which to base decisions.

Always compare new information with old. Make sure that you clearly understand the similarities and differences. Sometimes the long-established practice is not based on research, but rather is simply customary. If you do not understand the current practice, you will have difficulties making judgments about changing practices.

Critical Thinking Activity

Working with a small group of students, identify a nursing care question that is of interest to you. Using the EBP process discussed, seek evidence for the best nursing practices in relationship to this question. Be sure to document all references you used in your process. Based on the evidence you found, formulate a policy and/or protocol to address the nursing care question and present it to your class.

Sharing Information Retrieved

Information that has been retrieved and evaluated has value to other nurses as well as yourself. Twibell, Siela, Rook, et al. (2010) provide multiple suggestions on ways that nurses can share information for use in evidence-based care. These include bulletin boards, the designation of specific nurses as experts, posters on stands that can be moved about, and a cart or box containing information about a specific nursing care question. You and your colleagues may identify other effective strategies for your own work environment. Creating a climate of inquiry and responsiveness will support ongoing development of EBP.

TECHNOLOGY IN HEALTHCARE

Technology in healthcare is found in many places. It is found as an approach to managing general knowledge related to healthcare, as well as computerized patient care data. In 2009, the Board of Governors of the NLN published a position statement regarding the importance of preparing nursing students to practice in a technology-rich environment (NLN, 2009).

From e-mail and listservs to handheld computers (PDAs) and "smart phones," nurses are adopting personal technology to support their practice. Both individuals and institutions rely on information technology to access resources and references. Institutions are adopting computerized systems to gather data and manage the healthcare environment. The use of computerized systems in healthcare has increased steadily, and all information will eventually be managed by computer. This poses challenges to nursing to maintain a "high touch" relationship with the patient in the midst of the high tech environment of healthcare.

Information technology is being used to store research data, disseminate research and practice information, and retrieve information for use. The study and management of information technology is often referred to as the field of **informatics**. There is a national specialty group in nursing that focuses on nursing informatics.

Computerized Patient Records

Computerization of patient data began in most facilities with the computerization of payment and billing data. While forward-looking healthcare institutions began computerizing patient care records beginning in the early 1980s, the beginning of the 21st century was characterized by directives from Medicare and Medicaid to computerize patient records and communication. The Health Information Portability and Accountability Act of 1996 (HIPAA) mandated that all billing to the federal government be done electronically. In order to facilitate this, all providers submitting bills were required to use standardized documentation.

Early Computerization of Standardized Data

The International Classification of Diseases (ICD), which is now in its 10th edition and the Current Procedural Terminology 4th edition (CPT) both use a numbering system to enable the coding of diseases, treatment modalities, and procedures performed. Health information specialists became essential to manage these complex systems for data entry and retrieval. Billing of third-party payers is dependent on exact use of the correct codes. Deliberately using incorrect codes in order to generate increased income has been prosecuted as fraud. All statistical management became computerized with birth and death records, cancer registries, and other data-gathering requirements met by skilled coders taking each patient's handwritten chart and extracting and coding the data into computer systems.

As health information specialists became responsible for reviewing patient charts for billing purposes, they were given responsibility for monitoring charts for complete documentation. Their sphere of responsibility in most facilities also includes management of the patient privacy mandates such as HIPAA and may involve quality monitoring processes.

Pharmacy and laboratory records usually followed billing data in the process of computerization. Computerized records could then be accessed more quickly by those who needed them. Pharmacy and laboratory records are, by their nature, specific, concrete, and objective, thus making them adaptable to and suitable for computerization.

Nurses are able to access laboratory data more quickly and respond by providing the appropriate intervention that is based on data. Many hospitals have made laboratory data available to providers who are not in the hospital to enable them to respond more effectively to information as it becomes available. The availability of data on the computer has freed the nursing department from a major collection, filing, and notification role. Although this was often delegated to a unit secretary, the nursing staff was responsible for ensuring that this was accomplished.

Computerized pharmacy records have decreased the nurses' need to process large volumes of paperwork related to medication administration. Information regarding allergies, drug interactions, and other concerns are often immediately available.

Computerized Nursing Care Records

Computerizing the nursing patient care record has been a complex task. Many different people need to enter data into the record, and many need to extract it. Data that are non-standardized and more qualitative in nature are more difficult to computerize. The increase in checklists and charting by exception paved the way for an easier entry into computerized data for some aspects of nursing care. The need for detailed narrative was lessened by these various tables, checklists, and charts. Many institutions are turning to the various nursing terminology systems such as the NANDA-I nursing diagnoses, Nursing Intervention Classification (NIC), Nursing Outcomes Classification (NOC), the Omaha system, and others to systematize the language used in documentation. By systematizing the language, uniform data can be extracted for quality improvement purposes as well as for research.

For nurses, there are still problems with computerized data systems. Some have been designed without the input of direct caregivers and are time-consuming and cumbersome to use. The need for large numbers of computer entry stations for nursing units has been a problem in other settings. The move toward computerization of the nursing record will continue until all records are computerized. Learning a new computer system is becoming a standard part of any orientation to a new facility.

Computerized Physician/Provider Order Entry

Computerized physician/provider order entry (CPOE) systems, sometimes referred to as computerized order entry (COE), are gaining in use. To institute CPOE, prescribers, whether physicians, dentists, nurse practitioners, or physician assistants, must be willing to change their practice patterns. One major advantage of CPOE is that errors based on handwriting difficulties are eliminated. Nurses do not have to decipher handwritten orders or spend time trying to contact the provider to clarify the order. Computer prompts may be used to indicate such items as default doses and a range of potential doses for each medication, and to indicate a requirement to enter dosage, route, and frequency for each order. This has helped to eliminate the time-consuming process for nurses of contacting providers to obtain complete information when it was overlooked at the time of writing the order. There may also be prompts to suggest the need for laboratory monitoring, and the computer may be programmed to display values already in the patient record. Most systems provide for a cross-check with patient drug allergy data and drug–drug interactions for the medications already prescribed. The system may be set to reject the use of abbreviations that appear on a "do not use" list. All of these provide greater safety for the patient and have the potential to decrease nursing workload in a time of nursing shortage.

CPOE can be used to facilitate the use of standard protocols for care. When the standard protocol with options for individualization is offered on the screen, it becomes easy for a physician to use the standard protocol. Institutions seeking to systematize best practices find this a valuable asset.

In a systematic review, van Rosse, Maat, Rademaker, et al. (2009) noted that CPOE clearly reduces medication errors but that implementation strategies are important to its success. Nurses need to be aware that CPOE does not eliminate all problems and not become complacent. CPOE will not decrease the need for nursing knowledge and critical thinking in regard to the administration of medications.

Patient Privacy and Computerized Records

Concerns about privacy become magnified when information is available to many people in many sites far removed from where the patient is located. All systems require passwords for entry and contain tracking capabilities to determine who has accessed which record from which location. This is essential to enforce the restrictions that govern authorized access. Of even greater concern than the individual who violates confidentiality is the wholesale access to large databases for illegal purposes. As ambulatory care data are merged into overall systems with hospital data, the potential for misuse of information is expanded. HIPAA legislation has mandated that institutions using computerized records have safeguards for patient privacy in place. Agencies that fail to implement appropriate privacy policies are subject to substantial fines.

COMMUNICATION IN ACTION

Maintaining Integrity With Computerized Records

Jose Martinez an RN working on the evening shift was approached by one of the nursing assistants who said, "My sister was admitted to the Birth Room just before I came on the shift. Would you check the computer and see if she has had the baby yet? I think it will appear on the new admissions." Jose replied, "I wish I could help you. I know how anxious you have been about your sister. But remember, none of us can access the computer for information if we are not involved in that person's care. But I can watch your patients for you so that you can go to the mother–baby area and see if you can talk with her or a family member there."

Advantages of Computerized Patient Records

Computerized records have many advantages for patients and healthcare providers. Some of those were discussed in relationship to specific aspects of the record.

A major advantage of the computerized record is that it can be available at the point-of-care without the need to obtain a copy of the written record. Continuity of care is also facilitated when the information follows the patient from setting to setting. Many health systems are integrating ambulatory care data with hospital data so that wherever the patient is, the provider has access to the needed care information. According to the investigation done by Wilson (2010), integration of systems will greatly improve patient care. Even when the records are not integrated, it may be possible to send electronic forms of the record to the setting where it is required to facilitate continuity of care.

Computerizing Management of Patient Care

The use of technology for direct care has increased gradually throughout the past 30 years. Within nursing, computerized devices initially became available in ICUs as monitors for cardiac rhythms. Computerized pumps and controllers were introduced to monitor IV infusions. Automatic blood pressure–measuring devices provide for frequent measurements accompanied by alarms for readings outside preset parameters. Small blood glucose monitors that allow for more precise control of blood sugar for the patient with diabetes have become common. A wide variety of real-time patient monitoring systems provide continuous readouts of physiologic measurements such as blood oxygen saturation and neurologic status (Nahm, 2010). After beginning slowly in many places, the introduction of new technology for direct care has increased at a rapid pace. The issues around safety of these devices were discussed in Chapter 10.

Distance Monitoring Using Technology

The ability for someone to monitor a critically ill patient from another site has created the opportunity to develop what is being called the *electronic ICU (eICU)*. The eICU includes both monitoring equipment and video cameras connected to a separate monitoring center. In the monitoring center, an expert ICU nurse assumes the role of overseeing the electronic monitoring of patients, analyzing data, and recognizing patterns. The eICU nurse uses the video monitor to view a patient as well as review monitor information. The bedside nurse manages the direct care of two or three patients. The eICU nurse communicates with the bedside nurse to alert that individual to problems that occur and may initiate calling a physician if necessary. Working together, the bedside nurse and the eICU nurse form a strong team to ensure that the patient receives optimum care (Federwishch, 2006).

Expert ICU nurses typically rotate through the eICU role as one of their assignments, but work as bedside nurses on other days. This ensures that the eICU nurse remains skilled in bedside care. A critical role of the eICU nurse is in mentoring beginning ICU nurses. The eICU nurse assists the new nurse in developing toward an expert role.

While in its infancy, the concept of the distance monitoring is expanding. Long-distance monitoring is one suggested expansion. An expert ICU nurse at a distant site also could assist by monitoring patients in a smaller hospital where there are fewer ICU experts.

Handheld Electronic Devices for Nurses

Personal digital assistants (PDAs), smart phones, and devices such as the iPod touch, are all small, handheld computers that provide the technology for nurses and physicians to have information resources immediately available. A personal electronic device may be loaded with a drug reference book, a laboratory reference book, a resource on diseases and their management, a medical dictionary, a calculator, and nursing references. The technologically proficient nurse can access information immediately when it is needed. The literature supports the use of personal electronic devices as an effective teaching strategy for nursing education (Zurmehly, 2010). Some nursing education programs have developed projects in which all students must have a PDA and, rather than purchasing print versions of reference books, purchase versions to be loaded on the PDA. They may have developed ways for students to use their PDAs for record keeping and managing their clinical paperwork (Zurmehly, 2010). All of these strategies help students prepare for the demand to use technology to support nursing practice.

Another nursing use for handheld computers is to manage assessment data as they are collected and to track nursing actions taken. For nursing students, this might include using the handheld to develop all of the paper work required for clinical experiences. The instructor may use a handheld to manage student data. There are Web sites that offer programs for organizing and managing assessment data.

When used in these ways, concerns arise about privacy and the protection of information for both patients (in accord with HIPAA) and students (who are protected under federal Family Educational Rights and Privacy Act). A healthcare agency may have specific rules regarding entering patient data into a personal electronic device. However, in settings where these are still uncommon, the institution may not have developed policies and procedures around their use. The nurse who uses any such device to enter information has an obligation to use the available security provisions to protect the patient. This includes setting up effective passwords to access the information and deleting information as soon as it is not needed for care. PDA loss prevention is another important responsibility. For students, personal identifiable health information about a patient should not be entered into a handheld just as it should not be written on papers to be handed in.

Telehealth

Telehealth is "the use of electronic information and telecommunications technologies to support long-distance clinical healthcare, patient and professional health-related education, public health and health administration" (Office for the Advancement of Telehealth [OAT], n.d.).

Telehealth has the potential for supporting effective care of rural populations that have difficulty accessing certain types of healthcare. Through online technology, nurses and physicians may be available to patients who reside far from the provider. Cameras can be used to facilitate long-distance assessment, and specific laboratory and physical assessment information can be communicated to the provider through the Internet.

One area of practice for nurses in telehealth is in telephone triage. Patients and families call the telephone help line, and the nurse uses evidence-based protocols to assess and direct patients in self-care or in accessing medical care as needed. Telephone help lines are often supported by health plans to decrease the use of expensive emergency room care for less serious problems that could be managed in other ways. For patients, the consultation with the nurse provides expert advice and relieves anxiety over which steps appropriately may be taken.

Licensure and practice laws affect the practice of those in telehealth. One concern relates to the control of practice versus the control for patient safety. If the patient is in one legal jurisdiction and the provider is in another (which often occurs), to whom is the provider accountable for care? Many states are addressing this specifically within their licensure laws. Information on specific states may be accessed through the Center for Telemedicine Law Web site (n.d.).

The value of technology for the education of health professionals has become more apparent as opportunities arise. There are online degree programs, online continuing education for providers, and online conferences in which individuals may participate. Technology is overcoming the barriers to staying up to date that occur because of distance and funding for healthcare professionals living in smaller communities or rural areas.

Telehealth may also be used to facilitate improved screening and detection of illness, to improve patient self-management of chronic conditions, for short- and long-term symptom monitoring, and for the delivery of appropriate health interventions. To address all of these areas, the OAT is supporting research and projects that can be used to implement effective telehealth programs.

Clinical Decision Support Systems

Clinical decision support systems are computer programs designed to integrate a medical knowledge base and patient data and provide specific advice on how to manage the individual patient case. The goal of clinical decision support systems is to provide the best of EBP to care providers in an efficient and cost-effective manner that maintains patient safety. A wide variety of different computer systems have been developed for this purpose. A meta-analysis (integrative review of multiple resources) concluded that while computerized clinical decision support systems hold great promise, their benefits are yet to be realized (OpenClinical, n.d.).

 KEY CONCEPTS

- Nursing research has grown and developed since the middle of the 20th century and now is supported through the NINR, which is part of the NIH.
- Nursing research involves the development of a research question, a literature review, a plan for seeking answers, implementation of the plan, analysis of the data gathered, a discussion and evaluation of the results of the study, and recommendations for further research.
- Understanding research terminology and the types of research that can be conducted are essential to reading and using any nursing research.
- The staff nurse's role in relationship to conducting nursing research includes identifying research questions, safeguarding patients who participate in a study, and collecting data and performing treatments.
- "Evidence-based practice (EBP) is a problem-solving approach to the delivery of healthcare that integrates the best evidence from studies and patient care data with clinician expertise and patient preferences and values"

(Fineout-Overholt, Melnyk, Stillwell, et al., 2010). This definition provides an excellent foundation both for the individual nurse and for the institution to establish evidence-based nursing practice.
- A wide variety of evidence, including research reports, chart reviews, quality improvement, benchmarking, and data regarding risk management, infection control, pathophysiological information, cost-effectiveness, and patient preferences, may be used to support nursing practice.
- While many models for EBP exist, a simplified process is incorporated in the terms Ask, Acquire, Analyze, Apply, and Assess.
- Barriers to EBP include the availability of resources, time availability, educational preparation, and nursing commitment.
- Accessing information resources requires knowledge of information resources and the use of databases, as well as an understanding of data such as quality improvement and infection control data from the institution.
- Information must be evaluated in relationship to its source, the authors, its relevance to your

own practice setting, support from multiple resources, and how this relates to current practice and then shared with colleagues.

- Information technology is dramatically changing how individual patient care information and provider planning for care are entered into the record, stored, and retrieved. Personal electronic devices are allowing individual healthcare providers to manage large volumes of information more easily. Security and privacy of patient information remain both an ethical and legal challenge.

- Computerized devices increasingly are used to manage the direct care of patients, from automatic blood pressure measuring devices to IV controllers to monitoring equipment both locally and from a distance. They are changing the way nursing is practiced.

RELEVANT WEB SITES

 Web sites relevant to this chapter can be found at thePoint accessed through *http://thePoint. lww.com/Ellis10e* and by entering the code found on the inside cover of your text.

REFERENCES

Center for Telemedicine Law. (n.d.). *Licensure.* Retrieved June 29, 2010, from http://www.telehealthlawcenter.org/

Ellis, J. R., & Hartley, C. L. (2009). *Managing and coordinating nursing care* (5th ed.) Philadelphia, PA: Lippincott Williams & Wilkins.

Federwishch, A. (2006). From a distance. *Nurseweek: Mountain Edition, 7*(1), 10–11.

Fineout-Overholt, E., Melnyk, B. M., Stillwell, S. B., & Williamson, K. M. (2010). Evidence-based practice step by step: Critical appraisal of the evidence. *American Journal of Nursing, 110*(7), 47–52.

Melnyk, B. M. (2004). Integrating levels of evidence into clinical decision-making. *Pediatric Nursing, 30*(4), 323–326.

Melnyk, B. M., & Fineout Overholt, E. (2005). *Evidence based practice in nursing & healthcare. A guide to best practice.* Philadelphia, PA: Lippincott Williams & Wilkins.

Melnyk, B. M., Fineout Overholt, E., Stillwell, S. B., & Williamson, K (2010). Evidence-based practice step by step: Igniting a spirit of inquiry: An essential foundation for evidence-based practice. *American Journal of Nursing, 109*(11), 49–52.

Nahm, E. S. (2010). Innovations in patient-monitoring systems. *American Nurse Today, 4*(9), 29–30.

National Institute of Nursing Research. (n.d.). *A brief history of the NINR.* Retrieved July 21, 2010, from http://www.ninr.nih.gov/AboutNINR/

National League for Nursing, Board of Governors. (2009). *Preparing the next generation of nurses to practice in a technology-rich environment: An informatics agenda.* Retrieved July 20, 2010, from http://www.nln.org/aboutnln/PositionStatements/informatics_052808.pdf

Office for the Advancement of Telehealth. (n.d.). *What is telehealth?* Retrieved June 29, 2010, from http://www.hrsa.gov/telehealth/

OpenClinical. (n.d.). *DSS Success Factors.* Retrieved June 29, 2010, from http://www.openclinical.org/dssSuccessFactors.html

Stillwell, S. B., Fineout-Overholt, E., Melnyk, B. M., Williamson, K. M. (2010a). Evidence-based practice, step by step: Asking the clinical question. *American Journal of Nursing, 110*(3), 58–61.

Stillwell, S. B., Fineout-Overholt, E., Melnyk, B. M., Williamson, K.M. (2010b). Evidence-based practice, step by step: Searching for the evidence. *American Journal of Nursing, 110*(5), 41–7.

Thompson, C., Cullum, N., McCaughan, D., Sheldon, T., & Raynor, P. (2004). Nurses, information use, and clinical decision making: The real world potential for evidence based decisions in nursing, *Evidence Based Nursing, 7*(3), 68 72.

Titler, M. G., Kleiber, C., Rakel, B., Budreau, G., Everett, L. Q., Steelman, V., et al. (2001). *The Iowa Model of evidence based practice to promote quality care*. University of Iowa Hospitals. Retrieved July 20, 2010, from http://www.uihealthcare.com/depts/nursing/rqom/evidencebasedpractice/iowamodel.html

Twibell, R., Siela, D., Rook, G., Wrightsman, E., and Johnson, D. (2010). Pick up some research to go! *American Nurse Today, 5*(7), 25–27.

University of North Carolina. (n.d.). *Evidence based nursing*. Retrieved June 28, 2010 from http://www.hsl.unc.edu/Services/Tutorials/EBN/practice.htm

van Rosse, F., Maat, B., Rademaker, C. M., van Vught, A. J., Egberts, A. C., Bollen, C. W. (2009). The effect of computerized physician order entry on medication prescription errors and clinical outcome in pediatric and intensive care: A systematic review. *Pediatrics, 123*(4):1184–90.

Wilson, M. L. (2010). How integrated information systems will change health care. *American Nurse Today, 4*(9), 40–42.

Zurmehly, J. (2010). Personal digital assistants (PDAs): Review and evaluation. *Nursing Education Perspectives, 31*(3), 179–182.

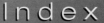

Index

Page numbers followed by d *indicate displays; those followed by* f *indicate figures; those followed by* t *indicate tables.*